# Basic Laboratory Calculations for Biotechnology

# Basic Laboratory Calculations for Biotechnology

Second Edition

Lisa A. Seidman

CRC Press
Taylor & Francis Group
Boca Raton London New York

CRC Press is an imprint of the
Taylor & Francis Group, an **informa** business

Second edition published 2022
by CRC Press
6000 Broken Sound Parkway NW, Suite 300, Boca Raton, FL 33487-2742

and by CRC Press
4 Park Square, Milton Park, Abingdon, Oxon, OX14 4RN


First edition published by Pearson 2008

CRC Press is an imprint of Taylor & Francis Group, LLC



*Library of Congress Cataloging-in-Publication Data*
Names: Seidman, Lisa A, author.
Title: Basic laboratory calculations for biotechnology / Lisa A Seidman.
Description: Second edition. | Boca Raton : CRC Press, 2022. | Includes bibliographical references and index.
Identifiers: LCCN 2021033477 | ISBN 9780367244804 (pbk) | ISBN 9780367244859 (hbk) | ISBN 9780429282744 (ebk)
Subjects: LCSH: Biotechnology—Laboratory manuals.
Classification: LCC TP248.24.S45 2022 | DDC 660.6—dc23
LC record available at https://lccn.loc.gov/2021033477

ISBN: 978-0-367-24485-9 (hbk)
ISBN: 978-0-367-24480-4 (pbk)
ISBN: 978-0-429-28274-4 (ebk)

DOI: 10.1201/9780429282744

Typeset in Warnock Pro
by codeMantra

# Contents

## UNIT II — Applications of Proportional Relationships

## UNIT IV — Introduction to Descriptive Statistics



## UNIT V — Biotechnology Applications

# Preface

STEM fields (science, technology, engineering, and mathematics) provide a myriad of rewarding career opportunities. However, the math calculations required in STEM jobs can be problematic. Employers often report that entering employees cannot "do math." Calculation mistakes in the workplace have, on many occasions, had serious consequences. In response, states and localities have added math course requirements to their high school curricula, and colleges and universities require advanced math courses for STEM majors. We would argue that these additional math course requirements will not solve the root "math" problem, at least not in biotechnology. Rather, these requirements erect a formidable barrier that prevents people, who otherwise would be successful, from entering STEM careers.

Yes, it is true that biotechnologists must perform a wide variety of math calculations as part of their routine work. However, the math required in a biotechnology setting for most jobs – including those of many research scientists – is relatively simple. In fact, studies have shown that for most incoming workers in a variety of fields, the math required is middle school or, at most, beginning high school math.[1] Most adults can "do" middle school math, with review and practice. Classes in advanced algebra or calculus will not increase their success in typical biotechnology settings. (There are, of course, careers in STEM that do require higher-level math, but that does not mean that every person entering STEM careers must have such skills.) The problem for many people is that they have learned middle school math techniques but cannot apply them to unfamiliar situations. For newcomers in a biotechnology setting, the vocabulary and context are complex and filled with math "story" problems, where the story is unfamiliar and where there are serious consequences for wrong answers.

This text and workbook is therefore intended to assist newcomers to biotechnology in two key ways. First, it contains an accessible introduction to common, basic laboratory calculations. It is not intended to replace a math textbook. Rather, these chapters review a few essential areas of math, discussing problems commonly encountered in biotechnology and providing strategies to solve those problems. Along with this review, there are practice problems to help students develop confidence and skill using the required calculation tools. Second, the text contains problems that, as much as is practically possible, model situations where math is encountered in the workplace. In these problems, the math is surrounded by context and students must extract the math required to solve the problem.

The book is primarily organized around laboratory applications, beginning with more general topics and moving to more specific biotechnology laboratory techniques at the end. Unit I provides a quick review of a few basic math tools that are used commonly in the laboratory. Unit II explores the many examples of proportional relationships in the biology laboratory. Units III and IV explore how data are manipulated, with equations, graphs, and introductory statistical methods. Unit V discusses specialized applications in biotechnology. It is assumed in this text that students are comfortable with addition, subtraction, multiplication, division, solving a linear equation with one unknown, and using a scientific calculator.

This book briefly describes a number of laboratory techniques, such as centrifugation and spectrophotometry, to show how math calculations are applied to these applications. For more information about basic laboratory techniques, refer to *Basic Laboratory Methods for Biotechnology: Textbook and Laboratory Reference*, by Lisa A. Seidman, Cynthia J. Moore, and Jeanette Mowery, CRC Press.

[1] This study, for example, provides data for the math required for entry in a variety of technical fields: National Center on Education and the Economy. *What Does It Really Mean to Be College and Work Ready? The Mathematics Required of First Year Community College Students.* May 2013.

# Acknowledgments

Thanks to all the students who have used this material and provided feedback. Thanks to Mary Ellen Kraus and Jeanette Mowery, instructors at Madison Area Technical College, who taught from the first edition of this text and made many important contributions to its development. Diana L. Brandner, Joseph Lowndes, Noreen Warren, Rebecca Dunn, Joy McMillan, Cynthia J. Moore, and Thomas Tubon contributed technical examples and provided support in a number of ways. Percy Mather provided editorial assistance. My appreciation also goes to the reviewers who made a number of significant contributions to the manuscript: Jane Breun, Madison Area Technical College; Linda Roselli Rehfuss, Montgomery County Community College; Gail Baughman, MiraCosta College; and Linnea Fletcher, Austin Community College. Thanks also to the many colleagues who have provided encouragement over the years and who have used parts of this manual, particularly Elaine A. Johnson, City College of San Francisco, and Linnea Fletcher, Austin Community College. Rodney Null from Rhodes State College and Wayne Sigelko from Madison Area Technical College, both math instructors, took the time to meticulously read and correct every page and problem of the first edition, and their efforts made it a much better book. Rodney Null heroically revisited every problem in the second edition and contributed ideas and inspiration that deepened the mathematical content of this text – thanks Rod!

Funding for the first edition of this text was provided in part by the National Science Foundation Advanced Technological Education Program, grants DUE 9752027, 0101093, and 0501520. Any opinions, findings, and conclusions or recommendations are those of the author and do not necessarily reflect the views of the National Science Foundation.

# Author

**Lisa Seidman** obtained her Ph.D. from the University of Wisconsin and has taught for more than 30 years in the Biotechnology Laboratory Technician Program at Madison Area Technical College. She is presently serving as Emeritus Faculty at the college.

# Glossary

**Abscissa.** In graphing, the X-coordinate of a point, the distance of a point along the X-axis.

**Absolute Value.** The distance of a number from zero, regardless of direction. The distance is always positive, so the absolute value cannot be a negative number.

**Absorbance (in spectrophotometry).** The negative log of the transmittance: $A = -\log_{10}$ transmittance. A measure of how much light is absorbed by an analyte.

**Absorptivity Constant (in spectrophotometry).** A measure of the inherent tendency of a specific compound to absorb light of a specific wavelength.

**Adenine, A.** One of the four types of nucleotide subunit that comprise DNA and RNA.

**Agarose Gel Electrophoresis.** A common molecular biology technique in which DNA fragments are separated from one another on the basis of their size under the influence of an electrical current.

**Aliquot.** The process of dividing a material into smaller volumes for storage. The reason for aliquoting reagents is that often once a vial is opened, the material inside it must be used immediately, and whatever is unused must be discarded.

**Amount.** How much of a substance is present. For example, 2 g or 4 cups.

**Amplicon.** The product of a successful PCR reaction consisting of millions of copies of the target sequence.

**Analyte.** A substance of interest that is analyzed in a sample.

**Angstrom, Å.** Unit of length that is $10^{-10}$ m, named after the Swedish physicist A.J. Angstrom. A human hair has a diameter of about 500,000 Å.

**Antibody.** A type of protein made by certain white blood cells in response to a foreign material in the body. Antibodies bind to the foreign substance and aid in its destruction.

**Antigen.** An agent that induces the production of antibodies and to which antibodies respond.

**Antilogarithm (antilog).** The number corresponding to a given logarithm. For example, $100 = 10^2$. The log of 100 is 2. The antilog of 2 is $10^2 = 100$. Thus, the antilog of a number, x, is 10 raised to that number, $10^x$.

**Assay.** A test of a property of a sample. For example, an assay might test the amount of protein in a sample, or the identity of a contaminant in a product.

**Bar Graph.** A graphical method to display data using rectangular bars.

**Base (for exponents).** A number that is raised to a power. In the expression $10^3$, the base is 10 and the exponent is 3.

**Base (in genetics).** The portion of a DNA or RNA subunit that distinguishes one type of subunit from another. The DNA bases are adenine, guanine, cytosine, and thymine. RNA has uracil in place of thymine.

**Base Pair, BP (in genetics).** A pair of opposing nucleotides in a DNA strand.

**Basic Properties (in the SI system).** The fundamental measured properties for which the SI system defines units. These properties are length, mass, time, electrical current, thermodynamic temperature, luminous intensity, and amount of substance.

**Beer's Law.** A rule that states the light absorbance of a homogeneous sample is directly proportional to both the concentration of the absorbing substance and to the thickness of the sample in the optical path.

**Best Fit Line.** A line drawn through the points on a graph that best expresses the relationship between those points.

**Beta-galactosidase.** An enzyme that splits lactose into glucose and galactose.

**Beta-mercaptoethanol, β-mercaptoethanol.** A chemical commonly used by biologists to protect the structure of proteins in laboratory solutions.

**Billion.** In common usage in the United States, 1,000,000,000. (This term is not used consistently in all countries.)

**Biopharmaceutical.** Any therapeutic drug product manufactured by living cells or organisms; or consisting of cells or tissues; or that is a large biological molecule, such as a protein, DNA, or RNA.

**Bit.** A unit of computer memory that is the amount of information in a system with two equally probable states, for example, "on" and "off," or 0 and 1.

**Blank (in spectrophotometry).** A preparation that contains no analyte but does contain the solvent and any reagents that are intentionally added to the sample, used to set the spectrophotometer to zero absorbance.

**Bovine Serum Albumin, BSA.** Soluble, globular proteins isolated from the serum of cattle that is used as an enzymatically inert protein in various biological procedures.

**Bring to Volume, BTV.** The procedure in which solvent is added to solute (typically in a volumetric flask or graduated cylinder) until the total volume of the solution is the final volume required.

**BTV.** See Bring to Volume.

**Buffer (as relates to laboratory solutions).** A compound that resists changes in pH, commonly used in biological solutions to protect the structure and function of biological molecules and cells. Many of the aqueous solutions used for biological molecules are termed buffers because they buffer (maintain) the proper pH, although they often have additional components (such as salts) that do not affect the pH.

**Byte.** A unit of computer memory equal to 8 bits. One byte is the amount of memory required to store one character.

**cDNA, complementary DNA.** A DNA copy of messenger RNA produced by the enzyme reverse transcriptase.

**Cell Culture.** The process in which living cells derived from the tissue of multicellular animals are maintained in nutrient medium inside petri dishes, flasks, or other vessels.

**Cell Division.** The method by which cells reproduce; one cell divides to form two cells.

**Cell Density (in cell culture).** A ratio that is the numbers of cells per a given volume of culture medium, or attached to a given surface area of a culture vessel.

**Cell Line.** Cells of a single type derived from a human or animal and grown in the laboratory.

**Centi-, c.** A prefix meaning 1/100.

**Centimeter, cm.** A unit of length that is 1/100 of a meter.

**Centrifugal Force.** A force that drives a spinning particle away from the center of rotation.

**Coefficient (as relates to scientific notation).** The first part of a number expressed in scientific notation. For example, the number 235 in scientific notation is expressed as $2.35 \times 10^2$ where "2.35" is the coefficient.

**Coefficient of Variation, CV (relative standard deviation, RSD).** A measure that expresses the standard deviation as a percentage of the mean.

**Colorimetric Assay.** A spectrophotometric method to determine the amount or concentration of an analyte by adding dyes that cause a color change in the analyte proportional to its amount or concentration.

**Common Logarithm, log or $\log_{10}$.** The power to which 10 must be raised to give that number. For example, $1{,}000 = 10^3$, so the log of 1000 is 3. The log of 5 is approximately 0.6990 which means that $10^{0.6990} \approx 5$.

**Complementary (in genetics).** The DNA subunits guanine and cytosine always reside across from one another in a DNA strand, as do adenine and thymine. Guanine and cytosine are complementary, as are adenine and thymine.

**Compound (as relates to chemistry).** Two or more atoms bonded together chemically in a fixed ratio.

**Concentration.** A ratio where the numerator is the amount of a material of interest and the denominator is the volume (or sometimes mass) of the entire solution or mixture. For example, if 1 g of table salt is dissolved in water so that the total volume is 1 L, the concentration is 1 g/L.

**Constant.** Number in a particular equation that always has the same value.

**Control Chart.** A graphical quality control method used to understand and monitor how a process changes over time.

**Confluent (in cell culture).** The situation when a culture vessel surface is entirely covered by a layer of cells.

**Coordinates.** The "address" for a point on a graph consisting of two values: one that describes the distance of the point from the origin horizontally and the other that describes the distance of the point from the origin vertically.

**Cubic Centimeter, cc, $cm^3$.** A unit of volume that is equal to 1 mL.

**Cuvette.** Holder for a sample in spectrophotometry.

**Cytosine, C.** One of the four types of nucleotide subunit that comprise DNA and RNA.

**Dalton.** A unit of molecular mass approximately equal to the mass of a hydrogen atom.

**Data.** Observations of a variable (singular, **datum**).

**Denominator.** The number written below the line in a fraction.

**Density.** The ratio between the mass and volume of a material.

**Deoxyribonucleic Acid, DNA.** The molecule that contains genetic information in a cell. DNA controls the structure and function of the cell.

**Deoxyribonucleotide triphosphate, dNTP.** Any of the four nucleotide building blocks of DNA.

**Dependent Variable.** A variable whose value changes depending on the value of the independent variable. For example, if an experimenter measures the growth of seedlings under different light intensities, the growth of the seeds is the dependent variable and the light intensity is the independent variable. (See also "Variable" and "Independent Variable.")

**Descriptive Statistics.** Statistical methods that are used to describe and summarize data.

**Detector.** An electronic transducer that generates an electrical signal in response to a physical or chemical property of a sample. The sensor in a digital camera that is sensitive to light is a familiar example of a detector.

**Deviation (of a data point).** The difference between a data point and the mean.

**Diluent.** A substance used to dilute another. For example, when concentrated orange juice is diluted, the diluent is water.

**Dilution.** Addition of one substance (often but not always water) to another to reduce the concentration of the original substance.

**Dilution Series.** A group of solutions that have the same components but at different concentrations.

**Dispersion (in statistics).** How widely the data in a data set are spread out from one another.

**Distribution (in statistics).** The pattern of variation for the values for a given variable.

**Dot Diagram.** Simple graphical technique to represent a data set in which each datum is represented as a dot along an axis of values.

**EDTA, Ethylene Diamine Tetraacetic Acid.** A chelating molecule that binds to heavy metals and prevents the metals from acting in a system.

**Electrophoresis.** A common molecular biology procedure used to separate fragments or types of DNA or proteins from one another, based on differential migration of molecules in an electrical field.

**Endpoint PCR.** The situation where a PCR reaction is allowed to go through enough cycles to reach a plateau, at which time the reactants are depleted and the maximum number of copies of target have been produced.

**Enzyme.** A type of protein that speeds up chemical reactions in cells.

**Enzyme Linked Immunosorbent Assay, ELISA.** A class of assays that rely on antibodies and their attraction to antigens. These assays can be used to detect and quantify specific proteins or specific antibodies in a sample.

**Equation.** A description of a relationship between two or more entities of equal value that uses mathematical symbols.

**Error Bars.** A graphical method to indicate the dispersion of data.

**Exponent.** A number used to show that a value (base) should be multiplied by itself a certain number of times. The expression $10^3$ means: $10\times10\times10$, which equals 1,000. The base is 10, and the exponent is 3.

**Exponential Equation.** A relationship between two or more entities whose equation includes a variable that is an exponent, for example, $y = 2^x$.

**Exponential Notation.** See "Scientific Notation."

**Frequency Histogram.** A graph where the X-axis is the relevant units of measurement, and the Y-axis is the frequency of occurrence of a particular value in a given interval or class.

**Frequency Polygon.** A graphical method for depicting the shape of a distribution of data. Typically it is constructed based on a frequency histogram.

**Gene.** The basic unit of heredity; genes are composed of DNA.

**Generation Time (for cells).** The time it takes for a population of cells to double in number.

**Genome.** The complete genetic material of an organism.

**Gram, g.** The basic SI unit for mass.

**Gram Atomic Mass (or weight).** The mass, in grams, of 1 mole of a given element. Note: weight and mass are not synonyms, and it is correct to use gram atomic or molecular *mass.* However, it is common practice to speak of "atomic weight," "molecular weight," and "formula weight," as we do in this book.

**Gram Formula Mass (or weight, FW).** The mass, in grams, of 1 mole of a given compound, the sum of the atomic masses of the atoms that make up that compound. See also note under "Gram Atomic Mass."

**Gram Molecular Mass (or weight, MW).** See "Gram Formula Mass."

**Guanine, G.** One of the four types of nucleotide subunit that comprise DNA and RNA.

**Half-Life.** The time it takes for half of the initial number of radioactive atoms in a given sample to undergo radioactive decay.

**Hemocytometer.** A modified microscope slide used for counting cells. The most common type is a Neubauer hemocytometer.

**Hydrates (in chemistry).** Compounds that contain chemically bound water.

**Incident Light (in spectrophotometry).** The light that is directed towards the sample or the blank.

**Independent Variable.** A variable whose value is controlled by the experimenter. (See also "Variable" and "Dependent Variable.")

**International Unit (IU) of Enzyme Activity.** The amount of enzyme required to catalyze transformation of 1.0 µmole of substrate to product per minute under specified conditions (such as a particular temperature and pH).

**Kilo-, k.** A prefix meaning 1,000.

**Kilogram, kg.** A unit of mass equal to 1,000 g. A kilogram is about 2.2 pounds.

**Kilometer, km.** A unit of length equal to 1,000 m.

**Lambda, λ.** (1) An older term sometimes used to mean 1 µL. (2) A kind of virus that in nature attacks bacteria and in the laboratory is commonly used by biotechnologists for various purposes.

**Least Squares Method.** A statistical method used to calculate the equation for the line of best fit.

**Limit of Detection.** The lowest level of an analyte that can be reliably discerned in an assay method.

**Line of Best Fit.** A line representing a series of data points on a graph in such a way that the points are collectively as close as possible to the line.

**Linear Relationship.** A relationship between two properties such that when they are plotted on a graph the points form a straight line.

**Liter, L.** A metric system unit of volume. $1\,L = 1\,dm^3$. A liter is slightly more than a quart. (See also "Volume.")

**Log, Logarithm, $Log_{10}$.** See "Common Logarithm."

**Log Reduction Value, LRV.** A calculated number that is usually used to express how effectively a method reduces the number of contaminants.

**Mean.** The average. The sum of all values divided by the number of values. Statisticians distinguish between the true mean of an entire population, represented by µ, and the mean of a sample from that population, represented by $\overline{X}$.

**Measurement.** Quantitative observation, numerical description.

**Measurement System.** A related group of units, such as inches, feet, and miles. (See also "United States Customary System," "Metric System," and "SI System.")

**Measures of Central Tendency.** Measures of the values about which a data set is centered, e.g. the mean, median, and mode.

**Measures of Dispersion (also called measures of variation or spread).** Measures of the variability in a set of numerical data, e.g., range, variance, and standard deviation.

**Median.** A statistic that is the middle value of a data set, the number that is greater than or equal to 50% of the values and less than or equal to 50% of the values.

**Meter, m.** The basic SI unit for length. A meter is a bit longer than 39 in.

**Metric System.** A measurement system used in most laboratories and in much of the world whose basic units include meters, grams, and liters. These basic units are modified by the addition of prefixes that designate powers of 10.

**Micro-, µ.** A prefix meaning 1/1,000,000 or $10^{-6}$.

**Microgram, µg.** A unit of mass that is 1/1,000,000 grams or $10^{-6}$ g.

**Microliter, µL.** A unit of volume that is 1/1,000,000 liters or $10^{-6}$ L.

**Micrometer, µm.** A unit of length that is 1/1,000,000 meters or $10^{-6}$ m.

**Micron.** A micrometer.

**Micropipette.** Device used to accurately dispense small volumes of liquids, typically in the 0.5 µL–1 mL range.

**Milli-, m.** A prefix meaning 1/1,000 or $10^{-3}$.

**Milligram, mg.** A unit of mass that is 1/1,000 g or $10^{-3}$ g.

**Milliliter, mL.** A unit of volume that is 1/1,000 L or $10^{-3}$ L.

**Millimeter, mm.** A unit of length that is 1/1,000 m or $10^{-3}$ m.

**Mitochondria.** The membrane-bound subunits of cells in which energy is produced.

**Mode (in statistics).** The value that is most frequently observed in a set of data.

**Molar.** A measure of the concentration of a substance, the number of moles of solute per liter of solvent.

**Mole (in chemistry).** A measure of the amount of a particular chemical substance, defined as the amount of substance that contains as many atoms or molecules as there are atoms in exactly 0.012 kg of $^{12}$Carbon. This quantity is called "Avogadro's number" and is about $6.022 \times 10^{23}$.

**Molecular Biology.** The study of the structure, function, and role of biologically important molecules, typically, DNA, RNA, and proteins.

**Nano-, n.** A prefix meaning 1/1,000,000,000 or $10^{-9}$.

**Nanogram, ng.** A unit of mass that is 1/1,000,000,000 g or $10^{-9}$ g.

**Nanoliter, nL.** A unit of volume that is 1/1,000,000,000 L or $10^{-9}$ L.

**Nanometer, nm.** A unit of length that is 1/1,000,000,000 m or $10^{-9}$ m.

**Natural Log, ln.** Logarithms whose base is a number called "e," whose value is approximately 2.7183.

**Normal Distribution (in statistics).** A description of data that occurs when most of the data cluster around a central peak (the mean) and the probabilities of obtaining a value further away from the mean taper off equally in both directions.

**Nucleotides.** The molecular building blocks of DNA and RNA.

**Numerator.** The number written above the line in a fraction.

**Nutrient Media.** Aqueous solutions that contain ingredients (such as salts, sugar, and vitamins) that cells require in order to grow and reproduce.

**Oligonucleotide.** A molecule made up of a small number of nucleotides, usually fewer than 25.

**Order of Magnitude.** One order of magnitude is $10^1$. For example, 100 is said to be "two orders of magnitude" less than 10,000 because $10,000 \div 100 = 100 = 10^2$.

**Ordinate.** In graphing, the Y-coordinate for a point, the distance of a point along the Y-axis.

**Origin.** The intersection of the X- and Y-axes on a two-dimensional graph whose coordinates are (0,0).

**Parts per Billion.** A concentration expression; the number of parts of a solute per 1 billion parts of total solution. The parts may have any units (such as grams) but must be the same in the numerator and denominator.

**Parts per Million.** A concentration expression; the number of parts of a solute per 1 million parts of total solution. The parts may have any units (such as grams) but must be the same in the numerator and denominator.

**Passage (in cell culture).** See "Subculture."

**Pellet (in centrifugation).** The material concentrated at the bottom of a centrifuge tube after centrifugation.

**Percent, %.** A fraction whose denominator is 100.

**Percent Yield.**

$$\frac{\text{Total Amount of a Protein of Interest at a Particular Step}}{\text{Total Amount of the Protein of Interest Initially}} \times 100\%.$$

**pH.** Expression of the concentration of $H^+$ ions (in units of moles/liter) in a solution where $pH = -\log [H^+]$.

**Pico-, p.** A prefix meaning 1/1,000,000,000,000 or $10^{-12}$.

**Picogram, pg.** A unit of mass that is 1/1,000,000,000,000 g or $10^{-12}$ g.

**Picoliter, pL.** A unit of volume that is 1/1,000,000,000,000 L or $10^{-12}$ L.

**Picometer, pm.** A unit of length that is 1/1,000,000,000,000 m or $10^{-12}$ m.

**Plasmids.** Small, circular DNA molecules that were originally isolated from bacteria and are commonly used as vectors.

**Plate Reader.** A type of spectrophotometer used to measure the absorbance of samples contained in plates with multiple wells (depressions) each of which contains a different sample.

**Polyacrylamide gel electrophoresis, PAGE.** A type of electrophoresis commonly used to separate proteins of different sizes from one another under the influence of an electrical current.

**Polymerase Chain Reaction, PCR.** A method of amplifying the amount of a specific sequence of DNA.

**Polymerase.** Enzyme that replicates DNA or RNA.

**Population.** A group of events, objects, or individuals where each member of the group has some unifying characteristic(s). Examples of populations are all of a person's red blood cells and all the enzyme molecules in a test tube.

**Population Variance (in statistics).** The sum of squares divided by the number of values.

**Primers.** During replication of DNA, short strands of DNA or RNA that attach to the template DNA and provide a starting point for the polymerase enzymes.

**Proportion.** Two ratios that have the same value but different numbers. For example, $1/2 = 5/10$.

**Proportionality Constant.** A value that expresses the relationship between the numerators and the denominators in a proportional relationship.

**Protein.** Diverse biological molecules that are composed of amino acid subunits and that control the structure, function, and regulations of cells.

**Protocol/Procedure.** These words are used to refer to the instructions to perform a specific task. A familiar example would be a recipe in a cookbook. The recipe includes a list of ingredients required and possibly equipment, such as a mixer. The recipe also includes the steps required to combine the ingredients and prepare the final food. Similarly, a protocol/procedure in the scientific literature usually includes a list of the materials required followed by step-by-step directions. The two terms protocol and procedure can have slightly different meanings in different situations, but we use them interchangeably in this text.

**Purification Factor.** A comparison of the specific activity at some point in a protein purification procedure to the specific activity at the beginning of the purification process.

**Quantitative Analysis.** The determination of how much of a particular material is present in a sample.

**Quantitative PCR, qPCR (also called "Real Time" PCR).** A PCR method that monitors a PCR reaction as it occurs and allows analysis of the amount of template originally present in the reaction mixture.

**Radioisotopes.** Materials that produce radiation.

**Radius of Rotation.** The distance from the center of rotation to the material being centrifuged.

**Range.** (1) A range of values, from the lowest to the highest, that a method or instrument can measure with acceptable results. (2) A statistical measure that is the absolute difference between the lowest and the highest values in a set of data.

**Ratio.** The relative sizes of two quantities, for example, "25 miles per 1 gallon" and "10 mg of NaCl per 1 liter." Ratios are often expressed in the laboratory as a quotient, for example, "10,000 cells/1 mL" and "10 mg NaCl/1 L."

**Reaction Mixture.** To a biologist, a reaction mixture is a solution containing an enzyme that catalyzes a reaction together with its substrate(s) and any required cofactors and buffers.

**Reagent/Solution/Biological Solution.** These terms have various usages in scientific literature. In this text, we use all three terms to refer to any material that is used as part of an experiment, laboratory test, or procedure to make a product. Almost all such materials used in biotechnology applications involve water, that is, are aqueous. For example, an enzyme used to break apart DNA would be dissolved in water (along with a suitable buffer).

**Reciprocal.** A number related to another so that when multiplied together their product equals 1. To calculate the reciprocal of a number, divide 1 by that number. For example, the reciprocal of 5 is 1/5 or 0.2.

**Regression Equation.** The equation for the line of best fit on a graph. This equation expresses the relationship between a dependent and an independent variable.

**Relative Centrifugal Field.** The force in a centrifuge relative to the earth's force of gravity.

**Relative Standard Deviation.** See "Coefficient of Variation."

**Restriction Digest.** An enzymatic reaction in which DNA is cut with specialized enzymes, called restriction endonucleases.

**Restriction Endonucleases.** Enzymes that recognize a specific DNA sequence and cleave the DNA at that site.

**Reverse Transcription, RT.** The enzyme-catalyzed translation of an RNA sequence into DNA with the same genetic information.

**Revolutions per Minute (RPM).** A measure of the speed of rotation in a centrifuge.

**Ribonucleic Acid, RNA.** A chemical whose structure is related to that of DNA, which is found in the nucleus and cytoplasm of cells and that plays a number of important roles in protein synthesis and other cellular activities.

**Ribosomes.** The cellular subunit responsible for manufacturing proteins.

**"Rise" (in graphing).** An expression that describes the amount by which the Y-coordinate changes on a two-dimensional graph, the vertical change in position.

**"Run" (in graphing).** An expression that describes the amount by which the X-coordinate changes on a two-dimensional graph, the horizontal change in position.

**Sample.** A subset of a population. For example, a person's blood sample is a subset of the population of all that person's blood.

**Sample Data Set.** When a sample is drawn from a population and the value for a particular variable is measured for each individual in the sample, the resulting values constitute a data set.

**Scientific Notation (also exponential notation).** The use of exponents to simplify handling numbers that are very large or very small. A value is expressed in scientific notation as a number between 1 and 10 multiplied by 10 raised to a power. For example, 4,500 in scientific notation is $4.5 \times 10^3$.

**Seeding (in cell culture).** To add cells to a culture vessel.

**Semilogarithmic Plot.** A type of graph that has a log scale on one axis and a linear scale on the other axis.

**Serial Dilutions.** Dilutions made in series (each one derived from the one before) and that all have the same dilution factor. For example, a series of 1/10 dilutions of an original sample would be 1, 1/10, 1/100, and 1/1,000.

**SI System (Système International d'Unités).** A standardized system of units of measurement adopted in 1960 by a number of international organizations, which is derived from the metric system.

**SI Unit of Enzyme Activity.** The amount of enzyme necessary to transform 1.0 mole of substrate to product per second under optimal conditions.

**Significant Figure.** The number of digits in a number that convey useful information.

**Slope (of a line).** Given a straight line plotted on a graph, the slope of the line is how steeply the line rises or falls. It is the ratio of vertical change to horizontal change between any two points on the line. Slope can be calculated by choosing any two points on the line and dividing the change in their Y values by the change in their X values.

**Solute.** A substance that is dissolved in some other material. For example, if table salt is dissolved in water, salt is the solute and water is the solvent.

**Solution (general chemical definition).** A homogeneous mixture of two or more substances, called solutes, dissolved in another substance, called solvent, where the molecules of each kind of substance are in direct contact with one another.

**Solvent.** A substance that dissolves another. For example, if salt is dissolved in water, then water is the solvent.

**Specific Activity.** The amount (or units) of a protein of interest divided by the total amount of all proteins in a sample.

**Spectrophotometer.** Laboratory instruments that measure how much light is absorbed as it passes through a liquid sample.

**Standard.** A physical embodiment of a unit of measure.

**Standard Curve.** A graph that shows the relationship between a response, for example, of an instrument, and a property that the experimenter controls, for example, the concentration of a substance.

**Standard Deviation.** The average amount by which each value in a set of values differs from the mean. Also, the square root of the variance.

**Stock Solution.** A concentrated solution that is diluted to a working concentration.

**Subculture (in cell culture).** The process of removing cultured cells from their culture vessel, suspending them in fresh medium, and placing them in a new culture vessel(s) such that the cell density is reduced. Each time this is done, it is called a "passage." The process is also called "passaging" the cells or "splitting" the cells.

**Sum of Squares (also called the total squared deviation).** The result obtained when adding the squares of a set of values.

**Supernatant.** The liquid material remaining above the pellet after centrifugation of a suspension.

**Suspension (in chemistry).** A mixture in which fine particles are suspended in a fluid (usually water in a biology laboratory) where they are supported by buoyancy.

**Target Sequence (in PCR).** The section of DNA that is replicated.

**Template DNA.** A piece of DNA that is of interest and that will be copied in PCR.

**Thermocycler.** A device used in PCR that subjects the reaction mixture to a series of repeated temperature cycles.

**Threshold (for a graph).** A change in a relationship plotted on a graph.

**Threshold Cycle, $C_t$, (in PCR).** The cycle number where the fluorescence labeling the DNA copies crosses a threshold such that it is bright enough to reliably detect.

**Thymine, T.** One of the four types of nucleotide subunit that comprise DNA.

**Transcription Factor.** A protein that turns a gene on or off at the proper time.

**Transfection (relating to genetics).** The introduction of genetic information from one higher order (i.e. not bacterial) cell to another.

**Transformation (relating to genetics).** The introduction of genetic information from one bacterial cell into another, usually involving a plasmid vector.

**Transformation Efficiency.** When introducing a gene of interest into bacteria using a plasmid vector, the number of transformed bacteria per µg of plasmid DNA.

**Transmittance (in spectrophotometry).** The ratio of light transmitted through the sample to that transmitted through the blank.

**Trillion.** An ambiguous term that in common usage often, but not always, means 1,000,000,000,000.

**Tris.** Tris(hydroxymethyl)aminomethane. A chemical often used in molecular biology to buffer laboratory solutions, purchased as a powder.

**Unit (of measure).** A precisely defined amount of a property.

**Unit Conversion Factor.** The number or formula required to convert a measurement from one unit to another, for example the value that relates pounds to kilograms.

**United States Customary System, USCS.** The measurement system common in the United States that includes miles, pounds, gallons, inches, and feet.

**Uracil, U.** One of the four types of nucleotide subunit that comprise RNA.

**Value (in math).** An assigned or calculated numerical quantity.

**Variable.** A property or a characteristic that can have various values (in contrast to a constant that always has the same value). (See also "Dependent Variable" and "Independent Variable.")

**Variance.** A measure of the variability in a set of data. The variance is an average of the squared deviation from the mean for all the points in a set of data.

**Vector (in molecular biology).** DNA molecule that has the ability to replicate and into which molecular biologists insert a fragment of DNA of interest to carry the DNA of interest into another cell.

**Volume.** The amount of space a substance occupies. Commonly, liter ($dm^3$) is used as the basic unit of volume in biological settings. See also "Liter."

**Volume per Volume Percent, v/v.** A concentration expression; mL of solute per 100 mL total solution.

**Weight per Volume Percent, w/v.** A concentration expression; the weight of the solute (in g) per 100 mL of total solution.

**Weight per Weight Percent, w/w.** A concentration expression; grams of solute per 100 grams of solution.

**X-Axis.** The main horizontal line on a graph.

**Y-Axis.** The main vertical line on a graph.

**Y-Intercept.** The point at which a graph intersects the Y-axis, where X=0, on a two-dimensional graph.

# Introduction

We have good and bad news. The bad news: Mathematical descriptions and operations permeate daily life in the biotechnology workplace, and many employers report that entry-level scientists and technicians cannot consistently and accurately perform the math required for their jobs. This is, indeed, bad news for both employer and employee. Now, the good news: The vast majority of people, with some instruction, can, in fact, perform the math that is required for the majority of jobs. Let us take a look at the key math tools and concepts used in biotechnology settings:

- Addition, subtraction, multiplication, and division
- Fractions
- Ratios and proportions
- Solving equations with one unknown
- Exponents and scientific notation
- Logarithms
- Linear equations
- Graphing data
- Exponential relationships

It is likely that the items on this list (with a couple of possible exceptions) are familiar to you and are things you studied in middle school. It is true that there are scientists and engineers who use advanced math (e.g., calculus) in their work, but those jobs are less common and are usually filled by specialists with advanced credentials. Some readers may discover that a math-rich career is right for them. However, most biotechnologists use only middle school or beginning high school math in their routine work.

If the math required to be successful in biotechnology is mainly middle school math, why do so many people have difficulty with it? Here are two important reasons:

1. Most people do not have enough practice with the math calculations required in a biotechnology setting. A related problem is that math often seems intimidating and beginners often do not feel confident about their mathematical abilities.
2. Another issue for beginning science professionals is that the math that is required in the workplace is often camouflaged. For example, here is a problem from later in this textbook:

***Show that 1 µg of lambda*** $DNA = 1.9 \times 10^{10}$ ***molecules. The length of a single lambda DNA molecule is 48,502 bp.***

This short question includes unfamiliar terms, "lambda" and "bp." To solve the problem, you must know a bit about the structure of DNA and must know where to find conversion factors that relate one unit to another. The appropriate conversion factors for this problem are specialized and are not found in every middle school text or cookbook. However, the underlying math skill that is required to solve this problem is simply ratios and proportions. Thus, the math required is not difficult for most people, but finding the math within the context takes experience.

This textbook is designed to help you in two ways. First, the most common types of calculations encountered in biotechnology workplaces are introduced along with ample practice problems. Second, there are problems provided where the required math tool is "hidden," and you will need to find it. With practice, most people develop the skills they need to enter the exciting biotechnology workplace.

# I

# Brief Review of Some Basic Math Techniques

**Chapters in This Unit**



DOI: 10.1201/9780429282744-1

## INTRODUCTION

In 1999, NASA, the US space agency, lost a $125 million robotic spacecraft in a spectacular mishap that could likely have been avoided if scientists had written down the units in their calculations. The errant spacecraft dipped 100 km lower than planned into the Martian atmosphere where it vanished. The problem apparently arose because of miscommunication between two teams working on the orbiter mission. One team was expressing force in metric units while the other team expressed force in units of pounds. Apparently, the teams did not write down the units of their calculations and as a result the orbiter went to the wrong place and was lost. According to Marcia S. Smith, space policy analyst of the Congressional Research Service in Washington D.C., "Truly, it is just dumbfounding, flabbergasting...that this could possibly happen." (Reported by R. Cowen in *Science News*, Volume 156, October 9, p. 229, 1999.)

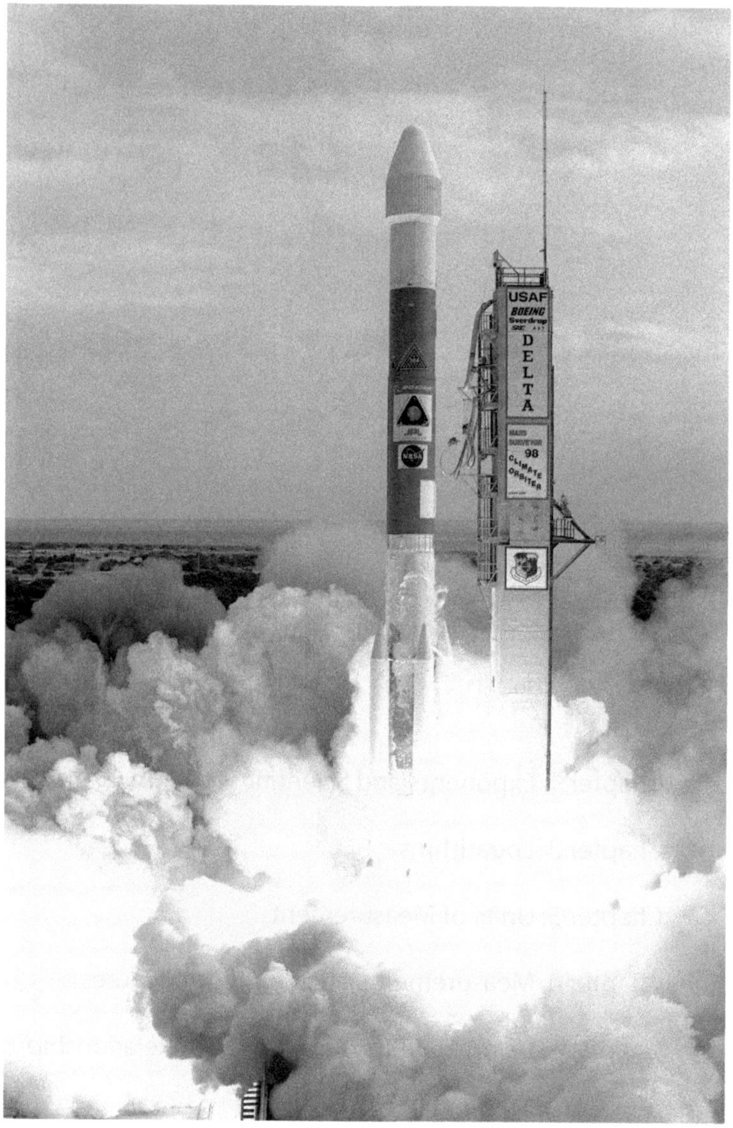


The Mars Robotic Spacecraft Being Launched in 1998. (Image Credit: NASA/KSC, Public domain, via Wikimedia Commons)

We can all learn from NASA's mistake. Their mistake was not due to an error in some complex, esoteric math calculation. It related to a simple failure to keep track of measurement units. The most obvious lesson is therefore to always record and keep track of units. Frequently in math classes problems are solved without units, or units are present but are not recorded. This may be acceptable in a math class but can lead to major problems in a workplace.

Biotechnologists do not lose spacecraft when we make a math error, but we can lose valuable reagents, cells, time, and money. Many biotechnologists work with products that have medical applications. Mistakes in making or administering medical products can be life-threatening. The good news is that with practice and attention, you can develop your ability to perform basic math calculations successfully.

The topics in this unit were selected because of their fundamental importance and because students frequently require a refresher in them. These topics, such as working with scientific notation or using metric units, are usually taught in middle school or introductory high school math courses. However, like anything that we do not use frequently, these skills may become rusty. This unit has a number of practice (drill) problems to help you become comfortable and skilled in basic calculations that are particularly relevant in biotechnology settings. For example, some units of measurement are familiar to everyone, but working with units like nm (nanometer) or µL (microliter) can feel uncomfortable at first. Practicing with these units will help them become familiar to you. Later units in this text will show you how these basic calculation skills apply to a wide variety of interesting and important biotechnology tasks.

# Exponents and Scientific Notation

1



## 1.1 EXPONENTS

Exponents and scientific notation are routinely used in the laboratory, and so it is important to be able to manipulate them easily. This chapter provides short sections that review these math tools. It also provides practice problems to help you become comfortable and efficient in calculations involving exponents and scientific notation. If the calculations in this chapter seem difficult at first, they will become easier with practice.

An **exponent** *is used to show that a number is to be multiplied by itself a certain number of times*. For example, $2^4$ is read "two raised to the fourth power" and means that 2 is multiplied by itself 4 times:

$$2^4 = 2 \times 2 \times 2 \times 2 = 16$$

Similarly,

$$10^2 \text{ means: } 10 \times 10, \text{ or } 100$$

$$4^5 \text{ means: } 4 \times 4 \times 4 \times 4 \times 4, \text{ or } 1{,}024$$

*The number that is multiplied is called the* **base** *and the power to which the base is raised is the* **exponent**. In the expression $10^3$, the base is 10 and the exponent is 3.

A negative exponent indicates that the reciprocal of the number should be multiplied times itself. For example,

$$10^{-3} = \frac{1}{10} \times \frac{1}{10} \times \frac{1}{10} = \frac{1}{1{,}000} = 0.001$$

Rules that govern the manipulation of exponents in calculations are summarized in Box 1.1.

DOI: 10.1201/9780429282744-2

**Box 1.1 Calculations Involving Exponents**

1. **To multiply two numbers with exponents where the numbers have the same base, add the exponents:**

$$a^m \times a^n = a^{m+n}$$

Two examples:

$$5^3 \times 5^6 = 5^9$$

$$10^{-3} \times 10^4 = 10^1 = 10$$

To convince yourself that this rule makes sense, consider the following example:

$$2^3 \times 2^2 = (2 \times 2 \times 2) \times (2 \times 2) = 2 \text{ multiplied 5 times } = 2^5 = 32$$

2. **To divide two numbers with exponents where the numbers have the same base, subtract the exponents:**

$$\frac{a^m}{a^n} = a^{m-n}$$

Two examples:

$$5^3/5^6 = 5^{3-6} = 5^{-3}$$

$$2^{-3}/2^{-4} = 2^{(-3)-(-4)} = 2^1 = 2$$

Convince yourself that this rule makes sense by rewriting the example this way:

$$\frac{5^3}{5^6} = \frac{\cancel{5} \times \cancel{5} \times \cancel{5}}{\cancel{5} \times \cancel{5} \times \cancel{5} \times 5 \times 5 \times 5} = \frac{1}{5 \times 5 \times 5} = \frac{1}{125} = 5^{-3}$$

3. **To raise an exponential number to another power, multiply the two exponents.**

$$\left(a^m\right)^n = a^{m \times n}$$

Two examples:

$$\left(2^3\right)^2 = 2^6$$

$$\left(10^3\right)^{-4} = 10^{-12}$$

To convince yourself that this rule makes sense, consider this example:

$$\left(2^3\right)^2 = 2^3 \times 2^3 = (2 \times 2 \times 2) \times (2 \times 2 \times 2) = 2^6$$

4. **To multiply or divide numbers with exponents that have different bases, convert the numbers with exponents to their corresponding values without exponents. Then, multiply or divide.**

Two examples:

$$\text{Multiply: } 3^2 \times 2^4$$

$$3^2 = 9 \text{ and } 2^4 = 16,$$

$$\text{so, } 9 \times 16 = 144$$

$$\textbf{Divide: } 4^{-3} / 2^3$$

$$2^3 = 8$$

$$4^{-3} = 0.015625$$

$$\frac{0.015625}{8} = 0.001953125$$

5. **To add or subtract numbers with exponents (whether their bases are the same or not), convert the numbers with exponents to their corresponding values without exponents.**
   For example,

$$4^3 + 2^3 = 64 + 8 = 72$$

6. **By definition, any number (other than zero) raised to the 0 power is equal to 1.**
   For example,

$$85^0 = 1$$

**Example Problem:**

Perform the operations indicated:

$$\frac{10}{43^2 + 13^3}$$

***Answer:***

The denominator involves addition of numbers with exponents. Convert the numbers with exponents to standard notation. Then perform the calculations.

$$\frac{10}{(43)^2 + (13)^3} = \frac{10}{1{,}849 + 2{,}197} = \frac{10}{4{,}046} = \frac{5}{2{,}023} \approx \mathbf{0.002472}$$

Why do we care about the manipulations in Box 1.1? Equations like this, $\frac{a^m}{a^n} = a^{m-n}$, might appear to have little use outside a math class, but this algebraic notation actually describes a math procedure that is used routinely in the laboratory. Let us look at an example from cell culture, a topic explored in more detail later in this text. Suppose you are working with cells growing in a nutritional liquid medium, and these cells have been genetically modified to manufacture a product of interest. You know that you have $10^4$ cells in each milliliter of liquid culture medium, and you need $10^3$ cells to run a test of the cells' characteristics. How many milliliters of culture do you need to remove to run your test? To solve this problem, you will need to divide $10^3$ by $10^4$. In this example, the symbol "a," which is the base, is 10. The symbol "m" is 3 and the symbol "n" is 4. So,

$$\frac{a^m}{a^n} = a^{m-n}$$

$$\frac{10^3}{10^4} = 10^{3-4} = 10^{-1} = 0.1$$

This means you need 0.1 mL of culture medium to obtain $10^3$ cells. Of course, your calculator can help you to solve this type of problem, but when using a calculator, it is important to understand what you are doing in order to ensure that your answers are correct. (We will practice this type of calculation in later sections of this text, so do not worry now if it seems difficult. The point is that algebra provides tools we use routinely to solve problems in a biotechnology workplace.)

**Practice Problems**

1. ***Give the whole number or fraction that corresponds to these exponential expressions.***
   a. $2^2$ b. $3^3$ c. $2^{-2}$
   d. $3^{-3}$ e. $10^2$ f. $10^4$
   g. $10^{-2}$ h. $10^{-4}$ i. $5^0$
   j. ***Explain how to solve 1d using your calculator.***
   k. ***Explain how to solve 1d without using your calculator.***
2. **Perform the operations indicated:**
   a. $(2^2)(3^3)$ b. $(14^3)(3^6)$ c. $5^5 - 2^3$
   d. $5^7/8^4$ e. $(6^{-2})(3^2)$ f. $(-0.4)^3 + 9.6^2$
   g. $(a^2)(a^3)$ h. $c^3/c^{-6}$ i. $(3^4)^2$
   j. $(c^{-3})^{-5}$ k. $\frac{13}{43^2 + 13^3}$ l. $10^2/10^3$

*Answers:*

1. a. $2^2 = \mathbf{4}$ b. $3^3 = \mathbf{27}$ c. $2^{-2} = 1/4 = \mathbf{0.25}$
   d. $3^{-3} = 1/27 \approx \mathbf{0.037}$ e. $10^2 = \mathbf{100}$ f. $10^4 = \mathbf{10{,}000}$
   g. $10^{-2} = 1/100 = \mathbf{0.01}$ h. $10^{-4} = 1/10{,}000 = \mathbf{0.0001}$ i. $5^0 = \mathbf{1}$
   j. Press 3; press $y^x$; press 3; press ±; press = (your calculator may be somewhat different)
   k. $(1/3)(1/3)(1/3) = 1/27 \approx \mathbf{0.037}$
2. a. $(2^2)(3^3) = (4)(27) = \mathbf{108}$ b. $(14^3)(3^6) = (2744)(729) = \mathbf{2{,}000{,}376}$
   c. $5^5 - 2^3 = (3{,}125) - 8 = \mathbf{3{,}117}$ d. $\frac{5^7}{8^4} = \frac{78{,}125}{4{,}096} \approx \mathbf{19.07}$

e. $(6^{-2})\,(3^2) = (1/36)\,(9) = 9/36 = 1/4 = \mathbf{0.25}$
f. $(-0.4)^3 + (9.6)^2 = (-0.064) + (92.16) = \mathbf{92.096}$

g. $(a^2)\,(a^3) = \mathbf{a^5}$ h. $\dfrac{c^3}{c^{-6}} = \mathbf{c^9}$

i. $(3^4)^2 = 3^8 = \mathbf{6{,}561}$ j. $(c^{-3})^{-5} = \mathbf{c^{15}}$

k. $\dfrac{13}{(43)^2 + (13)^3} = \dfrac{13}{1{,}849 + 2{,}197}$ l. $\dfrac{10^2}{10^3} = \dfrac{1}{10} = 10^{-1} = \mathbf{0.1}$

$= \dfrac{13}{4{,}046} \approx \mathbf{0.00321305}$

## 1.2 EXPONENTS WHERE THE BASE IS 10

In preparation for discussing scientific notation, consider the particular case of numbers written with exponents where the base is 10 as illustrated in Table 1.1.

**TABLE 1.1 Exponents Where the Base is Ten – "Powers of Ten"**

| Number in Standard Notation | Number Written with Exponent | Number Written in Words |
|---|---|---|
| 1,000,000 | $= 10^6$ | = one million |
| 100,000 | $= 10^5$ | = one hundred thousand |
| 10,000 | $= 10^4$ | = ten thousand |
| 1,000 | $= 10^3$ | = one thousand |
| 100 | $= 10^2$ | = one hundred |
| 10 | $= 10^1$ | = ten |
| 1 | $= 10^0$ | = one |
| 0.1 | $= 10^{-1}$ | = one tenth |
| 0.01 | $= 10^{-2}$ | = one hundredth |
| 0.001 | $= 10^{-3}$ | = one thousandth |
| 0.0001 | $= 10^{-4}$ | = one ten thousandth |
| 0.00001 | $= 10^{-5}$ | = one hundred thousandth |
| 0.000001 | $= 10^{-6}$ | = one millionth |

People commonly use the phrase "orders of magnitude" where **one order of magnitude** *is $10^1$*. Using this terminology, $10^2$ is said to be two orders of magnitude less than $10^4$. Similarly, $10^8$ is three orders of magnitude greater than $10^5$.

## 1.3 SCIENTIFIC NOTATION

**Scientific notation** is a tool that uses exponents to simplify handling numbers that are very big or very small. Consider the number:

**0.0000000000000000000000602**

In scientific notation, this lengthy number is compactly expressed as follows:

$$\mathbf{6.02 \times 10^{-23}}$$

A value in scientific notation is usually written as a number between 1 and 10 multiplied by 10 raised to a power. For example,

$$\mathbf{100}(\text{Standard Notation}) = \mathbf{10^2} = \mathbf{1 \times 10^2}\,(\text{Scientific Notation})$$

$$1\times10^{2} = 1\times10\times10 = 100$$

$$300 \text{(Standard Notation)} = 3\times10^{2} \text{(Scientific Notation)}$$

$$3\times10^{2} = 3\times10\times10 = 300$$

The number of bacterial cells in 1 L of culture might be

$$100{,}000{,}000{,}000 \text{(Standard Notation)} = 1\times10^{11} \text{(Scientific Notation)}$$

A number in scientific notation has two parts. *The first part, that is, a number between* 1 and 10, *is sometimes called the* **coefficient**. *The second part is* 10 *raised to some power,* **the exponential term**. For example,

| First Part (Coefficient) | Second Part (Exponential Term) |
|---|---|
| 1,000 = 1 | $\times 10^{3}$ |
| 235 = 2.35 | $\times 10^{2}$ |

As shown in Table 1.1, a negative exponent is used for a number less than one.
For example,

$$1\times10^{-5} = \frac{1}{10}\times\frac{1}{10}\times\frac{1}{10}\times\frac{1}{10}\times\frac{1}{10} = \frac{1}{100{,}000} = 0.00001$$

Observe that when the coefficient is 1, it is often omitted. For example, $1\times10^{2} = 10^{2}$.
Box 1.2 gives a procedure to convert a number from standard notation to scientific notation.

**Box 1.2 A Procedure to Convert a Number from Scientific Notation to Standard Notation**

Step 1.

**a.** If the number in standard notation is greater than 10, move the decimal point to the left so that there is one nonzero digit to the left of the decimal point. This gives the first part of the notation.

**b.** If the number in standard notation is less than 1, move the decimal point to the right so that there is one nonzero digit to the left of the decimal point. This gives the first part of the notation.

**c.** If the number in standard notation is between 1 and 10, then scientific notation is seldom used.

Step 2. Count how many places the decimal was moved in Step 1.

Step 3.

**a.** If the decimal was moved to the left, then the number of places it was moved gives the exponent in the second part of the notation.

**b.** If the decimal point was moved to the right, then place a negative (–) sign in front of the value. This is the exponent for the second part of the notation.

**Example:**

Express the number **5,467** in scientific notation.

**Step 1.** This number is greater than 10. Therefore, move the decimal point to the left so that there is only one non-zero digit to the left of the decimal point:

= **5,467.** move decimal point 3 places left

= **5.467**

**Step 2.** The decimal point was moved three places to the left.

**Step 3.** The exponent for the second part of the notation is therefore 3. This means the number in scientific notation is:

$$\mathbf{5.467 \times 10^3}$$

**Example Problem:**

Convert the number **0.000348** to scientific notation.

*Answer:*

**Step 1.** This number is less than 1. Move the decimal point to the right:

**0.000348**

= 3.48

**Step 2.** The decimal point was moved four places to the right.

**Step 3.** The exponent is –4, so the answer in scientific notation is: $\mathbf{3.48 \times 10^{-4}}$.

**Practice Problems**

1. ***In each pair, underline the number that is larger:***
   a. $1\times10^{-3}$ ***or*** $1\times10^{3}$ b. $1\times10^{-6}$ ***or*** $1\times10^{1}$ c. $4\times10^{3}$ ***or*** $4\times10^{-4}$
2. ***Fill in the blanks so that the numbers on both sides of the = sign are equal. For example,*** $100 = 1\times10^{2}$
   a. *1,000 = 1 × 10*__ b. *100,000 = 1 × 10*__ c. *0.1 = 1 × 10*__
   d. *0.001 = 1 × 10*__ e. *2,000 = 2 × 10*__ f. *0.003 = 3 × 10*__
   g. *5,000 = 5 × 10*__ h. *101 = 1.01 × 10*__ i. *0.32 = 3.2 × 10*__
   j. *0.004 = 4 × 10*__ k. *25 = 2.5 × 10*__ l. *0.023 = 2.3 × 10*__
3. ***Convert the following numbers to scientific notation.***
   a. *54.0* b. *4,567* c. *0.345000* d. *10,000,000*
   e. *0.009078* f. *540* g. *0.003040* h. *200,567,987*
4. ***Convert the following numbers to standard notation.***
   a. $12.3\times10^{3}$ b. $4.56\times10^{4}$ c. $4.456\times10^{-5}$
   d. $2.300\times10^{-3}$ e. $0.56\times10^{6}$ f. $0.45\times10^{-2}$

*Answers*

1. a. $1\times10^{-3}$ or $\underline{\mathbf{1\times10^{3}}}$ b. $1\times10^{-6}$ or $\underline{\mathbf{1\times10^{1}}}$ c. $\underline{\mathbf{4\times10^{3}}}$ or $4\times10^{-4}$

2. a. $1000 = 1 \times 10^{\underline{3}}$ b. $100{,}000 = 1 \times 10^{\underline{5}}$ c. $0.1 = 1 \times 10^{\underline{-1}}$
d. $0.001 = 1 \times 10^{\underline{-3}}$ e. $2{,}000 = 2 \times 10^{\underline{3}}$ f. $0.003 = 3 \times 10^{\underline{-3}}$
g. $5{,}000 = 5 \times 10^{\underline{3}}$ h. $101 = 1.01 \times 10^{\underline{2}}$ i. $0.32 = 3.2 \times 10^{\underline{-1}}$
j. $0.004 = 4 \times 10^{\underline{-3}}$ k. $25 = 2.5 \times 10^{\underline{1}}$ l. $0.023 = 2.3 \times 10^{\underline{-2}}$

3. a. $54.0 = \mathbf{5.40 \times 10^{1}}$ b. $4{,}567 = \mathbf{4.567 \times 10^{3}}$
c. $0.345000 = \mathbf{3.45000 \times 10^{-1}}$ d. $10{,}000{,}000 = \mathbf{1 \times 10^{7}}$
e. $0.009078 = \mathbf{9.078 \times 10^{-3}}$ f. $540 = \mathbf{5.4 \times 10^{2}}$
g. $0.003040 = \mathbf{3.040 \times 10^{-3}}$ h. $200{,}567{,}987 = \mathbf{2.00567987 \times 10^{8}}$

4. a. $12.3 \times 10^{3} = \mathbf{12{,}300}$ b. $4.56 \times 10^{4} = \mathbf{45{,}600}$
c. $4.456 \times 10^{-5} = \mathbf{0.00004456}$ d. $2.300 \times 10^{-3} = \mathbf{0.002300}$
e. $0.56 \times 10^{6} = \mathbf{560{,}000}$ f. $0.45 \times 10^{-2} = \mathbf{0.0045}$

## 1.4 MORE ABOUT SCIENTIFIC NOTATION

So far, we have shown the customary manner of writing numbers in scientific notation with the coefficient as a number between 1 and 10. However, it is not necessary to always write scientific notation this way*. For example, the 205 may be expressed as follows:

$$\mathbf{205. = 0.205 \times 10^{3}}$$

$$\mathbf{205. = 2.05 \times 10^{2}}$$

$$\mathbf{205. = 20.5 \times 10^{1}}$$

$$\mathbf{205. = 2{,}050 \times 10^{-1}}$$

$$\mathbf{205. = 20{,}500 \times 10^{-2}}$$

Similarly:

$$\mathbf{1.00 \times 10^{4} = 10.0 \times 10^{3} = 100. \times 10^{2}}$$

$$\mathbf{3.45 \times 10^{23} = 0.0345 \times 10^{25} = 345 \times 10^{21}}$$

There are situations where it is useful to manipulate coefficients and exponents without changing the value of the numbers. This is the case in addition and subtraction of numbers expressed in scientific notation, as will be shown in Section 1.5.

**Example Problem:**

Fill in the blank so that the numbers on both sides of the = sign are equal.

$$\mathbf{0.0055 \times 10^{4} = 5{,}500 \times 10^{—}}$$

***Answer:***

One way to think about this problem:

1. Convert the expression on the left to standard notation; it equals 55.

* In formal usage, it is not "scientific notation" unless the coefficient is a number between 1 and 10. However, for simplicity, we use the term "scientific notation" in this chapter where the coefficient is not a number between 1 and 10.

2. The number on the right side of the expression, 5500, is larger than the number on the left, 55. Therefore, the exponent that fills in the blank will need to be negative (to make 5500 smaller).
3. 5,500 times $10^{-2}$ equals 55. The answer is therefore −2.
4. You can check this answer with a calculator. First, enter the number on the left in scientific notation and have your calculator convert it to standard notation. Then, enter your answer on the right in scientific notation and have your calculator convert it to standard notation. Check that the two answers are the same.

Another way to think about this problem:

1. Observe that the coefficient on the left, 0.0055, is a smaller number than the coefficient on the right, 55,000.
2. To make 0.0055 equal to 55,000, the decimal point must move to the right six places; that is, 0.0055 must be multiplied by 10 over and over six times:

$$0.0055 \times 10^6 = 5{,}500$$

3. Since the coefficient on the left was *multiplied* by $10^6$, its exponent must be *divided* by $10^6$:

$$10^4 \div 10^6 = 10^{4-6} = 10^{-2} \text{ (see rule 2, Box 1.1)}$$

So, the new exponent is $\mathbf{10^{-2}}$.

4. You can again check the answer by entering both the left and right values into your calculator and converting both to standard notation to see if they are the same.

**Practice Problems**

1. ***Fill in the blanks so that the numbers on both sides of the = sign are equal. For example, $1\times10^2 = 10\times10^1$***

| | |
|---|---|
| a. $1\times10^3 = 10\times10^{\_\_}$ | b. $1\times10^4 = 10\times10^{\_\_}$ |
| c. $10\times10^4 = 1\times10^{\_\_}$ | d. $1\times10^1 = 0.1\times10^{\_\_}$ |
| e. $0.1\times10^3 = 10\times10^{\_\_}$ | f. $0.1\times10^4 = 10\times10^{\_\_}$ |
| g. $1\times10^2 = 0.10\times10^{\_\_}$ | h. $100\times10^1 = 1\times10^{\_\_}$ |
| i. $1\times10^3 = 1000\times10^{\_\_}$ | j. $10\times10^4 = 100\times10^{\_\_}$ |
| k. $1\times10^{-1} = 10\times10^{\_\_}$ | l. $1\times10^{-1} = 0.1\times10^{\_\_}$ |
| m. $1\times10^{-3} = 10\times10^{\_\_}$ | n. $1\times10^{-4} = 10\times10^{\_\_}$ |
| o. $1\times10^{-2} = 10\times10^{\_\_}$ | p. $1\times10^{-5} = 0.1\times10^{\_\_}$ |

2. ***Fill in the blanks so that the numbers on both sides of the = sign are equal. For example, $2.58\times10^{-2} = 25.8\times10^{-3}$***

a. $0.0050\times10^{-4} = 0.050\times10^{\_\_} = 0.50\times10^{\_\_} = 5.0\times10^{\_\_}$

b. $15.0\times10^{-3} = \_\_\_\_\times10^{-2} = \_\_\_\_\times10^{-1} = \_\_\_\_\times10^{1}$

| | |
|---|---|
| c. $5.45\times10^{-3} = 54.5\times10^{\_\_}$ | d. $100.00\times10^1 = 1.0000\times10^{\_\_}$ |
| e. $6.78\times10^2 = 0.678\times10^{\_\_}$ | f. $54.6\times10^2 = \_\_\_\_\times10^6$ |
| g. $45.6\times10^8 = \_\_\_\_\times10^6$ | h. $4.5\times10^{-3} = \_\_\_\_\times10^{-5}$ |
| i. $356.98\times10^{-3} = \_\_\_\_\times10^1$ | j. $0.0098\times10^{-2} = 0.98\times10^{\_\_}$ |

***Answers***

1. a. $1\times10^{3}=10\times10^{\underline{2}}$ b. $1\times10^{4}=10\times10^{\underline{3}}$
   c. $10\times10^{4}=1\times10^{\underline{5}}$ d. $1\times10^{1}=0.1\times10^{\underline{2}}$
   e. $0.1\times10^{3}=10\times10^{\underline{1}}$ f. $0.1\times10^{4}=10\times10^{\underline{2}}$
   g. $1\times10^{2}=0.10\times10^{\underline{3}}$ h. $100\times10^{1}=1\times10^{\underline{3}}$
   i. $1\times10^{3}=1000\times10^{\underline{0}}$ j. $10\times10^{4}=100\times10^{\underline{3}}$
   k. $1\times10^{-1}=10\times10^{\underline{-2}}$ l. $1\times10^{-1}=0.1\times10^{\underline{0}}$
   m. $1\times10^{-3}=10\times10^{\underline{-4}}$ n. $1\times10^{-4}=10\times10^{\underline{-5}}$
   o. $1\times10^{-2}=10\times10^{\underline{-3}}$ p. $1\times10^{-5}=0.1\times10^{\underline{-4}}$
2. a. $0.0050\times10^{-4}=0.05\times10^{\underline{-5}}=0.5\times10^{\underline{-6}}=5.0\times10^{\underline{-7}}$
   b. $15.0\times10^{-3}=\mathbf{1.5}\times10^{-2}=\mathbf{0.15}\times10^{-1}=\mathbf{0.0015}\times10^{1}$
   c. $5.45\times10^{-3}=54.5\times10^{\underline{-4}}$ d. $100.00\times10^{1}=1.0000\times10^{\underline{3}}$
   e. $6.78\times10^{2}=0.678\times10^{\underline{3}}$ f. $54.6\times10^{2}=\mathbf{0.00546}\times10^{6}$
   g. $45.6\times10^{8}=\mathbf{4,560}\times10^{6}$ h. $4.5\times10^{-3}=\mathbf{450}\times10^{-5}$
   i. $356.98\times10^{-3}=\mathbf{0.035698}\times10^{1}$ j. $0.0098\times10^{-2}=0.98\times10^{\underline{-4}}$

## 1.5 CALCULATIONS WITH SCIENTIFIC NOTATION

Box 1.3 summarizes how numbers in scientific notation are multiplied, divided, added, and subtracted.

**Box 1.3 Calculations Involving Numbers in Scientific Notation**

1. **To multiply numbers in scientific notation, use two steps:**

   Step 1. Multiply the coefficients together.
   Step 2. Add the exponents to which 10 is raised.

   For example,

$$\left(2.34\times10^{2}\right)\left(3.50\times10^{3}\right)=\underset{\text{(Multiply coefficients)}}{\left(2.34\times3.50\right)}\times\underset{\text{(Add exponents)}}{\left(10^{2+3}\right)}=8.19\times10^{5}$$

2. **To divide numbers in scientific notation, use two steps:**

   Step 1. Divide the coefficients.
   Step 2. Subtract the exponents.

   For example,

$$\left(5.4\times10^{5}\right)/\left(2.4\times10^{3}\right)=\underset{\text{(Divide coefficients)}}{\left(5.4/2.4\right)}\times\underset{\text{(Subtract exponents)}}{\left(10^{5-3}\right)}=2.25\times10^{2}$$

3. **To add or subtract numbers in scientific notation:**
   a. If the numbers being added or subtracted all have 10 raised to the same exponent, then the numbers can be simply added or subtracted as shown in these two examples:

$$\left(3.0\times10^{4}\right)+\left(2.5\times10^{4}\right)=?\qquad\left(7.56\times10^{21}\right)-\left(6.53\times10^{21}\right)=?$$

(Add coefficients) (Keep common power of 10) (Subtract coefficients) (Keep common power of 10)

$$\begin{array}{r}3.0\times10^{4}\\ +2.5\times10^{4}\\ \hline 5.5\times10^{4}\end{array}\qquad\begin{array}{r}7.56\times10^{21}\\ -6.53\times10^{21}\\ \hline 1.03\times10^{21}\end{array}$$

   b. If the numbers being added or subtracted do not all have 10 raised to the same exponent, then there are two strategies for adding and subtracting numbers:

Strategy 1: Convert the numbers to standard notation and then do the addition or subtraction:
For example,

$$\left(2.05\times10^{2}\right)-\left(9.05\times10^{-1}\right)=?$$

Convert both numbers to standard notation:

$$2.05\times10^{2}=205$$

$$9.05\times10^{-1}=0.905$$

Perform the calculation:

$$\begin{array}{r}205\\ -\;0.905\\ \hline 204.095\end{array}$$

Strategy 2: Rewrite the values so they all have 10 raised to the same power:
For example,

$$\left(2.05\times10^{2}\right)-\left(9.05\times10^{-1}\right)=?$$

To convert both numbers to a form such that they both have 10 raised to the same power:
Step 1. Decide what the common exponent will be. It should be either 2 or –1. Suppose we choose 2.
Step 2. Convert $9.05 \times 10^{-1}$ to scientific notation with an exponent of 2:

$$9.05\times10^{-1}=0.00905\times10^{2}.$$

Step 3. Perform the subtraction:

(Subtract coefficients) (Keep common power of 10)

$$\begin{array}{r}2.05\ \times10^{2}\\ -0.00905\ \times10^{2}\\ \hline 2.04095\ \times10^{2}\end{array}$$

**Example Problem:**

$$\left(3.45\times10^{23}\right)+\left(4.56\times10^{25}\right)=?$$

*Answer:*

The two numbers in this example would require many zeros if written in standard notation. Therefore, the strategy of expressing both values in scientific notation with the same exponent is preferred:

Step 1. Decide on a common exponent. Either one is acceptable. Suppose we choose 25.
Step 2. Express both numbers in a form with the same exponent.

$$3.45\times10^{23}=0.0345\times10^{25}$$

Step 3. Perform the addition.

$$\text{(Add coefficients)}\ \text{(Keep common power of 10)}$$

$$\begin{array}{rl} & 0.0345\times10^{25} \\ + & 4.56\quad\times10^{25} \\ \hline & 4.5945\times10^{25} \end{array}$$

Scientific calculators greatly facilitate calculations involving numbers in scientific notation. A calculator will hold a limited number of places and will not accept very large or very small numbers. But a scientific calculator works easily with large and small numbers expressed in scientific notation. On my basic calculator, to key in the number $1\times10^3$, I push the following keys:

[1]

[EE]

[3]

Note that I do **not** key in the number 10, the base in scientific notation. "EE" tells my calculator that the 10 is present. To key in the number $3\times10^{-4}$ on my calculator, I press:

[3]

[EE]

[4]

[+/−]

The [+/−] key (the "opposite" key) tells the calculator I want a negative exponent. Sometimes "exp" is used to indicate that 10 is being raised to a certain power. Consult your instruction manual to see how to key in a number in scientific notation. Once the numbers are keyed in, they can be added, subtracted, multiplied, and divided just like numbers in standard notation.

**Example Problem:**

Figure 1.1 is a poster from the website of the United States Department of Energy Genomics Science Program. What is a **genome**? Organisms are made of one or more cells. When an organism reproduces, its cells divide to form new cells. Parental cells pass information to their offspring cells telling them how to grow and develop to form a particular organism with that individual's unique traits. *Information is transmitted from a parent cell to its offspring cells in the form of* **genes**, which are represented in the illustration in the poster. A **genome** *is all the genes that are contained in each cell of an organism.*

a. Suppose a person consists of about 10 trillion highly coordinated cells. (A **trillion** *is 1,000,000,000,000.*) Express 10 trillion in scientific notation.
b. Each cell in a person (with a few exceptions) contains two copies of the genome: one copy from the person's mother and the other from his/her father. The human genome consists of about 3 billion base pairs of DNA (a "base pair" is a building block of which DNA is composed). A **billion** *is 1,000,000,000.* About how many DNA base pairs are there in a human cell? Express your answer using scientific notation.
c. About how many DNA base pairs are there altogether in the person with 10 trillion cells? Express your answer using scientific notation.

*Answer:*

a. A trillion in scientific notation is $1\times10^{12}=10^{12}$, so a person with 10 trillion cells has $\mathbf{10^{13}}$ **cells.**
b. Since a person has two copies of the genome in each cell, he/she has about:

$$\mathbf{6\ billion = 6,000,000,000 = 6\times10^{9}\ DNA\ base\ pairs\ in\ each\ cell}$$

c. $(1\times10^{13})\times(6\times10^{9})=6\times10^{22}=60,000,000,000,000,000,000,000$ DNA base pairs.
It is remarkable to consider that all of these $6\times10^{22}$ DNA base pairs are in a specific location in the genome!

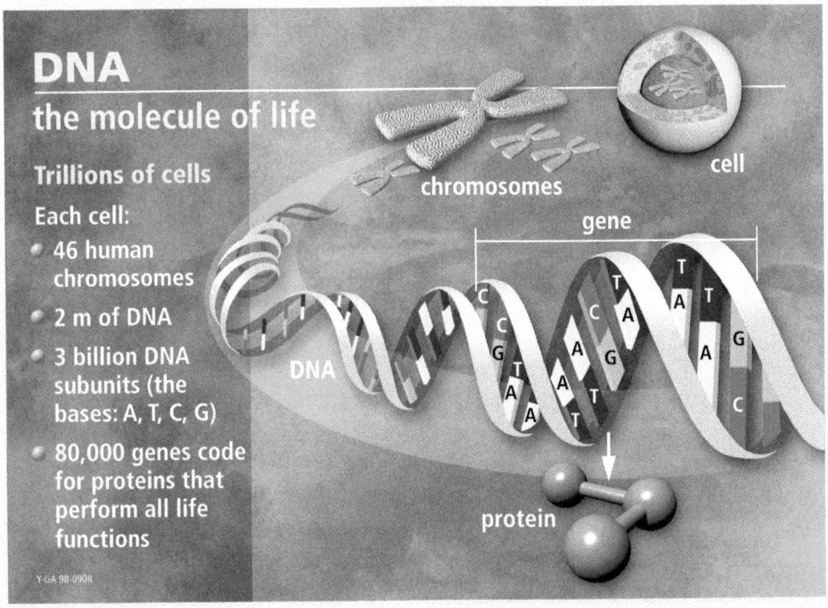


**FIGURE 1.1** The human genome. (Image credit: U.S. Department of Energy Genomic Science Program, https://genomicscience.energy.gov.)

## Practice Problems

1. ***Perform the following calculations.***

a. $\dfrac{\left(\mathbf{4.725\times10^{8}}\right)\left(\mathbf{0.0200}\right)}{\left(\mathbf{3700}\right)\left(\mathbf{0.770}\right)}$ b. $\dfrac{\left(\mathbf{1.93\times10^{3}}\right)\left(\mathbf{4.22\times10^{-2}}\right)}{\left(\mathbf{8.8\times10^{8}}\right)\left(\mathbf{6.0\times10^{-6}}\right)}$

c. $(4.5\times10^{3})+(2.7\times10^{-2})$ d. $(35.6\times10^{4})-(54.6\times10^{6})$

e. $(5.4\times10^{24})+(3.4\times10^{26})$ f. $(5.7\times10^{-3})-(3.4\times10^{-6})$

2. ***In common usage in the United States:***

***One million is 1,000,000***

***One billion is 1,000,000,000***

***One trillion is 1,000,000,000,000***

***Note that the meaning of the words "billion" and "trillion" is not the same in all countries, so it is best to avoid them in scientific writing. However, you will see these words in articles and news reports, and it is important to understand their meaning.***

***Convert each of the following numbers both to scientific notation and to a form using the word "million," "billion," or "trillion." For example, 1,000,500 is the same as 1.0005×10^6^. It is also the same as "1 million, five hundred." If the number is written with words, convert it to scientific notation.***

a. ***10,049,998***

b. ***10,050,000,000***

c. ***3,000,001***

d. ***Forty-one trillion dollars***

e. ***17,000,001***

f. ***Fourteen billion dollars***

## *Answers*

1. a. $$\frac{\left(4.725\times10^{8}\right)\left(0.0200\right)}{\left(3700\right)\left(0.770\right)}=\frac{\left(4.725\right)\times10^{8}\left(2.00\right)\times10^{-2}}{\left(3.7\times10^{3}\right)\left(7.7\times10^{-1}\right)}=\frac{9.45\times10^{6}}{28.49\times10^{2}}\approx\mathbf{3.317\times10^{3}}$$

b. $$\frac{\left(1.93\times10^{3}\right)\left(4.22\times10^{-2}\right)}{\left(8.8\times10^{8}\right)\left(6.0\times10^{-6}\right)}=\frac{8.1446\times10^{1}}{52.8\times10^{2}}\approx\mathbf{1.5425\times10^{-2}}$$

Alternatively, this problem can be rewritten as follows:

$$\frac{\left(1.93\times4.22\right)\times\left(10^{3}\times10^{-2}\right)}{\left(8.8\times6.0\right)\times\left(10^{8}\times10^{-6}\right)}=\frac{8.1446\times\left(10^{3}\times10^{-2}\right)}{52.8\times\left(10^{8}\times10^{-6}\right)}$$

$$\approx0.1542537\times\frac{\left(10^{3}\times10^{-2}\right)}{\left(10^{8}\times10^{-6}\right)}=0.1542537\times\frac{10^{3-2}}{10^{8-6}}$$

$$=0.1542537\times10^{1-2}=0.1542537\times10^{-1}\approx\mathbf{1.5425\times10^{-2}}$$

c. $(4.5\times10^{3})+(2.7\times10^{-2})=4{,}500+0.027=\mathbf{4{,}500.027}$

d. $(35.6\times10^{4})-(54.6\times10^{6})=(0.356\times10^{6})-(54.6\times10^{6})=\mathbf{-54.244\times10^{6}}$

e. $(5.4\times10^{24})+(3.4\times10^{26})=(0.054\times10^{26})+(3.4\times10^{26})=\mathbf{3.454\times10^{26}}$

f. $(5.7\times10^{-3})-(3.4\times10^{-6})=(5700\times10^{-6})-(3.4\times10^{-6})=\mathbf{5696.6\times10^{-6}}$

2. a. 10,049,998 = **$1.0049998 \times 10^7$ = ten million, forty-nine thousand, nine hundred ninety-eight**
   b. 10,050,000,000 = **$1.005 \times 10^{10}$ = ten billion, fifty million**
   c. 3,000,001 = **$3.000001 \times 10^6$ = three million, one**
   d. forty-one trillion dollars = **\$$4.1 \times 10^{13}$**
   e. 17,000,001 = **$1.7000001 \times 10^7$ = seventeen million, one**
   f. fourteen billion dollars = **\$$1.4 \times 10^{10}$**

# Logarithms

# 2



## 2.1 COMMON LOGARITHMS

Common logarithms (also called **logs, base-10 logarithms, or $\log_{10}$**) are closely related to scientific notation. *The* **common log** *of a number is the power to which 10 must be raised to give that number.*

For example,

$100 = 10^2$

**The log of 100 is 2 because 10 raised to the second power is 100:**

$\log 10^2 = 2$

$1{,}000{,}000 = 10^6$

**The log of 1,000,000 is 6 because 10 raised to the sixth power is 1,000,000:**

$\log 10^6 = 6$

$0.001 = 10^{-3}$

**The log of 0.001 is −3 because 10 raised to the −3 power is 0.001:**

$\log 10^{-3} = -3$

$1 = 10^0$

**The log of 1 is 0 because 10 raised to the zero power is 1 (by definition):**

$\log 10^0 = 0$

**So, by definition,** $\log(10^X) = X$.

DOI: 10.1201/9780429282744-3

**TABLE 2.1 Common Logs of Powers of Ten**

| Number in Standard Notation | Number Written with Exponent | Log |
|---|---|---|
| 1,000,000 | $= 10^6$ | $\text{Log } 10^6 = 6$ |
| 100,000 | $= 10^5$ | $\text{Log } 10^5 = 5$ |
| 10,000 | $= 10^4$ | $\text{Log } 10^4 = 4$ |
| 1,000 | $= 10^3$ | $\text{Log } 10^3 = 3$ |
| 100 | $= 10^2$ | $\text{Log } 10^2 = 2$ |
| 10 | $= 10^1$ | $\text{Log } 10^1 = 1$ |
| 1 | $= 10^0$ | $\text{Log } 10^0 = 0$ |
| 0.1 | $= 10^{-1}$ | $\text{Log } 10^{-1} = -1$ |
| 0.01 | $= 10^{-2}$ | $\text{Log } 10^{-2} = -2$ |
| 0.001 | $= 10^{-3}$ | $\text{Log } 10^{-3} = -3$ |
| 0.0001 | $= 10^{-4}$ | $\text{Log } 10^{-4} = -4$ |
| 0.00001 | $= 10^{-5}$ | $\text{Log } 10^{-5} = -5$ |
| 0.000001 | $= 10^{-6}$ | $\text{Log } 10^{-6} = -6$ |

Table 2.1 summarizes the common logs of powers of 10.

To what power must 10 be raised to equal the number 5? This is not obvious. We can reason that the number 5 is between 1 and 10, so the log of 5 must be greater than the log of 1 (which is 0) and less than the log of 10 (which is 1). The same is true for the numbers 2, 3, 4, 6, 7, 8, and 9; their logs are decimals between 0 and 1. There is no intuitive way to know the exact log of 5, although we know it is between 0 and 1. Rather, it is necessary to find it using a scientific calculator. There are also tables that list logs and are easily found on the Internet using a search engine. The log of 5 is approximately **0.699,** which means that $10^{0.699} \approx 5$. Thus,

$\mathbf{5 = 10^X}$

**Take the log of both sides:**
$\mathbf{\log 5 = \log 10^X}$
$\mathbf{\log 5 = X}$
**From a calculator, we find that:**
$\mathbf{X \approx 0.699}$
**which means that:**
$\mathbf{5 \approx 10^{0.699}}$

The same logic can be applied to numbers between 10 and 100. For example, what is the log of 48? The log of 10 is 1; the log of 100 is 2. Therefore, the log of the number 48 must fall between 1 and 2. It is, in fact, approximately **1.681**.

$\mathbf{\log 48 = X}$
**From a calculator, we find that:**
$\mathbf{X \approx 1.681}$
**which means that:**
$\mathbf{48 \approx 10^{1.681}}$

All numbers between 10 and 100 have a log between 1 and 2. We can continue and apply the same logic to all positive numbers. For example, the log of 4,987,000 must fall between 6 and 7 because 4,987,000 is between 1 million ($10^6$) and 10 million ($10^7$).

$\mathbf{\log 4{,}987{,}000 = X}$

$\mathbf{X \approx 6.698}$
**which means that:**
$\mathbf{10^{6.698} \approx 4{,}987{,}000}$

What about numbers between 0 and 1? Observe in Table 2.1 that the log of 1 is 0 and that the logs of numbers between 0 and 1 are negative numbers. Therefore, all numbers between 0 and 1 have a negative log. For example,

**The log of 0.130 is approximately −0.886**
**which means that:**
$\mathbf{10^{-0.886} \approx 0.130}$

**The log of 0.00891 is approximately −2.05**
**which means that:**
$\mathbf{10^{-2.05} \approx 0.00891}$

Note that zero and numbers less than zero do not have logs at all because there is no exponent that will make 10 to that number equal 0 or a negative value. Formally, we say that logarithms of 0 or negative numbers are undefined. (Your calculator will give you an error message if you try to take the log of zero or a negative number.)

## 2.2 ANTILOGARITHMS

An **antilogarithm (antilog)** *is the number corresponding to a given logarithm.* For example,

**The log of 100 is 2; therefore, 100 is the antilog of 2.**
**The log of 5 is approximately 0.699; therefore, 5 is approximately the antilog of 0.699.**

What is the antilog of 3? Remember that logs are exponents; therefore, to find the antilog of a number, n, use n as an exponent on a base of 10. If n = 3, then antilog 3 = $10^3$ = 1,000. 1,000 is the antilog of 3.

What is the antilog of 2.5?
**Antilog 2.5 =** $\mathbf{10^{2.5}}$

While it is not obvious what $10^{2.5}$ equals, we can reason that the antilog of 2.5 must be a number between 100 and 1000. (If this is not clear, think about the "2" in 2.5.) A scientific calculator is the simplest way to find antilogs. On many calculators, the "antilog key" is the second function of the "log key." (Consult your calculator directions to determine how to perform this function.) Using my basic calculator, I can find the antilog of 2.5 in two ways:

[2.5]

[2nd]

[log]

The answer **316.227766** appears.
Alternatively, I can press:

[10]

[$y^x$]

[2.5]

[=]

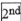

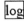

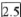

The answer **316.227766** appears.
Your calculator might work in a slightly different order; try it out.

**Example Problem:**

What is the antilog of 3.58?

***Answer:***

We can reason that the answer is between 1,000 and 10,000 because of the 3.

$$\textbf{Antilog (3.58)} = 10^{3.58} \approx 3,801.89$$

**Example Problem:**

What is the antilog of −0.780?

***Answer:***

The antilog of a negative number must be a value between 0 and 1.

$$\textbf{Antilog (−0.780)} = 10^{-0.780} \approx 0.166$$

## 2.3 NATURAL LOGARITHMS

Common logarithms have a base of 10, in mathematical notation:

$$\log_{10} n = \log\ n.$$

*There are also logarithms whose base is ≈ 2.7183, called "e." When e is the base, the log is called a* **"natural" log abbreviated "ln."** In mathematical notation:

$$\log_e n = \ln\ n$$

There are tables of natural logs and there are keys on scientific calculators to find the natural log. Note that the terms "log" and "ln" are not synonyms and should never be used interchangeably. In mathematical notation:

$$\log\ n \neq \ln$$

## 2.4 WHY DO WE CARE ABOUT THIS? AN APPLICATION OF LOGARITHMS: pH

The proper function of biological systems depends on their liquid environment having the correct concentration of hydrogen ions, Figure 2.1. pH is a convenient means to express the concentration of hydrogen ions in an aqueous solution.

The concentration of $H^+$ ions in aqueous solutions normally varies between 1.0 M and 0.00000000000001 M, where M, molarity, is a unit of concentration equivalent to moles/liter. (See Section 12.5 for an introduction to molarity.) The number 0.00000000000001 can also be written as $1 \times 10^{-14}$.

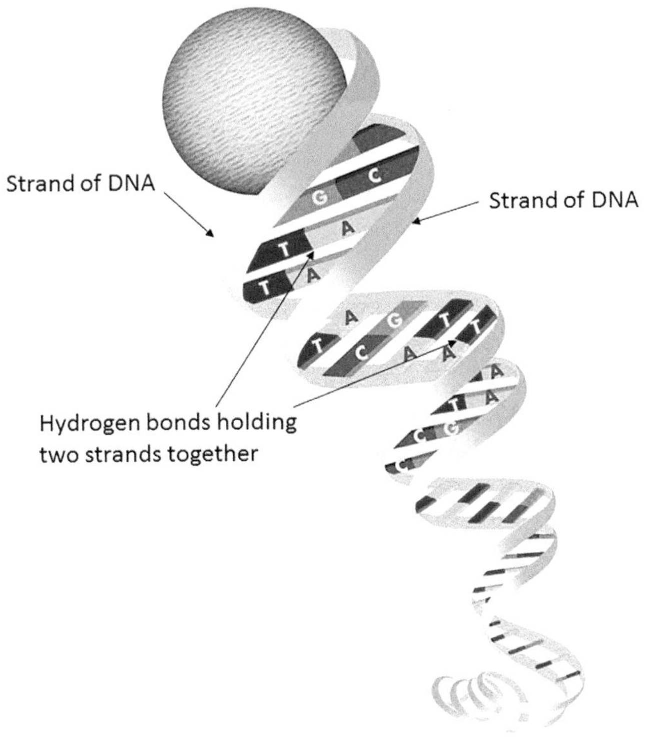


**FIGURE 2.1** DNA and pH. Biologists routinely work in the laboratory with biological molecules, such as DNA and proteins, that are suspended in an aqueous laboratory solution. The pH of these laboratory solutions must be rigorously controlled, otherwise the biological molecules of interest are altered. For example, DNA normally consists of two strands that lay side by side and are twisted into the famous double-helix shape. The two strands are held together by chemical hydrogen bonds. These hydrogen bonds can be disrupted if the pH of the solution containing the DNA is raised to about 11.0. (Image credit: U.S. Department of Energy Human Genome Project public.ornl.gov/site/gallery/gallery.cfm, labels added.)

Søren Sørenson devised a scale of pH units in which the wide range of hydrogen ion concentrations can be written as a number between 0 and 14. If the hydrogen ion concentration in a solution is $1 \times 10^{-14}$ M, then using Sørenson's method, its pH is **14**. If the hydrogen ion concentration of a solution is 0.0000001 M, or $1 \times 10^{-7}$ M, then its pH is **7**. If the hydrogen ion concentration of a solution is 1 M, then we say its pH is **0**. (Solutions with a pH less than 7 are said to be "acidic"; those with a pH greater than 7 are said to be "basic"; solutions with a pH of 7 are called "neutral.")

To find the pH of a solution:

*Step 1. Take the log of the hydrogen ion concentration.*
*Step 2. Take the negative of the log.*

For example,

**What is the pH of a solution with a $H^+$ concentration of 0.000234 M?**
Step 1. The log of 0.000234 is approximately −3.63.
Step 2. The negative of −3.63 is 3.63. So **3.63** is the pH of this solution.

We can express the relationship between pH and hydrogen ion concentration more formally using the following expression:

$$\mathbf{pH = -\log[H^+]}$$

*The symbol [ ] means "concentration."*

*In words, pH is equal to the negative log of the hydrogen ion concentration when concentration is expressed in units of molarity.*

If we know the pH and want to find the $[H^+]$ in a solution, then we apply antilogs. To do this:

*Step 1. Place a negative sign in front of the pH value.*
*Step 2. Find the antilog of the resulting number.*

For example,

What is the concentration of hydrogen ions in a solution whose pH is 5.60?
Step 1. Place a − sign in front of the pH: −5.60.
Step 2. The antilog of −5.60 is approximately $2.51 \times 10^{-6}$. Therefore, the concentration of hydrogen ions in this solution is about $\mathbf{2.51 \times 10^{-6}}$ **M.**

The relationship between hydrogen ion concentration (in units of moles/liter) and pH is expressed more formally using the following expression:

$$\mathbf{[H^+] = antilog\ (-pH)}$$

or

$$\mathbf{\left[H^+\right] = 10^{-(pH)}}$$

**Example Problem:**

The concentration of hydrochloric acid, HCl, secreted by the stomach after a meal is about $1.2 \times 10^{-3}$ M. What is the pH of stomach acid?

***Answer:***

The HCl dissociates to release $1.2 \times 10^{-3}$ M hydrogen ions. The log of $1.2 \times 10^{-3}$ is about −2.9. The negative of this log value is 2.9, so the pH of the stomach after a meal is about **2.9.**

**Practice Problems**

1. ***Answer the following without using a calculator*:**
   a. ***Is the log of 445 closer to 2 or 4?***
   b. ***Is the log of 1,876 closer to 3, 9, or 10?***
2. ***Give the common log of the following numbers.***
   a. ***100*** b. ***10,000*** c. ***1,000,000***
   d. ***0.0001*** e. ***0.001***

3. ***The log of 567 must lie between 2 and 3 because 567 is between 100 = $10^2$ and 1,000 = $10^3$. For each of the following numbers, state the values the log must lie between.***
   a. ***7*** b. ***65.9*** c. ***89.0***
   d. ***0.45*** e. ***0.0078***
4. ***Use a scientific calculator to find the log of the following numbers.***
   a. ***$1.50 \times 10^4$*** b. ***345*** c. ***0.0098***
   d. ***$2.98 \times 10^{-5}$*** e. ***1209*** f. ***0.345***
5. ***The log of 1,000 is 3. Therefore, 1000, or $10^3$, is the antilog of 3.***
   ***Fill in the blanks below without using your calculator:***
   ***The log of 100 is 2.0. Therefore, _______ is the antilog of 2.0.***
   ***The log of 200 is ≈ 2.301. Therefore, _______ is the approximate antilog of 2.301.***
6. ***Use a scientific calculator to find the antilog of the following numbers.***
   a. ***4.8990*** b. ***3.9900*** c. ***−0.5600***
   d. ***−0.0089*** e. ***9.8999*** f. ***1.0000***
   g. ***8.9000***

***pH is an application of logs that is of critical importance to biologists. Nearly every reagent that a biologist prepares – and biologists prepare a lot of reagents – must be prepared so it has the proper pH. The following problems relate to the preparation of reagents (also called "solutions").***

7. ***Use a scientific calculator to convert each of the following $\left[H^+\right]$ to a pH value.***
   a. ***[0.45 M]*** b. ***[0.045 M]*** c. ***[0.0045 M]***
   d. ***[0.00000032 M]***
8. ***pH meters are used to measure the pH of solutions. When using a pH meter, standards are commonly used to adjust the meter so that it reads correctly. Common standards include pH 7.00, 4.00, and 10.00. What is the hydrogen ion concentration of these standards?***
9. ***Use a scientific calculator to determine the hydrogen ion concentration of the reagents with the following pH values. (Express your answers in scientific notation.)***
   a. ***4.56*** b. ***5.67*** c. ***7.00***
   d. ***1.09*** e. ***10.1***
10. ***pH must be controlled in biological laboratory solutions. For example, buffer solution XYZ is specified to have a pH between 7.2 and 7.4. If the buffer solution XYZ is mistakenly prepared to have a pH of 8.0, how much is the hydrogen ion concentration "off"?***

### *Answers*

1. a. **2** b. **3**
2. a. log 100 = **2** b. log 10,000 = **4** c. log 1,000,000 = **6**
   d. log 0.0001 = **−4** e. log 0.001 = **−3**
3. a. log 7 between **0 and 1** b. log 65.9 between **1 and 2**
   c. log 89.0 between **1 and 2** d. log 0.45 between **0 and (−1)**
   e. log 0.0078 between **(−2) and (−3)**
4. a. **4.18** b. **2.54** c. **2.0** d. **4.53**
   e. **3.082** f. **−0.462**
5. <u>**100**</u> <u>**200**</u>

6. a. antilog 4.8990 ≈ **$7.925 \times 10^4$** b. antilog 3.9900 ≈ **$9.772 \times 10^3$**
   c. antilog −0.5600 ≈ **0.2754** d. antilog −0.0089 ≈ **0.9797**
   e. antilog 9.8999 ≈ **$7.94 \times 10^9$** f. antilog 1.0000 = **10**
   g. antilog 8.9000 ≈ **$7.9433 \times 10^8$**
7. a. **0.347** b. **1.35** c. **2.35** d. **6.49**
8. pH 7 = **$1 \times 10^{-7}$ M** pH 4 = **$1 \times 10^{-4}$ M** pH 10 = **$1 \times 10^{-10}$ M**
9. a. Antilog − 4.56 ≈ **$2.75 \times 10^{-5}$ M** b. Antilog − 5.67 ≈ **$2.14 \times 10^{-6}$ M**
   c Antilog − 7.00 ≈ **$1.00 \times 10^{-7}$ M** d. Antilog − 1.09 ≈ **$8.13 \times 10^{-2}$ M**
   e. Antilog − 10.1 ≈ **$7.94 \times 10^{-11}$ M**
10. At pH 7.4, the hydrogen ion concentration would be about $3.98 \times 10^{-8}$ M. At pH 8.0, the hydrogen ion concentration would be $1.0 \times 10^{-8}$ M. If you compare these two values, you can see that if buffer solution XYZ is mistakenly prepared to have a pH of 8.0, it will have a hydrogen ion concentration this is **only about 1/4 of what it should be**. This is a significant difference when working with proteins, nucleic acids, cells, and other biological materials and will likely have an adverse effect on the laboratory results.

## 2.5 WHY DO WE CARE ABOUT THIS? OTHER APPLICATIONS OF LOGARITHMS

Hydrogen ion concentration in aqueous solutions normally can be anywhere from 1.0 to 0.00000000000001 M. This is an example where there are vast differences in the order of magnitude between values in different situations. We saw that Søren Sørenson devised the pH scale to transform hydrogen ion concentration into a small number that scientists find more convenient than molarity. There are other situations where scientists use logarithms when working with values that span a wide range of orders of magnitude. The Richter scale, which measures earthquake force, is an example of a logarithmic scale that might already be familiar to you. An earthquake that is 4 on the Richter scale is 10 times stronger than an earthquake that is 3.

In a biotechnology setting, scientists sometimes use another logarithmic scale, the **log reduction value (LRV)**, *when reporting how effectively a product or procedure reduces pathogens*. For example, the numbers of microbial cells before and after a sterilizing procedure might span a wide range, from values such as $10^{12}$ down to $10^1$. The LRV simplifies reporting the results of such a procedure. As another example, LRVs might be used to express the number of viruses removed from a pharmaceutical preparation by a filtration procedure. Mathematically, the LRV is defined as Equation 2.1:

$$\text{Log reduction value} = \log\left(\frac{\text{beginning number}}{\text{ending number}}\right) \tag{2.1}$$

For example, suppose a test was performed to evaluate the effectiveness of autoclaving to kill bacteria. $10^6$ bacteria were added to a flask and the flask was autoclaved for 5 minutes. After autoclaving, $10^3$ bacteria were observed. What was the log reduction number?

$$\text{Log reduction value} = \log\left(\frac{10^6}{10^3}\right) = \log 10^3 \ = 3$$

In general, an LRV ≤ 1 shows that an agent is ineffective at eliminating pathogens, an LRV between 1 and 2 indicates some effectiveness, an LRV between 2 and 4 is moderately effective, and an LRV of ≥ 4 is considered to be highly effective. (Jing, Jane Lee Jia, et al. "Hand Sanitizers: A Review on Formulation Aspects, Adverse Effects, and Regulations." *International Journal of Environmental Research and Public Health*, vol. 17, no. 9, 2020, p. 3326. doi:10.3390/ijerph17093326.)

**Example Problem:**

**Biopharmaceuticals** are drug products that are produced by living cells (derived from bacteria, yeasts, insects, or mammals) or organisms (such as plants or sheep). These drugs are critically important in the treatment of many disorders such as cancer, diabetes, and stroke. Before a biopharmaceutical product can be released for treatment of people or other animals, viral contaminants in the product must be almost entirely eliminated. Manufacturers develop processes to remove viral contaminants and then test their processes by spiking (adding) known amounts of infectious virus into the beginning of their production process. They then analyze how much infectious virus is left at the end of each step. They express the results in terms of the LRV. Suppose that at the beginning of a processing step there are $10^7$ infectious viral particles and at the end of the step there are $3.25 \times 10^3$ infectious viral particles. What is the LRV?

***Answer:***

$$\text{Log reduction value} = \log\left(\frac{10^7}{3.25 \times 10^3}\right) \approx \log 3.077 \times 10^3 \approx \mathbf{3.49}$$

Later in this text, we will explore other situations where calculations are performed that involve logarithms. Chapter 16 discusses spectrophotometry, which is a technique routinely used to determine how much of a material of interest is present in a sample. Chapter 17 introduces concepts relating to the growth of populations or organisms. Biotechnologists routinely monitor the growth of populations of cells that are being used for producing products or performing experiments. Chapter 17 also introduces the concept of radioactive decay. Radioactive materials are sometimes used to monitor biological processes in the laboratory and medical clinic. In these situations, the concept of radioactive decay is important. Chapters 24 and 25 introduce a technique called the polymerase chain reaction (PCR), which is used to greatly amplify the amount of DNA or RNA present in a sample. PCR is an extremely important technique. For example, at the time of writing, thousands of PCR reactions are performed daily to diagnose the disease COVID-19. In all these situations, logarithms are used to solve practical laboratory problems.

**Practice Problems**

1. a. ***How much stronger is an earthquake of magnitude 6 on the Richter scale compared to an earthquake with a magnitude of 5?***
   b. ***How much stronger is an earthquake of magnitude 7 than an earthquake of magnitude 5?***
   c. ***How much less concentrated is the hydrogen ion concentration in a solution with a pH of 9 compared to one with a pH of 3?***

2. ***A filter was used to remove pyrogens (a type of contaminant derived from bacteria) from a pharmaceutical product being manufactured in cells. Initially, there were 10,000 pyrogen units/mL in the product. After filtration there were 0.00038 pyrogen units/mL. What was the LRV? How effective is this filtration step?***
3. ***Ultraviolet (UV) light is often used to inactivate pathogens. Every pathogen, depending on its biological features, has a different sensitivity to various wavelengths of UV light and will require a different amount of energy to be inactivated. It is necessary to determine this level of energy experimentally. The table below is excerpted from data found at: Randive, Rajul. "What is Log Reduction?"* Klaran. *www.klaran.com/what-is-log-reduction. (Do not worry about the units used to describe energy.)***

| Bacterium to be Inactivated | UV Dose Required to Achieve 2 LRV (in $mJ/cm^2$ at 254 nm) | UV Dose Required to Achieve 3 LRV (in $mJ/cm^2$ at 254 nm) |
|---|---|---|
| *E. coli* | 6.5 | 7 |
| *Pseudomonas aeruginosa* | 11 | 16.5 |
| *Salmonella typhi* | 4.1 | 5.5 |
| *Staphylococcus aureus* | 5.4 | 6.5 |

   a. ***Which bacterium is most resistant to UV light inactivation? Which is least resistant?***
   b. ***If a surface is contaminated with 25,000 infectious Salmonella typhi bacteria, about what UV dose would be required to reduce the number of infectious bacteria to not more than 30 infectious bacteria?***
4. ***Suppose a study was performed on the SARS-CoV-2 virus, the agent that causes COVID-19. In this (hypothetical) study, scientists tested the effect of UV light on viral inactivation in air samples. Samples were initially spiked with $10^6$ infectious virus particles. (To "spike" means to add something.) After UV treatment researchers detected 700 infectious viral particles in their sample. What was the log reduction value for this treatment? Is this treatment effective?***
5. ***In a real study, scientists investigated the effectiveness of seven hand sanitizers. They found that only two products (72% ethanol, pH 2.9) and one triclosan-based product had LRVs ≥ 2.***

   ***If they had spiked their samples with $10^4$ viruses, what is the maximum number of infectious virus that could have been present in the samples after treatment with the effective ethanol or triclosan-based product? (Park, Geun Woo, et al. "Comparative Efficacy of Seven Hand Sanitizers against Murine Norovirus, Feline Calicivirus, and GII.4 Norovirus." Journal of Food Protection, vol. 73, no. 12, 2010, pp. 2232–38. doi:10.4315/0362-028x-73.12.2232.)***
6. ***An LRV value of 1 means there are 10 times fewer (or 1/10th as many) pathogens or contaminants present after treatment than there were before treatment. To prove this to yourself, insert some numbers into the LRV equation. For example, suppose there are 1,000 contaminants before treatment and 100 pathogens after treatment. 1,000 is ten times greater than 100. If you plug the numbers 1000 and 100 into the LRV equation, you get:***

$$\text{Log Reduction Value} = \log\left(\frac{1{,}000}{100}\right) = \log 10 = 1$$

***Thus, an LRV of 1 corresponds to a ten-time reduction. We can also say that an LRV of 1 corresponds to a ten-fold or a 10× reduction in contaminant or pathogen. We can also say that there are 1/10th as many contaminants or pathogens after treatment as there were initially. Similarly, an LRV of 2 corresponds to a 100-fold reduction in contaminant/pathogen.***
***Fill in the blanks in this table:***

| LRV Value | Fold Reduction in Contaminant/Pathogen | Fold Reduction in Scientific Notation |
|---|---|---|
| 1 | 10 | $10^1$ |
| 2 | 100 | $10^2$ |
| 3 | _____ | _____ |
| 4 | _____ | _____ |
| 5 | _____ | _____ |
| 6 | _____ | _____ |
| 7 | _____ | _____ |

7. ***The graph in Figure 2.2 was developed as a planning tool for use during the COVID 19 pandemic. It displays the probability that one person attending an event is infected with COVID-19 and therefore a probability that other people might become infected if attending the same event. Two factors are considered to make this assessment: the number of people in a given area who are infected and the number of people attending the event. As the number of infections in a community increases, so does the probability that an infected person will attend the event. Similarly, the more people at the event, the higher the probability that one of them will be infected.***

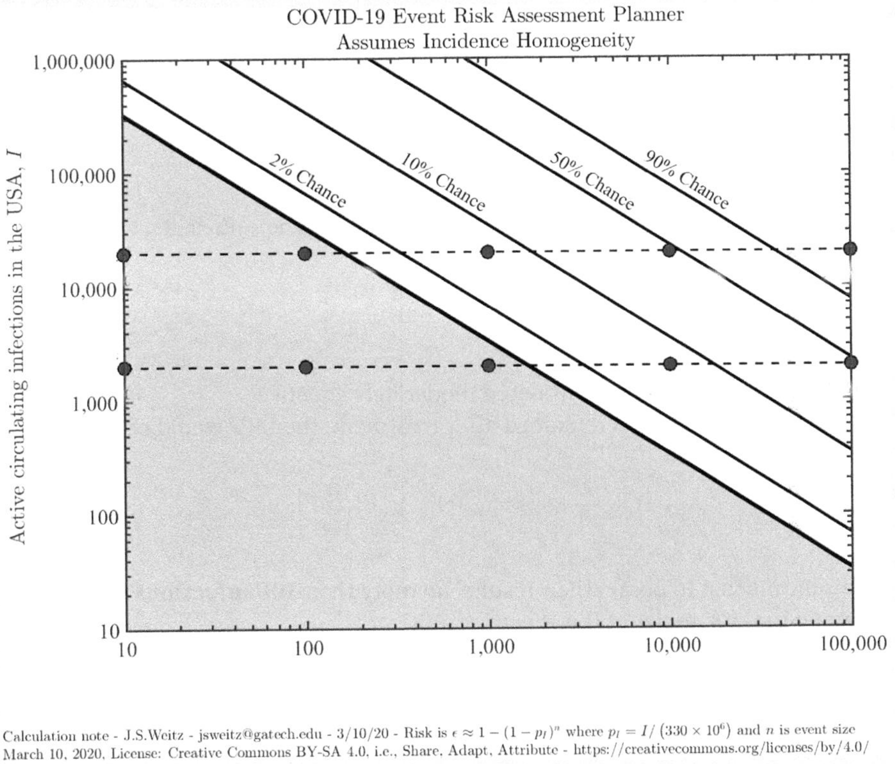


**FIGURE 2.2** A planning tool for estimating COVID-19 event risk.

***Both the X- and Y-axes on this graph are logarithmic meaning that the values on the Y-axis and the values on the X-axis increase by ten-fold. Thus, the Y-axis begins at 10, then goes to 10 × 10 = 100, then goes to 100 × 10 = 1,000 and so on. The X-axis also increases by 10 at each division. Why do you think the creators of this graph chose to use log scales? (We will further explore this type of graph in Chapter 17. Do not be alarmed if it seems somewhat confusing now, just consider why the researchers used logarithms on the graph.)***

## *Answers*

1. a. An earthquake of magnitude 6 on the Richter scale is **10×** stronger than an earthquake with a magnitude of 5.
   b. An earthquake of magnitude 7 is **100×** stronger than an earthquake of magnitude 5.
   c. A solution of pH 9 has a **$10^6$** lower hydrogen ion concentration than a solution with a pH of 3. (It has 1 million times fewer hydrogen ions, or we can say 1 millionth as many hydrogen ions.)
2. $$\text{Log reduction value} = \log\left(\frac{10^4}{0.00038}\right) \approx \mathbf{7.42}$$

   This treatment would be considered highly effective.
3. a. Which bacterium is most resistant to UV light inactivation? Which is least resistant?

   *Pseudomonas aeruginosa* requires the highest dose of UV light to be inactivated and is therefore the most resistant. *Salmonella typhi* is the least resistant.

   b. If the number of infectious bacteria is reduced from 25,000 to 30, the LRV is:

   $$\text{Log reduction value} = \log\left(\frac{25{,}000}{30}\right) \approx 2.9$$

   Therefore, a dose of **5.5 mJ/cm²** at 254 nm would be sufficient.
4. $$\text{Log reduction value} = \log\left(\frac{10^6}{700}\right) \approx \mathbf{3.15}$$

   This treatment would be considered moderately effective.
5. If 100 infectious viruses remained after treatment, the LRV would be 2:

   $$\text{Log reduction value} = \log\left(\frac{10^4}{100}\right) = 2$$

   This means that to obtain their results, no more than **100 infectious viruses** could remain in the samples of the effective sanitizers.

6. Table of LRV Values:

| LRV Value | Fold Reduction in Contaminant/Pathogen | Fold Reduction in Scientific Notation |
|---|---|---|
| 1 | 10 | $10^1$ |
| 2 | 100 | $10^2$ |
| 3 | **1,000** | $\mathbf{10^3}$ |
| 4 | **10,000** | $\mathbf{10^4}$ |
| 5 | **100,000** | $\mathbf{10^5}$ |
| 6 | **1,000,000** | $\mathbf{10^6}$ |
| 7 | **10,000,000** | $\mathbf{10^7}$ |

7. This is another situation where the values of interest span many orders of magnitude. Using logarithms allows these data to be displayed effectively on one graph.

# Units of Measurement

# 3



## 3.1 THE MEANING OF "MEASUREMENT"

**Measurements** are *quantitative observations or numerical descriptions*, such as the weight of an object, the amount of light passing through a solution, and the time required to run a race. Everyone has experience making measurements, for example, taking the temperature of a child, weighing oneself, or measuring ingredients when cooking.

Measuring properties of samples is an integral part of everyday work in any biology laboratory. For example, estimating the quantity of DNA in a test tube may involve measuring how much light passes through the solution. The pH of the medium in which bacteria grow during fermentation must be measured continuously.

**Measurement** *is basically a process of counting.* Consider, for example, an insect that is 1.55 centimeters in length. Length is the property that is measured, 1.55 is the **value** of the measurement, and centimeter (cm) is the **unit** of measurement. Another way to write this measurement is: $1.55 \times 1$ cm. This latter statement tells us that the length of the insect was determined by comparison with a standard of 1 cm in length and was found to be 1.55 times as long as the standard. Measuring length is therefore comparable to counting how many times the standard must be placed end-to-end to equal the length of the object. Another example is the characteristic of time, which can be measured by counting how many times the sun "rises" and "sets." The standard in this case is the apparent motion of the sun and the units are days.

## 3.2 UNITS OF MEASUREMENT

All measurements require the selection of a **standard** and then counting the number of times the standard is contained in the material to be measured. The terms **standard** and **unit** are related but can be distinguished from one another. A **unit of measure** *is a precisely defined amount of a property, such as length or mass.* A **standard** *is a physical embodiment of a unit.* Centimeters and millimeters are examples of units of measure; a ruler is an example of a standard. Because units are not physical entities, they are unaffected by environmental conditions such as temperature or humidity. In contrast, standards are affected by the environment. A strip of metal used to measure meters will differ in length with temperature changes and will therefore only be correct at a particular temperature and in a particular environment.

DOI: 10.1201/9780429282744-4

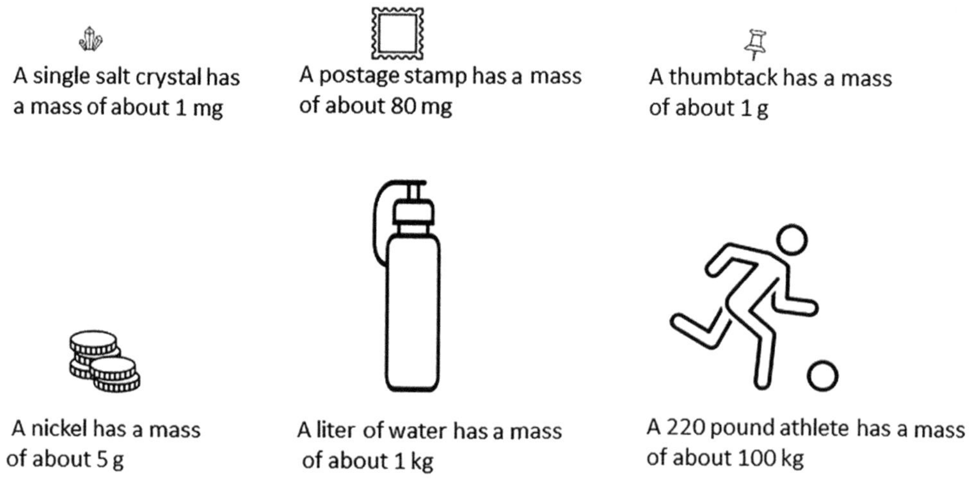


**FIGURE 3.1** The mass of some common objects in the metric system.

*A group of units together is a* **measurement system**. *The measurement system common in the United States, which includes miles, pounds, gallons, inches, and feet, is called* the **United States Customary System (USCS)**. In most laboratories and in most of the world, the **metric system**, *with units including meters, grams, and liters, is used*, Figure 3.1.

What we now call the US Customary System is a group of units that evolved over centuries, originating in the ancient Middle East, Greece, and Rome and further evolving in Europe during the Middle Ages. Some units of measurement are originally derived from body parts, for example, "foot" came from the length of a person's foot. The English government standardized this measurement system and spread it throughout their colonies, including the United States. As the system evolved, units were invented that are not related to one another in a systematic fashion. For example, for length, 12 in = 1 ft and 3 ft = 1 yard. There is no pattern to these relationships. The USCS formerly was called the "English system," but this name no longer applies because England (and most other countries in the world except the United States) has switched to the metric system and does not use units such as ounces or feet.

The metric system originated in France at the time of the French Revolution. It is designed systematically based on powers of 10 (and does not have units based on body parts). In contrast to the USCS, the metric system uses only one basic unit to measure length, the meter. The unit of a meter is then modified systematically by the addition of prefixes. For example, the prefix **"centi"** *means 1/100, so a* **centimeter** *is a meter/100.* **"Kilo"** *means 1000,* so a **kilometer** *is a meter × 1,000.* The same prefixes can be used to modify other basic units, such as grams or liters. The prefixes that modify a basic unit always represent a power of 10, Table 3.1.

In 1893, an international consortium, that included the United States, adopted metric standards for use around the world. Since then, the United States has defined its customary measurements – the foot, pound, etc. – in relation to the meter and the kilogram. Therefore, even though you will see the term a "pound of butter" in a US cookbook, the definition of a "pound" is based on the metric kilogram. (For an interesting explanation of the US and the metric system, see the blog posting: Benham, Elizabeth. "Busting Myths about the Metric System." *NIST*, 6 October 2020, https://www.nist.gov/blogs/taking-measure/busting-myths-about-metric-system.)

The most important basic metric units for biologists are: **meters (m)**, *for length*; **grams (g)**, *for mass;* and **liters (L)**, *for volume.* Table 3.2 shows how prefixes modify the basic units.

Biologists use some terms that are not part of the "regular" metric system or that are not common in other disciplines. These include:

- A microliter is 1/1,000,000 L and is normally abbreviated μL, but biologists sometimes refer to 1 μL as 1 "lambda" (λ).
- $10^{-10}$ m may be called an "angstrom" (Å).

**TABLE 3.1 Prefixes in the Metric System**

| Decimal | Prefix | Symbol | Power of 10 |
|---|---|---|---|
| 1,000,000,000,000,000,000 | exa- | E | $10^{18}$ |
| 1,000,000,000,000,000 | peta- | P | $10^{15}$ |
| 1,000,000,000,000 | tera- | T | $10^{12}$ |
| 1,000,000,000 | giga- | G | $10^{9}$ |
| 1,000,000 | mega- | M | $10^{6}$ |
| 1,000 | kilo- | k | $10^{3}$ |
| 100 | hecto- | h | $10^{2}$ |
| 10 | deca- | da | $10^{1}$ |
| 1 | Basic unit | No prefix | $10^{0}$ |
| 0.1 | deci- | d | $10^{-1}$ |
| 0.01 | centi- | c | $10^{-2}$ |
| 0.001 | milli- | m | $10^{-3}$ |
| 0.000001 | micro- | μ | $10^{-6}$ |
| 0.000000001 | nano- | n | $10^{-9}$ |
| 0.000000000001 | pico- | p | $10^{-12}$ |
| 0.000000000000001 | femto- | f | $10^{-15}$ |
| 0.000000000000000001 | atto- | a | $10^{-18}$ |

The prefixes used commonly in biology laboratories are underlined.

- A micrometer is often called a "micron," though micrometer is the preferred term.
- The terms "cc" and "$cm^3$" (in reference to volume) are the same as an mL. Both stand for "cubic centimeter," the space occupied by an mL of water.
- Micrograms may be abbreviated as μg or mcg where "mc" stands for "micro." The abbreviation mcg is often used when drug dosages are reported.

Table 3.3 shows some commonly used conversion factors that relate the USCS to the metric system. It is correct to convert between units that measure the same basic property. For example, length can be expressed in many units including miles, meters, centimeters, and nanometers, and these units may be converted from one to the other. It is not correct to convert units from one basic property to another. For example, time is a basic unit that is measured in seconds, minutes, etc. It is unreasonable to try to convert number of seconds to centimeters since these units measure different properties.

The **SI measurement system** *(Système International d'Unités) is an updated version of the metric system intended to standardize measurement in all countries.* The SI system was adopted in 1960 by a number of international organizations at the *Conférence Générale des Poids et Mesures.*

There are seven **basic properties** in the SI system: *length, mass, time, electrical current, thermodynamic temperature, luminous intensity, and amount of substance.* The units for these basic properties are shown in Table 3.4. To stay strictly within the SI system, the only units that can be used are those in Table 3.4 or those that are a combination of two or more units shown in this table. For example, the unit for **volume**, *the amount of space a substance occupies, is length×length×length in meters or* **meters³**. Units of liters are not part of the SI system, although liter remains the conventional metric unit for volume measurements in biology laboratories $(1\ L = 1\ dm^3)$.

It is critical to always record the units in any calculation and in any laboratory situation. Also, pay attention to the units in other people's work.

**TABLE 3.2 Some Commonly Used Metric Units**

| Multiple of Ten | | | Mass | Abbreviation | Volume | Abbreviation | Length | Abbreviation |
|---|---|---|---|---|---|---|---|---|
| **Basic Unit** | **Name** | **Symbol** | **Gram** | **g** | **Liter** | **L** | **Meter** | **m** |
| $\times 10^{12}$ | tera (trillion) | T | | | | | | |
| $\times 10^{9}$ | giga (billion) | G | Seldom used | | | | | |
| $\times 10^{6}$ | mega (million) | M | | | | | | |
| $\times 10^{3}$ | kilo (thousand) | k | Kilogram | Kg | Kiloliter | kL | Kilometer | km |
| $\times 10^{-1}$ | deci (tenth) | d | Decigram | dg | Deciliter | dL | Decimeter | dm |
| $\times 10^{-2}$ | centi (hundredth) | c | Centigram | cg | Centiliter | cL | Centimeter | cm |
| $\times 10^{-3}$ | milli (thousandth) | m | Milligram | mg | Milliliter | mL | Millimeter | mm |
| $\times 10^{-6}$ | micro (millionth) | μ | Microgram | μg | Microliter (formerly λ[a]) | μL | Micrometer | μm (formerly, micron[a]) |
| $\times 10^{-9}$ | nano (billionth) | n | Nanogram | ng | Nanoliter | nL | Nanometer | nm |
| $\times 10^{-10}$ | | | | | | | Angstrom[a] | Å |
| $\times 10^{-12}$ | pico (trillionth) | p | Picogram | pg | Picoliter | pL | Picometer | pm |
| $\times 10^{-15}$ | femto | f | Femtogram | fg | Femtoliter | fL | Femtometer | fm |
| $\times 10^{-18}$ | atto | a | Attogram | ag | Attoliter | aL | Attometer | am |

[a] Older term, not part of official SI system.

*Note:* There is inconsistency in capitalization. For example, you may see "Km" or "km" and "mL" or "ml."
The uppercase "L" for liter is used to avoid confusion with the number "1."

**TABLE 3.3 Commonly Used Conversion Factors for Units of Measurement**

| | |
|---|---|
| **Length** | |
| 1 mm = 0.001 m = 0.039 in | |
| 1 cm = 0.01 m ≈ 0.3937 in ≈ 0.0328 ft | 1 in = 2.540 cm (exactly) |
| 1 m ≈ 39.37 in ≈ 3.281 ft ≈ 1.094 yd | 1 ft = 12 in = 0.3048 m (exactly) |
| 1 km = 1000 m ≈ 0.6214 mi | 1 mi = 5,280 ft ≈ 1.609 km |
| **Mass** | |
| 1 g ≈ 0.0353 oz ≈ 0.0022 lb | 1 oz ≈ 28.35 g |
| 1 kg = 1000 g ≈ 35.27 oz ≈ 2.205 lb | 1 lb = 16 oz = 453.59237 g (exactly) |
| | 1 ton = 2000 lb |
| **Volume** | |
| 1 mL = 0.001 L ≈ 0.03381 fl oz | 1 fl oz ≈ 0.0313 qt ≈ 0.02957 L |
| 1 L ≈ 2.113 pt ≈ 1.057 qt ≈ 0.2642 gal (US) | 1 pt ≈ 0.4732 L |
| | 1 qt = 2 pt ≈ 0.9463 L |
| | 1 gal = 8 pt ≈ 3.785 L |
| **Temperature** | |
| °C = (°F − 32) 0.556 | °F = (1.8 × °C) + 32 |
| K = °C + 273 | °R ≈ °F + 460 |
| | (R is Rankine) |

*USCS abbreviations:* in, inch; ft, foot; yd, yard; mi, mile; lb, pound; oz, ounce; fl, fluid; pt, pint; qt, quart; gal, gallon.

**TABLE 3.4 The SI System**

| Basic Property Measured | Unit of Measurement | Abbreviation |
|---|---|---|
| Length | Meter | m |
| Mass | Gram | g |
| Time | Second | s |
| Electrical current | Ampere | A |
| Temperature | Kelvin | K |
| Amount of substance | Mole | mol |
| Luminous Intensity | Candela | cd |

It is important to be comfortable with the metric system. The first step is to begin memorizing the prefixes that are most commonly used in biology. The problems below relate to these prefixes.

**Practice Problems**

1. ***For each of the following abbreviations, fill in the full term. Do this from memory. Practice until these abbreviations are very familiar to you. For example, 1 cm = 1 centimeter***

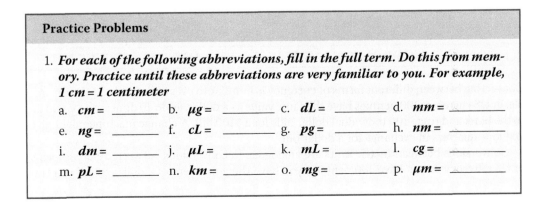

a. ***cm*** = ________ b. ***μg*** = ________ c. ***dL*** = ________ d. ***mm*** = ________
e. ***ng*** = ________ f. ***cL*** = ________ g. ***pg*** = ________ h. ***nm*** = ________
i. ***dm*** = ________ j. ***μL*** = ________ k. ***mL*** = ________ l. ***cg*** = ________
m. ***pL*** = ________ n. ***km*** = ________ o. ***mg*** = ________ p. ***μm*** = ________

2. ***Fill in the following blanks from memory. Practice until these are very familiar to you.***

a. *1 Kg* = _____ *g* b. *1 mL* = _____ *L* c. *1 dL* = _____ *L* d. *1 mg* = _____ *g*
e. *1 KL* = _____ *L* f. *1 dg* = _____ *g* g. *1 pg* = _____ *g* h. *1 nm* = _____ *m*
i. *1 pL* = _____ *L* j. *1 μL* = _____ *L* k. *1 Km* = _____ *m* l. *1 μm* = _____ *m*
m. *1 dm* = _____ *m* n. *1 nL* = _____ *L* o. *1 μg* = _____ *g* p. *1 mm* = _____ *m*
q. *1 ng* = _____ *g* r. *1 pm* = _____ *m* s. *1 cL* = _____ *L* t. *1 cm* = _____ *m*
u. *1 cg* = _____ *g*

3. ***Underline the larger value in each pair:***

a. *1 mm or 1 cm* b. *1 mcg or 1 ng* c. *1 pg or 1 ng*
d. *1 km or 1 m* e. *1 μL or 1 mL* f. *1 dL or 1 mL*
g. *1 μm or 1 nm* h. *1 nL or 1 μL* i. *100 fg or 100 pg*

### *Answers*

1. Fill in the full term from memory.

a. cm = centimeter b. μg = microgram c. dL = deciliter d. mm = millimeter
e. ng = nanogram f. cL = centiliter g. pg = picogram h. nm = nanometer
i. dm = decimeter j. μL = microliter k. mL = milliliter l. cg = centigram
m. pL = picoliter n. km = kilometer o. mg = milligram p. μm = micrometer

2. Fill in the following blanks from memory.

a. 1 Kg = $\mathbf{10^{3}\ g}$ b. 1 mL = $\mathbf{10^{-3}\ L}$ c. 1 dL = $\mathbf{10^{-1}\ L}$ d. 1 mg = $\mathbf{10^{-3}\ g}$
e. 1 KL = $\mathbf{10^{3}\ L}$ f. 1 dg = $\mathbf{10^{-1}\ g}$ g. 1 pg = $\mathbf{10^{-12} g}$ h. 1 nm = $\mathbf{10^{-9}\ m}$
i. 1 pL = $\mathbf{10^{-12}\ L}$ j. 1 μL = $\mathbf{10^{-6}\ L}$ k. 1 Km = $\mathbf{10^{3}\ m}$ l. 1 μm = $\mathbf{10^{-6}\ m}$
m. 1 dm = $\mathbf{10^{-1}\ m}$ n. nL = $\mathbf{10^{-9}\ L}$ o. 1 μg = $\mathbf{10^{-6}\ g}$ p. 1 mm = $\mathbf{10^{-3}\ m}$
q. 1 ng = $\mathbf{10^{-9}\ g}$ r. 1 pm = $\mathbf{10^{-12}\ m}$ s. 1 cL = $\mathbf{10^{-2}\ L}$ t. 1 cm = $\mathbf{10^{-2}\ m}$
u. 1 cg = $\mathbf{10^{-2}\ g}$

3. Underline the larger value in each pair:

a. 1 mm or <u>1 cm</u> b. <u>1 mcg</u> or 1 ng c. 1 pg or <u>1 ng</u>
d. <u>1 km</u> or 1 m e. 1 μL or <u>1 mL</u> f. <u>1 dL</u> or 1 mL
g. <u>1 μm</u> or 1 nm h. 1 nL or <u>1 μL</u> i. 100 fg or <u>100 pg</u>

## 3.3 CONVERTING FROM ONE METRIC UNIT TO ANOTHER METRIC UNIT

Converting between different forms of currency is familiar to everyone, Table 3.5. For example, in US currency, 100 pennies have the same value as a dollar, as do 10 dimes. You could go to the bank and trade 100 individual dollar bills for a $100 bill. A change machine might give you four quarters in exchange for a dollar bill.

Conversions between metric units are analogous to conversions between different forms of US currency. If you have 100 pennies, you have the equivalent of a dollar bill; if you run

**TABLE 3.5 Units of US Currency**

| Term | Multiple of Ten | Decimal Notation |
|---|---|---|
| | **Basic Unit = dollar = $1** | |
| Quarter | $2.5\times10^{-1}$ | $0.25 |
| Dime | $10^{-1}$ | $0.10 |
| Nickel | $5\times10^{-2}$ | $0.05 |
| Cent | $10^{-2}$ | $0.01 |

a km, you run 1,000 m. Metric conversions are briefly introduced in the problems below. In Chapter 7, unit conversions are covered in more detail, including conversions from the USCS. to the metric system. (Converting between the USCS and the metric systems is analogous to converting between dollars and Euros; a Euro is a unit of currency used in many European countries.)

**Example Problem:**

Which is larger, 1 cm or 100 µm?

***Answer:***

One strategy to solve this problem is to convert both values to the same units, for example, meters.

$$\mathbf{1\ cm} = 1/100\ \text{m} = \mathbf{0.01\ m}$$

$$\mathbf{100\ \mu m} = 100\times10^{-6}\ \text{m} = 1.00\times10^{-4}\ \text{m} = \mathbf{0.0001\ m}$$

Once both values are converted to meters, it is easy to see that the first number, 1 cm, is larger.

**Example Problem:**

The bacterial toxin, botulinum, is extremely toxic and acts by paralyzing muscles. Exposure to a few µg of toxin causes death. The toxin can, however, be used to treat patients with a rare disorder, blepharospasm. These patients are blind because their eyes are squeezed shut. Tiny doses of the botulinum toxin allow patients to open their eyes. If a patient is administered 100 pg of toxin, will the patient be able to see or will the patient die?

***Answer:***

A **pg = 1 ×10$^{-12}$ g** and **100 pg = 1 ×10$^{-10}$ g.**

A few micrograms would be about $3\times10^{-6}$ g. Therefore, 100 pg is thousands of times less than a few micrograms and this dose of botulinum toxin is likely to be safe. (Its effectiveness depends on the patient.)

$$(100\ \text{pg} = 0.0001\ \mu\text{g})$$

**Practice Problems**

1. ***Converting currency. Fill in the following:***
   a. ***$100=______ $10 bills=______ $1 bills***
   b. ***$500=______ $10 bills=______ $1 bills***
   c. ***$1,000=______ $100 bills=______ $10 bills=______ $1 bills***
   d. ***$10,000=______ $1,000 bills=______ $100 bills=______ $10 bills=______ $1 bills***
2. ***More currency conversions:***
   a. ***$1=what fraction of $10?______***
   b. ***$1=what fraction of $100?______***
   c. ***$1=what fraction of $1,000?______***
   d. ***One dime=what fraction of $1?______***
   e. ***How many dimes are in one dollar?______***
   f. ***How many dimes are in three dollars?______***
   g. ***One penny=what fraction of $1?______***
   h. ***How many pennies are in one dollar?______***
   i. ***How many pennies are in three dollars?______***
3. ***Fill in the blanks.***
   a. ***1 m=______ mm***
   b. ***1 m=______ µm***
   c. ***1 m=______ cm***
   d. ***1 m=______ nm***
   e. ***1 m=______ pm***
   f. ***1 L=______ µL***
   g. ***1 g=______ µg***
   h. ***1 mg=______ g***
   i. ***1 ng=______ g***
4. ***Underline the larger value in each pair. Underline both if they are equivalent:***
   a. ***1 µm, 1 nm***
   b. ***1 cm, 1 mm***
   c. ***10 cm, 1,000 mm***
   d. ***10,000 µm, 10 m***
   e. ***1,000 g, 1 kg***
   f. ***100 nm, 1,000 µm***
   g. ***100 µg, 1 mg***
   h. ***1 nm, 10 pm***
   i. ***10 nm, 1 Å***
   j. ***100 mg, 1 g***
   k. ***1,000 µL, 1 mL***
   l. ***100,000 µm, 1 m***
   m. ***1 L, 1,000 µL***
   n. ***1 m, 500 cm***
   o. ***1 pL, 0.001 nL***
   p. ***10 nm, 0.1 µm***
   q. ***100 cm, 0.1 m***
   r. ***0.0001 m, 10 µm***
5. ***Clifford was using Synthroid after his thyroid was removed. He entered the hospital for an unrelated ailment. The physician in the hospital prescribed 25 mcg orally each day. Prior to surgery, a pharmacist prepared an IV dose for Clifford of 25 mg. Clifford died. What happened?*** *(Based on real events posted by the ASMP Medication Safety Alert, 6 September 2000. www.ismp.org/MSAarticles/Levothy-Digoxin.html)*
6. ***If a veterinarian orders 0.5 L of 0.9% saline, how many mL would be administered?***
7. ***If a physician orders 0.75 mL of medication for a patient, how many microliters is administered?***
8. ***When talking about biological molecules, it is often necessary to use unfamiliar units. For example, the weight of a single HIV virus is reported to be about*** $1 \times 10^{-18}$ ***kg or 1 fg. What is its weight in units of attograms?***

*Answers*

1. Fill in the following:
   a. \$100 = **10** \$10 bills = **100** \$1 bills
   b. \$500 = **50** \$10 bills = **500** \$1 bills
   c. \$1000 = **10** \$100 bills = **100** \$10 bills = **1,000** \$1 bills
   d. \$10,000 = **10** \$1000 bills = **100** \$100 bills = **1,000** \$10 bills = **10,000** \$1 bills
2. More currency conversions:
   a. \$1 = what fraction of \$10? **1/10 = 0.1**
   b. \$1 = what fraction of \$100? **1/100 = 0.01**
   c. \$1 = what fraction of \$1,000 ? **1/1,000 = 0.001**
   d. One dime = what fraction of \$1? **1/10 = 0.1**
   e. How many dimes are in one dollar? **10**
   f. How many dimes are in three dollars? **30**
   g. One penny = what fraction of \$1? **1/100 = 0.01**
   h. How many pennies are in one dollar? **100**
   i. How many pennies are in three dollars? **300**
3. Fill in the blanks.
   a. 1 m = **1000 mm** b. 1 m = **1,000,000 µm** c. 1 m = **100 cm**
   d. 1 m = **$10^9$ nm** e. 1 m = **$10^{12}$ pm** f. 1 L = **$10^6$ µL**
   g. 1 g = **1,000,000 µg** h. 1 mg = **$10^{-3}$ g** i. 1 ng = **$10^{-9}$ g**
4. Larger:
   a. **1 µm** b. **1 cm** c. **1,000 mm** d. **10 m** e. **1,000 g = 1 kg**
   f. **1,000 µm** g. **1 mg** h. **1 nm** i. **10 nm** j. **1 g**
   k. **1,000 µL = 1 mL** l. **1 m** m. **1 L** n. **500 cm**
   o. **1 pL = 0.001 nL** p. **0.1 µm** q. **100 cm** r. **0.0001 m**
5. Clifford was administered 25 mg of drug when 25 µg was prescribed. He was therefore given 1,000 times too much drug and he died. The pharmacist misread the units.
6. If a veterinarian orders 0.5 L of 0.9% saline, this is the same as **500 mL.**
7. If a physician orders 0.75 mL of medication for a patient, this is the same as **750 mL.**
8. 1 fg = **1,000 ag**

## 3.4 SIZES OF BIOLOGICAL MOLECULES

As a biologist it is important that you have a feeling for the sizes of biological structures. This is easy for objects that we can see. For example, you probably have a sense of the length of a fingernail and the height of a giraffe and you can imagine how much bigger a giraffe is than a fingernail. In contrast, biologists think about cells, the structures within cells, and molecules and atoms. These structures are small and are not visible with the naked eye, so it is difficult to imagine their sizes.

Table 3.6 provides some examples of the sizes of "typical" biological structures expressed with metric units. (Note that for all of these structures there is variability in their sizes, for example, a mammalian cell might be anywhere from about 10 to 20 µm.) **Mitochondria** *are subunits of cells that help the cell use energy.* **Ribosomes** *are subunits of cells that help the cell make proteins.* **Proteins** *are molecules that perform many varied jobs in the cell,* for

**TABLE 3.6 Average Sizes of Biological Structures**

| Structure | In Units of Meters | In Units of Micrometers | In Units of Nanometers |
|---|---|---|---|
| Child's height | 1.5 | $1.5\times10^{6}$ | $1.5\times10^{9}$ |
| Bee (length) | $1.5\times10^{-2}$ | $1.5\times10^{4}$ | $1.5\times10^{7}$ |
| Pollen grain (diameter) | $3\times10^{-5}$ | 30 | $3\times10^{4}$ |
| Mammalian cell (diameter) | $1.5\times10^{-5}$ | 15 | $1.5\times10^{4}$ |
| Mammalian nucleus (diameter) | $5\times10^{-6}$ | 5 | $5\times10^{3}$ |
| Bacterial cell (length) | $1.5\times10^{-6}$ | 1.5 | $1.5\times10^{3}$ |
| Mitochondrion (length) | $5\times10^{-7}$ | $5\times10^{-1}$ | $5\times10^{2}$ |
| Virus | $1\times10^{-7}$ | $1\times10^{-1}$ | $1\times10^{2}$ |
| Ribosome | $1\times10^{-8}$ | $1\times10^{-2}$ | 10 |
| Protein | $5\times10^{-9}$ | $5\times10^{-3}$ | 5 |
| Glucose molecule | $1\times10^{-9}$ | $1\times10^{-3}$ | 1 |
| A water molecule | $1\times10^{-10}$ | $1\times10^{-4}$ | 0.1 |

example, antibodies and enzymes are proteins. Observe that the heights of people might be described conveniently in units of meters or perhaps centimeters. Most people would probably not find it convenient to express their height in units of micrometers, although it is possible to do so. Cells and their subunits are easily described with units of micrometers. Atoms and small molecules like water fall into the range that is easily described with units of nanometers. The burgeoning field of "nanotechnology" involves manufacturing machines and devices by manipulating atoms and small molecules.

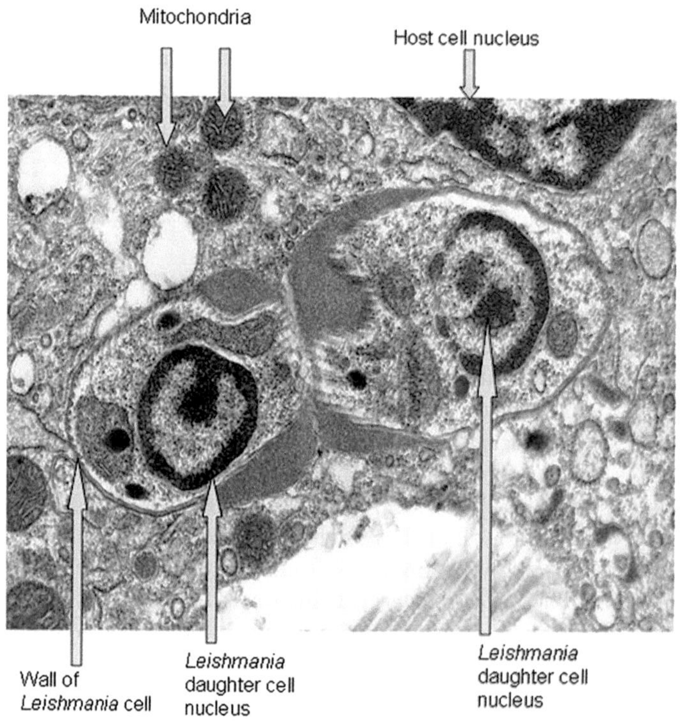


**FIGURE 3.2** Electron micrograph of ***Leishmania*** parasite reproducing inside of an animal cell. Magnification about 35,000x. Various subcellular structures are labeled.

Next examine Figure 3.2, which shows a picture of the interior of an animal cell taken with an electron microscope. The structures in the image are magnified to be about 35,000 times larger than their actual size. In the center of the picture there is a parasite (called *Leishmania*) that is in the process of reproducing by dividing into two daughter cells. The parasite is living and reproducing inside an animal's tissue. (This parasite causes a disease called leishmaniasis that afflicts animals and more than one million people, mainly in the tropics. The parasite can affect the skin, causing sores that may or may not be painful. It can also affect the internal organs causing fever, weight loss, and an enlarged spleen and liver.) Various structures are labeled in the photo. Begin by finding the parasite's two daughter cells. Then, find three nuclei: those of the two parasite daughter cells and the portion of the host animal cell's nucleus. After you find the nuclei, look for mitochondria. Some examples of mitochondria are labeled, but you can find more if you look. Next find the ribosomes, which look like very small, black dots in the photo, about the size of a period. Observe that nuclei and mitochondria are much larger than ribosomes.

**Practice Problems**

1. a. ***What is the diameter of a typical cell in μm?*** ___________
   b. ***What is the diameter of a typical protein?*** ___________
2. ***The child in Table 3.6 is 100 times taller than a bee.***
   a. ***About how many times bigger is a bee than a single mammalian cell?***
   b. ***About how many times shorter is a typical ribosome than a single mammalian cell?***
   c. ***About how many times taller is a child than a typical mammalian cell's diameter?***
   d. ***About how many times taller is a child than a water molecule?***
3. ***Without looking at Table 3.6, put the following items in order from the largest to the smallest:***
   ***A single*** **Serratia marcescens** ***cell (this is a type of bacterium)***
   ***Water molecule***
   ***Human blood cell***
   ***Grape***
   ***Sesame seed***
   ***Ant***
   ***A polio virus***
   ***An oxygen atom***
   ***A hemoglobin (a kind of protein) molecule***
   ***Ribosome***
   ***A football***
4. ***An electron micrograph of a portion of a liver cell is shown in Figure 3.3. A few of the mitochondria are labeled (these are the round or oblong structures on the left of the photo). Each mitochondrion is bordered by a membrane. Measure the lengths of some of the mitochondria with a ruler (in mm) and take the average. Based on this value, and assuming these mitochondria are average in length, how many times was this picture magnified?***
5. ***Assume that you can see an object that is about 1 mm. How many times would you need to magnify a water molecule to see it?*** ___________

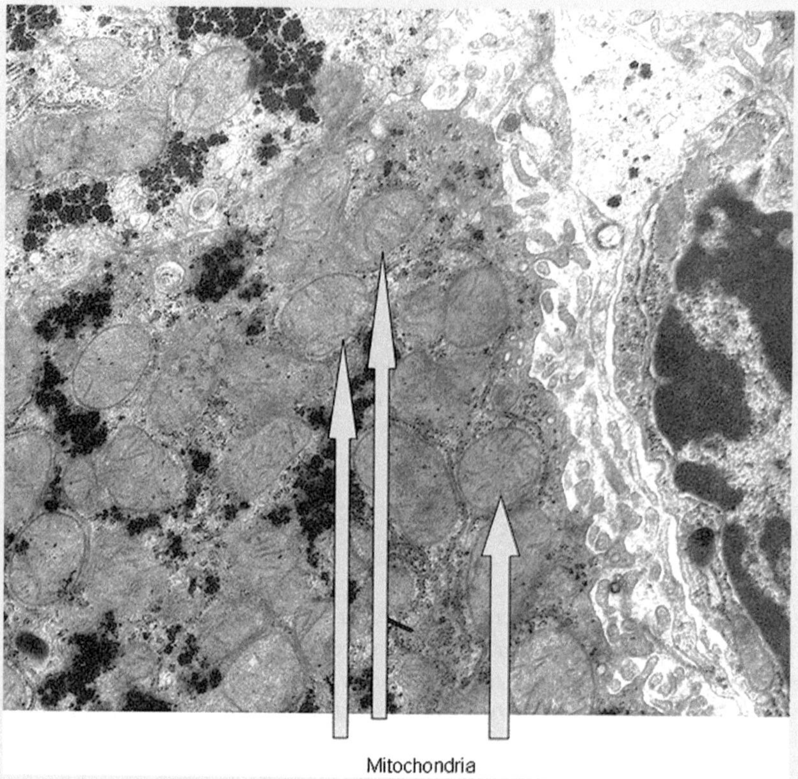


**FIGURE 3.3** Electron micrograph of a liver cell.

6. ***Suppose you decided to make cardboard models of biological structures. You begin by making a cardboard cell that is 0.1 m in diameter. Next, you want to make a cardboard model of a child that is to scale. How big should your model child be? Will this plan work?***
7. ***Imagine a filter with pores of about 0.10 μm.***
   a. ***Would sand pass through this filter?***
   b. ***Could you sterilize a solution by passing it through this filter, that is, will bacteria be retained by the filter or will they pass through it?***
   c. ***Could you use this filter to remove viruses from a solution?***
   d. ***Would glucose molecules pass through this filter?***
8. ***The COVID-19 pandemic has made everyone aware of the threat of pathogenic viruses. Even before COVID-19 entered the public's awareness, scientists in the biotechnology industry have known that viruses can cause disease and death and they have developed methods to remove viral agents from any medical products that will be administered to humans or other animals. Filtration is one of the most common methods to remove viral contaminants from biotechnology protein-based products. For filtration to work in this application, it is important to have a pore size that traps the viral contaminants while allowing the desired protein product to pass through. The largest viruses are about 0.5 μm and the smallest are about 0.012 μm. The largest proteins are about 12 nm and the smallest are around 4 nm in size. If you were to design a filter to remove viruses from a protein product, what pore size would you select for your filter? Express your answer in nm.***

*Answers*

1. a. What is the diameter of a typical cell in micrometers? **Around 15 μm**
   b. What is the size of a typical protein? **Around 5 nm**
2. a. About how many times bigger is a bee than a single mammalian cell? **1,000**
   b. About how many times smaller is a typical ribosome than a single mammalian cell? **1,500**
   c. About how many times taller is a child than a typical mammalian cell's diameter? **100,000**
   d. About how many times taller is a child than a water molecule? $\mathbf{1.5 \times 10^{10}}$
3. Put the following items in order from the largest to the smallest:
   Football
   Grape
   Ant
   Sesame seed
   Human blood cell
   A single *Serratia Marcescens* cell
   A polio virus
   Ribosome
   A hemoglobin molecule
   A water molecule
   An oxygen atom
4. The average length of the mitochondria in the image is about 14 mm (assuming a standard, printed page). Since the actual average length of a mitochondrion is about $5 \times 10^{-1}$ μm, the magnification is about $\left(14 \times 10^{-3}\text{ m}\right)/\left(0.5 \times 10^{-6}\text{ m}\right) = \mathbf{28,000\times}$
5. Assume that you can see an object that is about 1 mm. How many times would you need to magnify a water molecule in order to see it?
   1 mm = 1,000 μm A water molecule is about $1 \times 10^{-4}$ μm.
   $\left(1 \times 10^{-4}\ \mu\text{m}\right)(?) = 1000\ \mu\text{m}$ $? = 1 \times 10^{7}$, so you would need to magnify it about **10 million times.**
6. Suppose you decided to make cardboard models of biological structures. You begin by making a cardboard cell that is 0.1 m in diameter. Next, you want to make a cardboard model of a child that is to scale. How big should your model child be? Will this plan work? To solve this:
   From question 2, we know that a child is roughly 100,000 times bigger than a cell. So if the cell is 0.1 m, the child's cardboard model should be $1 \times 10^{4}$ m. 10,000 m is about 6.2 miles, so this is not practical.
7. Imagine a filter with pores of about 0.10 μm.
   a. Would sand pass through this filter?
      No, sand will be retained by the filter. Note that a sand grain is large enough to see with your eyes and to hold, but an object 0.10 μm is too small to see without a microscope.
   b. This size filter is often used to sterilize laboratory solutions because bacteria (with typical lengths around 1.5 μm) are too big to pass through its pores.
   c. Many viruses (with typical sizes around 0.1 μm) will pass through this filter's pores, so it cannot be used to remove them from a solution.
   d. Glucose molecules are much smaller than the pore size and will readily pass through this filter.

8. This is a real and challenging task in the biotechnology industry partly because the smallest viruses are about the same size as the largest proteins. The design of filters to remove viruses from protein products is actually quite complex. However, one can imagine that a pore size of about 10 nm will allow most proteins to pass through while retaining almost all viruses on the surface of the filter.

## 3.5 METRIC PREFIXES FOR LARGE NUMBERS

Cell and molecular biologists have traditionally been more familiar with metric system prefixes for small numbers than for large ones. For example, cells are in the micrometer size range, proteins in the nanometer range. A molecular biologist might add only picomoles of some reagent into a reaction mixture. Therefore, until recently, a molecular biologist could usually ignore metric system prefixes for very large numbers – such as mega, giga, and tera. This situation has changed, however, because computers require everyone to think about very large numbers. Also, the sequencing of the human genome has given molecular biologists billions of nucleotide base pairs (the subunits of DNA) to talk about, Figure 3.4.

Computers use "memory" that is described with units of **bits** and **bytes**. A **bit** *is the amount of information in a system with two equally probable states, for example, "on" and "off," or 0 and 1.* A **byte** *is 8 bits.* One byte is the amount of memory required to store one character. There are kilobytes (about 1000 bytes), megabytes (about 1 million bytes), gigabytes (about one billion bytes), and terabytes (about one trillion bytes). One kilobyte is roughly equivalent to one page of double-spaced text.

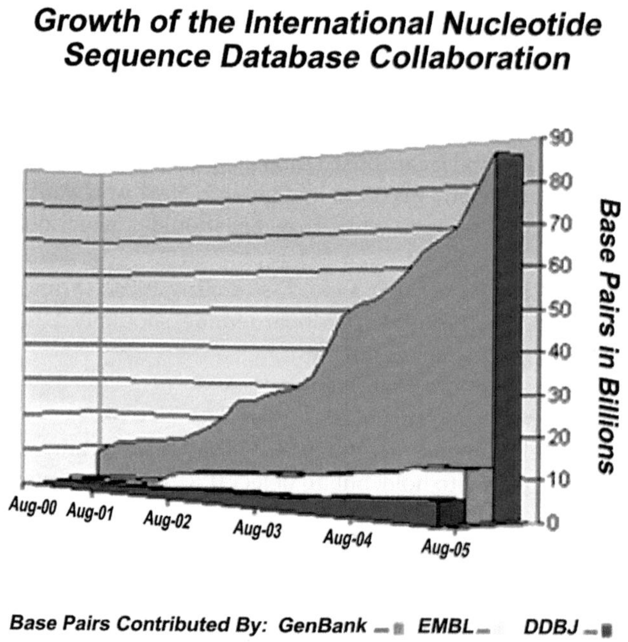


**FIGURE 3.4** Genome sequencing projects reach 100 gigabases. In August 2005, representatives of an international collaboration of genome sequencing projects announced that their combined databases contain information about more than 100 gigabases of DNA. (A base pair is a subunit of DNA. A gene is a specific sequence of DNA base pairs, on the order of about 10,000–15,000 base pairs long, that codes for a particular protein.) According to the press release, 100 billion base pairs is about equal to the number of nerve cells in the human brain and a bit less than the number of stars in the Milky Way. (Image credit: NCBI. www.ncbi.nlm.nih.gov/Genbank/.)

- *1 Byte = 8 bits = one character*
- *1 kilobyte = 1 KB = about 1,000 bytes = $10^3$ bytes = one thousand bytes*
- *1 Megabyte = 1 MB = about 1,000,000 bytes = $10^6$ bytes = one million bytes*
- *1 Gigabyte = 1 GB = about 1,000,000,000 bytes = $10^9$ bytes = one billion bytes*
- *1 Terabyte = 1 TB = about 1,000,000,000,000 bytes = $10^{12}$ bytes = one trillion bytes*

**Practice Problems**

1. a. *1 TB = ________ GB = ________ MB = ________ KB*
   b. *10 GB = ________ MB* c. *100 KB = ________ MB*
2. ***If your digital photos on the average require 20 MB*:**
   a. ***How many will fit on a 64 GB memory card?***
   b. ***How many will fit on a 1 TB memory card?***
3. ***Suppose as lab manager you need to back up the laboratory's data on an external hard drive. Each researcher in the laboratory wants at least 500 GB. There are seven researchers in the laboratory.***
   a. ***What is the minimum size hard drive that will be sufficient at the moment?***
   b. ***What is the maximum size external hard drive or other memory device that is available at the time you are reading this text?***
4. ***If you buy a 32 GB flash drive, how many 3 MB cell phone pictures will it store?***
5. ***On August 25, 2005, Science magazine announced that the number of nucleotide base pairs in the world's three major databases had topped 100 billion, about equal to the number of nerve cells in a human brain.***
   a. ***Express 100 billion in scientific notation.***
   b. ***Express 100 billion base pairs using the metric system prefix for "billion."***

*Answers*

1. a. **1 TB = $\underline{10^3}$ GB = $\underline{10^6}$ MB = $\underline{10^9}$ KB** b. 10 GB = **10,000 MB**
   c. 100 KB = **0.1 MB**
2. If your digital photos on average require 20 MB:
   a. How many will fit on a 64 GB memory card? **3,200**
   b. How many will fit on a 1 TB memory card? **50,000**
3. a. You need 3,500 GB to meet the needs of the researchers. This is **3.5 TB**. A **4 TB** hard drive would work.
   b. At the time of writing, there are 100 TB hard drives available. Presumably, hard drives with more memory will be available in the future. This is particularly important for bioinformaticians who work with huge data sets.
4. If you buy a 32 GB flash drive, how many 3 MB pictures will it hold? **10,666**
5. a. $\mathbf{1 \times 10^{11}}$ b. **100 gigabases**

# Measurements and Significant Figures

4



## 4.1 MEASUREMENT UNCERTAINTY AND SIGNIFICANT FIGURES

If you count the number of students sitting in a small classroom or the number of microscopes in a laboratory, you can be certain that your numbers would be exactly correct. We would say that there is little, if any, ***uncertainty*** in your counts. However, if you were to try and count the number of grains of sand on a beach, you would be very uncertain about the exact, true number of sand grains. There are many reasons why it would be difficult to get an exact count of sand grains: it would be easy to lose some grains; it would sometimes be difficult to decide what constitutes a single grain; it would be hard to keep track of the results; and the size of the beach would constantly change due to tides and wave action. Thus, when counting small numbers of discrete items, it is possible to be certain of our counts. But when we try to count very large numbers of items, there are many possible sources of error and we become less certain that our counts are correct.

Now, consider certainty/uncertainty and measurements. When we measure items, using any type of measuring device, there is always uncertainty in our measurements. This is partly because every measuring device has limitations in how finely it is marked or calibrated. For example, if you measure your height using a tape measure that is marked off every sixteenth of an inch, then you can only measure your height to the nearest sixteenth of an inch. It is not possible to get a more exact measurement than the tape measure permits. Every measuring device has a limit in its "exactness" or fineness of markings, and so every measurement has uncertainty. This leads to the topic of significant figures.

**Significant figure** *conventions guide us when we report the results of measurements so that what we report indicates the exactness of the measuring device.* (The same ideas apply to counts of very large numbers, such as the number of grains of sand on a beach.) Significant figures are the most basic way that scientists show the certainty in a measurement value. A **significant figure** *is a digit that is a reliable indicator of value.* It is easiest to understand significant figures by looking at practical examples from the laboratory and everyday life.

**Example 1: Rulers**

Consider the length of the arrow drawn in Figure 4.1a and 4.1b.

In Figure 4.1a, the ruler's markings divide each centimeter in half. We know the arrow (at its tip) is somewhat longer than 4 cm and it is reasonable to estimate the tenth place and report the arrow's length as "4.3 cm" or perhaps as "4.4 cm." Information is lost if we report the length as simply "4 cm" since it is possible to tell that the arrow is

DOI: 10.1201/9780429282744-5

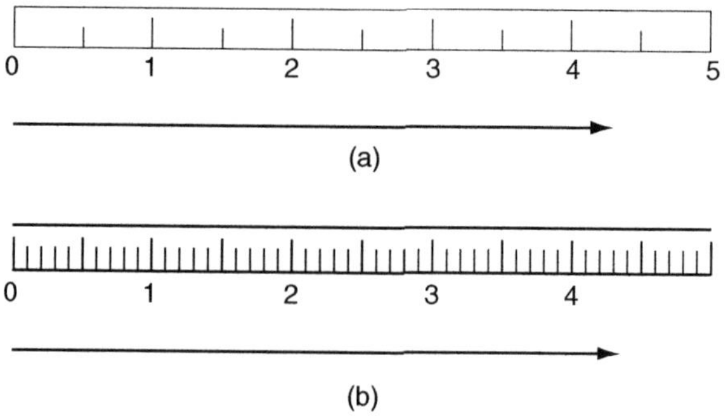


**FIGURE 4.1** Measurements of length with two rulers. (a) A ruler where each centimeter is subdivided in half. (b) A ruler where each centimeter is subdivided into tenths. (Drawing is not to scale.)

somewhat longer than 4 cm. It would be unreasonable to report that the arrow is "4.35" cm because the ruler gradations give no way to read the hundredths place. When measurements are recorded, it is customary to record all the digits of which we are certain plus one that is estimated. In this example, the 4 is certain and the 3 is estimated, so the measurement is said to have two significant figures. Thus, by reporting the measurement to be 4.3, we are telling the reader something about how certain we are of the length. We are sure about the 4 and not as sure about the .3.

The subdivisions in the second ruler, Figure 4.1b, are finer and divide each centimeter into tenths. With the second ruler, we can reliably say the arrow is "4.3" cm, and in fact, it is reasonable to estimate that the arrow is about "4.35" cm. The "4.3" is certain, the "5" is estimated and so there are three significant figures in the measurement. Thus, the arrow is the same length in both Figure 4.1a and 4.1b, yet the length *recorded* is different because the rulers are differently subdivided. The fineness of the measuring instrument, in this case, the rulers, determines our certainty in the length of the arrow. The measurement certainty is reflected by the number of significant figures used in recording the measurement.

**A NOTE ABOUT TERMINOLOGY:**

- Some would say the second ruler is more **accurate** than the first, because it gives values with more significant figures, that is, with more certainty. However, in this text we do not use the term "accurate" in this way. We reserve the term "accurate" to mean how close a value is to the true or correct value.
- Some would say the second ruler is more **precise** than the first because it can be read further past the decimal point. The word "precise" has two meanings. It may refer to the fineness of increments of a measuring device, the smaller the increments, the better the precision. Precision also can mean the consistency of values, the more consistent a series of measurements, the more precise.
- Some would say the second ruler has more **resolution** because it allows us to discriminate a smaller length change than the first ruler.
- Some would say the second ruler is more **exact** than the first ruler.

**Example 2: Balances**

Suppose a particular balance can weigh an object as light as 0.00001 g. On this balance, sample Q is found to weigh "0.12300 g." It would not be correct to report that sample Q weighs "0.123 g" because information about the certainty of the measurement is lost if the last zeros are discarded. In contrast, if sample Q is weighed on a balance that only reads three places past the decimal point, it is correct to report its weight as "0.123 g." It would not be correct to write "0.1230" g because the balance could not read the fourth place past the decimal point. The first balance gives more certainty about the sample weight. The difference in measurement certainty between the two balances is shown by the number of significant figures used: "0.12300" g has five significant figures while "0.123 g" has only three.

You can see in examples 1 and 2 that a basic principle in recording measurements from instruments is to report as much information as is reliable plus one last figure that is estimated and so might vary if the measurement were repeated. The number of figures reported by following this principle is the number of significant figures for the measurement, a rough estimate of its certainty.

Most modern electronic instruments have a digital display; there is no meter to read. With any digital display the last place is assumed to have been estimated by the instrument.

**Example 3: Budget**

As a final example, consider a company budget. Suppose that one newspaper reports the budget to be "$156,375,000" while another reports it as "$156,400,000." Let us assume that both reports are correct, but the second newspaper rounded the number to make it easier to read. The first number, $156,375,000, is a more exact figure for the budget and allows the reader to be more certain about the actual value than does the second number. We say that the number $156,375,000 has more significant figures (six) than the number 156,400,000 (which has four significant figures).

The budget example illustrates an important point regarding zeros. The zeros in the budget reports are essential, without them the budget would be reported as a paltry "$1,564" or "$156,375." The zeros are "place holders" that tell us we are talking about a multimillion dollar budget, but they are not correct indicators of value. Perhaps the budget was really $156,374,978 or $156,375,091 or any of a number of other possibilities. Sometimes zeros are "place holders," not indicators of value. In contrast, if you state "there are 10 microscopes in the lab" the zero is a reliable indicator of value. The zero shows that there are 10, not 9 or 11, microscopes. Zeros that are place holders are not significant figures while zeros that indicate value are significant.

## 4.2 INDICATING WHETHER ZEROS ARE SIGNIFICANT

Suppose the number given in a report is 45,000. The three zeros in this number each may be place holders or they may be indicators of value. There are various ways to tell the reader whether the zeros at the end of a number are significant. One method is to use scientific notation. For example, there are three zeros at the end of the number 45,000. If none of the zeros are significant, then the number could be reported as $4.5 \times 10^4$, two significant figures. If there are three significant figures the number could be reported as $4.50 \times 10^4$, and so on. If all the zeros in the number 45,000 are significant, this can be shown by placing a decimal point after the number. The number 45,000. and $4.5000 \times 10^4$ both have five significant figures.

Metric prefixes can also be used to indicate which digits of a numerical value are significant. For example, in the expression "length = 1,200 m," it is not possible to tell if the two zeros are significant. However, in the expression "length = 1.200 km," which uses the metric prefix for $10^3$, the two zeros are shown to be significant because if they were not, the expression would have been written as "length = 1.2 km."

Box 4.1 summarizes rules regarding how to record measurements with the accepted number of significant figures. These rules also show how to decide when a zero is significant and when it is a place holder.

### BOX 4.1 Rules to Record Measurements with the Correct Number of Significant Figures

1. **The number of significant figures is related to the certainty of a measurement or a count of great magnitude.** (Recall that exactly counted values, such as the number of microscopes in the laboratory, are exact and significant figure conventions do not apply.)
2. **When reporting a measurement, record as many digits as are certain plus one digit that is estimated.** When reading a meter or ruler, estimate the last place. When reading an electronic digital display, assume the instrument estimated the last place.
3. **All nonzero digits in a number are significant.** For example, all the digits in the number 98.34 are significant; this number has four significant figures. A reader will assume that the 98.3 is certain and the 4 is estimated.
4. **All zeros between two nonzero digits are significant**. For example, in the number 100.4, the zeros are reliable indicators of value and not just place holders.
5. **Zero digits to the right of a nonzero digit but to the left of an assumed decimal point may or may not be significant.** With the number "$156,400,000," the decimal point is assumed to be after the last zero. In this case, the zeros are ambiguous and may or may not be reliable indicators of value. Methods of clarifying ambiguous zeros are discussed in the text.
6. **All zeros to the right of a decimal point and to the right of a nonzero digit before a decimal place are significant.** The following numbers all have five significant figures: 340.00, 0.34000 (the zero to the left of the decimal point only calls attention to the decimal point), and 3.4000.
7. **All the digits to the left of a nonzero digit and to the right of a decimal point are not significant unless there is a significant digit to their left.** The number 0.0098 has two significant figures because the two zeros before the 98 are place holders. On the other hand, 0.4098 has four significant figures.

**Example Problem:**

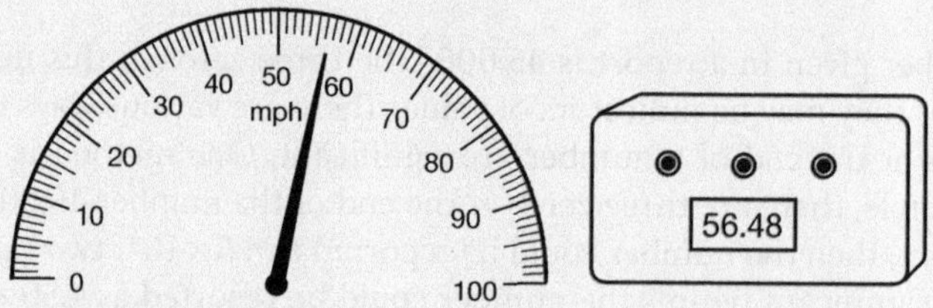


**FIGURE 4.2** Reading displays.

Read the meter and the digital display in the diagrams in Figure 4.2. How many significant figures does each measurement have?

*Answer:*

The meter reads "56.6," three significant figures; the operator estimates the last place. The digital display reads "56.48," four significant figures; the instrument estimates the last place.

## 4.3 CALCULATIONS AND SIGNIFICANT FIGURES

Calculations, such as addition or multiplication, bring together numbers from separate measurements. Each value in the calculation has a particular number of significant figures. The result from the calculation is limited to the certainty (number of significant figures) of the beginning number that is least certain. When calculations are performed that involve numbers from measurements, the significant figure conventions provide guidance on how to round the answer. The results of calculations should be rounded in such a way as to indicate the "exactness" with which the original measurements were made.

The result displayed on a basic calculator is seldom what should be recorded when a calculation is performed involving measurements because calculators do not give any indication of certainty*. The calculator result must be rounded to the proper number of significant figures. When numbers are brought together in calculations, it is often not obvious how many significant figures there are, and there are various rules to determine the correct number of significant figures. Box 4.2 summarizes rules that are often taught in chemistry classes and are likely to be adequate for situations in biology laboratories. (Sometimes these rules seem to give odd results because they simplify what is actually a more complex procedure.) **Remember, these rules are guides to decide where to round the result of a calculation(s) when measurements (or counts of great magnitude) are involved.**

**BOX 4.2 Rules for Recording Values from Calculations with the "Correct" Number of Significant Figures**

1. **It is assumed that the last digit of a result from a calculation is rounded.**
   For example, given the result "45.6," the .6 is assumed to have been rounded so the calculated value must have been greater than or equal to 45.55 and less than 45.65.
2. **When rounding:**
   a. **If the digit to be dropped is less than 5, the preceding digit remains the same.**
   b. **If the digit to be dropped is 5 or more, the preceding digit increases by 1.**
   For example:
   54.78 is rounded to 54.8
   54.83 is rounded to 54.8
   54.65 is rounded to 54.7
   (There are variant approaches when the digit to be dropped is 5. Some round a five to the nearest *even* number. 9.65 then is rounded to 9.6 and 4.75 to 4.8)
3. **Round after performing a calculation.**
   If a problem requires a series of calculations, round only after the final calculation.
4. **The rule for addition or subtraction is different than for multiplication or division.**
   The addition/subtraction rule focuses on the number of places to the right of the decimal point. The answer retains no more figures to the right of the decimal point than the number in the calculation having the least number of places past the decimal point.

* Note that some graphing calculators have an app that displays the significant figures after a calculation.

For example:

$$\begin{array}{r} 98.0008 \\ +\quad 7.9878 \\ 56.2 \\ \hline 162.1886 \end{array} \quad \text{Round to: } 162.2$$

The answer can be expressed only to the nearest tenth place because the value 56.2 has only that many places.

5. **In multiplication and division, keep as many significant figures as are found in the number with the least significant digits.**
   For example:

$$0.54678 \times 0.980 \times 7.899 =$$

   A calculator might display 4.232634916 but the answer should be reported as **4.23**, because 0.980 has three significant figures.

   Another example:

$$7{,}987 \times 12 = ?$$

   The answer has only two significant figures and is therefore not 95,844, but rather **96,000** (the zeros are place holders).

6. Constants are numbers whose value is exactly known.
   Constants are assumed to have an infinite number of significant figures. For example, given that "12 inches equal a foot," 12 in is a constant. So, for example:

$$7{,}987\ \text{ft} \times 12\ \text{in/ft} \approx \mathbf{95{,}840\ in}$$

**Example Problem:**

A laboratory recipe calls for you to weigh out 2.834g of NaCl. You need to double the recipe. How much NaCl should you weigh out?

***Answer:***

To double the recipe, you will need 2.834 g × 2 = **5.668 g** of NaCl. The answer has four significant figures and should *not* be rounded to 6. The "2" in the calculation is a number with no uncertainty, like a constant (see rule 6 above). This brings up an important caution: do not "throw away" significant figures by rounding when you should not.

**Example Problem:**

A catalog advertises a particular product to be 99% pure. A competitor advertises their version of the same product to be 98.8% pure. Which one is purer?

***Answer:***

First, assume that both competitors have followed the significant figures conventions. Second, assume that the value for purity is based on a calculation(s). Then the first product might reasonably be expected to be anywhere from 98.5% to just under 99.5% pure because anywhere in that range the value would be rounded to 99%. The second brand would be from 98.75% to just under 98.85% pure. It is unclear, therefore, which brand is actually most pure. The second manufacturer, however, has presumably been able to ascertain the purity of their product with more certainty.

**Example Problem:**

A biotechnology company specifies that the level of RNA impurities in a certain product must be less than or equal to 0.02%. If the level of RNA in a lot is 0.024%, does the lot meet the specification?

***Answer:***

The specification is set at the hundredth decimal place, therefore, the result is also reported to that place. 0.024% rounded to the hundredth place is 0.02%. Therefore, this lot meets its specification.

**Practice Problems**

1. ***For each illustration in Figure 4.3, what measurement should be reported? How many significant figures does the measurement have?***

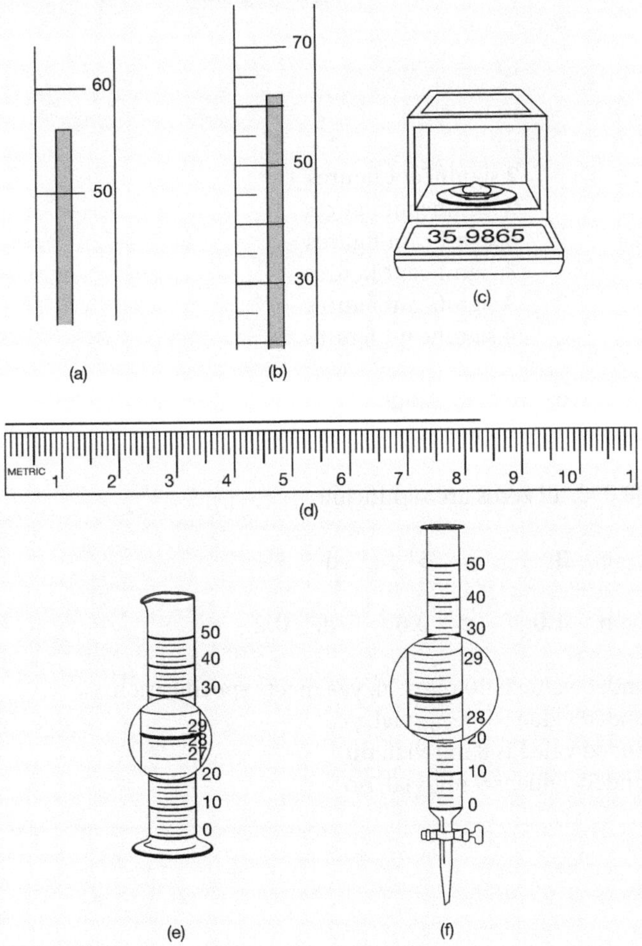


**FIGURE 4.3** Examples for Problem 1.

2. ***Put a line through each of the zeros in this problem that are place holders. Place a ? above each zero that is ambiguous, that is, may be a place holder or may convey value.***
   a. ***2,000*** b. ***1,000,000*** c. ***0.00677*** d. ***134,908,098***

3. ***How many significant figures does each of the following numbers have:***
   a. ***45.789*** b. ***0.00650*** c. ***10.009*** d. ***0.000878***

4. ***Round the following numbers to the nearest tenth decimal place.***
   a. ***0.0345*** b. ***0.98*** c. ***0.55*** d. ***0.2245***

5. ***A biotechnology company specifies that a product has at least 10. mg/vial. (The zero is significant.) Do the following lots meet the specification?***
   lot a. ***10.2 mg/vial*** lot b. ***9.899 mg/vial***
   lot c. ***7.82 mg/vial*** lot d. ***9.400 mg/vial***

6. ***A biotechnology company specifies that a product has ≤0.02% of impurities. Do the following lots meet the specification?***
   lot a. ***0.025%*** lot b. ***0.015%***
   lot c. ***0.027%*** lot d. ***0.024%***

7. ***A biotechnology company specifies that a product has less than 9.0 mg/vial of a contaminant. Do the following lots meet the specification?***
   a. ***9.227 mg/vial*** b. ***8.789 mg/vial***

*Answers*

1. a. 57 **2** significant figures
   b. 62 **2** significant figures
   c. 35.9865 **6** significant figures
   d. 8.25 **3** significant figures
   e. 28.4 **3** significant figures
   f. 28.44 **4** significant figures

2. a. All three zeros are ambiguous.
   b. All six zeros are ambiguous.
   c. ~~0~~.~~00~~677
   d. 134,908,098, all zeros are significant.

3. a. **5** b. **3** c. **5** d. **3**

4. a. **0.0** b. **1.0** c. **0.6** d. **0.2**

5. lot a. rounded value is 10 mg/vial, **yes** meets specification
   lot b. rounded value is 10 mg/vial, **yes**
   lot c. rounded value is 8 mg/vial, **no**
   lot d. rounded value is 9 mg/vial, **no**

6. lot a. rounded value is 0.03%, **no** does not meet specification
   lot b. rounded value is 0.02%, **yes**
   lot c. rounded value is 0.03%, **no**
   lot d. rounded value is 0.02%, **yes**

7. lot a. rounded value is 9.2 **Does not meet the specification.**
   lot b. rounded value is 8.8. **Does meet the specification**.

# Using Equations to Describe a Relationship

# 5



## 5.1 INTRODUCTION TO EQUATIONS

Much of scientific inquiry is about determining the relationship between two or more entities. For example, scientists might study how wolves affect deer populations, how size affects the rate of migration of DNA fragments in electrophoresis, or the relationship between resistance and current in an electrical circuit. Math provides various tools for describing such relationships, including equations, graphs, and statistics. This chapter introduces equations and later chapters discuss graphical and statistical methods of describing relationships.

**Equations** *are a way to describe relationships using mathematical symbols.* An equation is about a relationship in which two or more things are equal. Letters in a scientific equation represent the items involved in the relationship. Scientific equations with unfamiliar symbols may seem intimidating. However, even complicated equations with unfamiliar symbols can tell you about relationships in a system. There are equations in various places throughout this book, all of which convey information about relationships.

Consider, for example, the equation **V = I R**. This equation describes the relationship between voltage (V), current (I), and resistance (R) in an electrical circuit. Even if you have little understanding of electricity, you can learn from this equation that:

1. Voltage, current, and resistance in an electrical circuit are related to each other in a specific way.
2. If resistance increases, either the voltage must also increase or the current must decrease. Similarly, if current increases, then either voltage must increase or resistance must decrease.
3. If voltage goes down, then current and/or resistance must also go down.

For example,

**Suppose that initially the voltage = 12, resistance = 4, and current = 3.**

(Voltage, current, and resistance have units, but we will momentarily ignore them to simplify the example.)

$$\mathbf{V = I\,R}$$

$$\mathbf{12 = 3(4)}$$

DOI: 10.1201/9780429282744-6

What happens if the resistance increases to 5? Perhaps voltage increases and becomes 15. Or, perhaps current decreases and becomes 2.4:

| | |
|---|---|
| V = I R | V = I R |
| **15 = 3 (5)** | **12 = (2.4) (5)** |
| In this case, the current did not change, so voltage must increase | In this case, voltage remained constant |

You will encounter the V = IR equation when performing electrophoresis, a technique that uses electricity to separate various proteins and nucleic acids from one another. During electrophoresis, the resistance of the system increases as the separation of molecules occurs. Therefore, the current goes down – unless the operator increases the voltage.

Consider another equation:

$$\textbf{°F = 1.8 (temperature in °C) + 32}$$

where:

°F is degrees in the Fahrenheit scale
°C is degrees in the Celsius scale

Celsius and Fahrenheit are scales used to measure temperature. The size of a degree is different in the Celsius and Fahrenheit scales. Note that:

1. The numbers 1.8 and 32 in this equation are called **constants** *because they are always present in the equation and always have the same value.* The constant 1.8 is needed in the equation because a Celsius degree is 1.8 times larger than a Fahrenheit degree. The number 32 is necessary because the two scales put the zero point in a different place. Celsius places zero degrees at the temperature of frozen water. Zero degrees Fahrenheit is the lowest temperature that can be obtained by mixing salt and ice.
2. °F and °C are called **variables** *because their value can vary.* (In the previous example, V, I, and R are variables.)
3. Given either of the variables in the temperature equation, it is possible to calculate the other variable. Thus, if we know the temperature in either Celsius or Fahrenheit, the temperature can be converted to the other scale.

## 5.2 UNITS AND MATHEMATICAL OPERATIONS

Units can be manipulated in mathematical operations. Sometimes in math classes, measurement units are absent or ignored. In the "real world," however, units are essential and are not ignored.

Like numbers, units can have exponents. For example, the area of a rectangle is defined as "length times width." In equation form this is:

$$\mathbf{A = (L)\,(W)}$$

where:

A is area
L is length
W is width

For example, a room whose length is 15 ft and width is 10 ft has an area of 150 sq. ft:

$$\mathbf{(L)\;(W) = A}$$

$$(10\text{ ft})(15\text{ ft}) = 150\text{ ft}^2$$

The rules for the manipulation of exponents, as shown in Chapter 1, Box 1.1, apply to units with exponents. Exponents are added for multiplication and subtracted in division.

For example,

$$\frac{\mathbf{44\ cm^3}}{\mathbf{22\ cm^2}} = \frac{\mathbf{(44)}}{\mathbf{(22)}}\,\mathbf{cm}^{(3-2)} = \mathbf{2.0\ cm^1}$$

When working with equations, units can be canceled, multiplied, and divided. For example:

$$\left(2.00\frac{\mathbf{mg}}{\cancel{\mathbf{mL}}}\right)(13.0\ \cancel{\mathbf{mL}})(4.00) = 104\ \mathbf{mg}$$

Another example, which comes from a topic in statistics, is:

$$\mathrm{m} = \left[\frac{(4{,}716.20)(\mathrm{mg})(\mathrm{g}) - (161.03\,\mathrm{g})\dfrac{(170\ \mathrm{mg})}{7}}{5{,}750\ \mathrm{mg}^2 - \dfrac{170^2}{7}(\mathrm{mg})^2}\right]$$

At this point, the relationship expressed by this equation is not important, but watch the units as this equation is solved algebraically:

$$\mathbf{m} = \frac{\mathbf{(4{,}716.20)(mg)(g) - 3{,}910.728571(mg)(g)}}{\mathbf{5{,}750\ mg^2 - 4{,}128.571429\ mg^2}} = \frac{\mathbf{805.4714286(mg)(g)}}{\mathbf{1{,}621.428571\ mg^2}} \approx \mathbf{0.497}\frac{\mathbf{g}}{\mathbf{mg}}$$

**Example Problem:**

What is the volume of a box with a length of 3.45 cm, a width of 2.98 cm, and a height of 3.00 cm?

***Answer:***

V = (length) (width) (height)
V = (3.45 cm) (2.98 cm) (3.00 cm)
= (3.45) (2.98) (3.00) (cm) (cm) (cm) ≈ **30.8 cm³**

**Example Problem:**

Perform the following additions:

a. 23 cm + 56 cm =?
b. 2 cm + 4 s =?

***Answer:***

a. The correct answer is **79 cm** – not just 79
b. The correct answer is:
**2 cm + 4 seconds**

Seconds and cm are different units and cannot be added together.

This is a good time to emphasize that a unit of measurement is not the same thing as a variable. Consider the equation, V = IR. In this equation, there are three *variables*: voltage (V), current (I), and resistance (R). Voltage is measured in *units* of volts; volts are also abbreviated with the letter "V." Current is measured in units of amps; amps are abbreviated with the letter "A." Resistance is measured in units of ohms; ohms are abbreviated with the Greek letter omega, "Ω." Remember that a variable and a unit of measurement are quite different from one another – even in those cases (like volts) where the abbreviation is the same.

This is also a good time to note that the letter "X" has various meanings in mathematical calculations.

X is sometimes used to stand for a variable whose value is not yet known; it is the "unknown." We solve an equation in order to find the value of the unknown that makes the equation correct. For example, given the equation $2 + X = 4$, we can "solve for X." If we substitute the number 2 for X, then the equation is correct: $2 + 2 = 4$. However, we do not need to call the unknown "X." In this text, we often (though not always) use the symbol "?" to stand for the unknown.

Another meaning for the letter "X" is to indicate multiplication, that is, "X" can mean "times." We can avoid using the letter "X" to indicate multiplication by writing $(2)\ (2) = 4$ to indicate that we multiply 2 *times* 2. (You will have learned more about the use of parentheses in equations in an algebra class.) We can also use the related symbol "×" to indicate multiplication.

In Chapter 13, we will see how the letter "X" is also used to indicate that a biological solution is concentrated. As a familiar example of the term "concentrate," we might purchase frozen orange juice *concentrate* or frozen lemonade *concentrate*. These juices need to be diluted before we drink them. Concentration is an important concept that will be explored later in this text. For now, just note that the letter "X" will appear later with another, slightly different usage.

**Practice Problems**

1. ***Explain in words what the following relationships mean:***
   a. $A = 2C$ b. $C = A/D$ c. $Y = 2\,(X) + 1$
2. ***In a "short circuit" the resistance in the circuit suddenly decreases dramatically while the voltage remains the same. What must then happen to the current in the circuit?***
3. ***In the equation V= IR, the units of current must be expressed in amps (A), the units of voltage must be expressed in volts (V), and the units of resistance must be expressed in ohms (Ω). If the current in a circuit is 10 A and the voltage is 120 V, what is the resistance?***
4. ***A milliamp (mA) is one thousandth of an amp; a millivolt (mV) is one thousandth of a volt. If the current in a circuit is 100 mA and the resistance is 10 Ω, what is the voltage?***
5. ***Rewrite the equation that relates temperature in degrees F and degrees C (Section 5.1) so that it begins:***
   °C = ____________________
6. ***If the temperature in a room is 72°F, what is the temperature in °C?***
7. ***Insert numbers into each equation in Problem 1 that will satisfy the equation. For example, if the equation is A = 2 C, then 710 = 2 (355) will satisfy the equation. (So will many other answers.)***
8. ***Solve the following equations, that is, find the value of X. Pay attention to the units, if present.***
   a. $3X = 15$ b. $X = 25(5 - 4)$
   c. $-X = 3X - 1\ mg$ d. $5X = 3X - 5\ mL + 34\ mL$
   e. $\frac{X}{2} = 25(3)\ cm^2$ f. $X = \frac{25\ mg}{mL}(4.0\ mL)\frac{3.0\ oz}{mg}$

9. ***Perform the following calculations.***
   a. ***23.4 pounds × 34.1 pounds = ?*** b. ***15.2 g/3.1 g = ?***
   c. $\dfrac{\textit{25.2 cm} \times \textit{34.5 cm}}{\textit{3.00}} = ?$
10. ***Ruconest® is a biopharmaceutical drug that is manufactured in the milk of transgenic rabbits. It is used to treat a hereditary disease that can lead to dangerous and sometimes painful swelling. The following equation is used to determine the proper dose of this drug:***

$$\text{Volume to be administered} = \frac{\text{body weight (in kg)} \times 50\left(\dfrac{\text{Units}}{\text{kg}}\right)}{150\left(\dfrac{\text{Units}}{\text{mL}}\right)}$$

***The word "Units" is how the activity of the drug is expressed. You can consider "Units" to be like other measurement units, such as cm or g.***

***What is the proper dose for a person who weighs 68 kg?***

## *Answers*

1. a. A is equal to the value obtained if C is doubled.
   b. C is equal to the value obtained if A is divided by D.
   c. Y is equal to the value obtained if X is multiplied by 2 and then 1 is added.
2. The current goes up. (In fact, the current can become dangerously high in this situation.)
3. 120 V = 10 A (?) R = **12 ohms**
4. ? = 0.100 A (10 Ω) ? = **1 Volt**
5. °C = 5/9 (°F − 32)
6. °C = 5/9 (72 − 32) ≈ **22**
7. a. A = 2C **4 = 2(2)**
   b. $C = \dfrac{A}{D}$ $\mathbf{12 = \dfrac{36}{3}}$ c. Y = 2(x) + 1 **15 = 2(7) + 1**
8. a. 3X = 15 $X = \dfrac{15}{3} = \mathbf{5}$ b. X = 25(5 − 4) X = 25(1) = **25**
   c. −X = 3X − 1 mg 1 mg = 4X $X = \mathbf{\dfrac{1}{4}\ mg}$
   d. 5X = 3X − 5 mL + 34 mL 2X = (34 − 5) mL 2X = 29 mL
   X = **14.5 mL**
   e. $\dfrac{X}{2} = 25(3)\ \text{cm}^2$
   $\dfrac{X}{2} = 75\ \text{cm}^2$ $X = 2(75)\ \text{cm}^2$ $X = \mathbf{150\ cm^2}$
   f. $X = \dfrac{25\ \text{mg}}{\text{mL}}(4.0\ \text{mL})\dfrac{3.0\ \text{oz}}{\text{mg}}$
   $= \dfrac{300\ \cancel{\text{mg}}\ \cancel{\text{mL}}\ \text{oz}}{\cancel{\text{mg}}\ \cancel{\text{mL}}} = 300\ \text{oz}$ X = **300 oz**
9. a. ≈ $\mathbf{798\ lb^2}$ b. $\dfrac{15.2\ \cancel{\text{g}}}{3.1\ \cancel{\text{g}}} \approx \mathbf{4.9}$ c. $\dfrac{25.2\ \text{cm} \times 34.5\ \text{cm}}{3.00} \approx \mathbf{290\ cm^2}$

10. Plugging into the equation:

$$\text{Volume to be administered} = \frac{68\text{ kg} \times 50\left(\frac{\text{Units}}{\text{kg}}\right)}{150\left(\frac{\text{Units}}{\text{mL}}\right)}$$

The units of kg cancel, as do the "Units."

$$\text{Volume to be administered} = \frac{68\ \cancel{\text{kg}} \times 50\left(\frac{\cancel{\text{Units}}}{\cancel{\text{kg}}}\right)}{150\left(\frac{\cancel{\text{Units}}}{\text{mL}}\right)}$$

The equation becomes:

$$\text{Volume to be administered} = \frac{68 \times 50}{150/\text{mL}}$$

We can divide 50 by 150 to obtain:

$$\text{Volume to be administered} = \frac{68}{3/\text{mL}} \approx \frac{22.67}{1/\text{mL}}$$

Observe that there is a fraction in the denominator. When this is the case, recall from algebra that we must multiply the numerator by the reciprocal of the denominator:

$$\text{Volume to be administered} \approx 22.67 \times \frac{\text{mL}}{1} \approx \mathbf{23\ mL}$$

## 5.3 WHY DO WE CARE ABOUT THIS?

This section explores the use of an equation that relates to centrifugation. Biologists often use centrifuges to separate materials such as cells, organelles, bacteria, and viruses from a mixture of some kind. **Centrifuges** *accomplish this separation by rapidly spinning the samples, thus creating a centrifugal force many times that of gravity.* A centrifuge, Figure 5.1, contains a central drive shaft that rotates during centrifugation. A **rotor** *sits on top of the drive shaft and holds tubes, bottles, or other sample containers.* As the drive shaft rotates, the sample containers spin rapidly, creating the force that facilitates the separation of particles.

To appreciate the nature of the force in a centrifuge, imagine that you tie a stone to the end of a string and whirl it rapidly in a circle above your head. You will feel a pull on your hand as the stone rotates; this pull is centrifugal force. *Whenever an object is forced to move in a circular path (as in a centrifuge),* **centrifugal force** is generated.

Now, consider what would happen if you whirled the stone faster – you would feel more pull. Similarly, the faster a sample is spun in a centrifuge, the more force is experienced by that sample. *The speed of rotation in a centrifuge is expressed as* **revolutions per minute (RPM)**.

In addition to the speed of rotation, there is another (somewhat less obvious) factor that affects how much centrifugal force is experienced by a sample in a centrifuge. If you whirl a stone tied to a long string, there will be more force on the stone than if you use a shorter string, Figure 5.2a. In a centrifuge, the further a particle is from the center of rotation, the more force the particle experiences, Figure 5.2b. *The distance from the center of rotation to the particle of interest is called the* **radius of rotation**. In a centrifuge, the radius of rotation varies depending on the particular equipment being used.

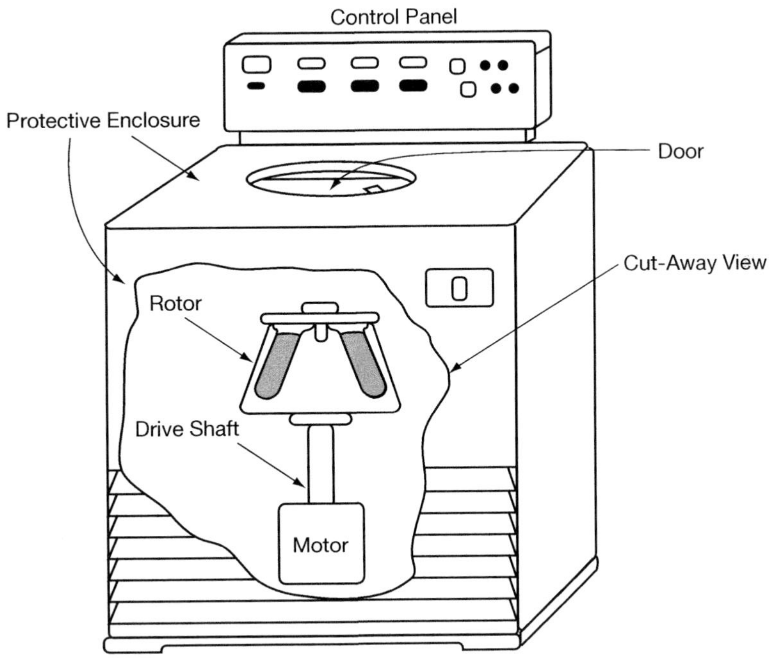


**FIGURE 5.1** A centrifuge. Tubes containing a sample are rapidly spun about a central shaft, creating a force many times that of gravity.

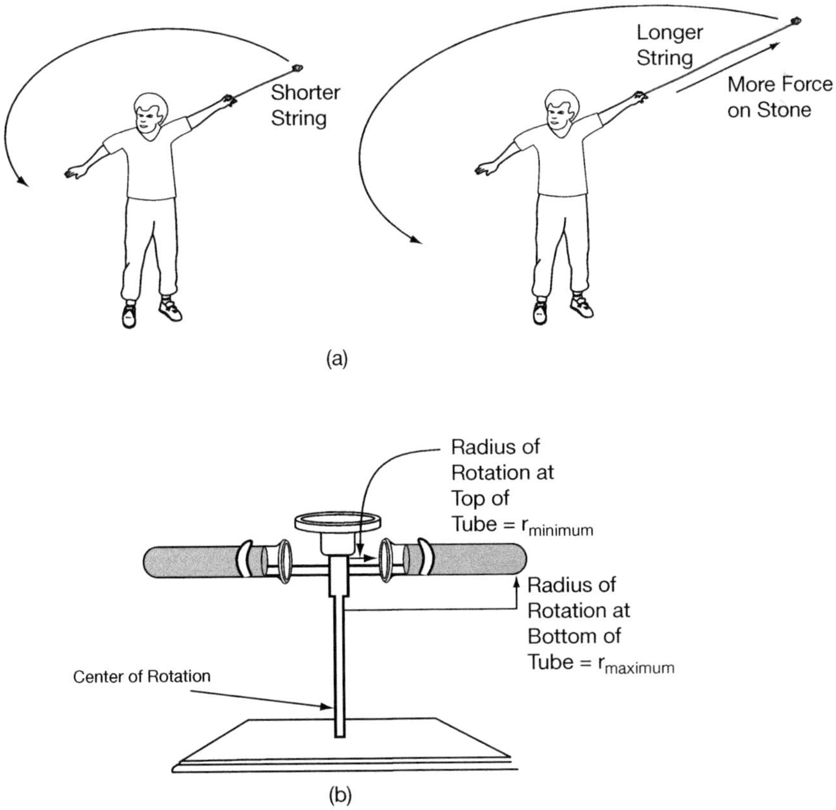


**FIGURE 5.2** The radius of rotation. (a) Assuming the same speed of rotation, the longer a string being whirled, the greater the radius of rotation and the more force that is experienced by the stone. (b) In a centrifuge, the further a particle is from the center of rotation, the more force it experiences.

*The name of the force acting on samples in a centrifuge is called the* **relative centrifugal field (RCF)**. The RCF has units that are multiples of the earth's gravitational field, g. Therefore, you may see the force in a centrifuge expressed as, for example, 10,000 × g or 10,000 RCF. Both these expressions mean that the force in the centrifuge is 10,000 times the normal force of gravity.

We have seen that there are two factors that determine the centrifugal force experienced by a particle in a centrifuge:

1. The speed of rotation, expressed as RPMs
2. The distance of the particle from the center of rotation, r

Here is an example of a situation where an equation can be used to express a relationship, in this case the relationship between the speed of rotation, the distance of the particle from the center of rotation, and the force on the particle generated by the centrifuge. The equation, Equation 5.1, is:

$$\mathbf{RCF = 11.2\,(r)\left(\frac{Speed}{1{,}000}\right)^2} \tag{5.1}$$

where:

RCF is the relative centrifugal field in units of ×g
Speed is the speed of rotation in units of RPM
r is the radius of rotation in units of centimeters

In this equation, the constant, 11.2, was derived in such a way that the units of "cm" (in the radius of rotation) "drop out." If the units of the radius of rotation were to be expressed in other units (for example, inches), then a different constant must be used. Similarly, the rotation rate (speed) must be expressed with units of "revolutions per minute," not, for example, "revolutions per second." This is generally true of constants in equations; they are dependent on using the correct units.

Observe that two centrifuges may be spinning at the same speed, yet they might each be subjecting their samples to a different centrifugal force. This will occur if the radius of rotation is different in the two centrifuges because of differences in their design. Because there are many styles of centrifuge, it is more useful to report to others the RCF rather than simply the speed of rotation.

Also observe in Figures 5.2b and 5.3 that the radius of rotation, r, for a particle varies depending on the particle's location in the tube. A particle at the top of the tube, closest to the center of rotation, is at the point where the radius of rotation is shortest, $r_{min}$.

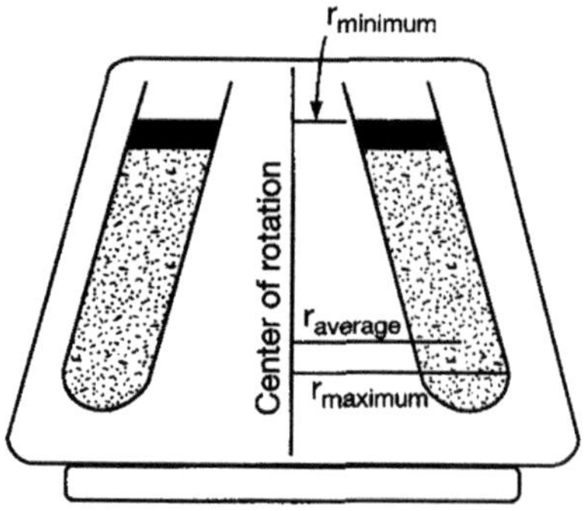


**FIGURE 5.3** Radius of rotation can vary depending on the position of a particle in a centrifuge tube.

At the bottom of the tube the radius is greatest and is called $r_{max}$ (maximum radius). There is also an average radius called $r_{ave}$. Therefore, particles at the bottom of a centrifuge tube (in most types of rotor) experience a higher g force than particles at the top of the tube. When calculating the g force experienced by a particle, it is necessary to consider its position in the tube. If the position is not known, use the average radius. The values for $r_{min}$, $r_{max}$, and $r_{ave}$ are provided by the rotor manufacturer.

**Example Problem:**

Your centrifuge equipment has a maximum radius of rotation of 9.2 cm. If you spin a sample at a speed of 15,000 RPMs, what is the maximum RCF?

***Answer:***

Substituting into Equation 5.1 gives:

$$RCF = 11.2(r)\left(\frac{speed}{1000}\right)^2$$

$$RCF = 11.2(9.2)\left(\frac{15,000}{1000}\right)^2$$

$$RCF = 11.2(9.2)(225)$$

$$RCF = \textbf{23,184 times the force of gravity}$$

**Example Problem:**

A colleague tells you that a sample was centrifuged for a certain length of time at a speed of 15,000 RPM and that the force of centrifugation was 16,000 times g. Your centrifuge equipment has a radius of rotation of 9.2 cm. What speed will you need to use to achieve a force of 16,000 times g?

***Answer:***

The unknown in this case is the speed of rotation. It is possible to algebraically rearrange Equation 5.1 to solve for speed as follows:

$$RCF = 11.2(r)\left(\frac{speed}{1,000}\right)^2$$

Divide both sides by 11.2 (r):

$$\frac{RCF}{11.2r} = \left(\frac{speed}{1,000}\right)^2$$

Take the square root of both sides:

$$\sqrt{\frac{\text{RCF}}{11.2\text{r}}} = \left(\frac{\text{speed}}{1{,}000}\right)$$

Multiply both sides by 1,000 to get Equation 5.2:

$$\mathbf{1{,}000\sqrt{\frac{RCF}{11.2r}} = speed} \tag{5.2}$$

Then, substituting into Equation 5.2 gives:

$$1{,}000\sqrt{\frac{16{,}000}{11.2(9.2)}} = \text{speed}$$

$$\mathbf{\approx 12{,}461 = speed\ in\ RPM}$$

Thus, to achieve a force of 16,000 RCF, you will need to use a speed of 12,461 RPM. Observe that to obtain the same force the two centrifuges must be run at different speeds. It is generally the speed of rotation that you, the operator, control on a centrifuge. However, it is the force in the centrifuge that matters in achieving a desired separation. This is why you need to be able to convert between speed in RPMs, and force.

**Practice Problems**

1. ***Given this equation,*** $\text{RCF} = 11.2(\text{r})\left(\frac{\text{speed}}{1000}\right)^2$
   a. ***What happens to RCF if the speed of rotation decreases?***
   b. ***What happens to RCF if r is decreased?***
   c. ***There are two constants in this equation. What are they?***
2. ***A portion of a table from a manufacturer's rotor manual is shown below. Calculate the RCFs to fill in the blanks. Refer to the diagram to determine the values for*** $r_{max}$, $r_{min}$, ***and*** $r_{average}$.

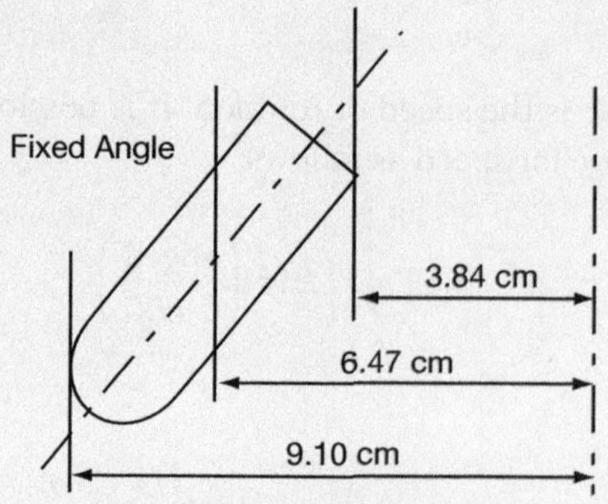


| Speed (in RPMs) | RCFs Generated $r_{max}$ | $r_{min}$ | $r_{average}$ |
|---|---|---|---|
| 20,000 | 40,800 | 17,200 | 29,000 |
| 30,000 | ____ | ____ | ____ |
| 40,000 | ____ | ____ | ____ |

3. ***The calculation shown below is incorrect. Why?***

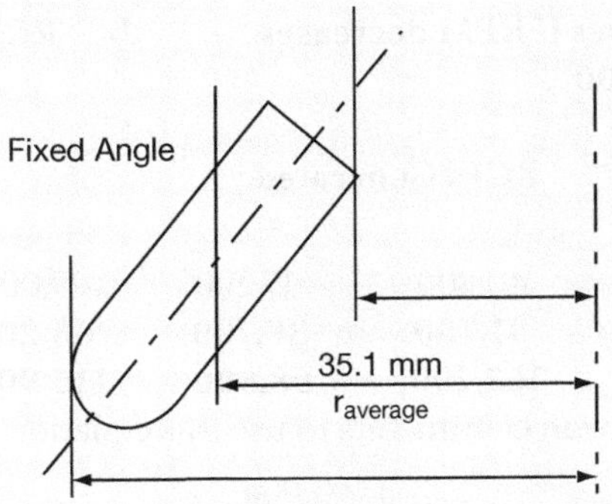


***Speed is 45,000 RPM***

$$RCF = 11.2(35.1)\left(\frac{45{,}000}{1{,}000}\right)^2$$

$$RCF = 796{,}068$$

***Incorrect answer!***

4. ***A journal article includes the statement below. If you have a fixed angle rotor with an $r_{ave}$ of 2.6 cm, how many RPMs will you need to use to duplicate the force used by these authors?***

   ***"The extract was centrifuged in a fixed angle rotor at 140,000 × g for three hours."***

5. ***Another equation from centrifugation is the following:***

$$v = \frac{d^2(\rho_p - \rho_m)RCF}{18\,\mu}$$

***where v = velocity of sedimentation***
***$\rho_p$ = density of the particle***
***d = the diameter of the particle***
***$\rho_m$ = density of the medium through which the particle is sedimenting.***
***RCF = the relative centrifugal force***
***$\mu$ = the viscosity of the medium***

***Although this equation may seem formidable because it has unfamiliar symbols, it is possible to obtain information from it fairly easily.***

a. ***What happens to the velocity of sedimentation as the viscosity of the medium increases?***
b. ***What happens to the velocity of sedimentation as the g force increases?***
c. ***What happens to the velocity of sedimentation when the particle and the medium are of the same density?***
d. ***What happens to the velocity of sedimentation when the particle is denser than the medium?***
e. ***What happens to the velocity of sedimentation when the particle is less dense than the medium?***

*Answers*

1. a. **RCF decreases if RPM decreases.** b. **RCF decreases if r decreases.**
   c. **11.2 and 1,000**
2. $r_{max} = 9.10$ cm $r_{min} = 3.84$ cm $r_{average} = 6.47$ cm

| Speed (in RPMs) | RCFs Generated $r_{max}$ | $r_{min}$ | $r_{average}$ |
|---|---|---|---|
| 20,000 | 40,800 | 17,200 | 29,000 |
| 30,000 | **91,700** | **38,700** | **65,200** |
| 40,000 | **163,100** | **68,800** | **115,900** |

3. The radius must be in centimeters to use this equation.
4. $1{,}000\sqrt{\dfrac{RCF}{11.2r}} = RPM \qquad 1{,}000\sqrt{\dfrac{140{,}000}{11.2(2.6)}}$

   $\approx$ **69, 338 RPM**
5. a. The viscosity of the medium is in the denominator – the more viscous the medium, the slower the velocity of sedimentation.
   b. The g force is in the numerator – the higher the g force, the faster the sedimentation velocity.
   c. When a particle and the medium are of the same density, $(\rho_p - \rho_m) = 0$ which means the velocity is zero – the particle does not move.
   d. If the particle is denser than the medium, the particle moves with a certain velocity toward the bottom of the tube.
   e. It is also possible for the particle to be less dense than the medium. In this case, the velocity is a negative number – that means the particle moves upward in the tube.

# II

# Applications of Proportional Relationships

**Chapters in This Unit**



DOI: 10.1201/9780429282744-7

## INTRODUCTION

This unit introduces one of the most powerful math tools used in a biotechnology setting. The good news is that you already know how to use this math tool and are probably adept at applying it in your daily life.

Suppose you are in a coffee shop. A latte costs \$3.00. You decide to buy a latte for yourself and your friend. How much will it cost for two lattes? Chances are you readily calculated that two lattes would cost \$6.00. Similarly, you would know that if another friend comes along and you buy three lattes, it will cost \$9.00.

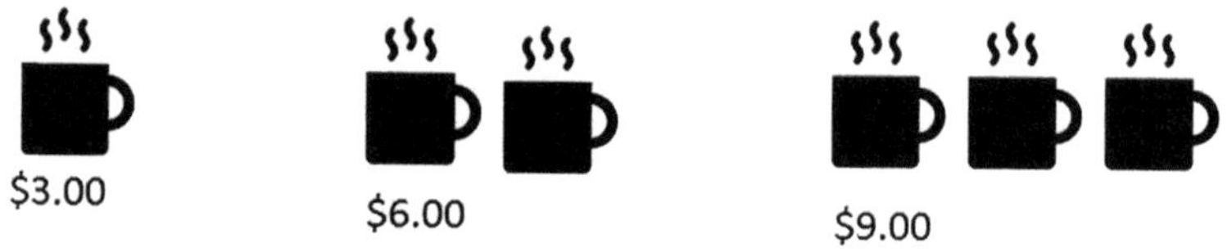


You just used a math tool called "ratios and proportions." We can rewrite this latte example in a way that looks a bit more like math:

$$\frac{\$3.00}{1\ \text{latte}} \qquad \frac{\$6.00}{2\ \text{latte}} \qquad \frac{\$9.00}{3\ \text{latte}}$$

Expressions like $\frac{\$3.00}{1\ \text{latte}}$ are called "ratios." This unit will introduce various ways in which ratios are encountered in a biotechnology setting. For example, we use ratios when converting between measurement units, such as between kilograms and pounds, or between microliters and milliliters. One of the most fundamental biotechnology laboratory tasks is preparing aqueous solutions with the right amounts of the proper components. Here again, ratios are involved. The following chapters explore these examples and other ways in which ratios are used to solve everyday problems in biotechnology.

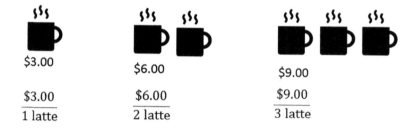

# Ratios and Proportions

# 6



## 6.1 RATIOS

***A ratio** is a comparison between two quantities using division.* For example, we might say that a car "gets 30 miles per gallon." This statement describes the relationship between gas consumption and miles traveled. The word "per" means "for every." Similarly, the preparation of a cake might require 10 oz of chocolate. The relationship between the cake and the amount of chocolate required is a ratio. Other commonplace examples of ratios are "revolutions per minute" (RPM) and "cost per pound." A ratio is expressed with a numerator and denominator, like a fraction. (However, a ratio is not a fraction. Fractions, for example, can be added together and ratios cannot.) Ratio examples:

$$\frac{30 \text{ miles}}{1 \text{ gallon}} \quad \text{or, it is also correct to say} \quad \frac{1 \text{ gallon}}{30 \text{ miles}}$$

$$\frac{1 \text{ cake}}{10 \text{ oz chocolate}} \quad \text{or} \quad \frac{10 \text{ oz chocolate}}{1 \text{ cake}}$$

**Example Problem:**

A laboratory solution contains 58.5 grams of NaCl per liter. Express this as a ratio.

***Answer:***

This relationship can be expressed either as:

$$\frac{58.5 \text{ g}}{1 \text{ L}} \quad \text{or} \quad \frac{1 \text{ L}}{58.5 \text{ g}}$$

DOI: 10.1201/9780429282744-8

**Practice Problems**

***Express each of the following as ratios in a fraction form. Be sure to have units in the numerator and denominator. For example:***

***A car is traveling 55 mph. Answer:*** $\frac{\text{55 miles}}{\text{1 hour}}$

***It would also be correct to say:*** $\frac{\text{1 hour}}{\text{55 miles}}$

a. ***A record is labeled "33 rpm."*** ___________
b. ***A laboratory centrifuge is spinning at 50,000 rpm.*** ___________
c. ***A cake requires 8 oz of chocolate.*** ___________
d. ***A jogger runs 3 miles in 38 minutes.*** ___________
e. ***45% of the class is female.*** ___________
f. ***The dosage for a drug is 38 mg for each kg of body weight.*** ___________
g. ***A person will die if exposed to ≥ 57 mg of mercury per kg of body weight.*** ___________
h. ***A laboratory solution requires 100 mg of NaCl for each liter of solution.*** ___________
i. ***The cost of a CD is $15.*** ___________
j. ***1 km = 1,000 m*** ___________
k. ***1 pound = 454 g*** ___________
l. ***1 mL = 1,000 μL*** ___________
m. ***A biotechnology production process can produce 3 g of product in each liter of culture.***

***Answers***

***(The reciprocals are also correct. For example, for problem a, you might say 33 revolutions/1 minute or 1 minute/33 revolutions.)***

a. ***33 revolutions/1 minute***
b. ***50,000 revolutions/1 minute***
c. ***8 oz of chocolate/1 cake***
d. ***3 miles/38 minutes***
e. ***45 females/100 students***
f. ***38 mg drug/1 kg body weight of patient***
g. ***57 mg of mercury/1 kg of body weight***
h. ***100 mg NaCl/1 L total solution***
i. ***$15/1 CD***
j. ***1 km/1,000 m***
k. ***1 pound/454 g***
l. ***1 mL /1,000 μL***
m. ***3 g/1 L***

One of the challenges in a professional setting is that calculations are often "camouflaged" by unfamiliar vocabulary and situations. It is therefore important to be able to "find" the math required in a situation. Ratios and proportions are very common, but sometimes they are not obvious. The Practice Problems below require that you "find" ratios within complex text. At this point, do not worry about understanding the text, just look for ratios.

**Example Problem:**

Underline or highlight any ratios you see in the following paragraph from the technical literature:

"The determination of the drug-to-antibody ratio (DAR) is typically performed using… chromatography. The eluents for this mild, nondenaturing analysis method contain high concentrations of corrosive salts, which challenge the liquid chromatography (LC) system. The number of free sulfhydryl groups limits the number of defined positions for the drug to be conjugated, resulting in a mixture of zero, two, four, six, and eight drugs per antibody..."

(Excerpted from: Schneider, Sonja. "Agilent Application Note: High Salt – High Reproducibility Analysis of antibody drug conjugates using hydrophobic interaction chromatography with the Agilent 1290 Infinity II Bio LC System.")

*Answer:*

The determination of the drug-to-antibody ratio (DAR) is typically performed using... chromatography. The eluents for this mild, nondenaturing analysis method contain high concentrations of corrosive salts, which challenge the liquid chromatography (LC) system. The number of free sulfhydryl groups limits the number of defined positions for the drug to be conjugated, resulting in a mixture of zero, two, four, six, and eight drugs per antibody...

**Practice Problems**

**Finding the Math**

Underline or highlight all the ratios in the following paragraphs or graphs.

1. The primary safety concern for DNA vaccines is their potential to integrate into the host cell genome. We describe an integration assay based on purification of high-molecular-weight genomic DNA away from free plasmid using gel electrophoresis, such that the genomic DNA can then be assayed for integrated plasmid using a sensitive PCR method. The assay sensitivity was approximately 1 plasmid copy/microg DNA (representing approximately 150,000 diploid cells). Using this assay, we carried out integration studies of three different plasmid DNA vaccines, containing either the influenza hemagglutinin, influenza matrix or HIV gag gene. Six weeks after intramuscular injection, free plasmid was detected in treated muscle at levels ranging from approximately 1,000 to 4,000 copies/microg DNA. At 6 months, the plasmid levels ranged between 200 and 800 copies/microg DNA. Gel purification of genomic DNA revealed that essentially all of the detectable plasmid in treated quadriceps was extrachromosomal....

   (Excerpted from: Ledwith, Brian J., et al. "Plasmid DNA Vaccines: Investigation of Integration into Host Cellular DNA Following Intramuscular Injection in Mice." *Intervirology*, vol. 43, nos. 4–6, 2000, pp. 258–72. doi:10.1159/000053993.)
2. A significant obstacle to the release of new medicines is the increasing complexity of drug molecules, which contributes to increased hydrophobicity and poorer water solubility. This is clear from the contrast between the solubility of drugs within the development pipeline and those that reach the market: 70–90% of pipeline drugs fall into the low solubility categories....

   The results of the study also demonstrated that a 20 mg/kg oral dose of nanoformed™ piroxicam possessed superior pharmacokinetic properties compared with piroxicam microparticles....

   (Excerpted from: Lakio, Satu. "Nanoparticle Engineering: Revolutionising Oral Drug Delivery – Whitepaper." *Pharmaceutical online*. 04 December 2020. nanoform.com/en/whitepaper-nanoparticle-engineering-revolutionising-oral-drug-delivery/)
3. Tempol protects mice from obesity and insulin resistance.

   Tempol is a member of a family of nitroxide compounds that promotes the metabolism of many reactive oxygen species. Although tempol was found to reduce body weight gain, the exact mechanism was unclear. Tempol treatment reduces body weight gain after 3 weeks of treatment with a HFD ... Body composition, measured by nuclear magnetic resonance (NMR), confirms that the fat mass, fat/body mass ratios and fat/lean mass ratios in tempol-treated mice are decreased significantly after 16 weeks of tempol treatment compared with vehicle-treated mice....

(Excerpted from: Li, Fei, et al. "Microbiome Remodelling Leads to Inhibition of Intestinal Farnesoid X Receptor Signalling and Decreased Obesity." *Nature Communications*, vol. 4, no. 1, 2013. doi:10.1038/ncomms3384.)

4. The NSF, a public health and safety organization, sets standards for water, food, and the environment. UV water disinfection systems that use 254 nm mercury lamps are classified as either Class "A" systems, for treating water that is assumed to be contaminated, or Class "B" systems, which provide only supplemental disinfection. As per the standards for this type of water disinfection, Class A systems need a UV dose of at least 40 $mJ/cm^2$ and Class B systems need a dose of at least 16 $mJ/cm^2$. Similar standards have not yet been established for disinfection systems that have upgraded to using 265 nm LEDs as the UV light source.

(Excerpted from: Crystal IS Application Note UVC LEDs for Disinfection. 30 August 2016.)

5.

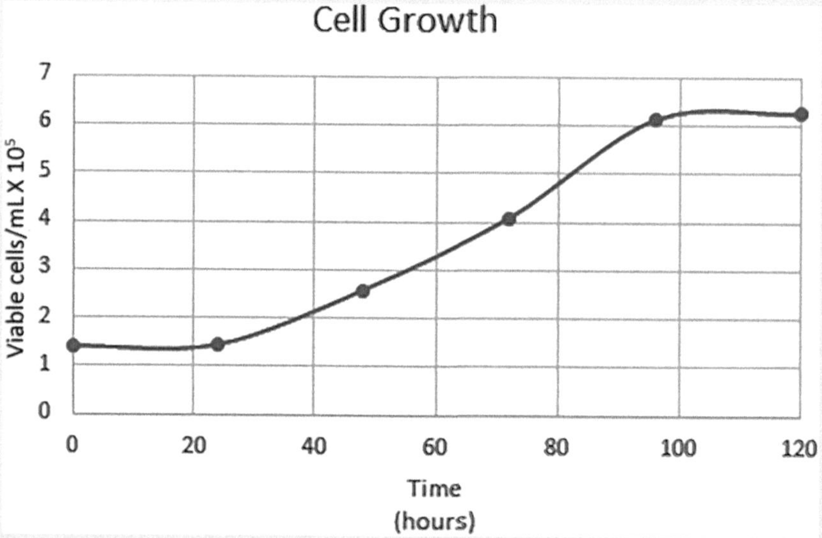


*Answers*

1. The primary safety concern for DNA vaccines is their potential to integrate into the host cell genome. We describe an integration assay based on purification of high-molecular-weight genomic DNA away from free plasmid using gel electrophoresis, such that the genomic DNA can then be assayed for integrated plasmid using a sensitive PCR method. The assay sensitivity was approximately 1 plasmid copy/microg DNA (representing approximately 150,000 diploid cells). Using this assay, we carried out integration studies of three different plasmid DNA vaccines, containing either the influenza hemagglutinin, influenza matrix or HIV gag gene. Six weeks after intramuscular injection, free plasmid was detected in treated muscle at levels ranging from approximately 1,000 to 4,000 copies/microg DNA. At 6 months, the plasmid levels ranged between 200 and 800 copies/microg DNA. Gel purification of genomic DNA revealed that essentially all of the detectable plasmid in treated quadriceps was extrachromosomal....
2. A significant obstacle to the release of new medicines is the increasing complexity of drug molecules, which contributes to increased hydrophobicity and poorer water

solubility. This is clear from the contrast between the solubility of drugs within the development pipeline and those that reach the market: 70–90% of pipeline drugs fall into the low solubility categories....

The results of the study also demonstrated that a 20 mg/kg oral dose of nanoformed™ piroxicam possessed superior pharmacokinetic properties compared with piroxicam microparticles....

3. Tempol protects mice from obesity and insulin resistance.

   Tempol is a member of a family of nitroxide compounds that promotes the metabolism of many reactive oxygen species. Although tempol was found to reduce body weight gain, the exact mechanism was unclear. Tempol treatment reduces body weight gain after 3 weeks of treatment with a HFD... Body composition, measured by nuclear magnetic resonance (NMR), confirms that the fat mass, fat/body mass ratios and fat/lean mass ratios in tempol-treated mice are decreased significantly after 16 weeks of tempol treatment compared with vehicle-treated mice....

4. The NSF, a public health and safety organization, sets standards for water, food, and the environment. UV water disinfection systems that use 254 nm mercury lamps are classified as either Class "A" systems, for treating water that is assumed to be contaminated, or Class "B" systems, which provide only supplemental disinfection. As per the standards for this type of water disinfection, Class A systems need a UV dose of at least 40 mJ/cm2 and Class B systems need a dose of at least 16 mJ/cm2. Similar standards have not yet been established for disinfection systems that have upgraded to using 265 nm LEDs as the UV light source.

5.

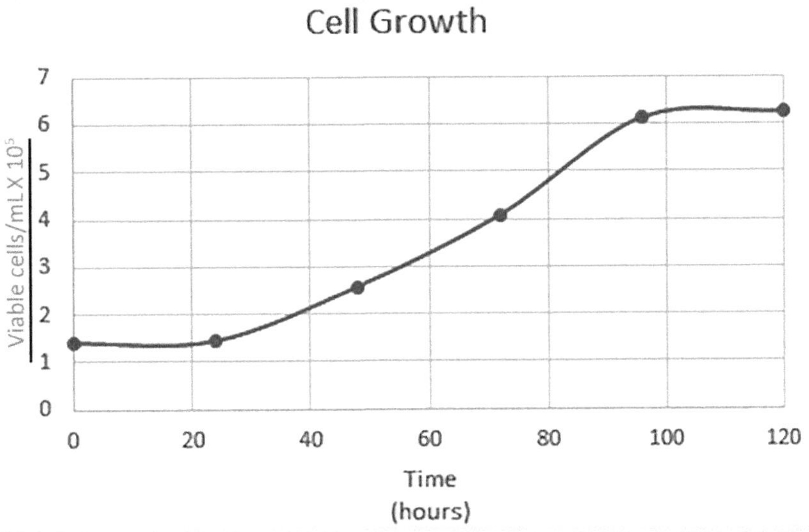


## 6.2 PROPORTIONS

*A* **proportion** *is a statement that two ratios are equivalent.* For example, suppose that baking a single cake requires 10 oz of chocolate. Then you know that 20 oz of chocolate are needed to bake two cakes, Figure 6.1. This can be expressed as a proportion equation:

$$\frac{1\text{ cake}}{10\text{ oz chocolate}} = \frac{2\text{ cakes}}{20\text{ oz chocolate}}$$

*Read as "1 cake is to 10 ounces of chocolate as 2 cakes is to 20 ounces of chocolate".*

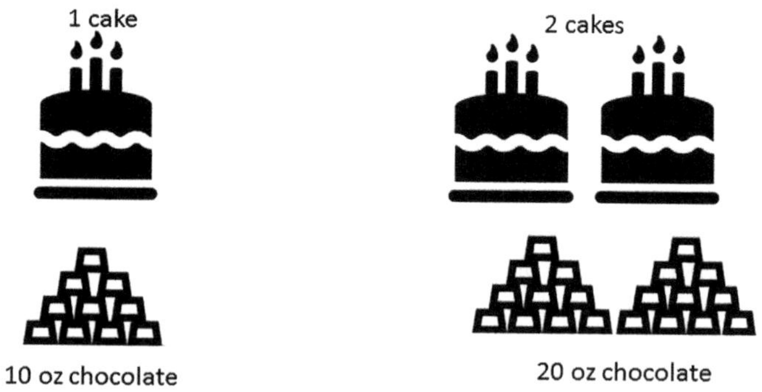


**FIGURE 6.1** The chocolate cake example.

A proportion statement is an equation because there is an = sign. Observe that numerically the two cake expressions have the same value, that is, $\frac{1}{10}$. Note also that it is important to include the units. So the relationship between cakes and required chocolate is $\frac{1 \text{ cake}}{10 \text{ oz chocolate}}$.

Many situations in the laboratory require the same reasoning as this "chocolate cake" example. For example, if 10 g of glucose is required to make 1 L of a nutrient solution, how many grams of glucose are needed to make 3 L of nutrient solution? Of course, 30 g is the answer.

Even if you are not a great baker, you probably "knew" that if 1 cake requires 10 oz of chocolate then 2 cakes require 20 oz. But suppose 16 oz of chocolate is needed for 3 cakes and you want to make 5 cakes. It may not be obvious in this case how much chocolate is necessary. It is possible to use an equation as a helpful tool to solve this problem:

**The Chocolate Cake Problem**

**Step 1.** The ratio "there are 16 oz of chocolate per 3 cakes" can be written as:

$$\frac{16 \text{ oz chocolate}}{3 \text{ cakes}}$$

**Step 2.** The unknown,?, is how much chocolate is required for 5 cakes.

**Step 3.** If 3 cakes require 16 oz of chocolate, then how many ounces of chocolate are required for 5 cakes? This proportional relationship is written:

$$\frac{16 \text{ oz chocolate}}{3 \text{ cakes}} = \frac{?}{5 \text{ cakes}}$$

Note that the units **must** be in the equation. The units in both numerators are the same and the units in both denominators are the same.

**Step 4.** To solve for the unknown, "cross multiply and divide."[1]

[1] Let us consider what the term "cross multiply" means. Recall from algebra that it is acceptable to multiply both sides of an equation by the same quantity. When "cross multiplying," *you are multiplying both sides of the equation by the product of the denominators.* In this case, that product is (3 cakes)(5 cakes). So, using this problem as an example:

$$\frac{16 \text{ oz chocolate}}{3 \text{ cakes}} = \frac{?}{5 \text{ cakes}}$$

Multiply both sides by the product of the denominators:

$$\frac{16 \text{ oz chocolate } \cancel{(3 \text{ cakes})}\ (5 \text{ cakes})}{\cancel{3 \text{ cakes}}} = \frac{?\ (3 \text{ cakes})\ \cancel{(5 \text{ cakes})}}{\cancel{5 \text{ cakes}}}$$

On the left, the 3 cakes cancel in the numerator and denominator, on the right the 5 cakes cancel:

$$\Rightarrow (16 \text{ oz chocolate})\ (5 \text{ cakes}) = (?)\ (3 \text{ cakes})$$

(Divide both sides by 3 cakes and continue with the rest of step 4.)

***Cross Multiply***

***Cross Multiply***

$$\frac{16 \text{ oz chocolate}}{3 \text{ cakes}} = \frac{?}{5 \text{ cakes}}$$

$$(16 \text{ oz chocolate})(5 \text{ cakes}) = (?)(3 \text{ cakes})$$

***Divide***

$$\frac{(16 \text{ oz chocolate})(5 \text{ cakes})}{3 \text{ cakes}} = ?$$

The units of "cake" cancel:

$$\frac{(16 \text{ oz chocolate})(5)}{3} = ?$$

Simplifying further and rounding the answer:

$$? \approx 27 \text{ oz chocolate} = \text{how much chocolate 5 cakes require}$$

Thus,

$$\frac{16 \text{ oz chocolate}}{3 \text{ cakes}} \approx \frac{27 \text{ oz chocolate}}{5 \text{ cakes}}$$

The fractions 16/3 and 27/5 are about equal although there is a slight difference due to rounding.

Some important points about proportional relationships include:

1. There are many problems in the laboratory that can be easily solved using the same reasoning as the "chocolate cake" example, even though the units may be less familiar and the numbers may be more complex.
2. It is necessary to keep track of units! The units in the chocolate cake example are "ounces" (oz) and "cake" (or "cakes"). In a proportion equation, the units in both denominators must be the same and the units in both numerators must be the same. For example, if one cake requires 10 oz of chocolate, how much chocolate is needed for two cakes? The ***wrong*** way to set this up is:

$$\frac{1 \text{ cake}}{10 \text{ oz}} = \frac{?}{2 \text{ cakes}}$$

Cross multiply and divide: $? = 0.2 \text{ cakes}^2/\text{oz}$

Clearly, these units are absurd, and the answer is wrong[2].

It is, however, correct to either write:

$$\frac{1 \text{ cake}}{10 \text{ oz}} = \frac{2 \text{ cakes}}{?} \quad \text{or} \quad \frac{10 \text{ oz}}{1 \text{ cake}} = \frac{?}{2 \text{ cakes}}$$

[2] To be thorough, we will also point out that another *incorrect* way to set up this proportion equation is to say $\frac{1 \text{ cake}}{?} = \frac{2 \text{ cake}}{10 \text{ oz}}$. Solving this equation, ? = 5 oz. In this case, the units do not tell you that the answer is wrong, but if you think about it, you will realize that it cannot require less chocolate for two cakes than it does to make 1 cake.

**Example Problem:**

Suppose human stem cells are being cultured for use as a medical treatment. If there are about 10,000 stem cells in each mL of culture, about how many stem cells are in each liter of culture?

***Answer:***

This is a proportion problem. Remember that the units in such an expression must be the same in both denominators and the same in both numerators. In this case, we are given both units of mL and L. We must make sure these units match. One way to handle this is to convert the unit "L" into its equivalent in mL.

$$1\text{ L} = 1{,}000\text{ mL}$$

So the proportion equation is:

$$\frac{10{,}000\text{ cells}}{1\text{ mL}} = \frac{?}{1{,}000\text{ mL}}$$

Cross multiply and divide:

$$(10{,}000\text{ cells})\ (1{,}000\text{ mL}) = (1\text{ mL})(?)$$

$$? = \frac{10{,}000\text{ cells}\ (1{,}000\ \cancel{\text{mL}})}{1\ \cancel{\text{mL}}} = \mathbf{1 \times 10^7\ cells}$$

**Practice Problems**

1. ***Calculate the following unknowns:***

   a. $\frac{?}{5} = \frac{2}{10}$ b. $\frac{?}{mL} = \frac{10\ cm}{5\ mL}$ c. $\frac{0.5\ mg}{10\ mL} = \frac{30\ mg}{?}$

   d. $\frac{50}{?} = \frac{100}{100}$ e. $\frac{?}{30\ in^2} = \frac{15\ lb}{100\ in^2}$

   f. ***? is to 15, as 30 is to 90*** g. ***100 is to 10, as 50 is to ?***

2. ***In the following problems, first state the unknown, set up the proportion equation with the units, then solve for the unknown.***

   a. ***If it takes 50 minutes to drive to Denver, how long does it take to drive to Denver and back?***
   b. ***If it requires 1 teaspoon of baking soda to make one loaf of bread, how many teaspoons of baking soda are required for 33 loaves?***
   c. ***If it costs $1.50 to buy one magazine, how much do 100 magazines cost?***
   d. ***If a recipe requires 1/4 cup of margarine for one batch, how much margarine is required to make five batches?***
   e. ***If a recipe requires 1/8 teaspoon of baking powder to make one batch, how much baking powder is required to make a half batch?***
   f. ***If one bag of snack chips contains 3 oz, how many ounces are contained in 4.5 bags of chips?***
   g. ***A person earns $12.00/hour. How much does that person earn in an 8-hour day?***

3. a. ***Burger Doodle Restaurant sells 500 hamburgers/day. How many do they sell in 7 days?***
   b. ***Burger Doodle Restaurant buys their hamburgers in cases of 1,000 hamburgers. How many cases do they need to buy to last one week?***
4. ***Burger Doodle Restaurant sells 150 ice cream cones a day. Each cone has 2 oz of soft serve ice cream. How many ounces of soft serve does Burger Doodle use each day?***
5. ***Each tablet of the drug, prednisone, contains 15 mg. How many tablets are required if you need to administer 45 mg?***
6. ***There are 12 in in a foot. How many inches are there in 3 ft?***
7. ***There are 24 hours in a day. How many hours are there in a year? (Assume this is not a leap year and there are 365 days.)***
8. ***There are 1,000 m in a kilometer. How many meters are there in 3 kilometers?***
9. ***There are 1,000 μL in a mL. How many μL are there in 3 mL?***
10. ***Enzymes catalyze chemical reactions in biological systems. Enzymes are rated on the basis of how active they are or how quickly they can catalyze reactions. Every preparation of enzyme has a certain activity expressed in Units of Activity. Suppose you buy a vial of an enzyme called beta-galactosidase. The vial is labeled: 3 mg solid, 500 Units/mg. How many Units are present in the vial?***
11. ***A vial of the enzyme horseradish peroxidase is labeled: 5 mg solid, 2,500 Units/mg. How many units are present altogether in this vial?***
12. ***An order is placed for 0.500 grams of the antibiotic drug, amoxicillin. The tablets on hand are 250 mg each. How many tablets are needed?***
13. ***If there are about $1 \times 10^2$ blood cells in a $1.0 \times 10^{-2}$ mL sample, about how many blood cells would be in 1.0 mL of this blood?***
14. ***10 mL of buffer are needed to fill a particular size test tube. How many mL are required to fill 37 of these test tubes?***
15. ***If there are about $5 \times 10^1$ paramecia (a microscopic one-celled animal) in a 20 mL water sample, about how many paramecia would be in $10^5$ mL of this water?***
16. ***If there are about 315 insect larvae in $1.0 \times 10^{-1}$ kg of river sediment, about how many larvae would be in $5.0 \times 10^4$ grams of this sediment?***
17. ***A fermenter is a vat in which microorganisms are grown. Fermenters come in many sizes, ranging from those that hold 1 L of microorganisms in culture broth to some that contain thousands of liters. Large fermenters may be as tall as a two or three story building. The microorganisms inside the fermenter produce a product, such as an enzyme or a drug, that has commercial value. Suppose a certain fermenter holds 1,000 L of broth and there are about $1 \times 10^9$ bacteria in each mL of the broth. About how many bacteria are present in the entire fermenter?***
18. ***A particular enzyme breaks down proteins by removing one amino acid at a time from the proteins. The enzyme removes 60 amino acids per minute from a protein. If a protein is initially 1,000 amino acids long and the enzyme is added to it, how long will the protein chain be after 10 minutes?***
19. ***A clinical trial was performed in which bone marrow stem cells were administered to patients at three different dosages: $5 \times 10^6$ cells, $10 \times 10^6$ cells, and $15 \times 10^6$ cells. Assuming that the stem cells are present in culture at a density of $8 \times 10^5$ cells/mL, what volume of culture medium will provide:***
    a. ***$5 \times 10^6$ cells***
    b. ***$10 \times 10^6$ cells***
    c. ***$15 \times 10^6$ cells***

    ***Note that cell density is a ratio where the number of cells is in the numerator and the volume is in the denominator.***

*Answers*

1. a. $\frac{?}{5}=\frac{2}{10}$ $\quad ?=\frac{2\times 5}{10}=\mathbf{1}$

   b. $\frac{?}{1\,\text{mL}}=\frac{10\,\text{cm}}{5\,\text{mL}}$ $\quad ?=\frac{10\,\text{cm}\,(1\,\cancel{\text{mL}})}{5\,\cancel{\text{mL}}}=\frac{10\,\text{cm}}{5}=\mathbf{2\,cm}$

   c. $\frac{0.5\,\text{mg}}{10\,\text{mL}}=\frac{30\,\text{mg}}{?}$ $\quad ?=\frac{(30\,\cancel{\text{mg}})(10\,\text{mL})}{0.5\,\cancel{\text{mg}}}=\mathbf{600\,mL}$

   d. $\frac{50}{?}=\frac{100}{100}$ $\quad ?=\frac{(50)\,100}{100}=\mathbf{50}$

   e. $\frac{?}{30\,\text{in}^2}=\frac{15\,\text{lb}}{100\,\text{in}^2}$ $\quad ?=\frac{15\,\text{lb}\,(30\,\cancel{\text{in}^2})}{100\,\cancel{\text{in}^2}}=\mathbf{4.5\,lb}$

   f. ? is to 15 as 30 is to 90

   $\frac{?}{15}=\frac{30}{90}$ $\quad ?=\frac{30\,(15)}{90}=\mathbf{5}$

   g. 100 is to 10 as 50 is to ?

   $\frac{100}{10}=\frac{50}{?}$ $\quad ?=\frac{50\,(10)}{100}=\mathbf{5}$

2. a. ? = time to drive to Denver and back

   $\frac{?}{2\,\text{way}}=\frac{50\,\text{min}}{1\,\text{way}}$

   $?\,(1\,\cancel{\text{way}})=(50\,\text{min})\,(2\,\cancel{\text{way}})$ $\quad ?=\mathbf{100\,min}$

   b. ? = amount of baking soda for 33 loaves

   $\frac{1\,\text{tsp}}{1\,\text{loaf}}=\frac{?}{33\,\text{loaf}}$

   $?=\frac{1\,\text{tsp}\,(33\,\cancel{\text{loaf}})}{\cancel{\text{loaf}}}$ $\quad$ **? = 33 tsp of baking powder**

   c. ? = cost of 100 magazines

   $\frac{\$1.50}{1\,\text{magazine}}=\frac{?}{100\,\text{magazine}}$

   $?=\frac{\$1.50\,(100\,\cancel{\text{magazine}})}{\cancel{\text{magazine}}}$ $\quad ?=\mathbf{\$150.00}$

   d. ? = margarine for 5 batches

   $\frac{1/4\,\text{cup}}{1\,\text{batch}}=\frac{?}{5\,\text{batch}}$

   $?=\frac{1/4\,\text{cup}\,(5\,\cancel{\text{batch}})}{\cancel{\text{batch}}}$ $\quad ?=\mathbf{\frac{5}{4}\,cup=1\frac{1}{4}\,cup}$

e. ?=Baking powder for a half batch

$$\frac{1/8\ \text{tsp}}{1\ \text{batch}} = \frac{?}{1/2\ \text{batch}}$$

$$? = \frac{1/8\ \text{tsp}\ (1/2\ \cancel{\text{batch}})}{1\ \cancel{\text{batch}}} = (1/8\ \text{tsp})(1/2)$$ **? = 1/16 tsp of baking powder**

f. ?=oz in 4.5 bags of chips

$$\frac{1\ \text{bag}}{3\ \text{oz}} = \frac{4.5\ \text{bag}}{?}$$ **? = 13.5 oz**

g. ?=earnings in a day

$$\frac{1\ \text{hour}}{\$12.00} = \frac{8\ \text{hour}}{?}$$ **? = $96.00**

3. a. $\frac{500\ \text{hamburgers}}{1\ \text{day}} = \frac{?}{7\ \text{day}}$ **? = 3,500 hamburgers**

b. $\frac{1{,}000\ \text{hamburgers}}{1\ \text{case}} = \frac{3{,}500\ \text{hamburgers}}{?}$ **? = 3.5 cases, so would buy four cases**

4. $\frac{1\ \text{cone}}{2\ \text{oz}} = \frac{150\ \text{cones}}{?}$ **? = 300 oz soft serve ice cream**

5. $\frac{15\ \text{mg}}{1\ \text{tablet}} = \frac{45\ \text{mg}}{?}$ **? = 3 tablets**

6. $\frac{12\ \text{in}}{1\ \text{ft}} = \frac{?}{3\ \text{ft}}$ **? = 36 in**

7. $\frac{24\ \text{hour}}{1\ \text{day}} = \frac{?}{365\ \text{day}}$ **? = 8,760 hours**

8. $\frac{1{,}000\ \text{m}}{1\ \text{km}} = \frac{?}{3\ \text{km}}$ **? = 3,000 m**

9. $\frac{1{,}000\ \mu\text{L}}{1\ \text{mL}} = \frac{?}{3\ \text{mL}}$ **? = 3,000 μL**

10. $\frac{500\ \text{Units}}{1\ \text{mg}} = \frac{?}{3\ \text{mg}}$ **? = 1,500 Units**

11. $\frac{2{,}500\ \text{Units}}{1\ \text{mg}} = \frac{?}{5\ \text{mg}}$ **? = 12,500 Units**

12. $\frac{250\ \text{mg}}{1\ \text{tablet}} = \frac{500\ \text{mg}}{?}$ **? = 2 tablets**

13. $\frac{10^2\ \text{cell}}{10^{-2}\ \text{mL}} = \frac{?}{1\ \text{mL}}$ **$? = 10^4$ blood cells**

14. $\frac{10\ \text{mL}}{1\ \text{tube}} = \frac{?}{37\ \text{tube}}$ **? = 370 mL**

15. $\frac{5 \times 10^1\ \text{paramecia}}{20\ \text{mL}} = \frac{?}{10^5\ \text{mL}}$ **$? \approx 2.5 \times 10^5$ paramecia**

16. $5 \times 10^4\ \text{g} = 50\ \text{kg}$

$$\frac{315\ \text{larvae}}{1.0 \times 10^{-1}\ \text{kg}} = \frac{?}{5.0 \times 10^1\ \text{kg}}$$ **$? \approx 1.6 \times 10^5$ insect larvae**

17. $\frac{1\times10^9 \text{ bacteria}}{1 \text{ mL}} = \frac{?}{1000\times10^3 \text{ mL}}$ **$? \approx 1\times10^{15}$ bacteria**

18. $\frac{60 \text{ amino acids}}{1 \text{ min}} = \frac{?}{10 \text{ min}}$ $? = 600$ amino acids removed in 10 minutes

1,000 amino acids − 600 amino acids = **400 amino acids left after 10 minutes**

19. a. $\frac{8\times10^5 \text{cells}}{1 \text{ mL}} = \frac{5\times10^6 \text{cells}}{?}$ $?$ = **6.25 mL**

b. **12.5 mL**

c. **18.75 mL**

# Unit Conversions

# 7



## 7.1 OVERVIEW

A given quantity, amount, or length can be measured in different units. For example, a candy bar that costs $1.00 also costs 100 cents. A dollar is a larger unit of currency than a cent. Therefore, it takes many cents (100) to equal the value of a single dollar. Similarly, a snake that is 1 ft long is also 12 in long and it is also 30.48 cm long. A foot is a larger unit of length than an inch or a centimeter. It takes more than 30 cm to equal the length of a single foot.

It is often necessary to convert numbers that have units in the United States Customary System (USCS) to numbers with metric units, for example, from pounds to kilograms. It is also often necessary to convert from one USCS unit to another USCS unit (for example, from feet to inches) or from one metric unit to another metric unit (for example, from centimeters to meters). This chapter discusses such conversions.

Converting between units requires relatively simple math: multiplication and division. Nonetheless, it is not unusual for people to make mistakes in unit conversions, perhaps becoming confused as to which number to divide by which, or when to multiply and when to divide. Even seasoned professionals occasionally make mistakes with unit conversions. (See, for example, the example of the lost Mars robotic spacecraft in the Unit I Introduction.) This chapter will provide you with strategies that, if applied consistently, will prevent such errors. These strategies can be used to perform commonplace conversions, such as converting between grams and pounds. The same strategies will be essential in later chapters when we introduce molecular biology applications that involve less familiar units.

There are two common strategies for performing unit conversions. The first approach is to think of conversion problems in terms of proportions and to use proportion equations to solve them. The second approach has various names including: "unit canceling method", "dimensional analysis", and "factor labeling." In this text, we use the term "unit canceling" method because it aptly describes the strategy. Some people prefer to use proportions to perform conversions, others prefer the unit canceling method. Either strategy will yield the right answers if it is used correctly. As you become experienced with laboratory calculations, you are likely to become comfortable with both strategies.

DOI: 10.1201/9780429282744-9

## 7.2 PROPORTION METHOD OF UNIT CONVERSION

Let us illustrate the proportion approach with an example of a conversion from the USCS system to metric units:

**If a student weighs 150 pounds, how much does she weigh in kilograms?**

First, we need a **unit conversion factor** *that relates pounds and kilograms*. There are unit conversion factors in Table 3.3 for this purpose. We find in the table that:

$$\mathbf{1\ kg \approx 2.205\ lb}$$

Any unit conversion factor can be written as a ratio. In this case, the ratio is either:

$$\frac{\mathbf{1\ kg}}{\mathbf{2.205\ pounds}} \quad \text{or} \quad \frac{\mathbf{2.205\ pounds}}{\mathbf{1\ kg}}$$

Observe that this ratio is equal to 1 since 1 kilogram is the same as 2.205 pounds. *All* unit conversion factors are equal to 1.

A proportion equation can now be used to convert from pounds to kilograms:

$$\frac{\mathbf{2.205\ lb}}{\mathbf{1\ kg}} = \frac{\mathbf{150\ lb}}{\mathbf{?}}$$

Read this as: "If there are 2.205 pounds in a kilogram, then 150 pounds is how many kilograms?"

Solving for the unknown:

$$? \approx \mathbf{68.03\ kg = the\ student's\ weight\ in\ kg}$$

Examine the answer to see if it makes sense. A kilogram is a larger unit than a pound (just as a dollar is a larger unit than a cent). Therefore, when the student's weight is converted from pounds to kilograms, it should take fewer kilograms to describe the student's weight. Does this make sense to you?

The above problem illustrates how proportion equations can be used to solve unit conversion problems. If we break the process into steps, Box 7.1 shows how it is done:

**BOX 7.1 Proportion Method of Unit Conversions**

Step 1. Find a conversion factor that relates the units of interest to one another.

Step 2. Express the conversion factor as a ratio (fraction form).

Step 3. Express the problem to be solved as a ratio with an unknown.

Step 4. Using the two ratios, set up a proportion equation such that the units in both numerators are the same and the units in both denominators are the same.

Step 5. Solve for the unknown.

Step 6. Check that the answer makes sense.

Here is another example to illustrate these steps:

**Example Problem:**

If a student weighs 80.0 kg, how much does he weigh in pounds?

***Answer:***

Step 1. Find a unit conversion factor that relates the units of interest:

$$\mathbf{1\ kg \approx 2.205\ pounds}$$

Step 2. Express the unit conversion factor as a ratio:

$$\mathbf{\frac{1\ kg}{2.205\ pounds}}$$

Step 3. Express the problem as a ratio with an unknown:

$$\frac{\mathbf{80.0\ kg}}{?}$$

Step 4. Set up a proportion equation such that the units in both numerators are the same and the units in both denominators are the same:

$$\mathbf{\frac{1\ kg}{2.205\ pounds} = \frac{80.0\ kg}{?}}$$

*Read as: "if one kg equals 2.205 pounds, then 80.0 kg equals how many pounds?"*
Step 5. Solve for the unknown (be sure the units cancel to leave the answer in the correct units):

$$? = \frac{80.0\ \cancel{kg}\ (2.205\ pounds)}{1\ \cancel{kg}}$$

$$? \approx \mathbf{176\ pounds}$$

Step 6. The answer makes sense. A pound weighs less than a kilogram (as a cent is smaller than a dollar) so it takes more pounds than kilograms to equal the student's weight (as it requires more pennies than dollar bills to pay for an item).

Here are two WRONG ways to set up the proportion equation:

$$\frac{\cancel{1\ \text{kg}}}{?} = \frac{80.0\ \text{kg}}{\cancel{2.205\ \text{lb}}} \qquad \frac{\cancel{1\ \text{kg}}}{2.205\ \text{lb}} = \frac{?}{\cancel{80.0\ \text{kg}}}$$

This way did not begin with the conversion factor as a ratio on one side.

This way gives absurd units.

Always check that your answer makes sense!

**Example Problem:**

A student is 6.00 ft tall. How tall is she in cm? Use these unit conversion factors:
1 in = 2.54 cm, 1 ft = 12 in

*Answer:*

This is a proportion problem that, with the unit conversion factors given, needs to be solved in two parts.

**Part 1. Use a proportion expression to convert her height in feet to inches.**
Steps 1 and 2 are to find a unit conversion factor and express it as a ratio:

$$\frac{\textbf{1 ft}}{\textbf{12 in}}$$

Steps 3 and 4 are to express the problem as a ratio and to set up a proportion expression:

$$\frac{\textbf{1 ft}}{\textbf{12 in}} = \frac{\textbf{6.00 ft}}{\textbf{?}}$$

*Read this as "if 1 foot is 12 inches, then 6 feet is how many inches?"*
Steps 5 and 6:

**? = 72.0 in = her height in inches** This makes sense.

**Part 2. Convert the height in inches to height in cm.**

Steps 1, 2, 3, and 4:

$$\frac{\textbf{1 in}}{\textbf{2.54 cm}} = \frac{\textbf{72.0 in}}{\textbf{?}}$$

*Read this as "if 1 in is 2.54 cm, then 72.0 in is how many cm"?*
Steps 5 and 6:

**? ≈ 183 cm = her height in cm**

Does this answer make sense? Yes, a centimeter is a smaller unit than a foot. Therefore, when the student's height is converted from feet to centimeters, the number will have to be larger; it will require more centimeters than feet to describe her height.

Proportions can also be used to convert from one metric unit to another:

**Example Problem:**

How many meters are 345 cm?

***Answer:***

There are 100 cm in a meter. So:

$$\frac{\mathbf{1\ m}}{\mathbf{100\ cm}} = \frac{\mathbf{?}}{\mathbf{345\ cm}} \quad \mathbf{? = 3.45\ m}$$

This answer makes sense. A meter is a larger unit than a centimeter. Therefore, when centimeters are converted to meters, the value is a smaller number; it takes fewer meters to describe the same distance.

**Example Problem:**

Convert 105 cm to nm.

$$\left(1\,\text{m} = 10^2\ \text{cm, and } 1\,\text{m} = 10^9\ \text{nm}\right)$$

***Answer:***

With the given unit conversion factors, this problem can be solved using two parts:

**Part 1.** $\frac{\mathbf{1\ m}}{\mathbf{10^2\ cm}} = \frac{\mathbf{?}}{\mathbf{105\ cm}} \quad \mathbf{? = 1.05\ m}$

**Part 2.** $\frac{\mathbf{1\ m}}{\mathbf{10^9\ nm}} = \frac{\mathbf{1.05\ m}}{\mathbf{?}} \quad \mathbf{? = 1.05 \times 10^9\ nm}$

This answer is reasonable. An nm is a very small unit of length. Therefore, it will take many nanometers to equal a length of 105 cm. The large answer obtained, $1.05 \times 10^9$ nm, makes sense.

## 7.3 UNIT CANCELING METHOD OF UNIT CONVERSION

The unit canceling method is a second strategy for doing conversion problems that can be thought of as a shortcut from the proportion method described above. In this method, the number to be converted is multiplied times the proper unit conversion factor(s). Multiplying the original number times one or more unit conversion factors does not change the *value* of the measurement because all unit conversion factors equal 1. Multiplying anything by one does not change its *value*. It does, however, change the *units*, which is the purpose of the procedure. The idea is to pick the unit conversion factor(s) that cancels out the units you do not want, leaving you with those you do want. (A proportion equation is not used in this strategy). Box 7.2 shows a stepwise overview of this strategy:

**BOX 7.2 Unit Canceling Method of Unit Conversions**

Step 1. Write the problem as an equation:

*Starting number with starting units = ending number with desired units*

Step 2. Find one or more unit conversion factors such that the units cancel, leaving only the desired units.

Step 3. Put the unit conversion factors(s), expressed as ratio(s), into the equation.

Step 4. Solve the equation.

Step 5. Check that the answer makes sense.

**Example Problem:**

Convert 2.80 kg to pounds.

*Answer:*

Step 1. Write the problem as an equation:

$$\mathbf{2.80\ kg = ?\,(expressed\ in\ pounds)}$$

Step 2. Find a unit conversion factor such that the units cancel. A pound is 0.454 kg. This unit conversion factor expressed as a ratio:

$$\frac{\mathbf{1\ lb}}{\mathbf{0.454\ kg}}$$

(Remember that all conversion factors = 1)

Step 3. Place the unit conversion factor into the equation:

$$\mathbf{2.80\ kg = 2.80\ \cancel{kg}\left(\frac{1\ lb}{0.454\ \cancel{kg}}\right) = ?}$$

Step 4. Solve the equation; multiply 2.80 kg by the unit conversion factor:

$$\mathbf{? \approx 6.17\ lb}$$

Step 5. Observe that the units of kilograms cancel, and the answer comes out with the correct units, pounds. If the units did not cancel, we would know the answer is incorrect.

Suppose you had another reference that told you not that 1 pound is 0.454 kg but rather that 1 kg is 2.205 pounds. If you use this factor directly, you will get the wrong answer:

$$\frac{\mathbf{2.80\ kg}}{\mathbf{1}}\left(\frac{\mathbf{1\ kg}}{\mathbf{2.205\ lb}}\right) \approx \mathbf{1.27\ kg^2/lb}$$

You can tell that this is the wrong answer because the units are wrong. But, if you "flip over" the unit conversion factor, the kg units cancel, resulting in the correct units at the end:

$$\frac{\mathbf{2.80\ \cancel{kg}}}{\mathbf{1}}\left(\frac{\mathbf{2.205\ lb}}{\mathbf{1\ \cancel{kg}}}\right) \approx \mathbf{6.17\ lb}$$

When using unit conversion factors, the units guide you in setting up equations. With the unit canceling method you can string together as many unit conversion factors as you want into one long equation. If the equation is correct, the units will cancel, leaving the answer in the desired units. The term "unit canceling method" is thus a good description for this strategy.

**Example Problem:**

A student is 6.00 ft tall. How tall is he in cm?

***Answer:***

Step 1. 6.00 ft =? (expressed in cm)

Step 2. Unit conversion factors are: $\frac{\mathbf{1\ in}}{\mathbf{2.54\ cm}}$ **and** $\frac{\mathbf{1\ ft}}{\mathbf{12\ in}}$

The inches will have to cancel, the feet will have to cancel, and centimeters must remain.

Steps 3 and 4. Let us try a couple of ways of setting this up:

$$6.00\ \text{ft}\left(\frac{1\ \text{ft}}{12\ \cancel{\text{in}}}\right)\left(\frac{1\ \cancel{\text{in}}}{2.54\ \text{cm}}\right) = ?$$

The units of feet do not cancel if the equation is set up this way and cm is in the denominator instead of the numerator. But, if the equation is set up differently, then the units of inches and feet cancel leaving the answer with units of centimeters:

$$6.00\ \cancel{\text{ft}}\left(\frac{12\ \cancel{\text{in}}}{1\ \cancel{\text{ft}}}\right)\left(\frac{2.54\ \text{cm}}{1\ \cancel{\text{in}}}\right) \approx \mathbf{183\ cm}$$

The answer is 183 cm, which is the same as the answer obtained previously using proportions.

Step 5. Remember to examine the answer to see that it makes sense.

Consider the conversion of metric units from one another.

**Example Problem:**

How many meters are 345 cm?

***Answer:***

Step 1. 345 cm =? (expressed in m)

Step 2. A unit conversion factor is: $\dfrac{1\text{ m}}{100\text{ cm}}$

Steps 3 and 4. $345\ \cancel{\text{cm}}\left(\dfrac{1\text{ m}}{100\ \cancel{\text{cm}}}\right) = \mathbf{3.45\ m}$

Step 5. The units of cm cancel, leaving the answer in the correct units. The answer makes sense.

**Example Problem:**

Convert 105 cm to nanometers.

***Answer:***

Step 1. 105 cm =? (expressed in nm)
Step 2. There are $10^9$ nm in 1 m and there are $10^2$ cm in 1 m. These are the unit conversion factors.
Steps 3 and 4. Then,

$$105\ \cancel{\text{cm}}\left(\frac{1\ \cancel{\text{m}}}{10^2\ \cancel{\text{cm}}}\right)\left(\frac{10^9\text{ nm}}{1\ \cancel{\text{m}}}\right) = ?$$

The cm and m cancel, leaving the answer in nm: **105 cm = $\mathbf{1.05 \times 10^9}$ nn**
Step 5. This answer makes sense.

## 7.4 COMPARING PROPORTIONS AND THE UNIT CANCELING METHODS OF UNIT CONVERSIONS

People sometimes think that either the proportion or the unit canceling method is superior to the other. In reality, both the proportion and the unit canceling strategies are equally effective ways to convert from one unit to another. Experienced laboratory workers often go back and forth between the two methods, selecting whichever seems best in a given situation. Both strategies require paying attention to the units. Observe that when using proportions to do conversion problems, there is always an equal (=) sign between two ratios. Also, when using proportions, the units must be the same in both denominators and the same in both numerators. In contrast, with the unit canceling method, there is not an equal sign between two ratios. There is multiplication between the number to be converted and the unit conversion factor(s).

The two methods are actually closely related to one another. Box 7.4 compares the two methods by solving the same problem with each side by side.

## BOX 7.4 A Comparison of the Proportion and Unit Canceling Methods of Unit Conversion

*A student weighs 130 pounds. How much is this weight in kg?*

**A unit conversion factor is:**

1 pound ≈ 0.454 kg

**Using the Proportion Method:**

Express the unit conversion factor as a ratio:

$$\frac{1 \text{ pound}}{0.454 \text{ kg}}$$

Set up a proportion expression:

$$\frac{1 \text{ pound}}{0.454 \text{ kg}} = \frac{130 \text{ pounds}}{?}$$

Cross multiply and divide:

1 pound (?) = 0.454 kg (130 pounds)

1 pound (?) = 59.02 kg (pounds)

$$? = \frac{59.02 \text{ kg (pounds)}}{1 \text{ pound}}$$

$$? = \frac{59.02 \text{ kg } \cancel{\text{(pounds)}}}{1 \cancel{\text{ pound}}}$$

$? \approx 59.0$ kg

This is the answer.

**A unit conversion factor is:**

1 pound ≈ 0.454 kg

**Using the Unit Canceling Method:**

130 pounds =? (expressed in kg)

$$130 \text{ pounds}\left(\frac{0.454 \text{ kg}}{1 \text{ pound}}\right) = ?$$

$$\frac{59.02 \text{ pounds (kg)}}{1 \text{ pound}} = ?$$

$$\frac{59.02 \cancel{\text{ pounds}} \text{ (kg)}}{1 \cancel{\text{ pound}}} = ?$$

59.0 kg ≈ ?

*Look at the highlighted steps from the proportion method and the dimensional analysis method. They are the same because the two methods are closely related!*

**Example Problem:**

A student weighs 130 pounds. Calculate her weight in kg using these two unit conversion factors: There are 454 g in a pound. There are 1,000 g in a kg.

***Answer:***

By proportions you need two parts:

**Part 1: Convert her weight in pounds to her weight in grams:**

Steps 1, 2, 3, and 4.

$$\frac{1 \text{ pound}}{454 \text{ g}} = \frac{130 \text{ pounds}}{?}$$

Step 5.

$$1 \text{ pound } (?) = 454 \text{ g } (130 \text{ pounds})$$

$$? = \frac{59{,}020 \text{ g } \cancel{\text{(pounds)}}}{1 \cancel{\text{ pound}}}$$

$$? = 59{,}020 \text{ g}$$

**Part 2: Convert her weight in grams to her weight in kilograms:**

Steps 1, 2, 3, and 4.

$$\frac{59{,}020\text{ g}}{?} = \frac{1{,}000\text{ g}}{1\text{ kg}}$$

Step 5.

$$?\,(1000\ \cancel{\text{g}}) = 59{,}020\ \cancel{\text{g}}\ (1\text{ kg})$$

$$? = \frac{59{,}020\text{ kg}}{1{,}000}$$

$$\mathbf{? \approx 59.0\ kg}$$

The proportion method was slow because two steps are required. Unit canceling provides a shortcut with one longer equation; the units cancel leaving the answer in kg:

Steps 1, 2, and 3.

$$130\text{ pounds}\left(\frac{454\text{ g}}{\text{pound}}\right)\left(\frac{1\text{ kg}}{1{,}000\text{ g}}\right) = ?$$

Step 4.

$$130\ \cancel{\text{pounds}}\left(\frac{454\ \cancel{\text{g}}}{\cancel{\text{pounds}}}\right)\left(\frac{1\text{ kg}}{1{,}000\ \cancel{\text{g}}}\right) = ? \quad \mathbf{? \approx 59.0\ kg}$$

Proportions and the unit canceling method both work. So if dimensional analysis is faster, why use proportions? The biggest problem with the unit canceling method is that people sometimes make errors as they try to cancel units without thinking about whether their string of unit conversion factors makes sense. With more complex problems (such as those you will see in Chapter 22), you may find that slowing down and using sequential proportions is more reliable. Also, the concept of proportions is extremely powerful. Proportions can help you understand calculations with percents, density, dosages of drugs, concentration of solutes in solutions, and other important laboratory applications. Another reason to use proportions is that most people have an intuitive understanding of proportions. Recall the latte example from the Unit Introduction for this chapter – we all use the logic of ratios and proportions in our daily lives. Finally, it is always good to know two strategies to check your answers. Whichever method you use, keep track of the units!

**Practice Problems**

1. ***Convert:***
   a. ***3.00 ft to cm***
   b. ***100 mg to g***
   c. ***12.0 in to miles (use scientific notation for your answer)***
   d. ***100 in to km***
   e. ***10.0555 pounds to oz***
   f. ***18.989 pounds to g***
   g. ***13 miles to km***
   h. ***150 mL to L***
   i. ***56.7009 cm to nm***
   j. ***500 nm to μm***
   k. ***10.0 nm to in***

2. ***How far is a 10-km race in miles?***

3. ***A marathon is 26.2 miles. Express this in km.***

4. ***How tall is a person who is 5 ft 4 in in meters?***

5. ***In kilometers, how far is a town that is 45 miles away?***

6. *A car is going 55 mph. How fast is it moving in km per hour?*

7. *How much does a 3.0 ton elephant weigh in the metric system?*

8. *Which jar of hot fudge is the best value?*
   a. *\$2.50 for 12 oz* b. *\$3.67 for 250 g* c. *\$4.50 for 0.300 kg*
   d. *\$2.35 for 0.75 pounds*

***Relationships (unit conversion factors)***

**52 weeks ≈ 1 year** **1 week = 7 days** **1 day = 24 hours**
**1 hour = 60 minutes** **1 minute = 60 seconds**

***Fill in the Blanks***

9. *1 week = _______ days = _______ hours = _______ minutes = _______ seconds*

10. _______ *year = 2 weeks = _______ hours = _______ minutes = _______ seconds*

11. *1 year = _______ weeks = _______ days = _______ minutes = _______ seconds*

***Relationships (unit conversion factors)***

**1,760 yd = 1 mi** **1 yd = 3 ft** **1 ft = 12 in**
**1 gal = 4 qt** **1 qt = 2 pt** **1 pt = 16 oz**
**1 km = 1,000 m = $10^3$ m** **1 m = 100 cm = $10^2$ cm** **1 cm = 10 mm**
**1 mm = 1,000 μm = $10^3$ μm** **1 μm = 1,000 nm = $10^3$ nm** **2.5 cm ≈ 1 in**

12. _______ *mi = _______ yd = 1 ft = _______ in*

13. _______ *gal = _______ pt = 2 oz*

14. *1 km = _______ m = _______ cm = _______ mm = _______ μm = _______ nm*

15. _______ *km = _______ m = _______ cm = _______ mm = _______ μm = 1 nm*

16. _______ *km = _______ m = 2.5 cm = _______ mm = _______ μm = _______ nm*

17. a. *6.25 mm = ___________ μm* b. *0.00896 m = _____________ mm*
    c. *9,876,000 nm = _______ mm*

18. _______ *km = 3.0 m = _______ cm = _______ in*

***Relationships (unit conversion factors)***

**1 g = $10^{-3}$ kg** **1 mg = $10^{-3}$ g** **1 μg = $10^{-3}$ mg**

19. *5 kg = _______ g = _______ mg = _______ μg*

20. _______ *kg = 0.0089 g = _________ mg = _______ μg*

21. _______ *kg = _______ g = _______ mg = 2 × $10^{-8}$ μg*

22. a. *0.8657 g = _______ mg* b. *526 kg = _______ mg*
    c. *63 g = _________ μg* d. *2.63 × $10^{-6}$ μg = _______ kg*

***Relationships (unit conversion factors)***

***(These units relate to the decay of radioactivity. Ci is a unit called a "Curie", named in honor of the physicists, Marie and Pierre Curie. A Becquerel is a unit named in honor of the physicist Antoine Henri Becquerel.)***

**1 Ci = $3.7 \times 10^{10}$ dps (disintegrations per second)** **1 Ci = 1000 mCi = $10^3$ mCi**

1 mCi = 1000 μCi = $10^3$ μCi **1 Bq (Becquerel) = 1 dps**

23. ***1 Ci =________ dps =________ dpm (disintegrations per minute)***

24. ***1 Ci =_______ mCi =_______ μCi =_______ dps***

25. _______ ***Ci =_______ mCi =_______ μCi = $10^5$ dps***

26. _______ ***Ci =_______ mCi = 100 μCi =_______ dps =_______ dpm***

27. ***1 Ci =_______ mCi =_______ μCi =_______ dps =_______ Bq***

28. _______ ***Ci =_______ mCi = 250 μCi =_______ dps =_______ Bq***

29. ***A physician orders 100 mcg of the drug levothyroxine (a synthetic form of thyroid hormone). The pharmacist mixes 0.1 mg levothyroxine. Is the dose correct?***

30. ***A physician orders 50 mcg of the drug Synthroid (a brand name for levothyroxine). The pharmacist mixes 0.5 mg Synthroid. Is the dose correct?***

## *Answers*

1. a. 3.00 ft to cm (proportion method):

$$\frac{?}{3.00\text{ ft}} = \frac{12\text{ in}}{1\text{ ft}} \qquad ? = \frac{(12\text{ in})(3.00\ \cancel{\text{ft}})}{1\ \cancel{\text{ft}}} \qquad ? = 36\text{ in}$$

$$\frac{?}{36\text{ in}} = \frac{2.54\text{ cm}}{1\text{ in}} \qquad ? = \frac{(2.54\text{ cm})(36\ \cancel{\text{in}})}{1\ \cancel{\text{in}}} \qquad ? \approx \mathbf{91.4\ cm}$$

3.00 ft to cm (unit canceling method):

$$3.00\ \cancel{\text{ft}}\left(\frac{12\ \cancel{\text{in}}}{\cancel{\text{ft}}}\right)\left(\frac{2.54\text{ cm}}{\cancel{\text{in}}}\right) \approx \mathbf{91.4\ cm}$$

b. 100 mg to g (proportion method):

$$\frac{?}{100\text{ mg}} = \frac{1\text{ g}}{1{,}000\text{ mg}} \qquad ? = \frac{(1\text{ g})(100\ \cancel{\text{mg}})}{1{,}000\ \cancel{\text{mg}}} = \mathbf{0.1\ g}$$

100 mg to g (unit canceling method)

$$100\ \cancel{\text{mg}}\left(\frac{1\text{ g}}{1{,}000\ \cancel{\text{mg}}}\right) = \mathbf{0.1\ g}$$

c. 12.0 in to miles (proportion method):

$$\frac{?}{12.0\text{ in}} = \frac{1\text{ ft}}{12.0\text{ in}} \qquad ? = \frac{(1\text{ ft})(12.0\ \cancel{\text{in}})}{12.0\ \cancel{\text{in}}} = 1\text{ ft}$$

$$\frac{?}{1\text{ ft}} = \frac{1\text{ mile}}{5280\text{ ft}} \qquad ? = \frac{(1\text{ mi})(1\ \cancel{\text{ft}})}{5280\ \cancel{\text{ft}}} = \frac{1\text{ mi}}{5280} \approx 0.000189\text{ mi}$$

$$? \approx \mathbf{1.89 \times 10^{-4}\ mile}$$

12.0 in to miles (unit canceling method)

$$12.0\ \cancel{\text{in}}\left(\frac{1\ \cancel{\text{ft}}}{12.0\ \cancel{\text{in}}}\right)\left(\frac{1\ \text{mile}}{5280\ \cancel{\text{ft}}}\right)\approx \mathbf{1.89\times10^{-4}\ mile}$$

d. 100 in to km (proportion method):

$$\frac{?}{100\ \text{in}}=\frac{2.54\ \text{cm}}{\text{in}}\quad ?=\frac{(2.54\ \text{cm})(100\ \cancel{\text{in}})}{1\ \cancel{\text{in}}}\quad ?=254\ \text{cm}$$

$$\frac{?}{254\ \text{cm}}=\frac{1\ \text{m}}{100\ \text{cm}}\quad ?=\frac{(254\ \cancel{\text{cm}})(1\ \text{m})}{100\ \cancel{\text{cm}}}\quad ?=2.54\ \text{m}$$

$$\frac{?}{2.54\ \text{m}}=\frac{1\ \text{km}}{1{,}000\ \text{m}}\quad ?=\frac{(2.54\ \cancel{\text{m}})(1\ \text{km})}{1{,}000\ \cancel{\text{m}}}\quad ?=\mathbf{2.54\times10^{-3}\ km}$$

100 in to km (unit canceling method):

$$100\ \cancel{\text{in}}\left(\frac{2.54\ \cancel{\text{cm}}}{\cancel{\text{in}}}\right)\left(\frac{1\ \cancel{\text{m}}}{100\ \cancel{\text{cm}}}\right)\left(\frac{1\ \text{km}}{1{,}000\ \cancel{\text{m}}}\right)=\mathbf{2.54\times10^{-3}\ km}$$

e. 10.0555 lbs to oz (proportion method):

$$\frac{?}{10.0555\ \text{lb}}=\frac{16\ \text{oz}}{1\ \text{lb}}\quad ?=\frac{(16\ \text{oz})(10.0555\ \cancel{\text{lbs}})}{1\ \cancel{\text{lb}}}\quad ?=\mathbf{160.888\ oz}$$

10.0555 lbs to oz (unit canceling method):

$$10.0555\ \cancel{\text{lb}}\left(\frac{16\ \text{oz}}{1\ \cancel{\text{lb}}}\right)=\mathbf{160.888\ oz}$$

f. 18.989 lbs to g (proportion method):

$$\frac{?}{18.989\ \text{lb}}=\frac{453.6\ \text{g}}{1\ \text{lb}}\quad ?=\frac{(18.989\ \cancel{\text{lb}})(453.6\ \text{g})}{1\ \cancel{\text{lb}}}\quad ?\approx\mathbf{8{,}613.4\ g}$$

18.989 lbs to g (unit canceling method):

$$18.989\ \cancel{\text{lb}}\left(\frac{453.6\ \text{g}}{1\ \cancel{\text{lb}}}\right)\approx\mathbf{8613.4\ g}$$

g. 13 mi to km (proportion method):

$$\frac{?}{13\ \text{mi}}=\frac{1.609\ \text{km}}{1\ \text{mi}}\quad ?=\frac{(1.609\ \text{km})(13\ \cancel{\text{mi}})}{\cancel{\text{mi}}}\quad ?\approx\mathbf{21\ km}$$

13 mi to km (unit canceling method):

$$13\ \cancel{\text{mi}}\left(\frac{1.609\ \text{km}}{1\ \cancel{\text{mi}}}\right)\approx\mathbf{21\ km}$$

h. 150 mL to L (proportion method):

$$\frac{?}{150\ \text{mL}}=\frac{1\ \text{L}}{1{,}000\ \text{mL}}\quad ?=\frac{(150\ \cancel{\text{mL}})(1\ \text{L})}{1{,}000\ \cancel{\text{mL}}}\quad ?=\mathbf{0.150\ L}$$

150 mL to L (unit canceling method):

$$150\ \cancel{mL}\left(\frac{1\ L}{1{,}000\ \cancel{mL}}\right) = \mathbf{0.150\ L}$$

i. 56.7009 cm to nm (proportion method):

$$\frac{?}{56.7009\ cm} = \frac{1\ m}{100\ cm} \quad ? = 0.567009\ m$$

$$\frac{?}{0.567009\ m} = \frac{10^9\ nm}{1\ m} \quad ? = \mathbf{5.67009 \times 10^8\ nm}$$

56.7009 cm to nm (unit canceling method):

$$56.7009\ \cancel{cm}\left(\frac{1\ \cancel{m}}{10^2\ \cancel{cm}}\right)\left(\frac{10^9\ nm}{1\ \cancel{m}}\right) = \mathbf{5.67009 \times 10^8\ nm}$$

j. 500 nm to μm (proportion method):

$$\frac{?}{500\ nm} = \frac{1\ \mu m}{1{,}000\ nm} \quad ? = \frac{(1\ \mu m)(500\ \cancel{nm})}{1000\ \cancel{nm}} \quad ? = \mathbf{0.500\ \mu m}$$

500 nm to μm (unit canceling method):

$$500\ \cancel{nm}\left(\frac{1\ \cancel{m}}{10^9\ \cancel{nm}}\right)\left(\frac{10^6\ \mu m}{1\ \cancel{m}}\right) = \mathbf{0.500\ \mu m}$$

k. 10.0 nm to in (proportion method):

$$\frac{?}{10.0\ nm} = \frac{1\ cm}{10^7\ nm} \quad ? = 1 \times 10^{-6}\ cm$$

$$\frac{?}{1 \times 10^{-6}\ cm} = \frac{1\ in}{2.54\ cm} \quad ? \approx \mathbf{3.94 \times 10^{-7}\ in}$$

10.0 nm to inches (unit canceling method):

$$10.0\ \cancel{nm}\left(\frac{1\ \cancel{m}}{10^9\ \cancel{nm}}\right)\left(\frac{100\ \cancel{cm}}{1\ \cancel{m}}\right)\left(\frac{1\ in}{2.54\ \cancel{cm}}\right) \approx \mathbf{3.94 \times 10^{-7}\ in}$$

2. 10 km to miles (proportion method):

$$\frac{?}{10\ km} = \frac{1\ mi}{1.609\ km} \quad ? = \frac{(1\ mi)(10\ \cancel{km})}{1.609\ \cancel{km}} \quad ? \approx \mathbf{6.2\ mi}$$

10 km to miles (unit canceling method):

$$10\ \cancel{km}\left(\frac{1\ mi}{1.609\ \cancel{km}}\right) \approx \mathbf{6.2\ mi}$$

3. $26.2\ \cancel{mi}\left(\frac{1.609\ km}{1\ \cancel{mi}}\right) \approx \mathbf{42.2\ km}$

4. 5 ft 4 in to meters (proportion method):

$$\frac{?}{5\ ft} = \frac{12\ in}{ft} \quad ? = \frac{(12\ in)(5\ \cancel{ft})}{\cancel{ft}} \quad ? = 60\ in,\ plus\ 4\ in = 64\ in$$

$$\frac{?}{64\text{ in}} = \frac{1\text{ m}}{39.37\text{ in}} \qquad ? = \frac{(1\text{ m})(64\ \cancel{\text{in}})}{39.37\ \cancel{\text{in}}} \qquad ? \approx \mathbf{1.6\ m}$$

5 ft 4 in to meters (unit canceling method):

$$5\ \cancel{\text{ft}}\left(\frac{12\text{ in}}{1\ \cancel{\text{ft}}}\right) = 60\text{ in} \quad 60\text{ in} + 4\text{ in} = 64\text{ in}$$

$$64\ \cancel{\text{in}}\left(\frac{1\text{ m}}{39.37\ \cancel{\text{in}}}\right) \approx \mathbf{1.6\ m}$$

5. 45 mi into km (proportion method):

$$\frac{?}{45} = \frac{1.609\text{ km}}{1\text{ mi}} \qquad ? = \frac{(1.609\text{ km})(45\ \cancel{\text{mi}})}{1\ \cancel{\text{mi}}} \qquad ? \approx \mathbf{72\ km}$$

45 mi into km (unit canceling method):

$$45\ \cancel{\text{mi}}\left(\frac{1\text{ km}}{0.6214\ \cancel{\text{mi}}}\right) \approx \mathbf{72\ km}$$

6. 55 mph to kph (proportion method):

1 mph = 1.609 kph

$$\frac{1\text{ mph}}{1.609\text{ kph}} = \frac{55\text{ mph}}{?} \qquad ? \approx \mathbf{88\ kph}$$

55 mph to kph (unit canceling method):

$$55\ \cancel{\text{mph}}\left(\frac{1\text{ kph}}{0.6214\ \cancel{\text{mph}}}\right) \approx \mathbf{89\ kph}$$

(The difference between methods is due to rounding of unit conversion factors)

Alternatively:

$$\frac{55\ \cancel{\text{mile}}}{1\text{ hour}}\left(\frac{1.609\text{ km}}{1\ \cancel{\text{mile}}}\right) \approx \frac{88\text{ km}}{1\text{ hour}} \approx \mathbf{88\ kph}$$

7. 3.0 ton to kg (proportion method):

$$\frac{?}{3.0\text{ ton}} = \frac{2{,}000\text{ lb}}{\text{ton}} \qquad ? = \frac{(2{,}000\text{ lb})(3.0\ \cancel{\text{ton}})}{\cancel{\text{ton}}} \qquad ? = 6{,}000\text{ lb}$$

$$\frac{?}{6000\text{ lb}} = \frac{1\text{ kg}}{2.205\text{ lb}} \qquad ? = \frac{(1\text{ kg})(6000\ \cancel{\text{lb}})}{2.205\ \cancel{\text{lb}}} \qquad ? = \mathbf{2{,}700\ kg}$$

3.0 ton to kg (unit canceling method):

$$3.0\ \cancel{\text{ton}}\left(\frac{2{,}000\ \cancel{\text{lb}}}{1\ \cancel{\text{ton}}}\right)\left(\frac{1\text{ kg}}{2.205\ \cancel{\text{lb}}}\right) \approx \mathbf{2{,}700\ kg}$$

8. a. $2.50 for 12 oz (proportion method):

$$\frac{?}{12\text{ oz}} = \frac{1\text{ lb}}{16\text{ oz}} \qquad ? = \frac{(1\text{ lb})(12\ \cancel{\text{oz}})}{16\ \cancel{\text{oz}}} \qquad ? = 0.75\text{ lb}$$

$$\frac{?}{0.75\text{ lb}} = \frac{453.6\text{ g}}{1\text{ lb}} \quad ? = \frac{(453.6\text{ g})(0.75\text{ }\cancel{\text{lb}})}{1\text{ }\cancel{\text{lb}}} \quad ? = 340.2\text{ g}$$

= 340.2 g/\$2.50 **136.1 g/\$1.00**

b. \$3.67 for 250 g (proportion method):

$$\frac{250\text{ g}}{\$3.67} \approx \mathbf{68.12\text{ g / \$1.00}}$$

c. \$4.50 for 0.300 kg:

$$\frac{?}{0.300\text{ kg}} = \frac{1000\text{ g}}{\text{kg}} \quad ? = \frac{(1000\text{ g})(0.300\text{ }\cancel{\text{kg}})}{\cancel{\text{kg}}} \quad ? = 300\text{ g}$$

$300\text{ g}/\$4.50 \approx \mathbf{66.7\text{ g}/\$1.00}$

d. \$2.35 for 0.75 lb:

$$\frac{?}{0.75\text{ lb}} = \frac{453.6\text{ g}}{\text{lb}} \quad ? = \frac{(453.6\text{ g})(0.75\text{ }\cancel{\text{lb}})}{\cancel{\text{lb}}} \quad ? = 340.2\text{ g}$$

$340.2\text{ g}/\$2.35 \approx \mathbf{144.8\text{ g}/\$1.00}$ = the most grams per dollar, is the best value

9. (proportion method)

$$\frac{?}{1\text{ week}} = \frac{7\text{ days}}{1\text{ week}} \quad ? = \mathbf{7\text{ days}}$$

$$\frac{?}{7\text{ days}} = \frac{24\text{ hours}}{1\text{ day}} \quad ? = 24 \times 7 = \mathbf{168\text{ hours}}$$

$$\frac{?}{168\text{ hours}} = \frac{60\text{ minutes}}{1\text{ hour}} \quad ? = 168 \times 60 = \mathbf{10,080\text{ minutes}}$$

$$\frac{?}{10,080\text{ minutes}} = \frac{60\text{ seconds}}{1\text{ minute}} \quad ? = 10,080 \times 60 = \mathbf{604,800\text{ seconds}}$$

(unit canceling method)

$$1\text{ }\cancel{\text{week}}\left(\frac{7\text{ days}}{1\text{ }\cancel{\text{week}}}\right) = \mathbf{7\text{ days}}$$

$$7\text{ }\cancel{\text{days}}\left(\frac{24\text{ hours}}{1\text{ }\cancel{\text{days}}}\right) = \mathbf{168\text{ hours}}$$

$$168\text{ }\cancel{\text{hours}}\left(\frac{60\text{ minutes}}{1\text{ }\cancel{\text{hours}}}\right) = \mathbf{10,080\text{ minutes}}$$

$$10,080\text{ }\cancel{\text{minutes}}\left(\frac{60\text{ seconds}}{\cancel{\text{minutes}}}\right) = \mathbf{604,800\text{ second}}$$

10. **2/52 years** = 2 weeks = **336 hours** = **20,160 minutes** = **1,209,600 seconds**

11. 1 year = **52 weeks** = **364 days** = **524,160 minutes** = **31,449,600 seconds**

12. **1/5,280 mi** = **1/3 yd** = 1 ft = **12 in**

or $\mathbf{0.000189\text{ mi}} \approx \mathbf{0.333\text{ yd}} \approx \mathbf{1\text{ ft}} = \mathbf{12\text{ in}}$

13. $\mathbf{0.015625\ gal} = \mathbf{0.125\ pt} = 2\ \mathrm{oz}$

14. $1\ \mathrm{km} = \mathbf{10^3\ m} = \mathbf{10^5\ cm} = \mathbf{10^6\ mm} = \mathbf{10^9\ \mu m} = \mathbf{10^{12}\ nm}$

15. $\mathbf{10^{-12}\ km} = \mathbf{10^{-9}\ m} = \mathbf{10^{-7}\ cm} = \mathbf{10^{-6}\ mm} = \mathbf{10^{-3}\ \mu m} = 1\ \mathrm{nm}$

16. $\mathbf{2.5 \times 10^{-5}\ km} = \mathbf{2.5 \times 10^{-2}\ m} = 2.5\ \mathrm{cm} = \mathbf{25\ mm} = \mathbf{2.5 \times 10^4\ \mu m} = \mathbf{2.5 \times 10^7\ nm}$

17. a. $6.25\ \mathrm{mm} = \mathbf{6.25 \times 10^3\ \mu m}$ b. $0.00896\ \mathrm{m} = \mathbf{8.96\ mm}$
    c. $9{,}876{,}000\ \mathrm{nm} = \mathbf{9.876\ mm}$

18. $\mathbf{3.0 \times 10^{-3}\ km} = 3.0\ \mathrm{m} = \mathbf{3.0 \times 10^2\ cm} \approx \mathbf{1.2 \times 10^2\ in}$

19. $5\ \mathrm{kg} = \mathbf{5 \times 10^3\ g} = \mathbf{5 \times 10^6\ mg} = \mathbf{5 \times 10^9\ \mu g}$

20. $\mathbf{8.9 \times 10^{-6}\ kg} = 8.9 \times 10^{-3}\ \mathrm{g} = \mathbf{8.9\ mg} = \mathbf{8.9 \times 10^3\ \mu g}$

21. $2 \times \mathbf{10^{-17}\ kg} = 2 \times \mathbf{10^{-14}\ g} = 2 \times \mathbf{10^{-11}\ mg} = 2 \times \mathbf{10^{-8}\ \mu g}$

22. a. $0.8657\ \mathrm{g} = 8.657 \times 10^{-1}\ \mathrm{g} = \mathbf{8.657 \times 10^2\ mg}$
    b. $526\ \mathrm{kg} = 5.26 \times 10^2\ \mathrm{kg} = \mathbf{5.26 \times 10^8\ mg}$
    c. $63\ \mathrm{g} = 6.3\ \mathrm{X}\ 10^1\ \mathrm{g} = \mathbf{6.3 \times 10^7\ \mu g}$
    d. $2.63 \times 10^{-6}\ \mu\mathrm{g} = \mathbf{2.63 \times 10^{-15}\ kg}$

23. $1\ \mathrm{Ci} = \mathbf{3.7 \times 10^{10}\ dps} = \mathbf{2.2 \times 10^{12}\ dpm}$

24. $1\ \mathrm{Ci} = \mathbf{1{,}000\ mCi} = \mathbf{10^6\ \mu Ci} = \mathbf{3.7 \times 10^{10}\ dps}$

25. $\mathbf{2.7 \times 10^{-6}\ Ci} = \mathbf{2.7 \times 10^{-3}\ mCi} = \mathbf{2.7\ \mu Ci} \approx 10^5\ \mathrm{dps}$

26. $\mathbf{1 \times 10^{-4}\ Ci} = \mathbf{0.1\ mCi} = 100\ \mu\mathrm{Ci} = \mathbf{3.7 \times 10^6\ dps} \approx \mathbf{2.2 \times 10^8\ dpm}$

27. $1\ \mathrm{Ci} = \mathbf{10^3\ mCi} = \mathbf{10^6\ \mu Ci} = 3.7\ \mathrm{X}\ \mathbf{10^{10}\ dps} = \mathbf{3.7 \times 10^{10}\ Bq}$

28. $\mathbf{2.5 \times 10^{-4}\ Ci} = \mathbf{2.5 \times 10^{-1}\ mCi} = 250\ \mu\mathrm{Ci} = \mathbf{9.25 \times 10^6\ dps} = \mathbf{9.25 \times 10^6\ Bq}$

29. 100 micrograms is the same as 0.1 mg, so the dose is correct.

30. No, because 50 mcg = 0.05 mg. The dose is ten times too high.

## 7.5 WORD PROBLEMS REQUIRING MULTIPLE STEPS

In the "real world" (outside of classes), the need to perform a math calculation always arises in a context or situation. For example, you might find yourself calculating interest rates, taxes, and repair bills when deciding whether to purchase a home. In the laboratory, you are likely to encounter calculations as you prepare the reagents to set up an experiment. In a biotechnology facility where a product is being produced, there may be nutritional media to prepare, or cells to count and culture. In the real world, math problems require first identifying the purpose of the calculation. For example, in the laboratory, the purpose of a calculation might be to determine how much of a particular compound must be weighed out. Once the purpose of a problem is understood, it is necessary to find the information required to solve it. For example, as we will see in Chapter 12, determining how much compound to weigh out in the laboratory often requires finding the formula weight of the compound.

"Word problems" in an educational setting are intended to model the real world, as much as possible. Word problems require that you extract the purpose of any required calculations from the words provided. Word problems also require that you find relevant information, either within the words of the problem itself or outside the word problem in tables or other resources. Unit conversion factors are an example of information that you frequently will need to find in a table, like Table 3.3 in this textbook, to perform the required calculations.

It is sometimes helpful to draw a quick sketch of a problem to collect the relevant information. It is often tempting to try and perform a calculation using one's calculator, without writing anything down on paper. This will likely work for simpler problems, but when a problem has multiple steps, using paper to keep track of where you are can help avoid confusion and mistakes.

Here are some examples of word problems with a biotechnology context.

**Example Problem:**

A transgenic animal is one that produces a protein or has a trait from another species as a result of incorporating a foreign gene(s) into its genome. In 1993, transgenic sheep were born that secrete a human protein, AAT (Alpha-1 Antitrypsin), into their milk. AAT is valuable in the treatment of emphysema. The concentration of AAT in the milk is 15 g/L. A sheep can produce 400 L of milk each year. AAT is worth $110/g. What is the value of a year's production of AAT from such transgenic sheep?

(Information from Amato, Ivan. "A Biotech Bonanza on the Hoof?" *Science*, 19 March 1993 vol. 259, p. 1698.)

*Answer:*

The question to be answered is: What is the value of a year's production of AAT from a transgenic sheep?

We are given three relationships in the form of ratios, as shown in Figure 7.1: This problem involves ratios, and we know that proportion equations can be used to solve such problems. With the relationships we are given, solving the problem by proportions requires more than one part.

**Part 1**:

First consider how much AAT a sheep can produce in a year. This is a proportional relationship: if the sheep secretes 15 g of AAT per liter of milk, how much will she secrete into 400 L? Using a proportion equation:

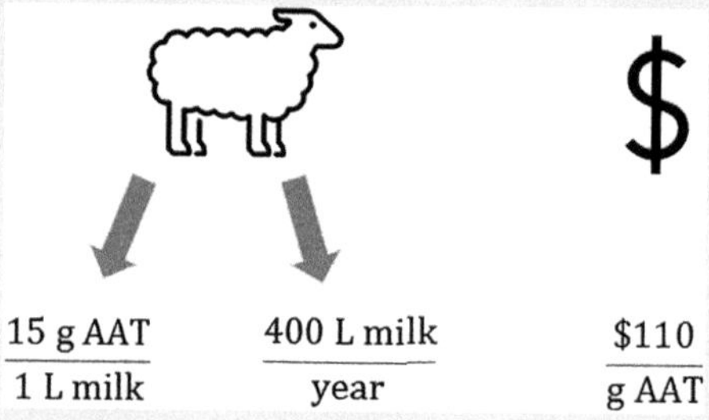


**FIGURE 7.1** Example problem sketch of sheep.

$$\frac{15\text{ g AAT}}{1\text{ L milk}} = \frac{?}{400\text{ L milk}}$$

$$? = \mathbf{6,000\ g}\text{ AAT}$$

This is the amount of AAT a single sheep might produce in a year.

**Part 2:**
Now that we know how much AAT a sheep can produce, it is straightforward to determine the value of this AAT. This is also a proportional relationship:

$$\frac{\$110}{\text{g AAT}} = \frac{?}{6000\text{ g AAT}}$$

$$? = \mathbf{\$660,000}$$

This is the answer to our question, what is the potential value of the AAT per year from one sheep?

For those who like the unit canceling method, here is the equation:

$$\frac{15\ \cancel{\text{g}}\ \cancel{\text{AAT}}}{1\ \cancel{\text{L milk}}}\left(\frac{400\ \cancel{\text{L milk}}}{1\text{ year}}\right)\left(\frac{\$110}{1\ \cancel{\text{g}}\ \cancel{\text{AAT}}}\right) = \frac{\mathbf{\$660,000}}{\mathbf{1\ year}}$$

**Example Problem:**

Phthalates are compounds that make plastics flexible and are used in many products including food wrap. Studies suggest that phthalates may activate receptors for estrogen, the primary female sex hormone. There is speculation that exposure to such estrogenic compounds may increase breast cancer incidence in women, reduce fertility in men, and adversely affect wildlife. One study suggested that margarine may pick up as much as 45 mg/kg of phthalates from plastic wrap. If you use 0.5 pound of margarine that has absorbed 45 mg/kg of phthalates to bake 3 dozen cookies, how much phthalate will three cookies contain?

***Answer:***

The question is: how much phthalate is in three cookies?

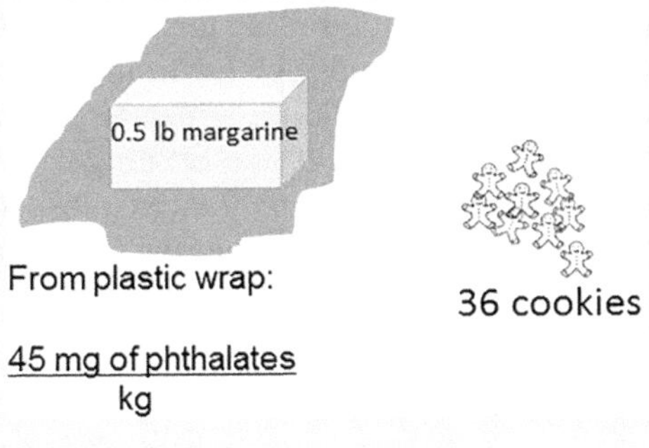


**FIGURE 7.2** Example problem sketch of phthalates.

**Part 1**:

Observe in the sketch in Figure 7.2 that the weight of the margarine is expressed in pounds but the ratio for phthalates is expressed in kg. The units must be consistent. Therefore, let us convert 0.5 lb of margarine to kg. This requires a unit conversion factor that is obtained from Table 3.3, 1 lb = 0.454 kg. Using proportions:

$$\frac{1\text{ lb}}{0.454\text{ kg}} = \frac{0.5\text{ lb}}{?} \quad ? = 0.227\text{ kg} = \text{weight of margarine in kg units}$$

**Part 2**:

Margarine can absorb 45 mg of phthalates per kg, so 0.227 kg of margarine can take up:

$$\frac{45\text{ mg}}{1\text{ kg}} = \frac{?}{0.227\text{ kg}}$$

$$? = 10.215\text{ mg} = \text{mg of phthalates that } 0.227\text{ kg of margarine can absorb}$$

This means that there are potentially **10.215 mg** of phthalates in 36 cookies.

**Part 3**:

To calculate the mg of phthalates in 3 cookies:

$$\frac{10.215\text{ mg}}{36\text{ cookies}} = \frac{?}{3\text{ cookies}} \quad ? \approx \mathbf{0.85\text{ mg} = \text{mg of phthalates in 3 cookies}}.$$

As you can see, this type of problem can be solved systematically with a series of proportional expressions.

**Example Problem:**

The pesticide DDT also has estrogenic effects. Although DDT is no longer used in the United States, it is still widely distributed worldwide. Humans have been shown to accumulate as much as 4.0 μg/g of body weight of DDT in their tissues. If a woman weighs 148 pounds, how much DDT might her body contain? (Let us simplify the situation by assuming that all tissues in her body accumulate the same maximum amount of DDT.) This is sketched in Figure 7.3.

*Information from*:

"Newest Estrogen Mimics the Commonest?" *Science News*, vol. 148, p. 47, 15 July 1995.

Raloff, Janet. "Beyond Estrogens: Why Unmasking Hormone-Mimicking Pollutants Proves So Challenging", *Science News*, vol. 148, 15 July 1995, pp. 44–46.

Guillette, L.J., Jr. "Endocrine-Disrupting Environmental Contaminant and Reproduction: Lessons from the Study of Wildlife." *Women's Health Today: Perspectives on Current Research and Clinical Practice*, 1994, pp. 201–207.

For a more recent review, see: Paumgartten, Francisco José Roma. "Commentary: 'Estrogenic and Anti-Androgenic Endocrine Disrupting Chemicals and Their Impact on the Male Reproductive System.'" *Frontiers in Public Health*, vol. 3, 2015. doi:10.3389/fpubh.2015.00165.

***Answer:***

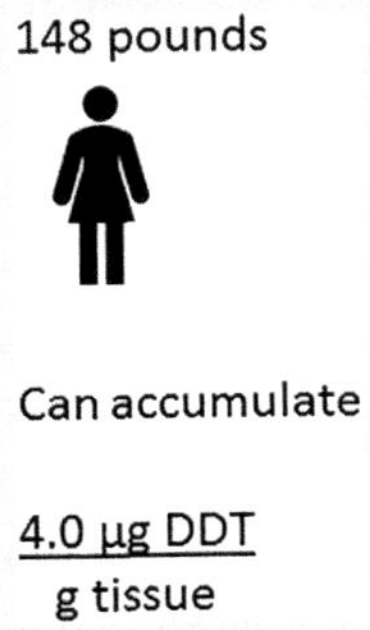


**FIGURE 7.3** Example problem sketch of DDT accumulation.

Let us use the unit canceling method. The question is: how much DDT might be present in the tissues of a woman who weighs 148 pounds?

We will string together ratios into one long equation. First, it is necessary to convert the woman's weight from pounds to grams. Then, a factor must be included to account for the fact that she accumulated 4.0 μg/g of DDT in all her tissues. Finally, it would be helpful to convert the answer from μg to grams. The resulting single equation is:

$$148\ \cancel{\text{lb}}\left(\frac{454\ \cancel{\text{g}}}{1\ \cancel{\text{lb}}}\right)\left(\frac{4.0\ \cancel{\mu\text{g}}}{\cancel{\text{g}}}\right)\left(\frac{1\ \text{g}}{10^6\ \cancel{\mu\text{g}}}\right) \approx \mathbf{0.269\ g = accumulated\ DDT}$$

Check the units and note that they cancel, leaving the answer in grams.

**Example Problem:**

Which is purer, a chemical that contains 0.025 g of contaminating material in $10^4$ g or a chemical that contains $10^2$ mg of contaminant in $10^2$ kg? Sketch this situation.

***Answer:***

A sketch is shown in Figure 7.4. The question is: which chemical is purer? Answering this requires converting the concentrations of contaminants in both chemicals into the same units so they can be compared more easily.

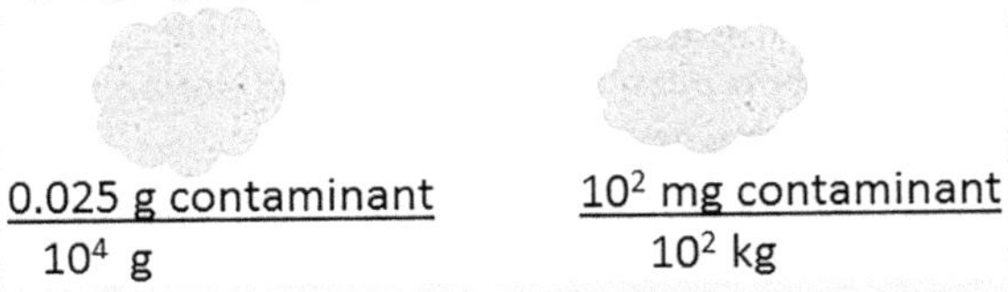


**FIGURE 7.4** Example problem sketch of contaminants.

Chemical 1: $\frac{0.025\text{ g of contaminant}}{10^4\text{ g}}$

Chemical 2: Convert $10^2$ mg to grams.

$$10^2\text{ mg} = 10^{-1}\text{ g}$$

Convert $10^2$ kg to g

$$10^2\text{ kg} = 10^5\text{ g}$$

Thus, chemical 2 has a contaminant concentration of

$$\frac{10^{-1}\text{g}}{10^5\text{ g}} = \frac{0.1\text{ g}}{10^5\text{ g}} = \frac{\mathbf{0.01\text{ g of contaminant}}}{\mathbf{10^4\text{ g}}}$$

When the purity of both chemicals is expressed in the same units, we can see that chemical 2 is purer because it has less contaminant per $10^4$ g than chemical 1.

**Practice Problems**

1. ***Body Mass Index (BMI) is a quick and inexpensive screening tool that is used to place people into a weight category – underweight, healthy weight, overweight, or obese. BMI should be interpreted cautiously because it does not exactly reflect a person's amount of body fat, but a high BMI does appear to be associated with various disorders, such as diabetes. A high BMI is also linked to a higher risk of severe disease if a person contracts COVID-19. BMI is calculated using Equation 7.1:***

$$\text{BMI} = \frac{\text{weight in kg}}{(\text{height in m})^2} \tag{7.1}$$

***Here is how BMI is interpreted.***

| ***BMI*** | ***Weight Status*** |
|---|---|
| ***Below 18.5*** | ***Underweight*** |
| ***18.5–24.9*** | ***Normal or Healthy Weight*** |
| ***25.0–29.9*** | ***Overweight*** |
| ***30.0 and Above*** | ***Obese*** |

   a. ***Calculate the BMI for a person who weighs 68 kg and is 165 cm tall. What weight status category is this person in?***
   b. ***What unit conversions are required for calculating a person's BMI if the person lives in the United States?***
   c. ***Calculate the BMI for a person who weighs 115 pounds and is 5 ft, 2 in tall. What weight status category is this person in?***
   d. ***Calculate the BMI for a person who weighs 193 pounds and is 6 ft, 1 in tall. What weight status category is this person in?***
   e. ***Calculate the BMI for a person who weighs 210 pounds and is 5 ft, 9 in tall. What weight status category is this person in?***

2. ***Bacteria are growing in a flask. The growth medium for the bacteria requires 5 g of glucose per liter. A technician has prepared some medium and added 0.24 pounds of glucose to 25 L. Did the technician make the broth correctly?***

3. ***A particular enzyme must be added to a nutrient solution (broth) used to grow bacteria. The enzyme comes as a freeze-dried powder. The manufacturer of the enzyme states that every gram of enzyme powder actually contains only***

*880 mg of enzyme, the rest is an inert filler that has no effect. If a recipe calls for 10 oz of this enzyme for every 100 L of broth and if you prepare 500 L of broth, how much of the enzyme powder will you need to add? Remember to compensate for the inert filler. Sketch this problem and then solve it.*

4. *Which is purer, a chemical that contains 1 gram of contaminating material in $10^6$ kg or a chemical that contains $10^{-2}$ mg of contaminant in $10^{-3}$ kg?*

5. *A prescription is placed for 0.25 g of amoxicillin three times a day. The tablets on hand are 250 mg. How many will be administered in 5 days?*

6. *It may come as a surprise to learn that all foods contain a small amount of naturally occurring radioactive material. This is because radioactivity has been present since the earth was formed and so minerals, rocks, and soil contain radioactive components, among them potassium 40, $^{40}K$. (Most of the potassium on earth is of a stable, non-radioactive form, but a small portion of naturally occurring potassium is radioactive.) Steak contains about 3,000 pCi/kg of $^{40}K$. If you eat four ounces of steak, about how many Bq of $^{40}K$ will you ingest? (Information from Idaho State University Radiation Information Network, www.physics.isu.edu/radinf/natural.htm.)*

   *1 kg = 1,000 g ≈ 35.27 oz    1 Ci = $3.7\times10^{10}$ dps (disintegrations per second)*
   *1 Bq (Becquerel) = 1 dps.*

8. ***Finding the math within unfamiliar terminology.***
   *You are a biotechnician operating a manufacturing process that makes antibodies to treat cancer patients. The antibodies are produced by cells that grow suspended in a nutrient medium inside of large vats that hold thousands of liters of cells. Your supervisor provides you with the following information from a scientific article:*

   *"A new process was developed for scale-up of an antibody that requires additional processing by a site-specific enzyme for correct functionality. Cell lines yielding high titers of highly processed antibodies were generated resulting in specific productivities of 50–75 pg/cell/day."*

   *Your supervisor would like you to calculate how much antibody could be produced in your facility using the new process described in the article. Suppose your vats each contain 2,000 L of suspended cells.*

   a. *There are $5\times10^6$ cells/mL in each vat. Using the new process, what is the maximum amount of antibody that one vat of your cells could produce in a production run that lasts 10 days? Express the answer in units of grams.*
   b. *How many grams does each liter of cells produce by the end of the production run?*

   *(These values are based on information from Bleck, G., et al., "Generating a Fully Processed Antibody." BioPharm Intl. August 2016. www.processdevelopmentforum.com/articles/generating-a-fully-processed-antibody/.)*

*Answer:*

1. a. $$\text{BMI} = \frac{68\text{ kg}}{(1.65\text{ m})^2} \approx 24.98$$

   This person is on the border between the healthy and overweight categories.

b. Because the United States does not customarily use the metric system, weight must be converted from pounds to kilograms and height from feet and inches to meters.

c. The person weighs 115 pounds and is 5 ft, 2 in tall. Calculating BMI requires unit conversions. There are various strategies that could be used. Here is one strategy:

First part: convert 115 pounds to kg.

$$\frac{115\text{ lb}}{?} = \frac{1\text{ lb}}{0.454\text{ kg}} \quad ? = 52.21\text{ kg}$$

Next: 5 ft 2 in needs to be converted to meters. One way to do this is to begin by converting height to inches:

$$1\text{ ft} = 12\text{ in}$$

Using a unit canceling strategy to convert 5 ft to in:

$$5\ \cancel{\text{foot}}\left(\frac{12\text{ in}}{\cancel{\text{foot}}}\right) = 60\text{ in}$$

Add the 2 in: = 62 in

Next: Convert 62 in to cm. From Table 3.3, 1 in = 2.54 cm

$$62\ \cancel{\text{in}}\left(\frac{2.54\text{ cm}}{\cancel{\text{in}}}\right) = 157.48\text{ cm}$$

$$157.48\text{ cm} = 1.5748\text{ m}$$

Next: Use the BMI equation:

$$\text{BMI} = \frac{52.21\text{ kg}}{(1.5748\text{ m})^2} \approx \mathbf{21.05}$$

This person is in the normal, healthy weight category.

d. The person weighs 193 pounds and is 6 ft, 1 in tall. What weight status category is this person in?

$$\text{Weight} = 87.622\text{ kg}$$

$$\text{Height} = 1.8542\text{ m}$$

$$\text{BMI} = \frac{87.622\text{ kg}}{(1.8542\text{ m})^2} \approx \mathbf{25.49}$$

This person is classified as slightly overweight.

e. The person weighs 210 pounds and is 5 ft, 9 in tall.

$$\text{Weight} = 95.34\text{ kg}$$

$$\text{Height} = 1.7526\text{ m}$$

$$\text{BMI} = \frac{95.34\text{ kg}}{(1.7526\text{ m})^2} \approx \mathbf{31.04}$$

This person is classified as obese based on BMI.

2. If the medium requires 5 g/1 L then 125 g of glucose are required for 25 L. The technician added:

$$\frac{?}{0.24\text{ lb}} = \frac{453.6\text{ g}}{1\text{ lb}} \quad ? = \frac{(453.6\text{ g})(0.24\text{ }\cancel{\text{lb}})}{\cancel{\text{lb}}} \quad ? = \mathbf{108.864\text{ g}}$$

Therefore, the technician added too little glucose.
Alternatively, you can think about it this way:

$$\frac{0.24\text{ }\cancel{\text{lb}}}{25\text{ L}}\left(\frac{453.6\text{ g}}{1\text{ }\cancel{\text{lb}}}\right) \approx \frac{\mathbf{4.35\text{ g}}}{\mathbf{1\text{ L}}} < \frac{\mathbf{5\text{ g}}}{\mathbf{1\text{ L}}}$$

3. An example sketch is shown below in Figure 7.5. First, 10 oz of enzyme are needed for every 100 L of broth and you want to make 500 L of broth. How many ounces of enzyme will you need?

$$\frac{10\text{ oz}}{100\text{ L}} = \frac{?}{500\text{ L}} \quad ? = 50\text{ oz}$$

Convert 50 oz to g; 1 oz is 28.35 g.

$$\frac{1\text{ oz}}{28.35\text{ g}} = \frac{50\text{ oz}}{?} \quad ? = 1{,}417.5\text{ g enzyme}$$

The manufacturer of the enzyme powder tells you that it is not pure enzyme. For every gram of powder weighed out, only 880 mg of it are enzyme. This means that if you weigh out a gram of the powder, you will only have 0.880 g of the enzyme. So, you need to do one more proportion equation to complete this problem.

$$\frac{0.880\text{ g enzyme}}{1\text{ g powder}} = \frac{1{,}417.5\text{ g enzyme}}{?}$$

$$\mathbf{? \approx 1{,}610.80\text{ g powder.}}$$

Observe that you want 1,417.5 g of enzyme, but you need *more* of the powder because some of what you weigh out is inert filler.

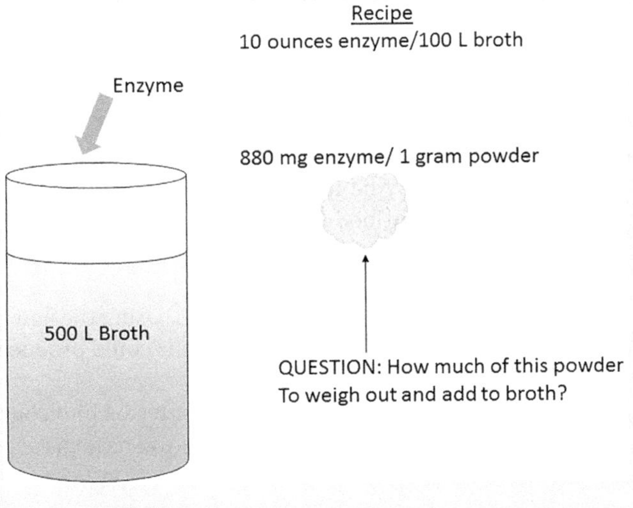


**FIGURE 7.5** Example sketch for Problem 3.

Note that different people might use different strategies to solve a problem like this – and also other problems we have seen in this section. For example, some people will always prefer a unit canceling strategy while others will prefer a strategy involving proportions. In this problem, some people might start by converting ounces to grams as the first step. The important thing is to keep track of where you are in the problem and check the answer to make sure it makes sense.

4. $1\text{ g}/10^6\text{ kg} = \dfrac{\mathbf{1\,g}}{\mathbf{10^9\,g}}$ **purer**

$$\frac{10^{-2}\text{ mg}}{10^{-3}\text{ kg}} = \frac{10^{-5}\text{ g}}{1\text{ g}} = \frac{1\text{ g}}{10^{5}\text{ g}}$$

5. 0.25 g/dose. Each tablet has 250 mg = 0.25 g. Need **15 doses total or 15 tablets**.

6. First, convert the amount of steak eaten from units of ounces to kg:

$$\frac{1\text{ kg}}{35.27\text{ oz}} = \frac{?}{4\text{ oz}} \quad ? = 0.1134108$$

Next, calculate how many Ci are in this amount of meat:

$$\frac{3{,}000\text{ pCi}}{1\text{ kg}} = \frac{?}{0.11341\text{ kg}} \quad ? = 340.23249\text{ pCi}$$

Convert 340.23249 pCi to Ci:

$$\frac{1\text{ Ci}}{10^{12}\text{ pCi}} = \frac{?}{340.23249\text{ pCi}} \quad ? = 3.402349\text{ X }10^{-10}\text{ Ci}$$

Convert $3.402349 \times 10^{-10}$ Ci to dps:

$$\frac{1\text{ Ci}}{3.7 \times 10^{10}\text{ dps}} = \frac{3.402349 \times 10^{-10}\text{ Ci}}{?} \quad ? \approx 12.588691\text{ dps}$$

Since 1 Bq = 1 dps this is **12.588691 Bq**

(This is actually a very low amount of radiation and organisms, including humans, have evolved to be able to repair damage caused by exposure to low, naturally occurring levels of radiation.)

7. Finding the math within unfamiliar terminology.
"A new process was developed for scale-up of an antibody that requires additional processing by a site-specific enzyme for correct functionality. Cell lines yielding high titers of highly processed antibodies were generated resulting in specific productivities of 50–75 pg/cell/day."

   a. Each of your 2,000 L vats contains $5 \times 10^6$ cells/mL. Using the new process, what is the maximum amount of antibody that your cells could produce in a production run that lasts one week?

   First, observe that productivity is expressed in terms of picograms **per cell** per day. So, you will need to know how many cells you have in each vat. Each vat is 2,000 L = $2{,}000 \times 10^3$ mL

Using a proportion strategy to calculate the number of cells/vat:

$$\frac{5\times10^{6}\text{ cells}}{1\text{ mL}}=\frac{?}{2{,}000\times10^{3}\text{mL}}$$

$$? = 1\times10^{13}\text{ cells}$$

Then, how much antibody could these cells produce in one day?

$$\frac{75\text{ pg}}{1\text{ cell}}=\frac{?}{1\times10^{13}\text{ cell}}$$

$$? = 7.5\times10^{14}\text{ pg} = 750\text{ g}$$

Then, how much antibody could the cells in one vat produce in 10 days?

$$750\text{ g/}\cancel{\text{day}}\times10\ \cancel{\text{days}}=\mathbf{7{,}500\ g}$$

b. On a per liter basis:

$$\frac{7{,}500\text{ g}}{2{,}000\text{ L}}=\mathbf{3.75\ g/L}$$

# Density

8

8.1 DENSITY IS ANOTHER TYPE OF RATIO

## 8.1 DENSITY IS ANOTHER TYPE OF RATIO

Density is another type of ratio. **Density, d,** *is the ratio between the mass and volume of a material*:

$$\textbf{density} = \frac{\textbf{mass}}{\textbf{volume}}$$

Observe that density is a ratio and therefore has a numerator and a denominator. Mass, in the numerator, is a measure of how much matter there is within a substance. Density expresses how much mass there is per a certain amount of volume. For example, 10 kg of granite and 10 kg of feathers have the same mass, but they will occupy very different volumes and therefore they have different densities.

For example, the density of benzene is:

$$\frac{\textbf{0.880 g}}{\textbf{mL}}$$

*This means that 1 mL of benzene has a mass of 0.880 g.*

Various materials have different densities. For example, balsa wood is less dense than lead. Therefore, a lead brick weighs more than a piece of balsa wood that occupies the same volume.

Density can be expressed in various units, so it is important to record the units. Also, the density of a material changes with temperature; most materials expand when heated and contract when cooled. This is because atoms vibrate and their vibration increases with higher temperature, moving the atoms further apart and therefore reducing the density value. It is therefore conventional to report the density of a material at a particular temperature. For example,

$$\text{benzene } d^{20^\circ} = 0.880 \text{ g/mL}$$

*This means that the density of benzene is 0.880 g/mL at 20°C.*

The densities of solids and liquids are often compared to the density of liquid water. If the density of a material is less than water, that material will float on water. If the material is denser than water, it will sink. In an oil spill in the ocean, the oil floats on the water's surface. This means that oil has a lower density than water. Similarly, the densities of gases are often compared to that of air. Materials that are less dense than air (such as balloons filled with helium) rise and materials that are denser than air do not rise.

DOI: 10.1201/9780429282744-10

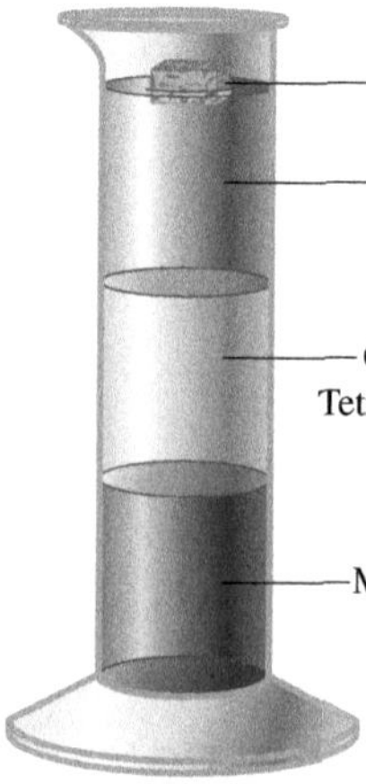


**FIGURE 8.1** Materials of different density. At room temperature, the density of mercury is 13.5 g/mL, carbon tetrachloride is 1.59 g/mL, and water is 0.998 g/mL. Since mercury is the densest, it is found on the bottom of the test tube. Cork is least dense and so floats on water.

Consider different substances that do not dissolve in one another. If these substances are mixed in a test tube, they will separate according to their densities with the densest substance on the bottom, Figure 8.1.

**Example Problem:**

The density for water is: $d^{4^\circ} = 1.000$ g/mL.
$d^{0^\circ} = 0.917$ g/mL
$d^{21^\circ} = 0.998$ g/mL

a. What is the volume occupied by 5.6 g of water at 4°C?
b. Why does ice float?

***Answer:***

a. This can easily be solved intuitively. The answer is simply 5.6 mL.
This can also be solved using a proportion equation:

$$\frac{1.000\text{ g}}{1\text{ mL}} = \frac{5.6\text{ g}}{?} \quad \mathbf{? = 5.6\ mL}$$

b. Water is less dense at 0°C than it is at 4°C. Therefore, ice (which is water at 0°C) floats on denser, unfrozen, water.

**Example Problem:**

What is the mass of 25.0 mL of benzene at 20°C? (Density=0.880 g/mL)

***Answer:***

**Strategy 1 Proportion method:**

$$\frac{0.880\text{ g}}{1\text{ mL}} = \frac{?}{25.0\text{ mL}} \quad \mathbf{? = 22.0\ g}$$

**Strategy 2 Unit canceling method:**

Since we know that 1 mL has a mass of 0.880 g, we can multiply by 25.0 to calculate the mass of 25.0 mL of benzene:

$$25\ \cancel{\text{mL}}\left(\frac{0.880\ \text{g}}{1\ \cancel{\text{mL}}}\right) = \mathbf{22.0\ g}$$

**Practice Problems**

1. ***The density of olive oil is 0.920 g/mL and of water is 0.997 g/mL at 25°C. Vinegar has a density similar to that of water. Which is the top layer in vinegar and oil dressing?***
2. ***The mass of a gold bar that is 3.00 cm$^3$ is 57.9 g at room temperature. What is the density of gold?***
3. ***The density of glycerol at 20°C is 1.26 g/mL. What is the volume of 20.0 g of glycerol?***
4. ***You need 20 mg of mercury (see Figure 8.1 for the density of mercury). How much volume will that amount occupy?***
5. ***You need to add 100 mg of the chemical, β-mercaptoethanol, to a laboratory reagent. The density of β-mercaptoethanol is 1.1 g/mL at room temperature and it comes as a liquid. How much should you measure out?***
6. a. ***What is the mass of 50 µL of pure water at room temperature?***
   b. ***What is the mass of 750 µL of pure water at room temperature?***

***Answers***

1. **Olive oil**
2. **19.3 g / cm$^3$**
3. Density = 1.26 g/mL $\quad \frac{1.26\ \text{g}}{1\ \text{mL}} = \frac{20.0\ \text{g}}{?} \quad ? \approx \mathbf{15.9\ mL}$
4. $\frac{13.5\ \text{g}}{\text{cm}^3} = \frac{0.020\ \text{g}}{?} \quad ? \approx \mathbf{0.0015\ cm^3}$
5. $0.100\ \cancel{\text{g}}\left(\frac{1\ \text{mL}}{1.1\ \cancel{\text{g}}}\right) \approx \mathbf{0.0910\ m}$
6. a. 0.050 mL (0.998 g/mL) = 0.0499 g ≈ **0.050 g**
   b. 0.750 mL (0.998 g/mL) = 0.7485 g ≈ **0.749 g**

# Dosages

9



## 9.1 CALCULATIONS OF DOSAGE

Dosages of drugs are another example of ratios. Drug dosages are commonly expressed as the amount of drug that is administered per unit of body weight of the patient. For example, a dose might be expressed as:

$$\frac{\mathbf{25\ mg}}{\mathbf{1\ kg}}$$

This means the patient is to receive 25 mg of the drug for every 1 kg that he or she weighs. Dosage calculations can be solved using either proportions or unit canceling, as illustrated in this Example Problem:

**Example Problem:**

Abby has flu and her parents want to give her ibuprofen to reduce her fever and help her feel better. Abby weighs 21 kg. She needs ibuprofen at a dose of 15 mg/kg. The ibuprofen comes as a liquid and the bottle reads "160 mg ibuprofen/5 mL." How much of the liquid ibuprofen does she get?

***Answer:***

The dosage is 15 mg/kg, which means that she gets 15 mg of ibuprofen for every kg of her weight. Since we know her weight in kg, we can easily figure out how much ibuprofen she gets using either proportions or the unit canceling method:

**Strategy 1 Proportion method:**

$$\frac{15\text{ mg ibuprofen}}{\text{kg weight}} = \frac{?}{21\text{ kg}} \qquad ? = 315\text{ mg}$$

This tells us how much ibuprofen she needs in terms of mg, however, the drug comes as a liquid and is administered by mL. So it is necessary to calculate how many mL to give Abby:

$$\frac{160\text{ mg ibuprofen}}{5\text{ mL}} = \frac{315\text{ mg}}{?} \qquad \mathbf{? \approx 9.8\ mL}$$

DOI: 10.1201/9780429282744-11

**Strategy 2 Unit canceling method:**

$$21\ \not{kg}\left(\frac{15\ \not{mg}\ \not{ibuprofen}}{\not{kg}}\right)\left(\frac{5\ \text{mL}}{160\ \not{mg}\ \not{ibuprofen}}\right) \approx \mathbf{9.8\ mL}$$

So Abby's parents give her 9.8 mL of ibuprofen.

**Example Problem:**

Herceptin is a drug that emerged from molecular biology/biotechnology research discoveries. In the 1970s, cancer researchers discovered that cancer cells often have genetic mutations that cause them to grow abnormally. Dr. Dennis Slamon and colleagues at UCLA found a genetic alteration in a gene called "Her2" in the cancer cells of about 25% of patients with breast cancer. The Her2 gene is responsible for making Her2 protein, which is found on the surface of cells where it receives and transmits growth signals. Every cell in a person normally contains the Her2 gene, but sometimes a mutation occurs that causes the Her2 gene to make too much receptor protein. When this happens, the cells divide and multiply more actively than normal, and women with this mutation develop an aggressive form of breast cancer. The Her2 gene is thus a normal gene that causes cancer when it becomes over-expressed (makes too much protein). Researchers designed a drug, named Herceptin, to bind to the Her2 receptor protein, thus blocking it from receiving growth signals. Clinical trials showed that Herceptin improves survival in women with Her2 positive breast cancer. Herceptin thus became one of the first novel cancer treatments to emerge from research into the fundamental mechanisms of cancer cell growth.

Here is a part of the dosage information provided for Herceptin (from "Package Insert Herceptin (Trastuzumab) Genentech Inc." *FDA*, www.accessdata.fda.gov/drugsatfda_docs/label/2000/trasgen020900lb.htm. Accessed 3 Apr. 2021.):

> Each carton contains one vial of 440 mg Herceptin® (Trastuzumab) and one 30 mL vial of Bacteriostatic Water for Injection [BWFI]l...
>
> Each vial of Herceptin should be reconstituted with 20 mL of BWFI... Immediately upon reconstitution with BWFI, the vial of Herceptin must be labeled in the area marked "Do not use after:" with the future date that is 28 days from the date of reconstitution.
>
> The recommended initial...dose is 4 mg/kg Trastuzumab...

a. What is the dosage strength (i.e., concentration) when a vial of Herceptin is reconstituted according to the directions given?

b. How much volume of the reconstituted Herceptin will be administered to a 150-pound patient to achieve the recommended initial dose?

*Answer:*

a. A vial contains 440 mg of drug and is reconstituted with 20 mL of BWFI, so the concentration of reconstituted drug is:

$$\frac{440\ \text{mg}}{20\ \text{mL}} = \frac{\mathbf{22\ mg}}{\mathbf{mL}}$$

b. How much volume of the reconstituted Herceptin will be administered to a 150-pound patient? Calculate the patient's weight in kg:

$$\frac{150\text{ lb}}{?} = \frac{2.205\text{ lb}}{1\text{ kg}} \quad ? \approx 68.0272\text{ kg}$$

The dose is 4 mg/kg:

$$\frac{4\text{ mg}}{\text{kg}} = \frac{?}{68.0272\text{ kg}} \quad ? \approx 272.109\text{ mg}$$

Calculate how many mL of reconstituted drug are required:

$$\frac{272.109\text{ mg}}{?} = \frac{22\text{ mg}}{\text{mL}} \quad \mathbf{? \approx 12.37\text{ mL}}$$

So the patient receives **12.37 mL** of reconstituted Herceptin.

Alternatively, by unit canceling:

$$\left(\frac{150\ \cancel{\text{lb}}}{1}\right)\left(\frac{1\ \cancel{\text{kg}}}{2.205\ \cancel{\text{lb}}}\right)\left(\frac{4\ \cancel{\text{mg drug}}}{1\ \cancel{\text{kg}}}\right)\left(\frac{1\text{ mL}}{22\ \cancel{\text{mg drug}}}\right) \approx \mathbf{12.37\text{ mL}}$$

**Practice Problems**

1. ***Tabby the puppy is sick and the veterinarian prescribes the antibiotic, Albon, at a dose of 25 mg/lb. The drug is supplied at 250 mg/5 mL. Tabby weighs eight pounds.***
   a. ***How many mg does Tabby require?***
   b. ***How many mL does Tabby get?***
2. ***Rusty the Amazon parrot needs the antibiotic, doxycycline, at a dose of 250 mg/kg. Rusty weighs 500 g. The tablets on hand are 25 mg each. How many tablets does Rusty get?***
3. ***A dose of the antibiotic, amoxicillin, is 10 mg/kg. How many mg are administered to a person who is 80 kg?***
4. ***Refer to the gentamicin sulfate (an antibiotic) label:***
   a. ***What is the total volume of this vial?*** _______
   b. ***What is the dosage strength (concentration)?*** _______
   c. ***If gentamicin 80 mg were required, how many mL would this be?*** _____
   d. ***If gentamicin 80 mcg were required, how many mL would this be?*** _______

**PHARM CO, INC.**

Store between 2 and 30 °C.
Each dose contains gentamicin sulfate USP equivalent to 40 mg gentamicin, 1.8 mg parabeben...

20 mL multiple dose sterile for use in preparation of large dose parenterals.

**GENTAMICIN SULFATE INJECTABLE USP**

40 mg/mL
20 mL, 800 mg

1234578910

5. ***Refer to the heparin label (heparin is used as a drug to prevent blood clotting).***
   a. ***How many units are in this vial altogether?***
   b. ***How many units are in 1.5 mL of this solution?***
   c. ***How would you prepare a dose of 55,000 U?***

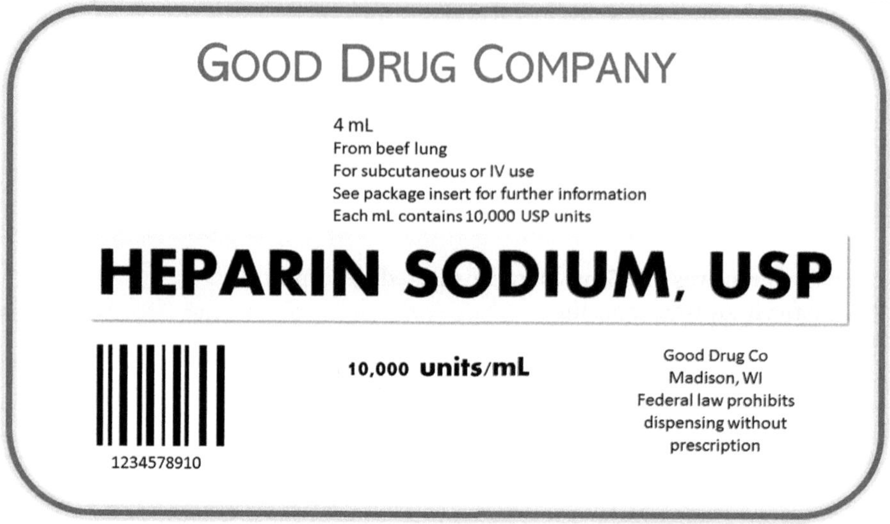
GOOD DRUG COMPANY
4 mL
From beef lung
For subcutaneous or IV use
See package insert for further information
Each mL contains 10,000 USP units
HEPARIN SODIUM, USP
10,000 units/mL
1234578910
Good Drug Co
Madison, WI
Federal law prohibits dispensing without prescription

6. ***Look at the sodium chloride label. How would you administer 40 mEq?***

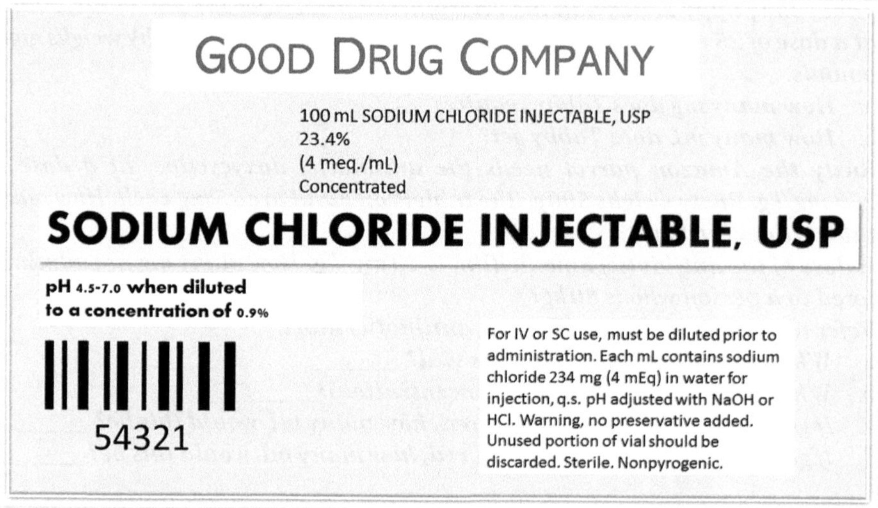
GOOD DRUG COMPANY
100 mL SODIUM CHLORIDE INJECTABLE, USP
23.4%
(4 meq./mL)
Concentrated
SODIUM CHLORIDE INJECTABLE, USP
pH 4.5-7.0 when diluted to a concentration of 0.9%
54321
For IV or SC use, must be diluted prior to administration. Each mL contains sodium chloride 234 mg (4 mEq) in water for injection, q.s. pH adjusted with NaOH or HCl. Warning, no preservative added. Unused portion of vial should be discarded. Sterile. Nonpyrogenic.

7. ***In 1998, Molly was diagnosed with thyroid cancer. Her thyroid was removed and she was put onto a synthetic hormone called Synthroid. In 2001, she was admitted to the hospital for an appendectomy. Prior to surgery, her doctor ordered 50 mcg of Synthroid. The pharmacist went to the shelf and found a vial of Synthroid labeled 500 mcg in a 10 mL vial. The drug was supplied in a lyophilized (dried powder) form. The pharmacist reconstituted the drug in 5 mL of diluent, and labeled the drug "Synthroid, 50 mcg/mL." One mL of the drug was administered to Molly during surgery. The physician was alarmed when she began showing signs of hypertension and tachycardia. Molly recovered, but a mistake had been made. What was it? (Based on real events posted by the "ASMP Medication Safety Alert," 6 September 2000, www.ismp.org/MSAarticles/Levothy-Digoxin.html)***

8. ***A study was performed to determine whether the administration of adipose-derived mesenchymal stromal cells is potentially useful as a treatment for severe cases of COVID-19. These cells are a type of human stem cell that are isolated from the connective tissue that surrounds tissues and organs. They have the capacity to differentiate into bone, cartilage, and fat cells and they play a normal role in injury healing. Additionally, this type of stem cell is thought to produce chemicals that might have a beneficial effect on the immune system and might reduce inflammation.***

***Ten patients received two doses of cells. Two patients received a single dose and another patient received three doses of these cells. The median number of cells per dose was $0.98 \times 10^6$ cells/kg body weight. Assuming that each patient weighed 160 pounds, how many cells did the patients who were administered one dose of cells receive? How many cells did the patients who were administered two doses receive? How many cells did the patient who was given three doses receive?***

(This study was reported in: Sánchez-Guijo, Fermín, et al. "Adipose-Derived Mesenchymal Stromal Cells for the Treatment of Patients with Severe SARS-CoV-2 Pneumonia Requiring Mechanical Ventilation. A Proof of Concept Study." *EClinicalMedicine*, vol. 25, 2020, p. 100454. doi:10.1016/j.eclinm.2020.100454.)

## *Answers*

1. a. $8 \cancel{\text{lb}}\left(\frac{25\text{ mg}}{1\cancel{\text{lb}}}\right) = \mathbf{200\ mg}$

   b. $200 \cancel{\text{mg}}\left(\frac{5\text{ mL}}{250\cancel{\text{mg}}}\right) = \mathbf{4\ mL}$

2. $0.500 \cancel{\text{kg}}\left(\frac{250\cancel{\text{mg}}}{\cancel{\text{kg}}}\right)\left(\frac{1\text{ tablet}}{25\cancel{\text{mg}}}\right) = \mathbf{5\ tablets}$

3. $\frac{10\text{ mg}}{\text{kg}} = \frac{?}{80\text{ kg}}$ $\quad ? = \mathbf{800\ mg}$

4. a. Total volume in vial: **20 mL** b. Dosage strength: **40 mg/mL**
   c. 80 mg requires: **2 mL**
   d. 80 mcg requires: **0.002 mL**. Note that this volume is probably too small to accurately measure, so more than this amount would need to be prepared.

5. a. Total units in vial: **40,000 units** b. In 1.5 mL: **15,000 Units**
   c. 55,000 U **requires 5.5 mL and requires two vials.**

6. There are 4 mEq/mL, so 40 mEq requires **10 mL**.
7. The pharmacist reconstituted 500 mcg in 5 mL = 100 mcg/1 mL; the order. said 50 mcg/mL. So she got twice the dose she should have.

8.

$$\frac{160\text{ lb}}{?} = \frac{2.205\text{ lb}}{1\text{ kg}} \quad ? \approx 72.56\text{ kg}$$

$$72.56 \cancel{\text{kg}}\left(\frac{0.98 \times 10^6\text{cells}}{\cancel{\text{kg}}}\right) \approx 7.11 \times 10^7\text{ cells}$$

The patients who received one dose received roughly $\mathbf{7.11 \times 10^7}$ **cells.**
The patients who received two doses received roughly $\mathbf{1.42 \times 10^8}$ **cells.**
The patient who received three doses received roughly $\mathbf{2.13 \times 10^8}$ **cells.**

# Percents

10



## 10.1 BASIC MANIPULATIONS INVOLVING PERCENTS

Percents are a familiar type of ratio. The **%** sign symbolizes a fraction, and the word **percent** *means "of every hundred."* Percents are "parts per hundred." For example,

**10% means 10/100 or "ten out of every hundred"**
**0.1% means 0.1/100 or "one tenth out of every hundred"**

A sample of 500 adults were surveyed to determine the amount of physical activity in which they engage each day. Of those surveyed, 450 reported less than 30 minutes of physical activity per day. Expressed as a ratio this is:

$$\frac{450 \text{ adults}}{500 \text{ adults}}$$

To convert this information to a percent, it is necessary to remember that percent means "out of every hundred." The ratio 450/500 can be converted to a percent using the logic of proportions:

$$\frac{450 \text{ adults}}{500 \text{ adults}} = \frac{?}{100}$$

$$\mathbf{? = 90}$$

This means "90 out of every hundred" or **90% of adults get less than 30 minutes of exercise each day**.

We can generalize from this example and say that the percent of individuals with a particular characteristic is:

$$\frac{\textbf{Number with the characteristic}}{\textbf{Total number}} \times \mathbf{100\% = \%\ with\ characteristic}$$

DOI: 10.1201/9780429282744-12

Thus, the percent of adults who get less than 30 minutes of exercise per day is:

$$\frac{450 \text{ adults}}{500 \text{ adults}} \times 100\% = 90\%$$

Observe that in a percent ratio, the numerator and denominator must have the same units.

Rules for manipulating percents are summarized in Box 10.1.

**BOX 10.1 Rules for Manipulating Percents**

1. **To convert a percent to its decimal equivalent, move the decimal point two places to the left and remove the percent sign.**
   Examples: 10% = 0.10 15% = 0.15 0.1% = 0.001
2. **To change a decimal to a percent, move the decimal point two places to the right and add a % sign.**
   Examples: 0.10 = 10% 0.87 = 87% 1 = 100%
3. **To change a percent to a fraction, write the percent as a fraction with a denominator of 100.**
   Examples: 30% = 30/100 1.5% = 1.5/100 100% = 100/100 = 1
4. **To change a fraction to a percent:**
   **Strategy 1 Use the logic of proportions.**
   For example, change 50/75 to a percent:
   a. Set the problem up as a proportion equation

$$\frac{50}{75} = \frac{?}{100}$$

   b. Cross multiply and divide

$$? = 66.66\ldots \text{ So, } 50/75 \approx \mathbf{66.67\%}$$

   **Strategy 2 Convert the fraction to its decimal equivalent and then move the decimal two places to the right and add a % sign.**
   Change 50/75 to a percent:
   a. Change the fraction to a decimal: 50/75 ≈ 0.6667
   b. Change the decimal to a percent: 0.6667 = **66.67%**
5. **To find a percentage of a particular number convert the percent to either its decimal equivalent or fractional equivalent and multiply times the number of interest.**
   For example:
   To find 45% of 900:
   a. Convert the percent to a decimal: 45% = 0.45
   b. Multiply the decimal times the number of interest: 0.45 (900) = **405.**
   To find 50% of 300:
   a. Convert the percent to a fraction: 50% = 50/100 = ½
   b. Multiply the fraction times the number of interest: ½ (300) = **150.**

**Example Problem:**

Show two strategies to convert the fraction 34/67 into a percent.

*Answer:*

**Strategy 1 Use proportions:**

$$\frac{34}{67} = \frac{?}{100}$$

Cross multiply and divide: ? ≈ 50.7

Therefore, the answer is **50.7%**

**Strategy 2 Convert the fraction to a decimal and then move the decimal point two places to the right and add a percent sign:**

$$\frac{34}{67} \approx 0.507$$

$$\Rightarrow 50.7\%$$

**Practice Problems**

1. ***Without using a calculator, give the approximate percent of each of the following. For example, 35 out of 354 is about 10% because it is close to 35 out of 350, which is close to 10/100, which is 10%.***
   a. ***98 out of 100*** b. ***110 out of 10,004***
   c. ***3 out of 15*** d. ***45 out of 45,002***
2. ***Express the following percents as fractions and as decimals.***
   a. ***34%*** b. ***89.5%***
   c. ***100%*** d. ***250%***
   e. ***0.45%*** f. ***0.001%***
3. ***Calculate the following.***
   a. ***15% of 450*** b. ***25% of 700***
   c. ***0.01% of 1,000*** d. ***10% of 100***
   e. ***12% of 500*** f. ***150% of 1,000***
4. ***Express the following fractions or decimals as percents.***
   a. ***15/45*** b. ***2/2*** c. ***10/100***
   d. ***1/100*** e. ***1/1,000*** f. ***6/40***
   g. ***0.1/0.5*** h. ***0.003/89*** i. ***5/10***
   j. ***0.05*** k. ***0.0034*** l. ***0.25***
   m. ***0.01*** n. ***0.10*** o. ***0.0001***
   p. ***0.0078*** q. ***0.50***
5. ***Calculate the following without using a calculator.***
   a. ***20% of 100*** b. ***20% of 1,000*** c. ***20% of 10,000***
   d. ***10% of 567*** e. ***15% of 1,000*** f. ***50% of 950***
   g. ***5% of 100*** h. ***1% of 876*** i. ***75% of 200***
6. ***State the following as percents:***
   a. ***1 part in 100 total parts*** b. ***3 parts in 50 total parts***
   c. ***15 parts in (15 parts + 45 parts)*** d. ***0.05 parts in 1 part total***
   e. ***1 part in 25 parts total*** f. ***2.35 parts in (2.35 parts + 6.50 parts)***

***Answers***

1. a. $98/100 = \mathbf{98\%}$

   b. $110/10{,}004 \approx \frac{1}{100} = \mathbf{1\%}$

   c. $\frac{3}{15} = \frac{1}{5} = \frac{20}{100} = \mathbf{20\%}$

   d. $\frac{45}{45{,}002} \approx \frac{1}{1{,}000} = \mathbf{0.1\%}$

2. a. $34\% = \frac{34}{100} = \mathbf{0.34}$
   b. $89.5\% = \frac{89.5}{100} = \frac{895}{1000} = \mathbf{0.895}$

   c. $100\% = \frac{100}{100} = \mathbf{1}$
   d. $250\% = \frac{250}{100} = \frac{2.5}{1} = \mathbf{2.5}$

   e. $0.45\% = \frac{0.45}{100} = \frac{45}{10{,}000} = \mathbf{0.0045}$
   f. $0.001\% = \frac{0.001}{100} = \frac{1}{100{,}000} = \mathbf{0.00001}$

3. a. $15\%$ of $450 = 0.15(450) = \mathbf{67.5}$
   b. $25\%$ of $700 = 0.25(700) = \mathbf{175}$

   c. $0.01\%$ of $1000 = 0.0001(1{,}000) = \mathbf{0.1}$
   d. $10\%$ of $100 = 0.1(100) = \mathbf{10}$

   e. $12\%$ of $500 = 0.12(500) = \mathbf{60}$
   f. $150\%$ of $1{,}000 = 1.5(1{,}000) = \mathbf{1{,}500}$

4. a. $\frac{15}{45} \approx 0.33 = \mathbf{33\%}$
   b. $\frac{2}{2} = 1 = \mathbf{100\%}$
   c. $\frac{10}{100} = 0.1 = \mathbf{10\%}$

   d. $\frac{1}{100} = 0.01 = \mathbf{1\%}$
   e. $\frac{1}{1{,}000} = 0.001 = \mathbf{0.1\%}$
   f. $\frac{6}{40} = 0.15 = \mathbf{15\%}$

   g. $\frac{0.1}{0.5} = 0.2 = \mathbf{20\%}$
   h. $\frac{0.003}{89} \approx 0.000034 = \mathbf{0.0034\%}$
   i. $\frac{5}{10} = 0.5 = \mathbf{50\%}$

   j. $0.05 = \mathbf{5\%}$
   k. $0.0034 = \mathbf{0.34\%}$
   l. $0.25 = \mathbf{25\%}$

   m. $0.01 = \mathbf{1\%}$
   n. $0.10 = \mathbf{10\%}$
   o. $0.0001 = \mathbf{0.01\%}$

   p. $0.0078 = \mathbf{0.78\%}$
   q. $0.50 = \mathbf{50\%}$

5. a. $20\%$ of $100 = \mathbf{20}$
   b. $20\%$ of $1{,}000 = \mathbf{200}$

   c. $20\%$ of $10{,}000 = \mathbf{2{,}000}$
   d. $10\%$ of $567 = \mathbf{56.7}$

   e. $15\%$ of $1{,}000 = \mathbf{150}$
   f. $50\%$ of $950 = \mathbf{475}$

   g. $5\%$ of $100 = \mathbf{5}$
   h. $1\%$ of $876 = \mathbf{8.76}$

   i. $75\%$ of $200 = \mathbf{150}$

6. a. $\frac{1\text{ part}}{100\text{ parts}} = \mathbf{1\%}$
   b. $\frac{3\text{ parts}}{50\text{ parts}} = \mathbf{6\%}$

   c. $\frac{15\text{ parts}}{(15+45)\text{ parts}} = \frac{15\text{ parts}}{60\text{ parts}} = \mathbf{25\%}$
   d. $\frac{0.05\text{ parts}}{1\text{ part}} = 0.05 = \mathbf{5\%}$

   e. $\frac{1\text{ part}}{25\text{ parts}} = 0.04 = \mathbf{4\%}$
   f. $\frac{2.35\text{ parts}}{(2.35+6.50)\text{ parts}} = \frac{2.35\text{ parts}}{8.85\text{ parts}} \approx 0.266 = \mathbf{26.6\%}$

**Percent Word Problems**

1. ***There are 55 students in a class. Of them, 25 work 20 hours a week or more at jobs outside school and 14 of them work 10–19 hours per week at jobs. The rest work 0–10 hours per week at outside jobs. What percent of the students work 20 hours or more per week at jobs? What percent work 19 hours or less at outside jobs?***
2. ***Suppose there is a population of insect in which 95% die over the winter, but the rest survive. Each surviving insect produces 100 offspring in the spring and then dies. Assuming there is no mortality during the summer and the population has 1,000 insects at the beginning of the first winter, how many insects will there be after two winters?***
3. ***Osteoporosis is a disease that leads to brittle bones and is partially caused by a lack of calcium. Each year, 250,000 people suffer osteoporosis-related hip fractures and about 15% of whom die after sustaining such fractures. How many people die each year after fracturing their hip?***
4. ***Double-stranded DNA consists of two long strands. An adenine on one strand is always paired with a thymine on the opposite strand and a guanine on one strand is always paired with a cytosine on the opposite strand. If a purified sample of DNA contains 24% thymine, what are the percentages of the other bases?***

*Answers*

1. $\frac{25}{55}$ work 20 + hours ≈ **45%**
   $\frac{30}{55}$ work 19 or less hours ≈ **55%**
2. 1,000 insects, 5% survive
   $1000\ (0.05) = 50$ insects survive the first winter
   50 insects (100) = 5,000 insects after the first summer
   $5{,}000\,(0.05) = \mathbf{250}$ insects after the second winter
3. 250,000 people $(0.15) = \mathbf{37{,}500}$ people die
4. Since thymine is **24%**, adenine must also be **24%** for a total of 48%. This leaves 52% that must be split equally between guanine and cytosine, at **26% each**.

## 10.2 AN APPLICATION OF PERCENTS: VACCINE EFFECTIVENESS

Before a vaccine can be released to the general public, it must be tested on volunteers to be sure that it is safe and that it works to substantially reduce illness in vaccinated individuals. When such testing is performed, typically half of the volunteers are given the vaccine and half are given a placebo. The **placebo** *is an injection that does not contain the active ingredient in the vaccine.* After administering the vaccine or the placebo to volunteers, researchers wait until a certain number of people in either group contract the disease. If a vaccine is effective, then substantially fewer of the vaccinated subjects should get sick, or, if they do, their disease should be mild. Observe that vaccines are seldom expected to be 100% effective; a certain number of vaccinated individuals do usually contract illness. Vaccines vary in effectiveness. For example, the flu vaccine that is available annually is frequently less than 50% effective. In contrast, the vaccine that prevents polio approaches 100% effectiveness.

To calculate the effectiveness of a vaccine (sometimes called its efficacy or VE), researchers use Equation 10.1:

$$VE = \frac{\text{percent infected in placebo group} - \text{percent infected in vaccinated group}}{\text{percent infected in placebo group}} \quad (10.1)$$

The Centers for Disease Control and Prevention says that "Vaccine efficacy/effectiveness is interpreted as the proportionate reduction in disease among the vaccinated group. So a VE of 90% indicates a 90% reduction in disease occurrence among the vaccinated group, or a 90% reduction from the number of cases you would expect if they have not been vaccinated."

Let us consider the calculation of VE based on data from one of the first vaccines to prevent the disease, COVID-19. This vaccine was tested in about 30,000 volunteers of whom we will assume half received the placebo and the others the vaccine. The first data were released when 95 volunteers contracted symptomatic COVID-19. Of those cases, 90 illnesses occurred in people who received the placebo and 5 cases occurred in those receiving the vaccine. Substituting these data into Equation 10.1:

$$VE = \frac{\frac{90}{15{,}000}100\% - \frac{5}{15{,}000}100\%}{\frac{90}{15{,}000}100\%} = \frac{0.6\% - 0.0333\%}{0.6\%} = 0.9445 = \mathbf{94.45\%}$$

This is an encouraging result that indicates the vaccine is likely to be extremely effective at preventing COVID-19 illness.

### Practice Problems

1. ***In a vaccine trial, 38,955 people received the vaccine and 6,583 were in the placebo group. There were 60 cases of illness in the placebo group and 34 cases in the vaccinated group. What was the vaccine efficacy based on these data?***
2. ***In a vaccine trial, 22,000 volunteers were vaccinated and 10,000 received the placebo. In the vaccinated group, 44 people contracted the illness being studied and in the placebo group 325 people contracted illness. Calculate the efficacy of the vaccine.***
3. ***There was an outbreak of chickenpox in Oregon in 2002. The following table provides data for children who were and were not vaccinated, and who did or did not get chickenpox. Calculate the vaccine's effectiveness.***

| | Contracted Chicken pox | Did Not Contract Chickenpox |
|---|---|---|
| Vaccinated | 18 | 134 |
| Unvaccinated – assume this is like a placebo group | 3 | 4 |

(Data are from: Centers for Disease Control and Prevention. *Principles of Epidemiology,* 3rd Ed. 2012. www.cdc.gov/csels/dsepd/ss1978/SS1978.pdf)

### *Answers*

1. Using Equation 10.1:

$$VE = \frac{\frac{60}{6,583}100\% - \frac{34}{38,955}100\%}{\frac{60}{6,583}100\%} = \frac{0.9114\% - 0.08728\%}{0.9114\%} \approx \mathbf{90.4\%}$$

2. Using Equation 10.1:

$$VE = \frac{\frac{325}{10,000}100\% - \frac{44}{22,000}100\%}{\frac{325}{10,000}100\%} = \frac{3.25\% - 0.200\%}{3.25\%} \approx \mathbf{93.8\%}$$

3. Using Equation 10.1:

$$VE = \frac{\frac{3}{7}100\% - \frac{18}{152}100\%}{\frac{3}{7}100\%} \approx \frac{42.857\% - 11.8421\%}{42.857\%} \approx \mathbf{72.49\%}$$

This means the vaccinated group experienced about 72% fewer chickenpox cases than they would have if they had not been vaccinated.

## 10.3 AN APPLICATION OF PERCENTS: PERCENT ERROR

This section considers an application of percents that is commonly used in the laboratory when analysts perform tests or assays of samples. For example, an assay might be used to test the level of glucose in a patient's blood, determine if there is lead in paint chips, or determine the effect of a gene therapy on cells.

Whenever a test or assay is performed, the analysts, of course, want to get the "right" answer. **Accuracy** *is the closeness of agreement between a measurement or test result and the true value or the accepted value for that measurement or test.* Two related ways to express the accuracy of measurements are:

Method 1:

$$\textbf{Error} = \textbf{true value} - \textbf{average measured value}$$

(This may also be called **absolute error**.)

Method 2:

$$\%\,\textbf{Error} = \frac{(\textbf{true value} - \textbf{average measured value})}{\textbf{true value}}(\textbf{100\%})$$

where "error" is an expression of accuracy (also called "inaccuracy") and the true value may be the value of an accepted standard material

Consider this example: Clinicians who use an assay to measure the amount of a drug in blood samples want to be sure that the method they use is accurate, that is, that it always delivers the "right" value for the drug. One way to determine the accuracy of the drug assay method is to periodically test a blood sample that contains a known amount of the drug. This sample with a known amount of drug is called a standard, accepted reference material, or control sample. The clinicians assay the level of drug in the control sample using the same assay method that is used for patient blood samples. They then compare the result obtained for the control with the expected result to determine the accuracy of the test procedure. Suppose that in one such test, they use a control sample with a known drug concentration of 1,000.00 mg/mL. The assay result is 1,000.03 mg/mL. The absolute error for this one test is:

$$\textbf{True value} - \textbf{average measured value} = \textbf{Error}$$

$$1{,}000.00 \text{ mg/mL} - 1{,}000.03 \text{ mg/mL} = \mathbf{-0.03 \text{ mg/mL}}$$

The percent error is:

$$\frac{(\text{True value} - \text{average measured value})}{\text{true value}} \times 100\%$$

$$\frac{\left(1{,}000.00 \dfrac{\text{mg}}{\text{mL}} - 1{,}000.03 \dfrac{\text{mg}}{\text{mL}}\right)}{1{,}000.00 \text{ mg/mL}} \times 100\% = \mathbf{-0.003\%}$$

Observe that there is a slight error in their measured value. It is likely that they will perform the test more than once and then determine, based on their knowledge of the assay, whether their results are sufficiently accurate for their purpose.

**Example Problem:**

Glucose, a sugar carried in our blood, is the major source of energy for cells. Normal blood glucose levels in a person fasting are between 70 and 99 mg/dL. Fasting glucose values greater than 126 mg/dL may be associated with diabetes and values between 100 and 126 mg/dL may indicate pre-diabetes.

Suppose a medical laboratory technician tests the glucose level in a control sample that is stated to contain 100.0 mg/dL of glucose. The technician performs a glucose test 10 times on this control sample and gets the following values:

99.6, 100.9, 100.8, 99.8, 100.1, 99.9, 99.7, 100.0, 100.8, 101.0 mg/dL

What are the absolute error and percent error based on these data?

***Answer:***

The average value from the ten tests is 100.26 mg/dL. The absolute error is:

$$100.0 \text{ mg/dL} - 100.26 \text{ mg/dL} = \mathbf{-\ 0.26 \text{ mg/dL}}$$

The percent error is:

$$\frac{(100.0 \text{ mg/dL} - 100.26 \text{ mg/dL})}{100.0 \text{ mg/dL}} \times 100\% = \mathbf{-0.26\%}$$

**Example Problem:**

An assay used to measure the amount of protein present in samples is giving erroneous results that are low by about 5 mg. What will be the percent error due to this problem if the *actual* amount of protein present in a sample is:

i. 30 mg ii. 50 mg iii. 100 mg iv. 550 mg

***Answer:***

i. $(30\text{ mg} - 25\text{ mg})/30\text{ mg} \times 100\% \approx$ **16.7%** ii. **10.0%** iii. **5.0%** iv. $\approx$ **0.91%**

Note that the impact of this error is more pronounced when protein is present in low amounts than when protein is present at higher levels; the 5 mg error is a larger percent of 30 mg than it is of 550 mg.

**Practice Problems**

1. ***An assay is performed in which the correct answer is known to be 200.8 mg. The assay gives a value of 200.1 mg. What is the percent error?***
2. ***An assay for the level of lead in paint chips is performed four times with a control that has a known lead concentration of 1.00 mg/cm$^2$. The results are:***

   ***0.99, 1.02, 1.01, and 0.97 mg/cm$^2$***

   ***What is the percent error of the assay based on these results?***
3. ***An assay used to measure the amount of protein present in samples is giving erroneous results that are low by about 2.5 mg/mL. What will be the percent error due to this problem if the actual protein present in a sample is 100 mg/mL?***
4. ***An environmental testing laboratory is about to begin testing water for chromium. The company's scientists learn to perform the chromium assay and test their skills by assaying commercially prepared standards with known chromium concentrations. They use four standards and obtain the results below. The scientists want to be able to guarantee their customers that they will be able to analyze chromium in samples with better than ±2% accuracy. Fill in the table to show the percent error for each measurement. Have the scientists met their goal for accuracy based on these results?***

| Actual Concentration of Chromium in the Standard | Assayed Concentration of Chromium Obtained in the Laboratory | % Error |
|---|---|---|
| *1.00 µg/L* | *0.91 µg/L* | |
| *5.00 µg/L* | *4.78 µg/L* | |
| *10.00 µg/L* | *9.89 µg/L* | |
| *15.00 µg/L* | *15.08 µg/L* | |

*Answers*

1. $\text{Percent error} = \frac{(200.8\text{ mg} - 200.1\text{ mg})}{200.8\text{ mg}} \times 100\% \approx \mathbf{0.349\%}$
2. $\text{Average} = 0.9975\text{ mg/cm}^2$

   $\text{Percent error} = \frac{(1.00\text{ mg/cm}^2 - 0.9975\text{ mg/cm}^2)}{1.00\text{ mg/cm}^2} \times 100\% \approx \mathbf{0.25\%}$
3. $\text{Percent error} = \frac{(100\text{ mg/mL} - 97.5\text{ mg/mL})}{100\text{ mg/mL}} \times 100\% \approx \mathbf{2.5\%}$
4. The percent errors are, in order: **9.00%, 4.40%, 1.10%, ≈ −0.533%**

   These data suggest that at the two lower concentrations they have not achieved the desired accuracy although they have at higher concentrations. Refinements in their technique are required.

## 10.4 PERCENT INCREASE AND PERCENT DECREASE

It is common to compare two data values by calculating their percent increase or decrease. For example, people in finance report the percent increase or decrease in a stock's value to understand how the stock has fared over time. Biotechnologists might talk about the percent increase or decrease in the numbers of organisms, cells, or microbes that are present at two timepoints. Researchers might report the increase or decrease in the amount of a specific protein present in cells with and without treatment. Suppose that at an initial timepoint, there are $2\times10^2$ cells/mL in a culture, and at a second timepoint, there are $3\times10^2$ cells/mL. What is the percent increase in cell number?

To calculate this, first find the difference (increase) between the two values:

$$\text{Increase} = \text{new value} - \text{original value}$$

$$\frac{3\times10^2\text{ cells}}{\text{mL}} - \frac{2\times10^2\text{ cells}}{\text{mL}} = 1\times10^2\text{ cells/mL}$$

Then, divide the increase by the original number and multiply by 100%

$$\%\text{ Increase} = \frac{\text{increase}}{\text{original value}} \times 100\%$$

For our example,

$$\%\text{ Increase} = \frac{1\times10^2\text{ cells/mL}}{2\times10^2\text{ cells/mL}} \times 100\% = 50\%$$

The percent increase is **50%.**

Now suppose that at an initial timepoint there are $2\times10^2$ cells/mL in a culture and at another timepoint there are $4\times10^2$ cells/mL. What is the percent increase in cell number?

$$\%\text{ Increase} = \frac{2\times10^2\text{ cells/mL}}{2\times10^2\text{ cells/mL}} \times 100\% = \mathbf{100\%}$$

Observe that when the number of cells doubles, it corresponds to a 100% increase.

Next consider a situation where we are concerned with a *decrease* in values, as is the case when we are trying to remove contaminants, such as microbes or viruses, from a product. For example, we perform a procedure to remove bacterial contaminants from a product. The original number of bacteria is $10^6$ and after the procedure there are 100 bacteria remaining. We can calculate the percent change in the same way as in the previous example:

$$\text{Decrease} = \text{new value} - \text{original value}$$

$$\text{Decrease} = 100 - 10^6 = -999{,}900 \quad (\text{Observe that the difference is a negative number})$$

$$\%\ \text{Decrease} = \frac{-999{,}900}{1 \times 10^6} \times 100\% = \mathbf{-99.99\%}$$

In general, the percent change between two values is:

$$\text{Percent increase or decrease} = \frac{\text{new value} - \text{original value}}{\text{original value}} \times 100\%$$

If the result is positive, then there was an increase, and if the result is negative, then there was a decrease between the two values.

## 10.5 PERCENTS AND LOG REDUCTION VALUES

Let us return to the example of bacterial contaminants that are removed from a product. In our example, we began with $10^6$ bacteria and ended with 100, for a 99.99% decrease. Recall from Section 2.5 that we can also express this change as a log reduction value (LRV). The LRV equation for this example is:

$$\text{LRV} = \log \frac{10^6}{10^2} = \log 10^4 = \mathbf{4}$$

Some analysts might report the results of this procedure in terms of percents, as a 99.99% reduction. Others might report a LRV of 4. These are two comparable ways to express the change between two values and both are used in the scientific literature.

Now consider a situation where the LRV value for a particular treatment is reported to be 1. This means there were 10 times fewer contaminants after treatment than before. (Review Section 2.5 if this is not clear.) What percent change does this represent? To find the answer to this question, consider an example. If we begin with $10^6$ contaminants and end with $10^5$ contaminants, the LRV value is 1.

The percent decrease is:

$$\frac{10^5 - 10^6}{10^6} \times 100\% = \mathbf{-90\%}$$

Thus, we can express this decrease in contaminants as an LRV of 1 or a 90% reduction or decrease.

## Application Problems

1. ***Suppose an experiment is performed to test the ability of UV light to reduce the number of infectious viruses present on a surface. $10^{10}$ infectious particles are applied to the surface and the UV light is turned on for a specified time. At the end of the UV light exposure there are $10^4$ infectious particles.***
   a. ***What is the percent reduction of infectious particles?***
   b. ***What is the LRV?***
2. ***A version of the following table was part of Practice Problem 6 in Section 2.5. In this particular example, there are 1,000,000 contaminants to begin with. Fill in the blanks in this table.***

| LRV Value | Fold Reduction in Contaminant/ Pathogen | Number of Contaminants Remaining After Treatment | % Contaminants Remaining After Treatment | Expressed as a % Decrease |
|---|---|---|---|---|
| 0 | Not applicable | 1,000,000 | 100% | 0% |
| 1 | 10 | 100,000 | 10% | –90% |
| 2 | ________ | ________ | ________ | ________ |
| 3 | ________ | ________ | ________ | ________ |
| 4 | 10,000 | 100 | 0.01% | –99.99% |
| 5 | ________ | ________ | ________ | ________ |
| 6 | ________ | ________ | ________ | ________ |
| 7 | 10,000,000 | Possibly all removed | 0.00001% | –99.99999% |

## *Answers*

1. ***$10^{10}$ infectious particles are applied to the surface and the UV light is turned on. At the end of the UV light exposure, there are $10^4$ infectious particles.***
   a. ***What is the percent reduction of infectious particles?***

$$\text{Percent decrease } = \frac{10^4 - 10^{10}}{10^{10}} \times 100\% = \mathbf{-99.9999\%}$$

   b. ***What is the log reduction?***

$$\text{LRV} = \log \frac{10^{10}}{10^4} = \log 10^6 = \mathbf{6}$$

2. ***Fill in the final column of this table***

| LRV Value | Fold Reduction in Contaminant/ Pathogen | Number of Contaminants Remaining After Treatment | % Contaminants Remaining After Treatment | Expressed as a % Decrease |
|---|---|---|---|---|
| 0 | Not applicable | 1,000,000 | 100% | Not applicable |
| 1 | 10 | 100,000 | 10% | –90% |
| 2 | **100** | **10,000** | **1%** | **–99%** |
| 3 | **1000** | **1,000** | **0.1%** | **–99.9%** |
| 4 | 10,000 | 100 | 0.01% | –99.99% |
| 5 | **100,000** | **10** | **0.001%** | **–99.999%** |
| 6 | **1,000,000** | **1** | **0.0001%** | **–99.9999%** |
| 7 | 10,000,000 | Possibly all removed | 0.00001% | –99.99999% |

# Introduction to Concentration Problems

# 11



## 11.1 CONCENTRATION IS A RATIO

One of the most important applications of biotechnology math is in making aqueous solutions and reagents. Preparing aqueous solutions is the first step in practically any biotechnology task. For example, growing cells for experimentation or making products requires an aqueous solution with nutrients and other components that living cells need. Aqueous solutions for growing cells are termed **nutrient media**. Molecular biology procedures begin with the preparation of aqueous solutions that provide biological molecules, notably DNA and RNA, with the proper pH and salt levels. Working with proteins, testing samples, and most other common biotechnology tasks all begin with the preparation of aqueous solutions to support the biological system of interest. There are calculations associated with the preparation of aqueous solutions; every biotechnologist must be comfortable with these calculations.

A **solution** *can be defined as a homogeneous mixture in which one or more substances is (are) dissolved in another.* **Solutes** *are the substances that are dissolved in a solution. The substance in which the solutes are dissolved is called the* **solvent**. In biological applications, the solutes are solids or liquids, and the solvent is a liquid, most often, water.

**Concentration** *is the amount of a particular substance (solute) in a stated volume (or mass) of a solution or mixture.* Concentration is a ratio where the numerator is the amount of the material of interest and the denominator is usually the volume (or sometimes mass) of the entire mixture. Observe that the terms "**amount**" and "**concentration**" are not synonyms. **Amount** *refers to how much of a component is present.* For example, 10 g, 2 cups, and 30 mL are amounts while concentration is a ratio. In our applications, amount is expressed either as a weight or as a volume of a component.

This is the first of four chapters relating to the preparation of laboratory solutions. This chapter introduces the concept of **solute concentration**. Each successive chapter delves more deeply into calculations relating to the concentration(s) of solute(s) in a solution. Because concentration is a ratio, throughout these chapters you will find that the logic of ratios and proportions often provides an effective tool for solving a laboratory problem.

DOI: 10.1201/9780429282744-13

## 11.2 AMOUNT AND CONCENTRATION ARE NOT SYNONYMS

In Figure 11.1, six "solutions" are sketched. The stars represent solute molecules. Observe that solutions (a) and (b) have different numbers of "stars" and different volumes, but their concentration of "stars" is the same. Solutions (c) and (d) have the same numbers of "stars," yet the concentration of "stars" is different in the two solutions; stars are more concentrated in solution (d) than they are in (c). Solutions (e) and (f) have the same volumes but different concentrations of "stars."

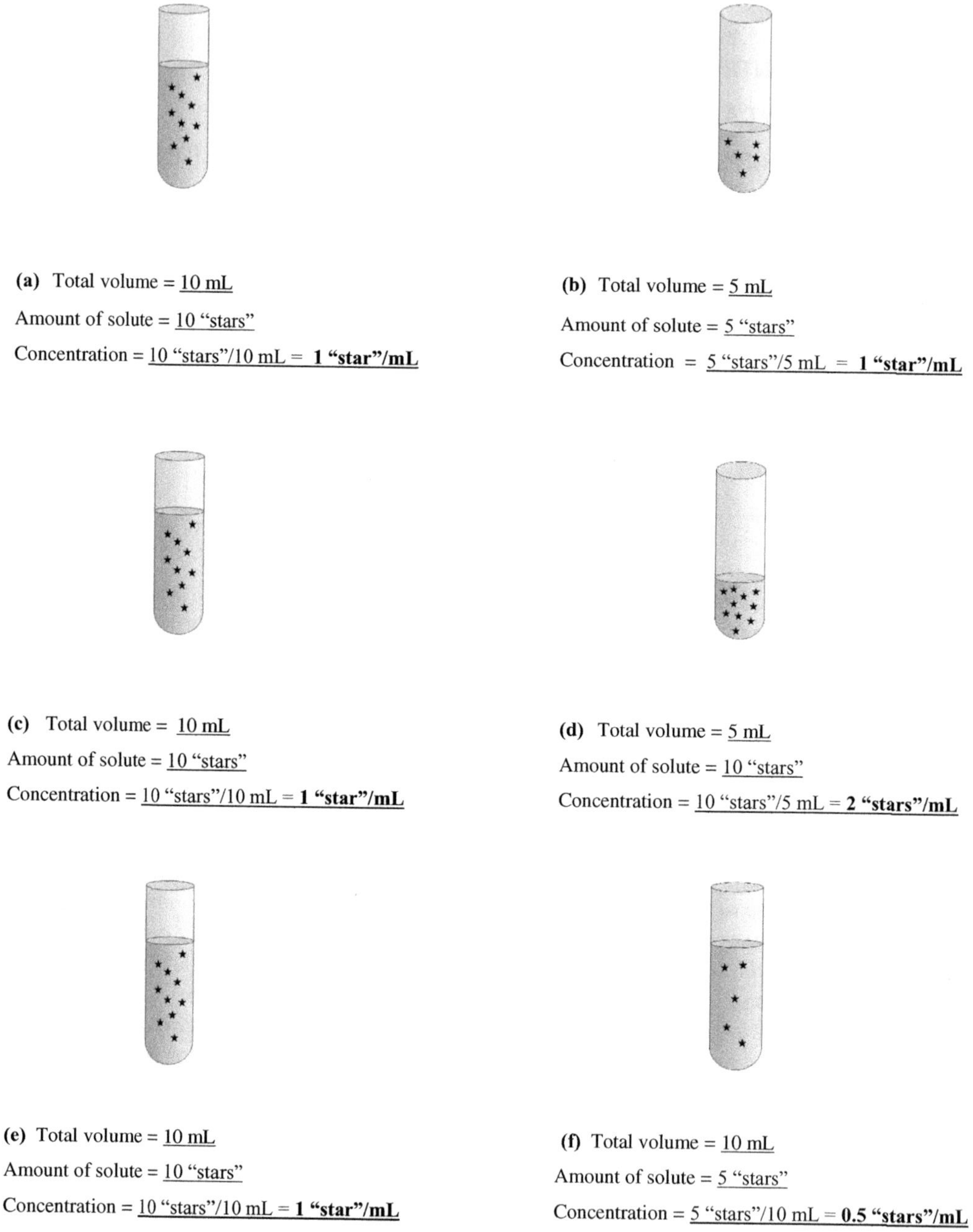


**FIGURE 11.1** Amount and concentration are not the same. Concentration is a ratio where the numerator is the amount of the substance of interest and the denominator is usually the volume of the entire mixture. See text for more explanation.

**Practice Problems**

1. ***State whether each of the following expressions is a concentration or an amount:***
   a. ***1 g enzyme*** b. ***1 mL solution*** c. ***1 g NaCl/mL*** d. ***1 pound of salt***
   e. ***1 mg of salt*** f. ***1 mg KCl/mL*** g. ***15 µg of NaCl*** h. ***18 pg NaCl***
   i. ***1 pg NaCl/L***
2. ***4 g of KCl is dissolved in water to a volume of 1 L. What is the solute? What is the solvent? What is the concentration of KCl in this solution?***
3. ***You have a solution of NaCl at a concentration of 15 mg/L. What is the solute? What is the solvent? What is the concentration of NaCl in this solution?***
4. ***Express each of the following as a concentration.***
   a. ***1 mg of enzyme out of 10 mL total solution***
   b. ***1 g of NaCl in water for a total of 1,000 mL***
   c. ***4 mL of ethanol dissolved in water for a total of 1 L***
5. a. ***If you take 5 g of solute and dissolve it in water to get a total volume of 10 mL, what is the concentration of solute in the solution? What is the amount of the solute in the solution?***
   b. ***If you take 5 g of solute and dissolve it in water to get a total volume of 100 mL, what is the concentration of solute in the solution? What is the amount of the solute in the solution?***

***Answers***

1. State whether each of the following expressions is a concentration or an amount:
   a. 1 g enzyme, **amount** b. 1 mL solution, **amount**
   c. 1 g NaCl/mL, **concentration** d. 1 pound of salt, **amount**
   e. 1 mg of salt, **amount** f. 1 mg KCl/mL, **concentration**
   g. 15 µg of NaCl, **amount** h. 18 pg NaCl, **amount**
   i. 1 pg NaCl/L, **concentration**
2. KCl is the solute and water is the solvent. The concentration of KCl is **4 g/L.**
3. NaCl is the solute and water is (assumed to be) the solvent. The concentration of NaCl is **15 mg/L.**
4. a. **1 mg enzyme/10 mL** b. **1 g NaCl/1,000 mL** c. **4 mL ethanol/1 L**
5. a. The *concentration* of solute in the solution is: $\frac{\textbf{5 g}}{\textbf{10 mL}}$

   The *amount* of solute in this solution is **5 g**.

   b. The *concentration* of solute in the solution is: $\frac{\textbf{5 g}}{\textbf{100 mL}}$

   The *amount* of solute in this solution is **5 g**.
   (Observe that the amount of solute, 5 g, is the same in a and b, but the concentrations are different.)

## 11.3 PREPARING A SOLUTION WITH THE RIGHT CONCENTRATION OF SOLUTE

Recall the following problem from Chapter 6:

If it requires one teaspoon of baking soda to make one loaf of bread, how many teaspoons of baking soda are required for 33 loaves?

Answer:

$$? = \text{amount of baking soda for 33 loaves}$$

$$\frac{1\ \text{tsp}}{1\ \text{loaf}} = \frac{?}{33\ \text{loaf}}$$

$$? = \frac{1\ \text{tsp}\left(33\ \cancel{\text{loaf}}\right)}{\cancel{\text{loaf}}}$$

$$? = \mathbf{33\ tsp}$$

The same sort of logic applies to problems where we need to calculate the amount of solute to make a solution at a particular concentration.

For example,

If it requires 1 g of enzyme to make 1 L of a particular solution, then how many grams of enzyme are required to make 3 L of this solution at the same concentration? (The enzyme is the solute.)

Answer:

$$? = \text{amount of enzyme for 3 L of this solution}$$

$$\frac{1\ \text{g enzyme}}{1\ \text{L}} = \frac{?}{3\ \text{L}}$$

$$? = \frac{1\ \text{g enzyme}\left(3\ \cancel{\text{L}}\right)}{1\ \cancel{\text{L}}}$$

$$? = 3\ \mathbf{g\ enzyme}$$

**Example Problem**

How could you make 300 mL of a solution at a concentration of 10 g NaCl per 100 mL?

***Answer***

The solute is NaCl. To answer the question, you must calculate how much solute is required to make a solution at the right volume and with the right concentration of the solute. This is easily solved with proportions:

$$\frac{10\ \text{g NaCl}}{100\ \text{mL total solution}} = \frac{?}{300\ \text{mL total solution}}$$

$$\mathbf{? = 30\ g}$$

The 30 g of NaCl in 300 mL is the same concentration as 10 g of NaCl in 100 mL.

To prepare this solution, weigh out 30 g of NaCl and dissolve it in <300 mL of water. After the solute is dissolved, bring the solution to a final volume of 300 mL by adding water until a volume of exactly 300 mL is reached. The 30 g is NOT added to 300 mL of water because the final volume (NaCl+water) might be more than 300 mL. The process of bringing a solution to the correct final volume is called "bringing to volume," or BTV. You might also see the term q.s. to mean bring to volume. q.s. stands for quantum sufficit, which is Latin, for "as much as suffices."

**Practice Problems**

1. a. ***How would you make 10 mL of a solution of NaCl at a concentration of 1 mg/mL?***
   b. ***How would you make 20 mL of a solution of NaCl at a concentration of 1 mg/mL?***
   c. ***How would you make 100 mL of a solution of NaCl at a concentration of 1 mg/mL?***
   d. ***How would you make 5 mL of a solution of NaCl at a concentration of 1 mg/mL?***

2. a. ***How would you make 1 L of a solution of KCl at a concentration of 4 g/L?***
   b. ***How would you make 0.5 L of a solution of KCl at a concentration of 4 g/L?***
   c. ***How would you make 2 L of a solution of KCl at a concentration of 4 g/L?***
   d. ***How would you make 10 mL of a solution of KCl at a concentration of 4 g/L?***

3. a. ***How would you make 100 mL of a solution of KCl at a concentration of 10 µg/mL?***
   b. ***How would you make 200 mL of a solution of KCl at a concentration of 10 µg/mL?***
   c. ***How would you make 50 mL of a solution of KCl at a concentration of 10 µg/mL?***
   d. ***How would you make 1 L of a solution of KCl at a concentration of 10 µg/mL?***

***Answers***

1. a. To make 10 mL of a solution of NaCl at a concentration of 1 mg/mL:

$$\frac{1\ \text{mg NaCl}}{1\ \text{mL total solution}} = \frac{?}{10\ \text{mL total solution}} \qquad ? = \mathbf{10\ mg}$$

   So you would weigh out 10 mg of NaCl, dissolve it in water, and bring it to a volume of 10 mL.

   b. To make 20 mL of a solution of NaCl at a concentration of 1 mg/mL:

$$\frac{1\ \text{mg NaCl}}{1\ \text{mL total solution}} = \frac{?}{20\ \text{mL total solution}} \qquad ? = \mathbf{20\ mg}$$

   Weigh out 20 mg of NaCl, dissolve it in water, and bring it to a volume of 20 mL.

   c. To make 100 mL of a solution of NaCl at a concentration of 1 mg/mL:

$$\frac{1\ \text{mg NaCl}}{1\ \text{mL total solution}} = \frac{?}{100\ \text{mL total solution}} \qquad ? = \mathbf{100\ mg}$$

   Weigh out 100 mg of NaCl, dissolve it in water, and bring it to a volume of 100 mL.

   d. To make 5 mL of a solution of NaCl at a concentration of 1 mg/mL:

$$\frac{1\ \text{mg NaCl}}{1\ \text{mL total solution}} = \frac{?}{5\ \text{mL total solution}} \qquad ? = \mathbf{5\ mg}$$

   Weigh out 5 mg of NaCl, dissolve it in water, and bring it to a volume of 5 mL.

2. a. To make 1 L of a solution of KCl at a concentration of 4 g/L:

$$\frac{4\text{ g KCl}}{\text{L}} = \frac{?}{1\text{ L}} \qquad ? = \mathbf{4\ g}$$

Weigh out 4 g of KCl, dissolve it in water, and bring it to a volume of 1 L.

b. To make 0.5 L of a solution of KCl at a concentration of 4 g/L:

$$\frac{4\text{ g KCl}}{\text{L}} = \frac{?}{0.5\text{ L}} \qquad ? = \mathbf{2\ g}$$

Weigh out 2 g of KCl, dissolve it in water, and bring it to a volume of 0.5 L.

c. To make 2 L of a solution of KCl at a concentration of 4 g/L:

$$\frac{4\text{ g KCl}}{\text{L}} = \frac{?}{2\text{ L}} \qquad ? = \mathbf{8\ g}$$

Weigh out 8 g of KCl, dissolve it in water, and bring it to a volume of 2 L.

d. To make 10 mL of a solution of KCl at a concentration of 4 g/L:
The units of volume must match; either convert 1 L to units of mL or convert 10 mL to units of L. 1 L = 1,000 mL.

$$\frac{4\text{ g KCl}}{1{,}000\text{ mL}} = \frac{?}{10\text{ mL}} \qquad ? = \mathbf{0.04\ g}$$

Weigh out 0.04 g of KCl, dissolve it in water, and bring it to a volume of 10 mL.

3. a. To make 100 mL of a solution of KCl at a concentration of 10 µg/mL:

$$\frac{10\ \mu\text{g}}{1\text{ mL}} = \frac{?}{100\text{ mL}} \qquad ? = 1{,}000\ \mu\text{g} = \mathbf{1\ mg}$$

Let us also use a unit canceling strategy for this problem:

$$\frac{10\ \mu\text{g}}{1\ \cancel{\text{mL}}}(100\ \cancel{\text{mL}}) = 1{,}000\ \mu\text{g} = \mathbf{1\ mg}$$

This means you would weigh out 1 mg of KCl, dissolve it in water, and bring it to a volume of 100 mL.

b. To make 200 mL of a solution of KCl at a concentration of 10 µg/mL:

$$\frac{10\ \mu\text{g}}{1\ \cancel{\text{mL}}}(200\ \cancel{\text{mL}}) = 2{,}000\ \mu\text{g} = \mathbf{2\ mg}$$

Weigh out 2 mg of KCl, dissolve it, and bring it to a volume of 200 mL.

c. To make 50 mL of a solution of KCl at a concentration of 10 µg/mL:

$$\frac{10\ \mu\text{g}}{1\ \cancel{\text{mL}}}(50\ \cancel{\text{mL}}) = 500\ \mu\text{g} = \mathbf{0.5\ mg}$$

Weigh out 0.5 mg of KCl, dissolve it, and bring it to a volume of 50 mL.

d. To make 1 L of a solution of KCl at a concentration of 10 µg/mL:

$$\frac{10\ \mu\text{g}}{1\ \cancel{\text{mL}}}(1{,}000\ \cancel{\text{mL}}) = 10{,}000\ \mu\text{g} = \mathbf{10\ mg}$$

Weigh out 10 mg of KCl, dissolve it, and bring it to a volume of 1 L.

## 11.4 SOLUTIONS WITH THE SAME CONCENTRATION OF SOLUTE

Look back at Figure 11.1 and observe that tubes (a) and (b) have the same *concentration* of solute (stars), but different volumes and different amounts of solute. Similarly, observe in the Practice Problems above, Section 11.3, that all the solutions in Problem 1 have the same *concentration* of solute (1 mg/mL), but they have different volumes and different *amounts* of solute:

$$\frac{1\text{ mg NaCl}}{1\text{ mL}} = \frac{10\text{ mg NaCl}}{10\text{ mL}} = \frac{20\text{ mg NaCl}}{20\text{ mL}} = \frac{100\text{ mg NaCl}}{100\text{ mL}} = \frac{5\text{ mg NaCl}}{5\text{ mL}}$$

Similarly, all the solutions in Section 11.3, Practice Problem 2, have a concentration of KCl of 4 g/L:

$$\frac{4\text{ g KCl}}{1\text{ L}} = \frac{2\text{ g KCl}}{0.5\text{ L}} = \frac{8\text{ g KCl}}{2\text{ L}} = \frac{0.04\text{ g KCl}}{0.01\text{ L}}$$

All the solutions in Problem 3 have a concentration of KCl of 10 µg/mL:

$$\frac{10\ \mu\text{g KCl}}{1\text{ mL}} = \frac{1{,}000\ \mu\text{g KCl}}{100\text{ mL}} = \frac{2{,}000\ \mu\text{g KCl}}{200\text{ mL}} = \frac{500\ \mu\text{g KCl}}{50\text{ mL}} = \frac{10{,}000\ \mu\text{g KCl}}{1{,}000\text{ mL}}$$

**Example Problem:**

Which of the following solutions have the same *concentration* of solute?

a. $\frac{1\text{ mg solute}}{2\text{ mL}}$ b. $\frac{30\text{ mg solute}}{60\text{ mL}}$ c. $\frac{100\text{ mg solute}}{300\text{ mL}}$ d. $\frac{780\text{ mg solute}}{1{,}560\text{ mL}}$

***Answer:***

Observe that the expression of concentration for solution b can be simplified by dividing both the numerator and denominator by 30 to get:

$$\frac{1\text{ mg solute}}{2\text{ mL}}$$

This means that solutions a and b have the same *concentration* of solute, even though they have different volumes and different amounts of solute.

If the concentration expression for solution c is simplified by dividing both the numerator and denominator by 100, it is:

$$\frac{1\text{ mg solute}}{3\text{ mL}}$$

This is not the same as the concentration of solution a or solution b.

If the concentration expression for solution d is simplified by dividing both the numerator and denominator by 780, it is:

$$\frac{1\text{ mg solute}}{2\text{ mL}}$$

**Solutions a, b, and d all have the same concentration of solute, that is, 1 mg/2 mL.**

**Practice Problems**

1. ***Which of the following solutions have the same concentration of solute?***

a. $\frac{\textit{1 g solute}}{\textit{2 L}}$ b. $\frac{\textit{300 g solute}}{\textit{600 L}}$ c. $\frac{\textit{100 g solute}}{\textit{500 L}}$ d. $\frac{\textit{0.1 g solute}}{\textit{200 mL}}$

2. ***Which of the following solutions have the same concentration of solute?***

a. $\frac{\textit{1 µg solute}}{\textit{20 mL}}$ b. $\frac{\textit{0.5 µg solute}}{\textit{10 mL}}$ c. $\frac{\textit{0.1 µg solute}}{\textit{2 mL}}$ d. $\frac{\textit{3 µg solute}}{\textit{60 mL}}$

***Answers***

1. b. $\frac{\text{300 g solute}}{\text{600 L}}$ Simplify by dividing numerator and denominator by 300.

$= \frac{\text{1 g solute}}{\text{2 L}}$ So this is the same as the concentration in a.

c. If the expression in c is simplified by dividing the numerator and denominator by 100, it is:

$\frac{\text{1 g}}{\text{5 L}}$ So this is not the same as either a or b.

d. If the numerator and denominator are multiplied by 10, the result is:

$\frac{\text{1 g}}{\text{2,000 mL}}$ Since 2,000 mL=2 L, this expression is the same as a and b.

**a, b, and d are the same concentrations of solute.**

2. If the numerator and denominator in b are multiplied by 2, then the expression is 1 µg solute/20 mL, which is the same as a.

If the numerator and denominator in c are multiplied by 10, then the expression is 1 µg solute/20 mL, which is the same as a and b.

If the numerator and denominator in d are divided by 3, then the expression is 1 µg solute/20 mL, which is the same as a, b, and c. So **all these solutions have the same concentration of solute.**

## 11.5 HOW MUCH SOLUTE IS IN A SOLUTION?

Consider the situation diagramed in Figure 11.2. This tube has a volume of 5 mL and solute at a concentration of 10 mg/mL. This means that every mL of the solution contains 10 mg of solute. If there is 10 mg of solute in each mL, how many mg of solute is present in the entire 5 mL? There is 50 mg of solute altogether in this test tube.

Consider Figure 11.3. In this figure, 1 mL of solution is removed from test tube a and placed into test tube b. Therefore, test tube b contains 10 mg of solute.

**Example Problem:**

If you have 100 mL of a solution with an enzyme concentration of 1 mg/mL, how much enzyme is present in the entire solution?

***Answer:***

You can use either proportions or a unit canceling strategy to solve this problem. Be sure you understand both strategies for solving this common type of problem.

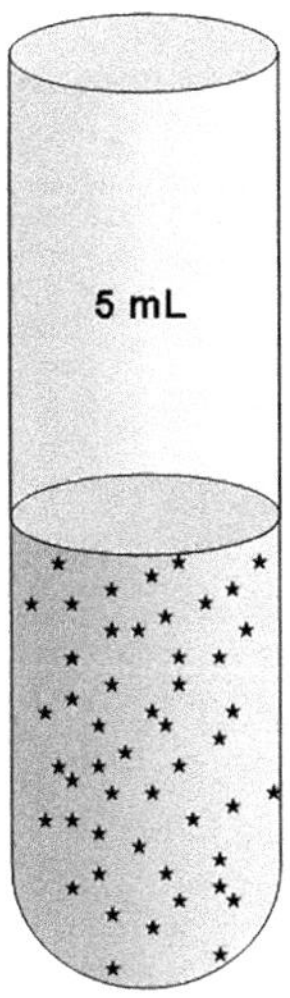


**FIGURE 11.2** Concentration and amount of solute in a solution. The concentration of solute is 10 mg/mL in this tube. Therefore, there is 50 mg altogether of solute in this test tube.

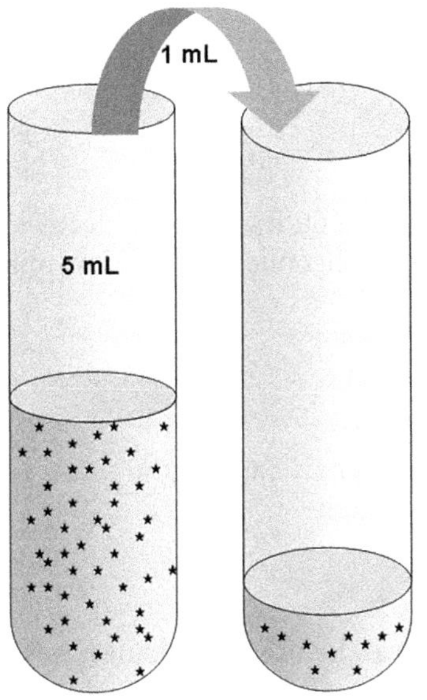


**FIGURE 11.3** Concentration and amount of solute in a solution. The concentration of solute is 10 mg/mL in the original tube. Therefore, if 1 mL of solution is removed and placed in another tube, the second tube will contain 10 mg of solute.

**Strategy 1: Proportions**

$$\frac{1\text{ mg}}{1\text{ mL}} = \frac{?}{100\text{ mL}} \qquad ? = \mathbf{100\ mg\ enzyme}$$

Read as: If there is 1 mg in each mL of the solution, then how many mg are in 100 mL?

**Strategy 2: Unit canceling**

$$\frac{100\ \cancel{\text{mL}}}{1}\left(\frac{1\text{ mg}}{1\ \cancel{\text{mL}}}\right) = \mathbf{100\ mg\ enzyme}$$

This means there are 100 mg of enzyme total in the solution.

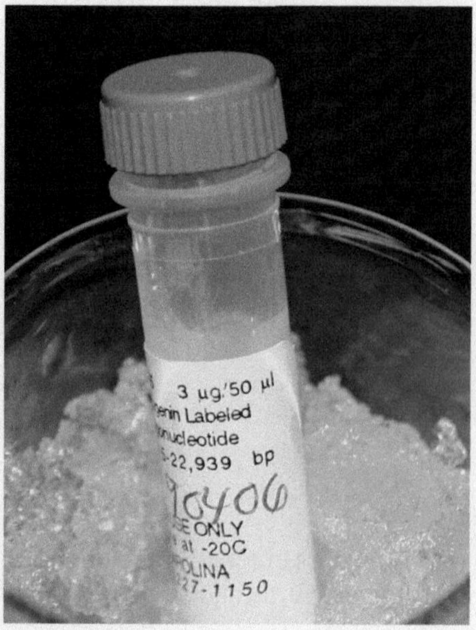


**FIGURE 11.4** A vial of oligonucleotides.

**Example Problem:**

You remove the vial of oligonucleotides (short molecules of DNA) from the freezer, Figure 11.4. You need 400 ng of oligonucleotides. How much should you pipette from the vial?

***Answer:***

The label on the vial says that there is 3 µg/50 µL.

First make sure the units match:

$$400\ \text{ng} = 0.400\ \mu\text{g}$$

Next, a proportion equation can be used to calculate how much volume is needed to get 400 ng of nucleotide:

$$\frac{3\ \mu\text{g}}{50\ \mu\text{L}} = \frac{0.400\ \mu\text{g}}{?} \qquad ? \approx \mathbf{6.7\ \mu L}$$

Alternatively, by unit canceling:

$$\left(\frac{400\ \cancel{\text{ng}}}{1}\right)\left(\frac{1\ \cancel{\mu\text{g}}}{1{,}000\ \cancel{\text{ng}}}\right)\left(\frac{50\ \mu\text{L}}{3\ \cancel{\mu\text{g}}}\right) \approx \mathbf{6.7\ \mu L}$$

So you would pipette 6.7 µL from the vial to get the correct amount of oligonucleotides.

**Practice Problems**

1. ***You have 2,000 mL of a solution with a concentration of protein of 1 g/mL. How much protein do you have altogether in the 2,000 mL?***
2. ***You have 100 mL of a solution with solute at a concentration of 5 mg/mL. How much solute do you have in the entire solution?***

3. ***You have a liter of a solution with 1 mg/mL of enzyme.***
   a. ***You need 2 mg of enzyme, how much of the solution should you take?***
   b. ***You need 0.5 mg of enzyme, how much of the solution should you take?***
   c. ***You need 3 mg of enzyme, how much of the solution should you take?***
   d. ***You need 1 mg of enzyme, how much of the solution should you take?***
4. ***You have a solution with a concentration of 0.4 g/L of enzyme.***
   a. ***You need 2 g of enzyme, how much of the solution should you take?***
   b. ***You need 0.5 g of enzyme, how much of the solution should you take?***
   c. ***You need 3 g of enzyme, how much of the solution should you take?***
   d. ***You need 1 mg of enzyme, how much of the solution should you take?***
5. ***You have a solution with 10 mg/mL of enzyme.***
   a. ***You need 2 g of enzyme, how much of the solution should you take?***
   b. ***You need 0.5 g of enzyme, how much of the solution should you take?***
   c. ***You need 3 g of enzyme, how much of the solution should you take?***
   d. ***You need 1 mg of enzyme, how much of the solution should you take?***
6. ***Which is a more concentrated solution, one that contains 10 mg NaCl/L or one that contains 100 mg NaCl/L?***
7. ***Which is a more concentrated solution, one that contains 20 mg NaCl/mL or one that contains 20 mg NaCl/L?***

### *Answers*

1. By proportions:

   $$\frac{1\text{ g}}{\text{mL}} = \frac{?}{2{,}000\text{ mL}} \qquad ? = \mathbf{2{,}000\ g}$$

   which means there is 2,000 g of protein total in this solution.

   By unit canceling:

   $\frac{1\text{ g}}{\cancel{\text{mL}}} \times 2{,}000\ \cancel{\text{mL}} = \mathbf{2000\ g}$ The same answer as by the proportion method.

2. By proportions:

   $\frac{5\text{ mg}}{1\text{ mL}} = \frac{?}{100\text{ mL}} \qquad ? = \mathbf{500\ mg}$ So there is 500 mg of solute in this solution.

   By unit canceling:

   $\frac{5\text{ mg}}{\cancel{\text{mL}}} \times 100\ \cancel{\text{mL}} = \mathbf{500\ mg}$ The same answer as by the proportion method.

3. a. $\frac{1\text{ mg}}{1\text{ mL}} = \frac{2\text{ mg}}{?} \qquad ? = \mathbf{2\ mL}$

   So you need 2 mL of the solution to get 2 mg of enzyme.

   b. $0.5\ \cancel{\text{mg}} \times \frac{1\text{ mL}}{1\ \cancel{\text{mg}}} = \mathbf{0.5\ mL}$

   So you need 0.5 mL of the solution to get 0.5 mg of enzyme.

   c. $\frac{1\text{mg}}{1\text{ mL}} = \frac{3\text{ mg}}{?} \qquad ? = \mathbf{3\ mL}$

   So you need 3 mL of the solution to get 3 mg of enzyme.

   d. $1\ \cancel{\text{mg}} \times \frac{1\text{mL}}{1\ \cancel{\text{mg}}} = \mathbf{1\ mL}$ So you need 1 mL of the solution to get 1 mg of enzyme.

4. a. $\frac{0.4\text{ g}}{1\text{ L}} = \frac{2\text{ g}}{?} \qquad ? = \mathbf{5\ L}$ So you need 5 L of the solution to get 2 g of enzyme.

   b. $0.5\ \cancel{\text{g}} \times \frac{1\text{ L}}{0.4\ \cancel{\text{g}}} = \mathbf{1.25\ L}$ So you need 1.25 L of the solution to get 0.5 mg of enzyme.

c. $\frac{0.4\text{ g}}{1\text{ L}} = \frac{3\text{ g}}{?}$ $\quad ? = \mathbf{7.5\text{ L}}$

So you need 7.5 L of the solution to get 3 g of enzyme.

d. $0.001 \cancel{\text{g}} \times \frac{1\text{ L}}{0.4 \cancel{\text{g}}} = 0.0025\text{ L} = \mathbf{2.5\text{ mL}}$ So you need 2.5 mL of the solution.

5. a. $\frac{10\text{ mg}}{1\text{ mL}} = \frac{2{,}000\text{ mg}}{?}$ $\quad ? = \mathbf{200\text{ mL}}$

b. $500 \cancel{\text{mg}} \times \frac{1\text{ mL}}{10 \cancel{\text{mg}}} = \mathbf{50\text{ mL}}$

c. $\frac{10\text{ mg}}{1\text{ mL}} = \frac{3{,}000\text{ mg}}{?}$ $\quad ? = \mathbf{300\text{ mL}}$

d. $1 \cancel{\text{mg}} \times \frac{1\text{ mL}}{10 \cancel{\text{mg}}} = \mathbf{0.1\text{ mL}}$

6. 100 mg/L is more concentrated – has more solute per unit of volume – than 10 mg/L.
7. 20 mg/mL is more concentrated than 20 mg/L. When 20 mg is dissolved in 1 mL, the solute molecules are closer together, that is, are more concentrated than when they are dissolved in 1 L. Similarly, 100 people in a classroom would be more "concentrated" than 100 people in a football stadium.

## 11.6 THE TERM "PARTS"

This section introduces concentration expressed in terms of **parts**. The most familiar form of this expression is parts per hundred, that is percent (%). Scientists speak also of parts per thousand, parts per million, and parts per billion.

Consider a container, Figure 11.5, that contains one million beads that are mostly blue. One of the beads is red, five are green, and 1,000 are yellow. We can express the concentration of colored beads in this container using the word "parts." We would say that the concentration of red beads is one part per million, abbreviated 1 ppm. What is the concentration of green beads in this container? What is the concentration of yellow beads in this container?

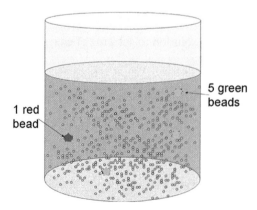


**FIGURE 11.5** A container with one million beads. The majority of the beads are blue, but one is red, five are green, and 1,000 are yellow. The concentration of red beads is one out of a million, or 1 ppm; green beads are present at five out of one million, or 5 ppm; yellow is present at 1,000 ppm.

Next, consider a container that has 1,000 beads, most of which are blue, 10 however are red, one is green, and three are yellow. We could use the word parts and say that the concentration of red is 10 parts per thousand, or 10 ppt. What are the concentrations of green and yellow?

*(The concentration of green beads is 1 out of 1,000, or 1 ppt; yellow is present at 3 ppt.)*

Next, consider a container that has 100 beads, most of which are blue, four are red, three are yellow, and one is green. We could say that the concentration of red beads is 4 parts per hundred, abbreviated 4%. The concentration of green beads is 1 out of 100 or 1%, and of yellow beads 3 out of 100 or 3%.

Let us consider this in terms of proportions. Suppose there are 10,000 red beads out of a total of a million, this is 10,000 ppm:

$$\frac{10{,}000\text{ red}}{1{,}000{,}000\text{ total beads}} = 10{,}000\text{ ppm}$$

Using proportions, this is the same as:

$$\frac{10{,}000\text{ red}}{1{,}000{,}000\text{ total beads}} = \frac{1{,}000\text{ red}}{100{,}000\text{ total}} = \frac{100\text{ red}}{10{,}000\text{ total}} = \frac{10\text{ red}}{1{,}000\text{ total}} = \frac{1\text{ red}}{100\text{ total}}$$

**Observe that 10,000 ppm = 10 ppt = 1 part per hundred or 1%.**

The expression of parts per hundred, or percent, is widely applied, both in the laboratory and in everyday life. The expression "parts per thousand" is rare in biological applications, but parts per million and parts per billion are commonly used, for example, by environmental scientists. Environmental scientists might speak of pollutants as being present at 10 ppm in air or 50 ppb in water, and so on. We will further explore the use of ppm and ppb in Chapter 12.

**Practice Problems**

1. ***There are 100 parts of solute per million parts of total solution.***
   ***Express this in terms of ppm _____________.***
   ***Express this in terms of parts per thousand _____________.***
   ***Express this in terms of percent _____________.***
2. ***There are 100,000 parts of solute per billion parts of total solution.***
   ***Express this in terms of parts per billion, ppb _____________.***
   ***Express this in terms of ppm _____________.***
   ***Express this in terms of ppt _____________.***
   ***Express this in terms of per cent _____________.***
3. ***There are 50,000 parts of solute per million parts of total solution.***
   ***Express this as ppm _____________.***
   ***Express this as parts per thousand _____________.***
   ***Express this as parts per hundred _____________.***
4. ***Cadmium is a heavy metal that can become a contaminant in water supplies. If there are ten parts of cadmium per thousand parts of water, what is the concentration in parts per million? _____________ What is the concentration expressed as a percent? _____________***
5. ***Assume that 1 mL of water weighs one gram. If there is one gram of cadmium per million mL of water, express this in terms of ppm _____________.***
6. ***If there are 45 g of PCBs (another type of pollutant) per liter of water, express this in terms of ppt _____________. Express this in terms of ppm _____________.***

*Answer:*

1. The concentration of solute is 100 out of one million, or **100 ppm, 0.1 ppt, 0.01%.**
2. There are **100,000 ppb, 100 ppm, 0.1 ppt, 0.01%.**
3. There are **50,000 ppm, 50 ppt, 5 parts per hundred.**
4. The concentration in parts per million is **10,000 ppm and 1%.**
5. **1 ppm**
6. **45 ppt, 45,000 ppm.**

## 11.7 FINDING THE MATH: THE CONCEPT OF CELL CONCENTRATION (DENSITY)

This section introduces the concept of cell concentration, also called cell density. In this section, we are deviating from the topic of preparing biological solutions. Instead, we are talking about working with living cells that are growing in culture medium inside of culture vessels. (Cell culture calculations are discussed in more detail in Chapter 21.) The reason for this deviation from the main theme of Chapter 11 is that many calculations relating to the concentration of cells in culture are analogous to the calculations relating to the concentration of solutes in a solution. It is essential to become adept at "finding the math," that is, recognizing what calculation tools apply to a particular situation. Therefore, this section illustrates when the same concepts that we discussed relating to solutes also apply to cultured cells.

Cultured cells often grow suspended in nutrient (culture) medium, Figure 11.6. In this case, for calculation purposes, the cells are like the solutes in a biological solution.

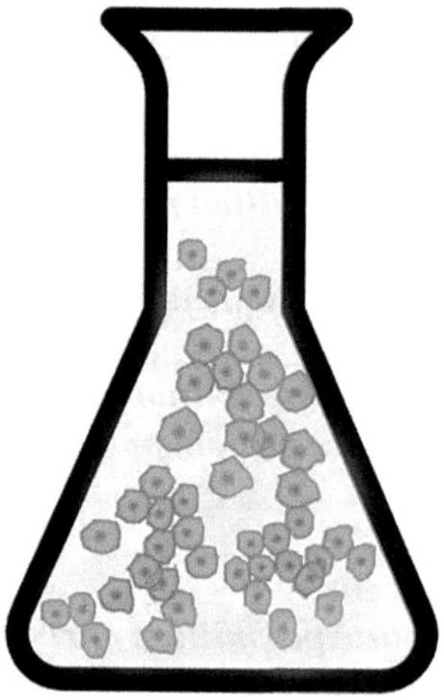

**FIGURE 11.6** Cells growing suspended in culture medium.

**Example Problem:**

If you have a flask with 100 mL of a culture medium and a cell concentration of about $10^3$ cells/mL, about how many cells are present in the entire flask?

*Answer:*

You can use either proportions or a unit canceling strategy to solve this problem. Be sure you understand both strategies for solving this common type of problem.

**Strategy 1: Proportions**

$$\frac{10^3 \text{ cells}}{\text{mL}} = \frac{?}{100 \text{ mL}}$$

$$? = \mathbf{10^5 \text{ cells}}$$

**Strategy 2: Unit canceling**

$$100 \cancel{\text{mL}} \left( \frac{10^3 \text{ cells}}{1 \cancel{\text{mL}}} \right) = \mathbf{10^5 \text{ cells}}$$

This means there are about $10^5$ cells in the flask.

Observe that the calculations here are analogous to Practice Problems 1 and 2 in Section 11.5.

**Practice Problems**

1. ***You have 2,000 mL of culture medium with 1,000 cells/mL. How many cells do you have altogether in the 2,000 mL?***
2. ***You have 100 mL of culture medium with $5 \times 10^4$ cells/mL. How many cells do you have altogether in the 100 mL?***
3. ***You have 1,000 mL of a culture with $5 \times 10^4$ cells/mL.***
   a. ***You need $2 \times 10^2$ cells. How many mL of culture should you take?***
   b. ***You need $3 \times 10^3$ cells. How many mL of culture should you take?***

*Answer:*

1. By proportions:

   $$\frac{1{,}000 \text{ cells}}{\text{mL}} = \frac{?}{2{,}000 \text{ mL}}$$ $? = \mathbf{2 \times 10^6 \text{ cells}}$, which means there are $2 \times 10^6$ cells total in this flask.

   By unit canceling:

   $$\frac{1{,}000 \text{ cells}}{\text{mL}} \times 2{,}000 \text{ mL} = \mathbf{2 \times 10^6 \text{ cells}}.$$

   The same answer as by the proportion method.

2. By proportions:

   $$\frac{5 \times 10^4 \text{ cells}}{1 \text{ mL}} = \frac{?}{100 \text{ mL}}$$ $? = \mathbf{5 \times 10^6 \text{ cells}}$ total.

   By unit canceling:

   $$\frac{5 \times 10^4 \text{ cells}}{\cancel{\text{mL}}} \times 100 \cancel{\text{mL}} = \mathbf{5 \times 10^6 \text{ cells}}.$$

   The same answer as by the proportion method.

3. a. $$\frac{5 \times 10^4 \text{ cells}}{1 \text{ mL}} = \frac{2 \times 10^2}{?}$$ $? = \mathbf{0.004 \text{ mL}}$,

   so you need **4 µL** of the culture medium.

By unit canceling:

$$\frac{2 \times 10^2 \ \cancel{\text{cells}}}{1}\left(\frac{1\,\text{mL}}{5\times10^4 \ \cancel{\text{cells}}}\right) = \mathbf{0.004\ mL} = \mathbf{4\ \mu L}$$

b. $\frac{5\times10^4\ \text{cells}}{1\,\text{mL}} = \frac{3\times10^3}{?}$ $? = \mathbf{0.06\ mL}$, so you need $\mathbf{60\,\mu L}$ of the culture medium.

By unit canceling:

$$\left(\frac{3\times10^3 \ \cancel{\text{cells}}}{1}\right)\left(\frac{1\,\text{mL}}{5\times10^4 \ \cancel{\text{cells}}}\right) = \mathbf{0.06\ mL} = \mathbf{60\ \mu L}$$

# Preparing Aqueous, Biological Solutions That Contain One Solute

# 12



## 12.1 PREPARING BIOLOGICAL SOLUTIONS

Chapter 11 introduced the concept of concentration as it relates to the preparation of biological solutions. This chapter further explores calculations that relate to the concentration of solutes in biological solutions.

Preparing biological solutions can be compared to baking. Suppose you decide to bake a batch of apple crisp. The first step is to find a recipe, such as that in Figure 12.1, which states:

1. The *components* of apple crisp.
2. *How much* of each component is needed.
3. *Advice for preparing* (mixing and baking) the components properly.

To successfully make apple crisp you need to understand the terminology in the recipe and to measure, combine, and prepare the ingredients in the proper fashion.

DOI: 10.1201/9780429282744-14

Preparing a laboratory solution has much in common with baking. You need a recipe (procedure) for preparing the solution. You follow the procedure and combine the right *amount(s)* of each *component* (solute) in the right volume of solvent to get the correct *concentration* of each solute at the end. You may also need to adjust the solution to the proper pH, sterilize it, or perform other manipulations. There are, however, differences between baking and preparing laboratory solutions. One important difference is that it is often appropriate to creatively modify a recipe when baking but laboratory procedures should be strictly followed.

Observe that the recipe for apple crisp in Figure 12.1 lists the *amount* of each component needed. A procedure to make a laboratory solution may similarly list the amount of each solute to use. For example, Laboratory Recipe I, Figure 12.1 lists the amount of each of the four solutes required: $Na_2HPO_4$, $KH_2PO_4$, NaCl, and $NH_4Cl$. Purified water is the solvent. The total solution has a volume of 1 liter. In overview, the procedure for preparing Laboratory Recipe I is:

Step 1: Weigh out the needed amount of each solute.
Step 2: Dissolve the solutes in <1 L of water.
Step 3: Add enough purified water so that the final volume is 1 L. (Recall from Chapter 11 that this process of adding purified water to bring a solution to the desired final volume is called "bringing to volume," or BTV.)

Laboratory Recipe I in Figure 12.1 is easy to interpret because it lists the *amount* of each solute required. However, many recipes for laboratory solutions do not show the *amount* of each solute required; rather, they specify the *concentration* of each. Recall from Chapter 11 that **concentration** *is the amount of a particular substance in a stated volume (or mass) of a solution or mixture.* Concentration is a ratio where the numerator is the amount of the material of interest and the denominator is usually the total volume (or sometimes mass) of the entire mixture.

There are various ways to express the concentration of solute in a solution, each of which involves somewhat different math calculations. This chapter describes four commonly used methods of expressing the concentration of a solute and calculations associated with that method. The key question that is solved by calculation in this chapter is:

**How much solute (an amount) is required to prepare a solution with a given concentration of this solute?**

Every time a solution is prepared, you must determine the amount of solute required to obtain a desired concentration; this is an important type of calculation in the laboratory.

KITCHEN RECIPE I
APPLE CRISP

Preheat oven to 375°F
12 oz can frozen lemonade
3 lb sliced apples
Reconstitute juice with water.
Cover apples with juice and refrigerate.

Blend together: 3 c rolled oats
1/2 c honey
1 c flour
3/4 c butter
1/2 tsp cinnamon

Place apples in bottom of 9 x 13 inch baking pan. Crumble oat mixture over apples. Pour juice over apples. Bake 1 hour.

LABORATORY RECIPE I

| | |
|---|---|
| $Na_2HPO_4$ | 6 g |
| $KH_2PO_4$ | 3 g |
| NaCl | 0.5 g |
| $NH_4Cl$ | 1 g |

Dissolve in water
Bring to a volume of 1 L

**FIGURE 12.1** Comparison of a kitchen recipe and a laboratory recipe.

**A NOTE ABOUT PRACTICAL CONSIDERATIONS**

The ranges of weights and volumes that can be accurately measured depends on the equipment available in a particular facility. For example, a research laboratory might not have glassware for holding and measuring volumes greater than a few liters while a production facility might have equipment for measuring hundreds of liters at a time. A biotechnology laboratory is likely to have micropipettes that can measure volumes as low as 1 µL, or even 0.5 µL, while some other types of facilities might not have these types of pipettes. Analytical balances that are common in laboratories can weigh substances as light as 0.0001 g (although it is difficult to handle such small quantities of chemicals). Research scientists are unlikely to weigh more than a kilogram of solute at a time. For the purposes of the problems in this chapter, assume that a practical range of volumes is 0.5 µL to a few liters, although it is more accurate to measure volumes >1 µL. A practical range for weight is from 0.0001 g to a kg or so.

## 12.2 METHOD 1: CONCENTRATION EXPRESSED AS A "WEIGHT/VOLUME" RATIO

A straightforward way to express concentration was shown in Chapter 11, as a "weight/volume" ratio, like this:

$$\frac{\textbf{2 g of NaCl}}{\textbf{1 L}}$$

This means that 2 g of NaCl is dissolved in enough liquid so that the total volume of the solution is 1 L. NaCl is the solute and water is the solvent.

Since concentration is a ratio, problems involving concentrations use the same reasoning as other proportion problems. For example, a concentration of 1 mg NaCl in 10 mL of solution is equivalent to a concentration of 10 mg NaCl in 100 mL of solution, 20 mg in 200 mL, and so on. We can write this as proportions:

$$\frac{1\text{ mg}}{10\text{ mL}} = \frac{10\text{ mg}}{100\text{ mL}} = \frac{20\text{ mg}}{200\text{ mL}}$$

The example problem and practice problems below deal with calculations of the amount of solute required to make a solution of a particular concentration (strength) and volume when concentration is expressed as a simple "weight/volume" ratio.

**Example Problem:**

a. How much NaCl (the solute) is required to make 500 mL of solution with a concentration of 3.0 g of NaCl per liter total solution?
b. How would you prepare this solution?

*Answer:*

a. Determining the amount of solute can be accomplished using a proportion equation, but remember to make sure the units match:

$$\frac{3.0\text{ g}}{1{,}000\text{ mL total volume}} = \frac{?}{500\text{ mL total volume}}$$

$$? = \mathbf{1.5\text{ g}}$$

1.5 g of NaCl in 500 mL is the same concentration as 3.0 g of NaCl in 1,000 mL.

This can also be solved using a unit canceling approach:

$$\left(\frac{500\ \cancel{\text{mL}}}{1}\right)\left(\frac{3.0\text{ g}}{1{,}000\ \cancel{\text{mL}}}\right) = \mathbf{1.5\text{ g}}$$

Observe that the answer, 1.5 g, is an *amount*. The *concentration* of solute is: 3.0 g/1,000 mL or 1.5 g/500 mL.

**b.** Weigh out 1.5 g of NaCl, dissolve it in <500 mL, and combine it with enough purified water so that the total volume of the solution is 500 mL. We could also say BTV 500 mL.

**Practice Problems**

1. ***How would you prepare 100 mL of an aqueous solution of $AgNO_3$ with a strength of 0.1 g $AgNO_3$/mL?***
2. ***How many mg of NaCl are present in 50 mL of a solution that is 2 mg/mL NaCl?***
3. ***How would you prepare 50 mL of the enzyme, Proteinase K (used to break down proteins), at a concentration of 100 µg/mL?***
4. ***A solution has 5 µg/L of enzyme Q. How much enzyme Q is present in:***
   a. ***50 mL of solution*** b. ***500 mL of solution***
   c. ***100 mL of solution*** d. ***100 µL of solution***
5. ***A solution has 0.5 mg/mL of the enzyme lysozyme (used to break apart the cell walls of bacteria). How much lysozyme is present in:***
   a. ***5 mL of solution*** b. ***0.5 mL of solution***
   c. ***100 µL of solution*** d. ***1000 µL of solution***
6. ***You have a solution of 0.5 mg/mL of the enzyme lysozyme.***
   a. ***You need 0.1 mg of enzyme, how much of the solution should you take?***
   b. ***You need 1 mg of enzyme, how much of the solution should you take?***
   c. ***You need 0.2 g of enzyme, how much of the solution should you take?***
   d. ***You need 350 µg of enzyme, how much of the solution should you take?***

### *Answers*

1. $\frac{0.1\text{ g}}{1\text{ mL}} = \frac{?}{100\text{ mL}}$ $\quad ? = \frac{0.1\text{ g}(100\ \cancel{\text{mL}})}{1\ \cancel{\text{mL}}}$ $\quad \mathbf{? = 10\ g}$

   Dissolve 10 g of $AgNO_3$ in purified water and bring it to 100 mL of total solution.

2. $\frac{2\text{ mg}}{1\text{ mL}} = \frac{?}{50\text{ mL}}$ $\quad \mathbf{? = 100\ mg}$

   100 mg of NaCl is dissolved in 50 mL total solution.

3. $\frac{100\ \mu\text{g}}{1\text{ mL}} = \frac{?}{50\text{ mL}}$ $\quad \mathbf{? = 5{,}000\ \mu g = 0.005\ g}$

   Dissolve 0.005 g of Proteinase K in purified water and BTV 50 mL.

4. $\frac{5\ \mu\text{g}}{1\text{ L}} = \frac{5\ \mu\text{g}}{10^3\text{ mL}}$ $\quad 1\text{ L} = 10^3\text{ mL}$

   a. $\frac{5\ \mu\text{g}}{10^3\text{ mL}} = \frac{?}{50\text{ mL}}$ $\quad ? = \frac{(5\ \mu\text{g})\,50\ \cancel{\text{mL}}}{10^3\ \cancel{\text{mL}}}$ $\quad ? = \frac{250\ \mu\text{g}}{10^3} = \mathbf{0.25\ \mu g}$

   b. $\frac{5\ \mu\text{g}}{10^3\text{ mL}} = \frac{?}{500\text{ mL}}$ $\quad ? = \frac{(5\ \mu\text{g})\,500\ \cancel{\text{mL}}}{10^3\ \cancel{\text{mL}}}$ $\quad ? = \frac{2{,}500\ \mu\text{g}}{10^3} = \mathbf{2.5\ \mu g}$

   c. $\frac{5\ \mu\text{g}}{10^3\text{ mL}} = \frac{?}{100\text{ mL}}$ $\quad ? = \frac{(5\ \mu\text{g})\,100\ \cancel{\text{mL}}}{10^3\ \cancel{\text{mL}}}$ $\quad ? = \frac{500\ \mu\text{g}}{10^3} = \mathbf{0.5\ \mu g}$

   d. $\frac{5\ \mu\text{g}}{10^6\ \mu\text{L}} = \frac{?}{100\ \mu\text{L}}$ $\quad ? = \frac{(5\ \mu\text{g})\,100\ \cancel{\mu\text{L}}}{10^6\ \cancel{\mu\text{L}}} = \frac{500\ \mu\text{g}}{10^6} = \mathbf{5 \times 10^{-4}\ \mu g}$

5. a. $\frac{0.5\text{ mg}}{1\text{ mL}} = \frac{?}{5\text{ mL}}$ $\quad ? = \frac{(0.5\text{ mg})\,5\ \cancel{\text{mL}}}{1\ \cancel{\text{mL}}}$ $\quad \mathbf{? = 2.5\ mg}$

   b. $\frac{0.5\text{ mg}}{1\text{ mL}} = \frac{?}{0.5\text{ mL}}$ $\quad ? = \frac{(0.5\text{ mg})\,0.5\ \cancel{\text{mL}}}{1\ \cancel{\text{mL}}}$ $\quad \mathbf{? = 0.25\ mg}$

   c. $1\text{ mL} = 10^3\ \mu\text{L}$

   $\frac{0.5\text{ mg}}{10^3\ \mu\text{L}} = \frac{?}{100\ \mu\text{L}}$ $\quad ? = \frac{(0.5\text{ mg})\,100\ \cancel{\mu\text{L}}}{10^3\ \cancel{\mu\text{L}}}$ $\quad \mathbf{? = 0.05\ mg}$

   d. $1{,}000\ \mu\text{L} = 1\text{ mL}$

   $\frac{0.5\text{ mg}}{1\text{ mL}} = \frac{?}{1\text{ mL}}$ $\quad \mathbf{? = 0.5\ mg}$

6. a. You need 0.1 mg of enzyme, how much of the solution should you take?

   $\frac{0.5\text{ mg}}{1\text{ mL}} = \frac{0.1\text{ mg}}{?}$ $\quad \mathbf{? = 0.2\ mL = 200\ \mu L}$

   b. You need 1 mg of enzyme, how much of the solution should you take?

   $\frac{0.5\text{ mg}}{1\text{ mL}} = \frac{1\text{ mg}}{?}$ $\quad \mathbf{? = 2\ mL}$

   c. You need 0.2 g of enzyme, how much of the solution should you take?
   Make sure the units match before setting up the proportion equation.

   $\frac{0.5\text{ mg}}{1\text{ mL}} = \frac{200\text{ mg}}{?}$ $\quad \mathbf{? = 400\ mL}$

   d. You need 350 μg of enzyme, how much of the solution should you take?
   Make sure the units match before setting up the proportion equation.

   $\frac{0.5\text{ mg}}{1\text{ mL}} = \frac{0.350\text{ mg}}{?}$ $\quad \mathbf{? = 0.7\ mL = 700\ \mu L}$

## 12.3 METHOD 2: CONCENTRATION EXPRESSED AS A PERCENT

Concentration is often expressed in terms of **percent**; the numerator is the amount of solute and the denominator is 100 units of total solution. Technically, the units should be the same in the numerator and denominator. If the amount of solute is expressed in milliliters, then the total volume in the denominator should also be expressed in milliliters. If solute is expressed in grams, then the total amount of solution should be expressed in grams. This way the units cancel. However, in practice, biologists often express percent solutions with different units in the denominator and numerator. This leads to three types of percent expressions that vary in their units.

### 12.3.1 TYPE I: WEIGHT PER VOLUME PERCENT

#### GRAMS OF SOLUTE PER 100 ML OF SOLUTION

A **weight per volume** *expression is the weight of the solute (in g) per 100 mL of total solution,*[1] Figure 12.2. This is the most common way to express a percent concentration in biology manuals. If a recipe uses the term % and does not specify type, assume it is a weight per volume percent. This type of expression is abbreviated as **w/v**. For example:

***20 g of NaCl in 100 mL of total solution is a 20%, w/v, solution.***

Box 12.1 shows the procedure for preparing a w/v solution.

### 12.3.2 TYPE II: VOLUME PERCENT

#### MILLILITERS OF SOLUTE PER 100 ML OF SOLUTION

In a **percent by volume expression**, abbreviated **v/v**, *both the amount of solute and the total solution are expressed in volume units.* This type of percent expression may be used when two compounds that are liquid at room temperature are being combined. For example,

***100 mL of methanol in 1,000 mL of total solution is a 10% by volume solution.***

Box 12.2 shows the procedure for making a v/v solution.

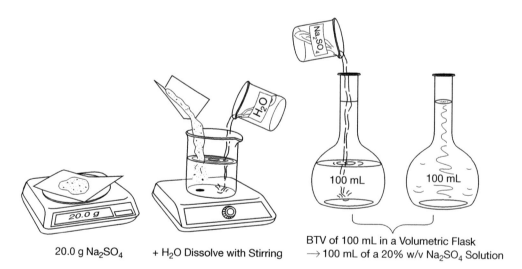

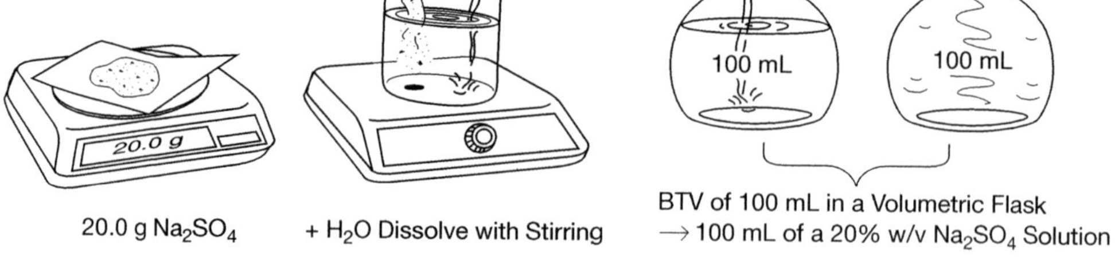


**FIGURE 12.2** A 20% weight per volume (w/v) solution of sodium sulfate ($Na_2SO_4$). The 20 g of $Na_2SO_4$ is dissolved in water and brought to a volume of 100 mL.

---

[1] This expression works for aqueous solutions because 1 mL of water weighs very close to 1 g – so the units in the numerator and denominator in essence are the same.

### 12.3.3 TYPE III: WEIGHT PERCENT

#### GRAMS OF SOLUTE PER 100 G OF SOLUTION

**Weight (mass) percent, w/w,** *is an expression of concentration in which the weight of solute is in the numerator and the weight of the total solution is in the denominator.* This type of expression is uncommon in biology manuals, but you may encounter it if you work with thick, viscous solvents whose volumes are difficult to measure. For example,

**5 g of NaCl plus 20 g of water is a 20%, w/w, solution.**

Because, the weight of the NaCl is 5 g.

The total weight of the solution = 20 g + 5 g = 25 g

$$\text{Weight percent} = \frac{\text{Weight of solute}}{\text{Total weight of solution}} \times 100\%$$

$$\frac{(5\text{ g NaCl})}{25\text{ g}} \times 100\% = \mathbf{20\%}$$

Box 12.3 shows the procedure for preparing a w/w solution.

**BOX 12.1: Procedure for Preparing a Weight per Volume (w/v) Percent Solution**

Step 1. Determine the percent concentration and volume of solution required.

Step 2. Express the percent concentration desired as a fraction (g/100 mL).

Step 3. Determine the amount of solute required to make a solution of the desired concentration and volume.

Step 4. Dissolve the amount of material calculated in step 3 in a volume of solvent less than the total, final volume. (Assume water is the solvent if solvent is not specified.)

Step 5. Bring the solution to the desired final volume.

**Note:**

To determine the amount of solute required, Step 3, use either proportions or unit canceling.

**Strategy 1: Proportion method**

Set up a proportion equation where the unknown (numerator) is the grams of solute required and the volume required is in the denominator.

**Strategy 2: Unit canceling method**

Multiply the total volume desired (step 1) by the fraction in step 2.

**Example Problem:**

How would you prepare 500 mL of a 5% (w/v) solution of NaCl?

*Answer:*

Step 1: Percent strength (concentration) is 5% (w/v). Total volume required is 500 mL.

Step 2: Expressed as a fraction, $5\% = \frac{5\text{ g}}{100\text{ mL}}$

Step 3: Determine the amount of solute required to make a solution of the desired concentration and volume:

**Strategy 1: Proportion method**

$$\frac{5\text{ g}}{100\text{ mL}} = \frac{?}{500\text{ mL}} \qquad ? = \mathbf{25\text{ g}} = \text{amount of solute (NaCl) needed}$$

**Strategy 2: Unit canceling method**

$$\left(\frac{500\ \cancel{\text{mL}}}{1}\right)\left(\frac{5\text{ g}}{100\ \cancel{\text{mL}}}\right) = \mathbf{25\text{ g}} = \text{Amount of NaCl needed}$$

Step 4: Weigh out 25 g of NaCl. Dissolve it in <500 mL of water.

Step 5: In a graduated cylinder or volumetric flask, bring the solution to a final volume of 500 mL by adding water.

**BOX 12.2: Procedure for Preparing a Percent by Volume (V/V) Solution**

Step 1. Determine the percent concentration and volume of solution required.

Step 2. Express the percent concentration desired as a fraction (mL/100 mL).

Step 3. Determine the amount of solute required to make a solution of the desired concentration and volume.

Step 4. Dissolve the amount of material calculated in step 3 in a volume of solvent less than the total, final volume. (Assume water is the solvent if solvent is not specified.)

Step 5. Bring the solution to the desired final volume.

**Note:**

To determine the amount of solute required, Step 3, use either proportions or unit canceling.

**Strategy 1: Proportion method**

Set up a proportion equation where the unknown (numerator) is the mL of solute required and the volume required is in the denominator.

**Strategy 2: Unit canceling method**

Multiply the total volume desired (step 1) by the fraction in step 2.

**Example Problem:**

How would you make 300 mL of a 10% by volume solution of ethanol in water (v/v)?

***Answer:***

Step 1: Percent strength is 10% (v/v). Total volume wanted = 300 mL.

Step 2: $10\% = \frac{10\text{ mL ethanol}}{100\text{ mL total volume}}$

Step 3: Determine the amount of solute required to make a solution of the desired concentration and volume:

**Strategy 1: Proportion method**

$$\frac{10\text{ mL}}{100\text{ mL}} = \frac{?}{300\text{ mL}} \qquad ? = \mathbf{30\text{ mL}} = \text{amount of ethanol needed}$$

**Strategy 2: Unit canceling method**

$$\left(\frac{300\ \cancel{\text{mL}}}{1}\right)\left(\frac{10\text{ mL}}{100\ \cancel{\text{mL}}}\right) = \mathbf{30\text{ mL}} = \text{Amount of ethanol needed}$$

Step 4: Place 30 mL of ethanol in a graduated cylinder. Add water to a final volume of 300 mL.

Note: You cannot assume that 30 mL of ethanol + 270 mL of water will give 300 mL total volume; their combined volume may be slightly <300 mL. Therefore, the correct way to prepare this solution is to bring it to the final volume in a graduated cylinder or volumetric flask (if a suitably sized volumetric flask is available).

**BOX 12.3: Procedure for Preparing a Percent by Weight Solution**

Step 1. Determine the percent concentration and weight of solution required.

Step 2. Express the percent concentration desired as a fraction (g/100 g).

Step 3. Multiply the total weight of the solution from step 1 by the fraction in step 2 to get the weight of the solute needed to make the solution.

Step 4. Subtract the weight of the solute from the total weight of the solution (step 1) to get the weight of the solvent needed to make the desired solution.

Step 5. Dissolve the amount of the solute found in step 3 in the amount of solvent from step 4 to make the desired solution.

**Example Problem:**

How would you make 500 g of a 5% NaCl solution by weight (w/w)?

*Answer:*

Step 1: Percent strength is 5% (w/w). Total weight of solution desired is 500 g.

Step 2: $5\% = \frac{5\text{ g}}{100\text{ g}}$

Step 3: $\frac{5\text{ }\cancel{\text{g}}}{100\text{ }\cancel{\text{g}}}(500\text{ g}) = 25\text{ g} =$ the amount of NaCl needed.

Step 4: $500 - 25\text{ g} = 475\text{ g} =$ the amount of water needed.

Step 5: Dissolve **25 g of NaCl in 475 g of water** to get a 5% NaCl solution by weight.

Observe that when we make either a w/v or a v/v solution, the solute is first mixed in less than the desired total volume, then the mixture is brought to its final volume in a graduated cylinder or volumetric flask. This is not done with a w/w solution because both solute and solvent are weighed, and their combined weights add up to the desired final weight.

## Practice Problems

1. *A particular laboratory solution contains 5mL of propanol per 100mL solution. Express this as a percent propanol solution. (Propanol is a clear, colorless liquid used as a solvent and mild antiseptic.)*
2. *A solution contains 15.0mL of ethanol (alcohol) per 700mL total volume. Express this as a percent ethanol solution.*
3. *A solution contains 10µL of dissolved enzyme in 1mL of water. Express this as a percent enzyme solution.*
4. *A solution contains 15mL of acetone per liter. Express this as a percent solution. (Acetone is a clear colorless liquid, commonly used as a solvent in the laboratory.)*
5. *How would you prepare 600mL of a 15% (w/v) solution of NaCl?*
6. *A laboratory solution is made of water and ethylene glycol. How could one prepare 250mL of a 30% (v/v) ethylene glycol solution?*
7. *A laboratory solution is required that is 10% (v/v) acetonitrile, 25% (v/v) methanol, and the rest is water. (Acetonitrile is a solvent commonly used in the laboratory.) How could you prepare this solution? (Note that the total volume is unspecified, so you can prepare any volume you want. Also, these components come as liquids.)*
8. *Suppose you have 100mg of solute in 1L of solution.*
   a. *Express this as a % solution.*
   b. *Is this a w/w, w/v, or v/v solution?*
9. *Suppose you have 50g of solute in 500mL of solution.*
   a. *Express this solution as a % solution.*
   b. *Is this a w/w, w/v, or v/v solution?*
10. *How would you prepare 200g of a 75% (w/w) solution of resin in acetone?*
11. *The label on a container of lidocaine, a drug used as a local anesthetic, states that the drug is present at a "dosage strength of 2%, or 20mg/mL." Are 2% and 20mg/mL the same dosage strength or is the container mislabeled?*

### *Answers*

1. $\frac{5\text{ mL}}{100\text{ mL}}$ = **5%** by volume propanol solution

2. $\frac{15.0\text{ mL EtOH}}{700\text{ mL}} = \frac{?}{100\text{ mL}}$ **? ≈ 2.14** so this is a 2.14% by volume (v/v) ethanol solution.

3. $\frac{10\ \mu\text{L}}{1\text{ mL}} = \frac{10\ \cancel{\mu\text{L}}}{1{,}000\ \cancel{\mu\text{L}}} = \frac{1}{100} = \mathbf{1\%\ by\ volume}(\text{v / v})\text{ enzyme solution}$

4. $\frac{15\text{ mL acetone}}{1\text{ L}} = \frac{15\text{ mL}}{1{,}000\text{ mL}} = \frac{1.5}{100} = \mathbf{1.5\%\ by\ volume}\ (\text{v / v})\text{ acetone solution}$

5. $\left(\frac{600\ \cancel{\text{mL}}}{1}\right)\left(\frac{15\text{g}}{100\ \cancel{\text{mL}}}\right) = 90\text{ g}$

   **Dissolve 90g of NaCl in water and bring to a volume of 600mL.**

6. 30% of 250 mL = 0.3×250 mL = **75mL ethylene glycol**

   Measure out the ethylene glycol and add purified water until the total volume is 250mL.

7. To make 100mL:

   10% acetonitrile **10mL**

   25% MeOH (methanol) **25mL**

   Measure out acetonitrile and MeOH, combine them, and add purified water until the volume is 100mL.

8. 100 mg = 0.1 g and 1 L = 1,000 mL
$\frac{0.1\text{ g}}{1{,}000\text{ mL}} = \frac{?}{100\text{ mL}}$ **? = 0.01 g** **a.** so this is a **0.01%** solution **b. w/v**
9. $\frac{50\text{ g}}{500\text{ mL}} = \frac{?}{100\text{ mL}}$ **? = 10 g** **a.** so this is a **10%** solution **b. w/v**
10. 75% of 200 g = 0.75 (200 g) = 150 g. Combine **150 g of resin and 50 g of acetone.**
200 − 150 g = 50 g
11. 2% = 2 g/100 mL = 0.02 g/1 mL = **20 mg/1 mL**

## 12.4 METHOD 3: CONCENTRATION EXPRESSED USING THE WORD "PARTS"

Parts expressions describe how many parts of each component to mix together. The parts may have any units but must be the same for all components. For example,

***A solution that is 3:2:1 ethylene:chloroform:isoamyl alcohol is:***
***Three parts ethylene, two parts chloroform, and one part isoamyl alcohol.***

There are many ways to prepare this solution. Two examples are:

***Combine: 3 L of ethylene + 2 L of chloroform + 1 L of isoamyl alcohol***
***Combine: 3 mL of ethylene + 2 mL of chloroform + 1 mL of isoamyl alcohol***

**Example Problem:**

How could you prepare 50 mL of 3:2:1 ethylene: chloroform: isoamyl alcohol? (These three chemicals come as liquids.)

*Answer:*

1. Add up all the parts required. In this case, there are 3+2+1 parts = 6 parts.
2. Use a proportion to calculate how much of each component is required.

If there are three parts of ethylene out of six parts total, then:

Ethylene: $\frac{3}{6} = \frac{?}{50\text{ mL}}$ ? = 25 mL **so 25 mL of ethylene is needed**

If there are two parts of chloroform out of six parts total, then:

Chloroform: $\frac{2}{6} = \frac{?}{50\text{ mL}}$ ? ≈ 16.7 mL **so 16.7 mL of chloroform is needed**

If there is one part of isoamyl alcohol out of six parts total, then:

Isoamyl alcohol: $\frac{1}{6} = \frac{?}{50\text{ mL}}$ ? ≈ 8.3 mL **so 8.3 mL of isoamyl alcohol is needed**

Thus, this solution requires: 25 mL of ethylene
16.7 mL of chloroform
8.3 mL of isoamyl alcohol

For a total of 50 mL

Note that a recipe expressed as it is in this example is not brought to volume rather the components are added to one another, as shown.

### 12.4.1 PARTS PER MILLION AND PARTS PER BILLION

The concentration expression "parts per million (ppm)" is a variation on the theme of parts. Recall from Chapter 11 that **parts per million** *is the number of parts of solute per one million parts of total solution.* Any unit may be used but must be the same for the solute and total solution. **Parts per billion (ppb)** *is the number of parts of solute per billion parts of total solution.* (Percent is the same class of expression as ppm and ppb. Percents are "parts per hundred.") For example, *5 ppm chlorine might be:*

***5 g of chlorine in $1 \times 10^6$ g of solution or***
***5 mg chlorine in $1 \times 10^6$ mg of solution or***
***5 pounds of chlorine in $1 \times 10^6$ pounds of solution, and so on***

### 12.4.2 CONVERSIONS BETWEEN PPM/PPB AND OTHER EXPRESSIONS

Concentration is often expressed in terms of ppm (or ppb) in environmental applications. This expression of concentration is useful when a very small amount of something (such as a pollutant) is dissolved in a large volume of solvent. For example, an environmental scientist might speak of a pollutant in a lake as being present at a concentration of 5 ppm.

To prepare a 5 ppm solution in the laboratory, you can convert the term 5 ppm to a simple fraction expression such as g/L, or mg/mL, or mg/L to determine how much of the solute to weigh out and dissolve. However, g/L, mg/mL, and mg/L all have units of weight in the numerator and volume in the denominator while ppm and ppb expressions have the same units in the numerator and denominator. To get around this problem, convert the weight of the water into mL based on the conversion factor that 1 mL of pure water at 20°C weighs 1 g. For example:

$$5\text{ ppm solute} = \frac{5\text{ g solute}}{1\text{ million g solution}} = \frac{5\text{ g solute}}{1\text{ million mL solution}} = \frac{5\text{ g solute}}{1{,}000\text{ L solution}}$$

In principle, you could make a 5 ppm solution by dissolving 5 g of solute with water for a total volume of 1,000 L. However, most laboratories do not have equipment for measuring out 1,000 L (nor would they waste purified water). So you might divide both the numerator and denominator by 1,000:

$$\frac{5\text{ g solute}}{1{,}000\text{ L solution}} = \frac{5\text{ mg}}{1\text{ L}}$$

It is easy to measure out 1 L in the laboratory. It is also possible to weigh out 5 mg with a high quality analytical balance, so you could prepare a 5 ppm solution by placing 5 mg of solute in a total volume of a liter.

Another way to think about the same problem is to divide the numerator and denominator both by 1 million:

$$5\text{ ppm solute} = \frac{5\text{ g solute}}{1\text{ million g solution}} = \frac{5 \times 10^{-6}\text{ g solute}}{1\text{ mL solution}}$$

$5 \times 10^{-6}$ g is the same as 5 µg, so 5 ppm solute in water is the same as $\frac{5\ \mu\text{g}}{1\text{ mL}}$ of solute in water.

For any solute:

$$\mathbf{1\ ppm\ in\ water} = \frac{\mathbf{1\ \mu g}}{\mathbf{1\ mL}} = \frac{\mathbf{1\ mg}}{\mathbf{1\ L}}$$

**Also,**

$$\mathbf{1\ ppb\ in\ water} = \frac{\mathbf{1\ ng}}{\mathbf{1\ mL}} = \frac{\mathbf{1\ \mu g}}{\mathbf{1\ L}}$$

**Example Problem:**

How would you prepare a 500 ppm solution of compound A?

***Answer:***

Recall that: 1 ppm in water $= \frac{1\text{ mg}}{1\text{ L}}$

So 500 ppm must be equal to $\frac{500\text{ mg}}{1\text{ L}} = \frac{\mathbf{0.500\text{ g}}}{\mathbf{1\text{ L}}}$

An acceptable method to prepare 500 ppm of compound A is to weigh out 0.500 g of the compound, dissolve it in water, and bring it to a volume of 1 L.

**Practice Problems**

1. ***Suppose you have a recipe that calls for one part salt solution to three parts water. How would you mix 10 mL of this solution?***
2. ***Suppose you have a recipe that calls for 1:3.5:0.6 chloroform/phenol/isoamyl alcohol. How would you prepare 200 mL of this solution?***
3. ***How would you mix 45 µL of a solution that is 5:3:0.1 Solution A: Solution B: Solution C? Assume water is the solvent.***

   Assume water is the solvent in Problems 4–6.
4. ***Convert 3 ppm to:***
   a. ***units of mg/mL***
   b. ***units of mg/L***
5. ***Convert 10 ppb to units of mg/L.***
6. ***How would you prepare a solution that has 100 ppm cadmium?***
7. ***Convert 600 ppb to units of g/L.***

***Answers***

1. 1 part + 3 parts = 4 parts total

   $\frac{1}{4} = \frac{?}{10\text{ mL}}$   $? = \mathbf{2.5\text{ mL}}$   $\frac{3}{4} = \frac{?}{10\text{ mL}}$   $? = \mathbf{7.5\text{ mL}}$

   Combine 2.5 mL of salt solution with 7.5 mL of water.
2. 1 part + 3.5 parts + 0.6 parts = 5.1 parts total

   | Chloroform | Phenol | Isoamyl alcohol |
   |---|---|---|
   | $\frac{1}{5.1} = \frac{?}{200\text{ mL}}$ | $\frac{3.5}{5.1} = \frac{?}{200\text{ mL}}$ | $\frac{0.6}{5.1} = \frac{?}{200\text{ mL}}$ |
   | $? \approx \mathbf{39.2\text{ mL}}$ | $? \approx \mathbf{137.3\text{ mL}}$ | $? \approx \mathbf{23.5\text{ mL}}$ |

   Combine the above volumes of each component.
3. 5 parts + 3 parts + 0.1 parts = 8.1 parts total

   | Solute A | Solute B | Solute C |
   |---|---|---|
   | $\frac{5}{8.1} = \frac{?}{45\,\mu\text{L}}$ | $\frac{3}{8.1} = \frac{?}{45\,\mu\text{L}}$ | $\frac{0.1}{8.1} = \frac{?}{45\,\mu\text{L}}$ |
   | $? \approx \mathbf{27.8\,\mu L}$ | $? \approx \mathbf{16.7\,\mu L}$ | $? \approx \mathbf{0.56\,\mu L}$ |

   Combine the above volumes of each component. Note that it would be difficult to accurately pipette 0.56 µL of a solution. Probably in practice you would mix a larger volume that would be easier to pipette accurately and remove 45 µL from it.

4. a. $3\text{ ppm} = \frac{3\text{ g}}{1\times10^{6}\text{ g}} = \frac{3\text{ g}}{1\times10^{6}\text{ mL}} = \frac{3{,}000\text{ mg}}{1\times10^{6}\text{ mL}} = \frac{\mathbf{3\times10^{-3}\ mg}}{\mathbf{mL}}$

Another way to think about this is to recall that:

$1\text{ ppm in water} = \frac{1\,\mu\text{g}}{1\text{ mL}}$ so $3\text{ ppm in water} = \frac{3\,\mu\text{g}}{1\text{ mL}} = \frac{3\times10^{-3}\text{ mg}}{1\text{ mL}}$

b. $3\text{ ppm} = \mathbf{3\ mg/L}$

5. $10\text{ ppb} = \frac{10\text{ g}}{1\times10^{9}\text{ g}} = \frac{10\text{ g}}{1\times10^{9}\text{ mL}} = \frac{10\times10^{3}\text{ mg}}{1\times10^{9}\text{ mL}} = \frac{10\times10^{-3}\text{ mg}}{1{,}000\text{ mL}} = \frac{\mathbf{0.01\ mg}}{\mathbf{1\ L}}$

6. $100\text{ ppm} = \frac{100\text{ g}}{1\times10^{6}\text{ mL}} = \frac{\mathbf{100\ mg}}{\mathbf{L}}$

Therefore, one could dissolve 100 mg of cadmium in water and BTV 1 L.

7. $600\text{ ppb} = \frac{600\text{ g}}{10^{9}\text{ mL}} = \frac{6\text{ g}}{10^{7}\text{ mL}} = \frac{6\text{ g}}{10^{4}\text{ L}} = \frac{\mathbf{6\times10^{-4}\ g}}{\mathbf{1\ L}}$

## 12.5 METHOD 4: CONCENTRATION EXPRESSED IN TERMS OF MOLARITY

**Molarity** *is a concentration expression that is equal to the number of moles of a solute that is dissolved per liter of solution.* Molarity is used to express concentration when the number of molecules in a solution is important. For example, in an enzyme-catalyzed reaction, the numbers of molecules of each reactant and the enzyme are important. If there is too little enzyme relative to the number of molecules of reactants present, the reaction may be incomplete, while adding too much enzyme is costly.

A brief review of terminology: A **mole** *of any element always contains* $6.02\times10^{23}$ *(Avogadro's number) atoms.* The word mole is often abbreviated as mol. Since some atoms are heavier than others, a mole of one element weighs a different amount than a mole of another element. *The weight of a mole of a given element is defined to be equal to its atomic weight in grams, or its* **gram atomic weight.**[2] Consult a periodic table of elements to find the atomic weight of an element. For example, one mole of the element carbon weighs 12.0 g.

**Compounds** *are composed of atoms of two or more elements bonded together.* A mole of a compound contains $6.02\times10^{23}$ molecules of that compound. The **gram formula weight (FW)** or **gram molecular weight (MW)** *of a compound is the weight in grams of 1 mole of the compound,* Figure 12.3.

For a compound, we can determine its FW by adding up the atomic weights of the atoms that make up the compound. For example, the FW of sodium sulfate ($Na_2SO_4$) is 142.04 g per mole:

| | | |
|---|---|---|
| 2 sodium atoms | 2×22.99 g = | 45.98 g |
| 1 sulfur atom | 1×32.06 g = | 32.06 g |
| 4 oxygen atoms | 4×16.00 g = | 164.00 g |
| | Total = | **142.04 g** |

**By definition, a 1 molar solution of a compound** *contains 1 mole of that compound dissolved in 1 L of total solution.* We also say that a "1 molar" solution has a "molarity of 1." For example, a 1 molar solution of sodium sulfate contains 142.04 g of sodium sulfate in 1 L of total solution, Figure 12.4.

[2] Weight and mass are not synonyms and it is correct to speak of gram molecular mass in the context of molarity. However, it is common practice to speak of "atomic weight," "molecular weight," and "formula weight," as we do in this book.

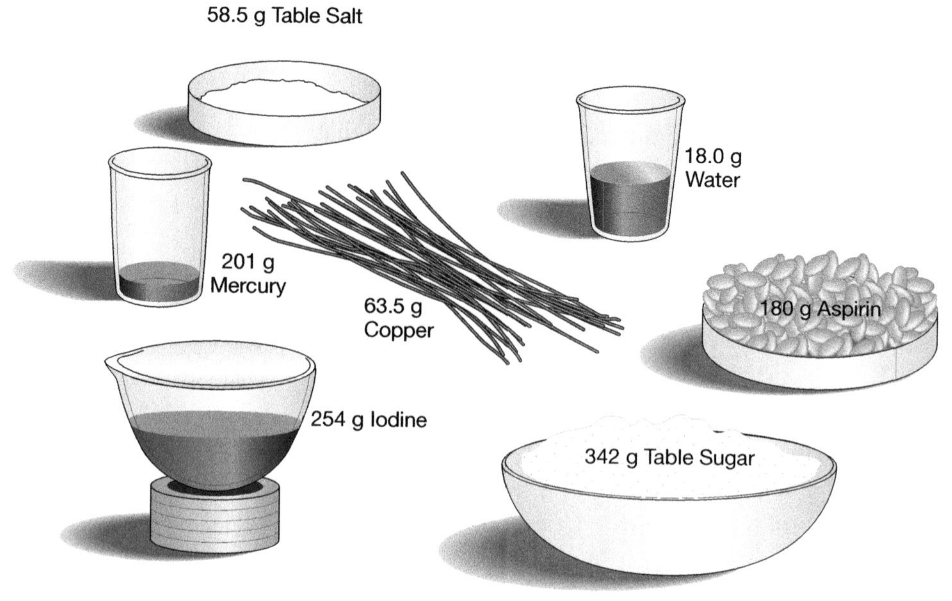


**FIGURE 12.3** A 1 mole of various substances. Different compounds have different FWs. Observe that a mole is an *amount* of molecules.

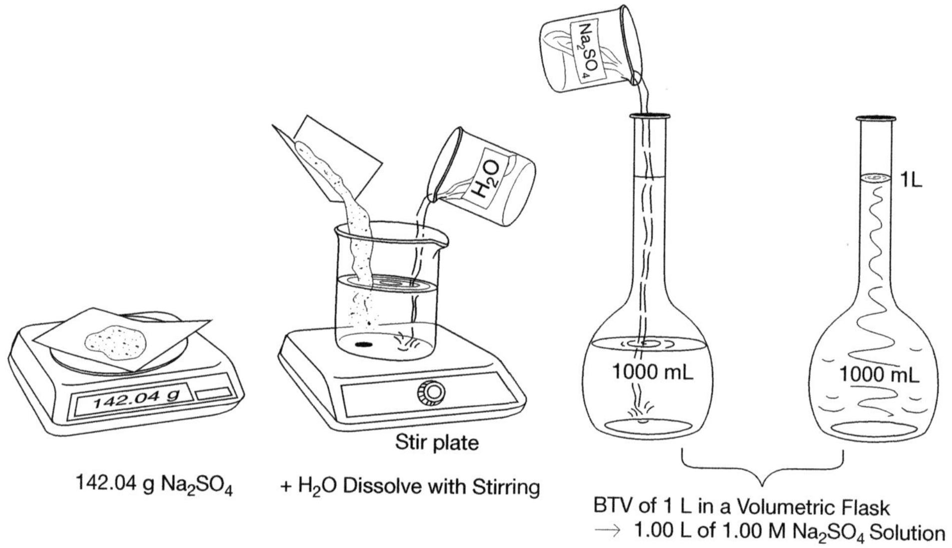


**FIGURE 12.4** A 1 M solution of sodium sulfate ($Na_2SO_4$). The FW of $Na_2SO_4$ is 142.04 g. This amount is dissolved in water so that the total volume is 1 L.

Note that a "mole" is an expression of ***amount*** and "molarity" and "molar" are words referring to the ***concentration*** of a solution. Let us consider how to calculate the amount of solute required when concentration is expressed in terms of molarity.

**Example Problem:**

How much solute is required to prepare 1 L of a 1 M solution of $CuSO_4$ solution?

By definition, a 1 molar solution of a compound contains 1 mole of that compound dissolved in 1 liter of total solution. This means that 1 L of a 1 M solution of copper sulfate contains 1 mole of copper sulfate. So the question is, how much does 1 mole of copper sulfate weigh?

*Answer:*

Calculate the FW of copper sulfate or find it on the label of the chemical's container. By calculation:

$$\begin{aligned} \text{1 copper} &= 1 \times 63.55\text{ g} = 63.55\text{ g} \\ \text{1 sulfur} &= 1 \times 32.06\text{ g} = 32.06\text{ g} \\ \text{4 oxygens} &= 4 \times 16.00\text{ g} = 64.00\text{ g} \\ \text{FW} &= 159.61\text{ g} \end{aligned}$$

**So 159.61 g of $CuSO_4$ is required to make 1 L of 1 M $CuSO_4$.**

Molarity is a concentration expression; concentration expressions are ratios. Therefore, we can determine how to prepare solutions of different molarities or different volumes by using straightforward proportional relationships.

**Example Problem:**

How much solute is required to prepare a 1 L solution of NaCl of molarity 0.25? The FW of NaCl is 58.44, which means that 1 mole of NaCl weighs 58.44 g.

*Answer:*

By definition, 1 L of a 1 M solution of sodium chloride requires 1 mole, 58.44 g, of NaCl, so:

$$\frac{58.44\text{ g}}{1\text{ M}} = \frac{?}{0.25\text{ M}} \qquad ? = \mathbf{14.61\text{ g}} = \text{solute required for 1 L of 0.25 M NaCl}$$

Sometimes it is necessary to make more or less than 1 L of a given solution. In these cases, proportions again can be used to determine how much solute is required.

**Example Problem:**

How much solute is required to make 500 mL of a 0.25 M solution of NaCl?

*Answer:*

We know from the previous example that 14.61 g of solute is required to make 1 L of 0.25 M NaCl.

$$\frac{?}{500\text{ mL}} = \frac{14.61\text{ g NaCl}}{1{,}000\text{ mL}}$$

$$? \approx \mathbf{7.31\text{ g}} \text{ NaCl} = \text{amount solute to make 500 mL of 0.25 M NaCl.}$$

Thus, it is possible to use proportions to calculate how much solute is needed to make a solution with a molarity other than 1 M and a volume other than 1 L. However, in practice, most often people use an equation, Equation 12.1, to calculate the amount of solute required to make a solution of a particular volume and a particular molarity. This equation can be written as follows:

**EQUATION 12.1: Calculation of How Much Solute Is Required for a Solution of a Particular Molarity and Volume**

$$\textbf{Solute required in grams} = (\textbf{grams / 1 mole})(\textbf{molarity})(\textbf{volume})$$

**This equation can also be written as:**

$$\textbf{Solute required in grams} = \left(\frac{\textbf{grams}}{\textbf{1 mole}}\right)\left(\frac{\textbf{mole}}{\textbf{liter}}\right)\left(\frac{\textbf{liter}}{\textbf{1}}\right)$$

where:

Solute required is the amount of solute needed, in grams

Grams per 1 mole is the number of grams in 1 mole of solute (the gram FW, or gram MW, for the solute)

Mole per liter is the desired molarity of the solution, expressed in moles/L

Volume is the final volume of the solution, in liters

**Note: To use Equation 12.1, volume must be expressed in units of liters. To convert a volume expressed in mL to L, simply divide the volume in mL by 1,000. For example,**

Convert 100 mL to L

Divide by 1,000

$$\frac{100}{1000} = 0.1$$

Therefore, 100 mL = 0.1 L.

As another example, convert 3,420 mL to L:

$$3,420 \text{ mL} = \frac{3,420}{1,000} = 3.420 \text{ L}$$

Note: If you wonder why dividing by 1,000 works, converting mL to L is a unit conversion, like those discussed in Chapter 7. For example, using the proportion method of unit conversions, as we did in Chapter 7, convert 3,420 mL to L:

$$\frac{1,000 \text{ mL}}{1 \text{ L}} = \frac{3,420 \text{ mL}}{?} \qquad ?(1,000 \text{ mL}) = 3,420 \text{ mL}(1 \text{ L})$$

$$? = \frac{3,420 \cancel{\text{mL}}(1 \text{ L})}{1,000 \cancel{\text{mL}}} \qquad ? = \frac{3,420 \text{ L}}{1,000} = 3.420 \text{ L}$$

We have now shown how to calculate the amount of solute required to prepare a solution of a given molarity and volume using two different strategies: proportions and Equation 12.1. Either strategy, when performed correctly, will give the right answer. The following example problem illustrates both the proportion strategy and the use of Equation 12.1 to calculate how much solute is required to make a solution of a particular molar concentration and volume. Box 12.4 outlines the procedure for making a solution of a particular volume and molarity.

**Example Problem:**

How much solute is required to prepare 300 mL of a 0.800 M solution of $CaCl_2$? (FW = 111.0 g)

*Answer:*

**Strategy 1: Proportion method**

First, determine how much solute is needed to make 1 L of 0.800 M $CaCl_2$

$$\frac{?}{0.800\text{ M}} = \frac{111.0\text{ g}}{1\text{ M}} \qquad ? = 88.80\text{ g}$$

Second, determine how much solute is needed to make 300 mL.

$$\frac{?}{300\text{ mL}} = \frac{88.80\text{ g}}{1{,}000\text{ mL}} \qquad ? = \mathbf{26.64\ g}$$

**= grams of $CaCl_2$ required to make 300 mL of 0.800 M solution**

**Strategy 2: Using Equation 12.1**

First, convert 300 mL to liters by dividing by 1,000:

$$\frac{300}{1{,}000} = 0.300 \quad \text{Therefore, } 300\text{ mL} = 0.300\text{ L}$$

Plug values into Equation 12.1:

$$\text{Solute required} = (\text{grams/mole})(\text{molarity})(\text{volume})$$

$$\frac{(111.0\text{ g})}{\cancel{\text{mole}}} \quad \frac{(0.800\ \cancel{\text{mole}})}{\cancel{\text{L}}} \quad (0.300\ \cancel{\text{L}})$$

**= 26.64 g = grams of solute required.**

Observe that the units cancel leaving the answer expressed in grams.

**BOX 12.4: Procedure to Make a Solution of a Particular Volume and Molarity**

Step 1. Find the FW of the solute.

Step 2. Determine the molarity required.

Step 3. Determine the volume required.

Step 4. Determine how much solute is necessary either by using proportions or Equation 12.1.

Step 5. Weigh out the amount of solute required as calculated in Step 4.

Step 6. Dissolve the weighed-out solute in less than the desired final volume of solvent.

Step 7. Place the solution in a volumetric flask or graduated cylinder and add solvent until exactly the right volume is reached.

**Notes:**

It is possible to calculate the FW of a compound by adding the atomic weights of its constituents. In practice, it is most common to find the FW by looking at the chemical container's label. This is the easiest method and avoids errors when the chemical is complex or comes in more than one form.

Compounds that come as liquids can be weighed out, but it may be easier to measure their volume with a pipette or graduated cylinder. Convert the required weight to a volume based on the density of the compound. (See Chapter 8 for a discussion of density.)

**Example Problem:**

How would you prepare 150 mL of a 0.010 M solution of $Na_2SO_4{\cdot}10H_2O$ using the procedure outlined in Box 12.4?

*Answer:*

Step 1: Find the solute's FW, preferably from the label on its container. FW is 322.04 g.
Step 2: Determine the molarity required. The molarity is 0.010 M.
Step 3: Determine the volume required. The volume is 150 mL, which equals 0.150 L.
Step 4: Determine how much solute is necessary:

**Strategy 1: Proportion method**

If it requires 322.04 g to make 1 L of a 1 M solution, then:

$$\frac{322.04\text{ g}}{1.000\text{ M}} = \frac{?}{0.010\text{ M}} \qquad ? = 3.2204\text{ g} = \text{solute to make 1 L of 0.010 M solution.}$$

To make 150 mL:

$$\frac{?}{150\text{ mL}} = \frac{3.2204\text{ g}}{1{,}000\text{ mL}} \qquad ? \approx \mathbf{0.4831\text{ g}} = \text{solute to make 150 mL of 0.010 M solution.}$$

**Strategy 2: Using Equation 12.1**

$$\text{Solute required} = (\text{grams/1 mole})\,(\text{molarity})\,(\text{volume})$$

$$\left(\frac{322.04\text{ g}}{1\ \cancel{\text{mole}}}\right)\left(\frac{0.010\ \cancel{\text{mole}}}{\cancel{\text{L}}}\right)(0.150\ \cancel{\text{L}}) \approx \mathbf{0.4831\text{ g}}$$

Step 5: Weigh out the amount of solute required, that is, 0.4831 g, of $Na_2SO_4{\cdot}10H_2O$.
Step 6: Dissolve the solute in less than the final volume of solvent.
Step 7: In a volumetric flask or graduated cylinder, add solvent to 150 mL.

**Example Problem:**

How many moles of NaCl are present in 50 mL of a 0.2 M NaCl solution?

*Answer:*

This is a variant of the more common problem of calculating how many grams of solute are needed to make a solution of a particular molarity and volume. It is solved by remembering the definitions of molarity and moles. By definition, a 0.2 M solution of a particular solute has 0.2 moles of that solute per liter. If there are 0.2 moles in 1 L, how many moles are contained in 50 mL (0.050 L)?

$$\frac{0.2\text{ moles}}{1\text{ L}} = \frac{?}{0.050\text{ L}} \qquad ? = \mathbf{0.01\text{ moles}}$$

## Practice Problems

*Assume purified water is the solvent for all questions.*

1. ***If you have 3 L of a solution of potassium chloride at a concentration of 2 M, what is the solute?__________ What is the solvent?________ What is the volume of the solution?_______ Express 2 M as a fraction. ____________***
2. ***Here are the FWs for three compounds often used in molecular biology:***
   ***NaCl, 58.44***
   ***Tris Base, 121.1***
   ***EDTA, 372.2***
   a. ***For each of these three compounds, how much solute is required to make 1 L of a 1 M solution?***
   b. ***For each of these three compounds, how much solute is required to make 0.5 L of a 1 M solution?***
3. ***How much solute is required to prepare 250 mL of a 1 molar solution of KCl? Atomic weight of K = 39.10, atomic weight of Cl = 35.45.***
4. ***How would you prepare 10 L of 0.3 M*** $KH_2PO_4$***? FW of*** $KH_2PO_4$ ***= 136.09.***
5. ***How much solute is required to make 600 mL of a 0.4 M solution of Tris buffer? FW of Tris base = 121.1.***
6. ***How would you make 500 mL of a 2 M solution of sodium hydroxide, NaOH? The reagent bottle is shown in Figure 12.5.***

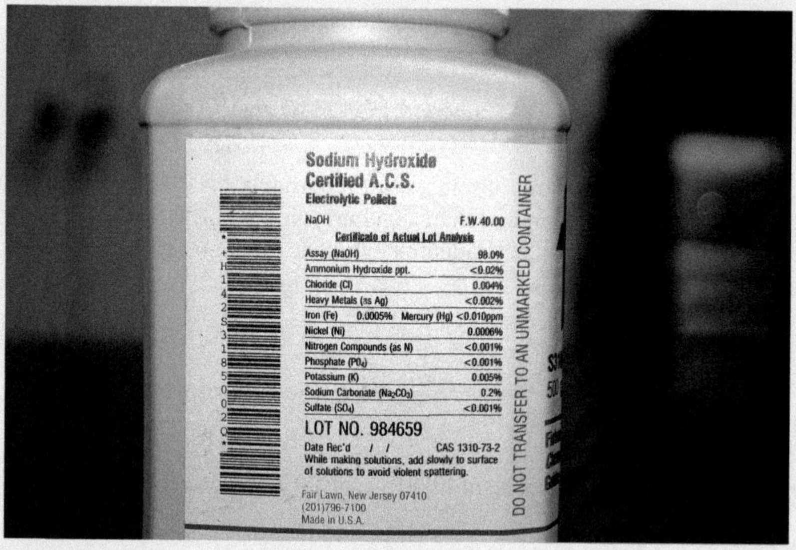


**FIGURE 12.5** Sodium hydroxide reagent bottle.

7. ***How would you make 250 mL of a 0.1 M solution of potassium phosphate, anhydrous, monobasic? The label from the reagent bottle is shown in Figure 12.6.***

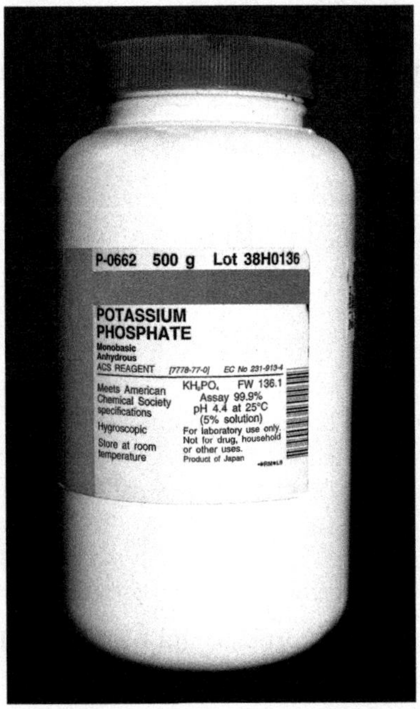


**FIGURE 12.6** Potassium phosphate reagent bottle.

## *Answers*

1. If you have 3 L of a solution of potassium chloride at a concentration of 2 M, what is the solute? potassium chloride What is the solvent? water (purified) What is the volume of the solution? 3 L Express 2 M as a fraction: $\frac{\text{2 moles of potassium chloride}}{\text{1 liter of solution}}$
2. a. By definition, 1 L of a 1 M solution of any compound contains 1 mole of that solute. One mole of NaCl is **58.44 g**, of Tris Base is **121.1** g, and of EDTA is **372.2 g**.
   b. 0.5 L of a 1 M solution of NaCl requires **29.22 g**, of Tris Base requires **60.55** g, and of EDTA requires **186.1 g.**
3. K = 39.10 g, Cl = 35.45 g. Therefore, the FW of KCl is: 39.10 g + 35.45 g = 74.55 g.
   Using Equation 12.1:

$$\left(\frac{74.55\text{ g}}{1\text{ }\cancel{\text{mole}}}\right)\left(\frac{1\text{ }\cancel{\text{mole}}}{\cancel{\text{L}}}\right)\left(\frac{0.250\text{ }\cancel{\text{L}}}{1}\right) = \textbf{18.64 g solute requir}$$

4. FW of $KH_2PO_4$ = 136.09 g.
   (136.09 g/mole) (0.3 mole/L) (10 L) = **408.27 g** = solute required.
   Dissolve the solute in <10 L of purified water and bring to the final volume.

5. Let us solve this using a proportion strategy: If 1 L of 1 M Tris buffer requires 121.10 g of solute, then 600 mL of 1 M solute requires:

$$\frac{?}{600\text{ mL}} = \frac{121.10\text{ g}}{1{,}000\text{ mL}} \qquad ? = \mathbf{72.66\text{ g}}$$

If 600 mL of 1 M Tris buffer requires 72.66 g of solute, then 0.4 M requires:

$$\frac{?}{0.4\text{ M}} = \frac{72.66\text{ g}}{1\text{ M}} \qquad ? \approx \mathbf{29.06\text{ g}}$$

6. From the label, we find that the FW is 40.00. Using Equation 12.1:

$$\left(\frac{40.00\text{ g}}{1\ \cancel{\text{mole}}}\right)\left(\frac{2\ \cancel{\text{mole}}}{\cancel{\text{L}}}\right)\left(\frac{0.5\ \cancel{\text{L}}}{1}\right) = \mathbf{40.00\text{ g solute requir}}$$

So take **40.00 g** of NaOH and bring to a volume of 500 mL with purified water.

7. From the label, we find that the FW is 136.1. Using Equation 12.1:

$$\left(\frac{136.1\text{ g}}{1\ \cancel{\text{mole}}}\right)\left(\frac{0.1\ \cancel{\text{mole}}}{\cancel{\text{L}}}\right)\left(\frac{0.250\ \cancel{\text{L}}}{1}\right) = \mathbf{3.4025\text{ g solute requir}}$$

So take **3.4025 g** of potassium phosphate and **BTV 250 mL**.

## Assorted Problems, Various Concentration Expressions

1. ***Underline the following that are expressions of concentration.***

| | | |
|---|---|---|
| *2% milk* | *34 mg/mL enzyme* | *12 teaspoons sugar* |
| *45 g NaCl* | *3 picomoles buffer* | *3 molar buffer* |
| *25 M Proteinase* | *K 75 ppm chlorine* | |

2. ***Which (if any) of the following solutions have the same concentration?***
   a. ***10 mg/mL*** b. ***1,000 g/L*** c. ***10 g/L*** d. ***0.01 µg/µL***
   e. ***10 µg/µL*** f. ***100 g/mL***
3. ***The density of B-mercaptoethanol is 1.1 g/mL. It comes as a liquid. If you need to add 5 g of this chemical to a solution, how much** <u>volume</u> **should you measure out?***
4. ***You have a solution of 100 µg/mL of the enzyme, Proteinase K.***
   a. ***You need 2 mg of enzyme, how much of the solution should you take?***
   b. ***You need 35 µg of enzyme, how much of the solution should you take?***
   c. ***You need 0.3 mg of enzyme, how much of the solution should you take?***
   d. ***You need 50 µg of enzyme, how much of the solution should you take?***

***For Problems 5–8:***

- Read each problem and identify those that are % type problems. Write % next to each. (Remember that for typical % problems, you do not need to know the FW of the solute to calculate how much of it is needed.)
- Read each problem below and identify those that are easily solved using a simple proportion and where you do not need to know the FW of the solute. Write PROPORTION next to these.
- Read each problem below and identify those that require you know FW of the solute to be solved. Write FW next to each such problem.
- Read each problem below and identify those that are ppm or ppb questions. Write PARTS next to these.

***Then, after identifying which type it is, solve each problem.***

5. ***How would you prepare 10 L of an aqueous solution of $AgNO_3$ of strength 0.1 mg $AgNO_3$ / mL?*** ***PROBLEM TYPE*** _________
6. ***Convert 50 ppm to g/L.*** ***PROBLEM TYPE*** _________
7. ***How would you prepare a 350 ppm solution of dioxin in water? (Dioxin is a by-product of industrial processes and is known to have adverse effects on organisms.)***
   ***PROBLEM TYPE*** _________
8. ***You are working in a microbiology laboratory. In order to make the medium in which to grow bacteria, you need 0.25 M NaCl (FW 58.44). How would you make 500 mL of this solution?***
   ***PROBLEM TYPE*** _________

### *Answers*

1. <u>2% milk</u> | <u>34 mg/mL enzyme</u> | 12 teaspoons sugar
   45 g NaCl | 3 picomoles buffer | <u>3 molar buffer</u>
   <u>25 M Proteinase K</u> | <u>75 ppm chlorine</u>
2. To determine which (if any) of the following solutions have the same concentration, convert all of them to the same units, for example, g/mL. **a, c, and e are the same.**
   a. 10 mg/mL = <u>0.01 g/mL</u> b. 1,000 g/L = 1 g/mL c. 10 g/L = <u>0.01 g/mL</u>
   d. 0.01 µg/µL = 0.01 mg/mL = 0.00001 g/mL e. 10 µg/µL = <u>0.01 g/mL</u>
   f. 100 g/mL
3. The density of B-mercaptoethanol is 1.10 g/mL. If you need to add 5 g of this chemical to a solution, how much <u>volume</u> should you measure out?

$$\frac{1.10\text{ g}}{1\text{ mL}} = \frac{5\text{ g}}{?} \qquad ? \approx \mathbf{4.55\ mL}$$

Or by unit canceling:

$$\left(\frac{5\ \not{\text{g}}}{1}\right)\left(\frac{1\text{ mL}}{1.10\ \not{\text{g}}}\right) \approx \mathbf{4.55\ mL}$$

4. a. $\frac{100\ \mu\text{g}}{1\text{ mL}} = \frac{2{,}000\ \mu\text{g}}{?} \qquad ? = \mathbf{20\ mL}$

   Or by unit canceling:

$$\left(\frac{2\ \not{\text{mg}}}{1}\right)\left(\frac{1{,}000\ \not{\mu\text{g}}}{1\ \not{\text{mg}}}\right)\left(\frac{1\text{ mL}}{100\ \not{\mu\text{g}}}\right) = \mathbf{20\ mL}$$

   b. $\frac{100\ \mu\text{g}}{1\text{ mL}} = \frac{35\ \mu\text{g}}{?} \qquad ? = \mathbf{0.35\ mL = 350\ \mu L}$

   c. $\frac{100\ \mu\text{g}}{1\text{ mL}} = \frac{300\ \mu\text{g}}{?} \qquad ? = \mathbf{3\ mL}$

   d. $\frac{100\ \mu\text{g}}{1\text{ mL}} = \frac{50\ \mu\text{g}}{?} \qquad ? = \mathbf{0.5\ mL = 500\ \mu L}$

5. $\frac{0.1\text{ mg AgNO}_3}{1\text{ mL}} = \frac{?}{10{,}000\text{ mL}}$ **? = 1,000 mg = 1 g PROBLEM TYPE** <u>proportion</u>
   Weigh out **1,000 mg = 1 g**, and **BTV of 10 L**

6. Convert 50 ppm to g/L. 50 ppm = 50 g/$10^6$ g (by definition)
   50 g/$10^6$ g = 50 g/$10^6$ mL (convert g water to mL)
   50 g/$10^6$ mL = 0.050 g/1,000 mL (divide both numerator and denominator by 1,000)
   **0.050 g/1 L** (rewrite 1,000 mL as 1 L) **PROBLEM TYPE** parts
7. How would you prepare a 350 ppm solution of dioxin in water?
   **PROBLEM TYPE** parts
   350 ppm = 350 g/$10^6$ mL (by definition, and convert g to mL)
   350 g/$10^6$ mL = 0.350 g/1,000 mL (divide numerator and denominator by 1,000)
   0.350 g/1 L (rewrite 1,000 mL as 1 L)
   Take **0.350 g** and **bring to a final volume (BTV) of 1 L**; other answers are possible if you plan for a different volume.
8. (0.25 moles/L) (58.44 g/mole) (0.5 L) = **7.305 g of NaCl BTV 500 mL PROBLEM TYPE** FW

## 12.6 VARIATIONS ON A THEME: MILLIMOLAR AND MICROMOLAR SOLUTIONS

The next sections deal with assorted concentration calculations that you will see in the biotechnology laboratory. Although these problems may seem unfamiliar at first, they are solved using the same strategies we have discussed so far in this chapter and are variations on the same themes.

A **millimole**, abbreviated mmol, *is 1/1,000 of a mole. A* **micromole**, abbreviated µmol, *is 1/1,000,000 of a mole.* If one millimole of a solute is dissolved in 1 L of solution, this is a **1 millimolar** solution, abbreviated 1 mM. Similarly, if 1 µmol of a solute is dissolved in 1 L of solution, this is a **1 µM solution**. Molecular biologists commonly work with solutions in the mM and µM ranges, and in fact, as we will see in Chapters 22–25, they also work with nanomolar and picomolar solutions.

Consider, as an example, the solute required to make 1 L of NaCl solution at various molar concentrations:

***1 M NaCl is 1 mole or 58.44 g of NaCl in 1 L of solution.***
***1 mM NaCl is 1 mmole or 0.05844 g of NaCl in 1 L of solution.***
***1 µM NaCl is 1 µmole or 0.00005844 g of NaCl in 1 L of solution.***

**Example Problem:**

How much solute is required to prepare 1 L of a 1 mM solution of $CuSO_4$?

*Answer:*

The FW of copper sulfate is 159.61 g. Therefore,

$$1\text{ mmole} = \frac{159.61\text{ g}}{1{,}000} = 0.15961\text{ g}$$

**So 1 L of 1 mM $CuSO_4$ requires 0.15961 g.**

You can also use Equation 12.1, but you must convert 1 mM to units of molar:

$$\text{Solute required} = (\text{grams/1 mole})(\text{molarity})(\text{volume})$$

$$= (159.61\text{ g/}\cancel{\text{mole}})(0.001\ \cancel{\text{moles}}/\cancel{\text{L}})(1\ \cancel{\text{L}}) \qquad ? = \mathbf{0.15961\ g}$$

**Example Problem:**

How many micromoles are there in 17.4 mg of NAD, FW 663.4? (NAD, nicotinamide adenine dinucleotide, is an organic compound that is important in metabolism.)

*Answer:*

Convert 17.4 mg to g. 17.4 mg = 0.0174 g.

Using a proportion, calculate how many moles are present:

$$\frac{1\text{ mole}}{663.4\text{ g}} = \frac{?}{0.0174\text{ g}} \qquad ? \approx 2.623 \times 10^{-5}\text{ moles}$$

Convert the answer in moles to micromoles by multiplying by $10^6$:

$$2.623 \times 10^{-5}\text{ moles} = \mathbf{26.23\ \mu moles\ NAD}$$

Or, by unit canceling:

$$\left(\frac{17.4\ \cancel{\text{mg}}}{1}\right)\left(\frac{1\ \cancel{\text{g}}}{1{,}000\ \cancel{\text{mg}}}\right)\left(\frac{1\ \cancel{\text{mole}}}{663.4\ \cancel{\text{g}}}\right)\left(\frac{10^6\ \mu\text{mole}}{1\ \cancel{\text{mole}}}\right) \approx \mathbf{26.23\ \mu moles\ NAD}$$

## 12.7 VARIATIONS ON A THEME: HYDRATES

***Hydrates** are compounds that contain chemically bound water.* (The bound water does not make the compounds liquid; they remain as powders or granules.) The weight of the bound water is included in the hydrate's FW. For example, calcium chloride can be purchased either as "anhydrous" (no bound water) or as a dihydrate. Anhydrous calcium chloride, $CaCl_2$, has a FW of 111.0. The dihydrate form, $CaCl_2{\cdot}2H_2O$, has a FW of 147.0 (111.0 g + the weight of two waters, 18.0 g each). When hydrated compounds are dissolved, the water is released and becomes indistinguishable from the water that is added as solvent.

**Example Problem:**

A recipe for preparing a calcium chloride solution calls for 11.1 g of anhydrous $CaCl_2$ to be dissolved in water to a final volume of 100 mL. You look in your chemical stockroom and find $CaCl_2 \cdot 2H_2O$, that is, calcium chloride dihydrate. The reagent bottle tells you that the FW of the hydrated calcium chloride is 147.0. It is not correct to use 11.1 g because the anhydrous and dihydrate forms are not the same. How can you prepare a calcium chloride solution that will have the concentration required for your recipe?

*Answer:*

**Strategy 1: Calculate the molarity required**

It is possible to determine the molarity of the calcium chloride solution that the recipe requires. Once you know the molarity required, you can determine how much of the hydrated form is needed.

To calculate the molarity required in the recipe, you must know the FW of the anhydrous calcium chloride. It must be 147.0 minus the weight of two waters, or $18.0 \times 2 = 36$.

$$147.0 - 36.0 = 111.0$$

This means that a 1 M solution of anhydrous $CaCl_2$ is 111.0 g/L. The recipe calls for 11.1 g in 100 mL.

$$\frac{11.1\text{ g}}{100\text{ mL}} = \frac{111.0\text{ g}}{1{,}000\text{ mL}} = 1\text{ M}$$

This means that the recipe is having you prepare a 1 M solution of $CaCl_2$.

Now, we can use Equation 12.1 to calculate how much of the hydrated form is required:

$$\text{Solute required} = (\text{grams/1 mole})(\text{molarity})(\text{volume})$$

$$? = (147.0\text{ g/mole})(1\text{ mole/L})\ (0.1\text{ L})$$

$$? = \mathbf{14.7\ g.}$$

This is how much you need to make your solution with the dihydrate form of calcium chloride. Dissolve this amount of the dihydrate and BTV 100 mL.

**Strategy 2: Using proportions**

Step 1: This problem can be solved with proportions, but to do so we must know the FW of both forms of calcium chloride. The FW of the dihydrate is 147.0 and of the anhydrous form is 111.0.

Step 2: You can now use a proportion to calculate how much dihydrate is required. You know you need 11.1 g of the form whose formula weight is 111.0, so how much is required of the form with the FW of 147.0?

$$\frac{11.1\text{ g}}{111.0} = \frac{?}{147.0} \qquad ? = \mathbf{14.7\ g.}$$

So use 14.7 g of the calcium chloride in your stockroom and BTV of 100 mL.

Observe that both strategies provide the same answer but using proportions is probably faster.

## 12.8 VARIATIONS ON A THEME: CONVERTING BETWEEN DIFFERENT CONCENTRATION EXPRESSIONS

Occasionally it is necessary to convert between one form of concentration expression and another. For example, you might be comparing two procedures to see if they are the same when the concentration of solutes in the required solutions is expressed differently.

**Example Problem:**

One solution recipe calls for 10% SDS. (SDS is a detergent commonly used in molecular biology procedures.) A second recipe calls for 0.5 M SDS. Are they the same? The FW of SDS is 288.37.

***Answer:***

$$\text{A 10\% solution of SDS has } \frac{10\text{ g SDS}}{100\text{ mL}} = \frac{100\text{ g SDS}}{1{,}000\text{ mL}} = \frac{100\text{ g SDS}}{\text{L}}$$

$$\text{A 0.5 M solution of SDS has } \frac{144.185\text{ g SDS}}{\text{L}}$$

So the two solutions do not have the same concentration of SDS.

**Example Problem:**

Convert 20% (w/v) NaCl to molarity. The FW of NaCl is 58.44

***Answer:***

20% NaCl = 20 g/100 mL = 200 g/1,000 mL = 200 g/L

By definition, 1 M of NaCl solution contains 58.44 g NaCl/L. If 58.44 g NaCl/L is 1 M, then what is the molarity of 200 g NaCl/L?

Using a proportion equation:

$$\frac{58.44\text{ g NaCl/L}}{1\text{ M}} = \frac{200\text{ g NaCl/L}}{?} \qquad ? \approx \mathbf{3.422\ M\ NaCl}$$

So for NaCl, a 20% solution is equivalent to a 3.422 M solution.

## 12.9 VARIATIONS ON A THEME: REAGENTS THAT ARE NOT PURE

**Example Problem:**

A particular recipe for medium used to grow bacterial cells calls for 500 μg/mL of G418 Sulfate. (G418 Sulfate is an antibiotic that will kill bacterial cells that are not resistant to it, leaving only resistant cells in the medium.) You are preparing a liter of growth medium but discover the following label on the G418 Sulfate bottle. How much of the antibiotic should you add? Will you have enough for 1 L of medium?

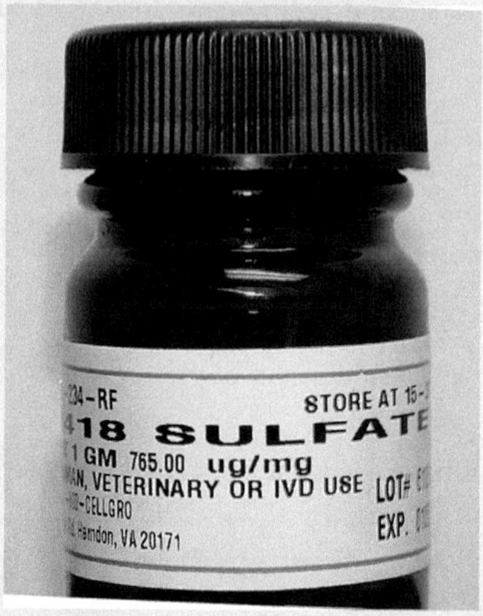


**FIGURE 12.7** G418 reagent bottle.

*Answer:*

From the label in Figure 12.7, we find that the bottle contains 1 g of antibiotic, but it is not pure. The label says "765 μg/mg," which means the bottle contains 765 μg of antibiotic in each mg of substance (the rest is an unidentified impurity). Sometimes each lot of a product will have a slightly different purity, and this will be indicated on the label or documentation that comes with the product.

In this case, your recipe calls for 500 μg/mL of antibiotic and you need 1,000 mL:

$$500\ \mu\text{g/mL} \times 1{,}000\ \text{mL} = 500{,}000\ \mu\text{g} = 0.5\ \text{g}.$$

If you just weigh out 0.5 g, you will not have enough antibiotic, because the material is not pure. You can use a proportion equation to calculate how much of the G418 Sulfate to weigh out:

$$\frac{765\ \mu\text{g antibiotic}}{1\ \text{mg}} = \frac{500{,}000\ \mu\text{g antibiotic}}{?} \qquad ? \approx 653.59\ \text{mg} = \mathbf{0.65359\ g}$$

This means you need to add ≈ **0.654 g** of the antibiotic from this bottle to your medium. Observe that if the antibiotic were pure, you would only need 0.5 g of it. Since it is not pure, you need more. You will have enough, since there is one gram in the bottle.

**Practice Problems**

1. ***Write out what each of these abbreviations stands for:***
   a. *1 M* b. *1 mM* c. *1 mmol* d. *1 pmol*
   e. *1 μmol* f. *1 μM*
2. ***State whether each of the following expressions is a concentration or an amount:***
   a. *1 mole* b. *1 mmol* c. *1 mM* d. *1 picomole*
   e. $2.5 \times 10^{-3}$ *M* f. *1 M NaCl* g. *1 μmol NaCl*
3. ***1 mole = ____________ millimoles = ____________ micromoles***
4. ***1.5 μmol = ____________ mmol = ____________ mol***
5. ***Convert 25 mmol to units of:***
   a. *mol* b. *μmol*
6. ***A reaction mixture contains 100 mmol of DNA. How much does it contain in units of:***
   a. *mol* b. *μmol*
7. ***Here are the formula weights for three compounds often used in molecular biology:***
   *NaCl, 58.44*
   *Tris Base, 121.1*
   *EDTA, 372.2*
   a. ***For each of these compounds, how much solute is required to prepare 1 L of a 1 mM solution?***
   b. ***For each of these compounds, how much solute is required to prepare 500 mL of a 1 mM solution?***
8. ***How many micromoles are there in 150 mg of D-ribose 5-phosphate, FW = 230.11?***
9. ***How would you prepare 500 mL of 5 mM NaCl (FW = 58.44)?***
10. ***How many millimoles of solute are present in 150 mL of a 0.1 mM solution?***
11. ***A molecular biology solution contains 150 μg of dissolved enzyme in a total volume of 1 mL. Express this as a percent (w/v) enzyme solution.***
12. ***Determine the molar concentration of 100 g of NaCl per liter of solution (FW = 58.44).***
13. ***A recipe calls for you to make 500 mL of 20% solution of anhydrous*** $CuSO_4$ ***but your stockroom only has*** $CuSO_4 \cdot H_2O$***. How much of the hydrated form of copper sulfate do you need? FW for anhydrous*** $CuSO_4$ ***is 160, and for*** $CuSO_4 \cdot H_2O$***, it is 178.***
14. ***Suppose you are preparing a solution whose recipe calls for 25 g of*** $FeCl_3{\cdot}6H_2O$***. You look on the shelf in your laboratory and find anhydrous ferric chloride,*** $FeCl_3$***. What should you do? (The FW of the hydrated form is 270.3 and the FW of the anhydrous form is 162.2.)***
15. ***Convert 3 M NaCl to a percent (w/v) expression (FW = 58.44).***
16. ***Convert a concentration of 10 mg/mL glucose to an expression of molarity. The FW of glucose is 180.16.***
17. ***What molarity is a 25% solution of NaCl (FW = 58.44)?***
18. ***You are going to prepare 500 mL of a cell culture medium that requires 100 μg/mL of a particular antibiotic. Your antibiotic arrives from the manufacturer in a powder form and it is labeled 891 μg/mg. How much of the antibiotic powder should you add?***

*Answers*

1. a. 1 molar b. 1 millimolar c. 1 millimole d. 1 picomole
   e. 1 micromole f. 1 micromolar
2. State whether each of the following expressions is a concentration or an amount:
   a. 1 mole, amount b. 1 mmol, amount c. 1 mM, concentration
   d. 1 picomole, amount e. $2.5\times10^{-3}$ M concentration
   f. 1 M NaCl, concentration g. 1 µmol NaCl, amount
3. 1 mol = **<u>1,000</u> mmol = <u>1,000,000</u> µmol**
4. 1.5 µmol = $\mathbf{\underline{1.5\times10^{-3}}}$ **mmol** = $\mathbf{\underline{1.5\times10^{-6}}}$ **mol**
5. a. 25 mmol $= 25\times10^{-3}$ mol $= \mathbf{2.5\times10^{-2}}$ **mol**
   b. 25 mmol $= 25\times10^{3}$ µmol $= \mathbf{2.5\times10^{4}}$ **µmol**
6. a. 100 mmol $= 100\times10^{-3}$ mol $= \mathbf{1\times10^{-1}}$ **mol**
   b. 100 mmol $= 100\times10^{3}$ µmol $= \mathbf{1\times10^{5}}$ **µmol**
7. a. By definition, 1 L of a 1 mM solution of a compound contains 1 mmole of that compound. 1 mmole is 1/1,000 of a mole. So 1 L of a 1 mM solution of NaCl requires **0.05844 g**, of Tris Base requires **0.1211 g**, and of EDTA requires **0.3722 g.**
   b. 500 mL of a 1 mM solution requires: NaCl, **0.02922 g;** Tris Base, **0.06055 g;** EDTA, **0.1861 g**.
8. 150 mg = 0.150 g
   Using a proportion:
   $$\frac{1\text{ mole}}{230.11\text{ g}} = \frac{?}{0.150\text{ g}} \qquad ? \approx 6.52\times10^{-4}\text{ moles} = \mathbf{652\,\mu moles}$$
   Or by unit canceling:
   $$\left(\frac{150\ \cancel{\text{mg}}}{1}\right)\left(\frac{1\ \cancel{\text{g}}}{1{,}000\ \cancel{\text{mg}}}\right)\left(\frac{1\ \cancel{\text{mole}}}{230.11\ \cancel{\text{g}}}\right)\left(\frac{10^{6}\ \mu\text{mole}}{1\ \cancel{\text{mole}}}\right) \approx \mathbf{652\ \mu moles}$$
9. Using Equation 12.1:
   Convert 5 mM to units of molarity: 5 mM = 0.005 M
   Plug into Equation 12.1
   $$0.005\frac{\cancel{\text{mole}}}{\cancel{\text{L}}}\times\frac{58.44\text{ g}}{\cancel{\text{mole}}}\times0.5\ \cancel{\text{L}} = 0.1461\text{ g NaCl}$$
   Weigh out **0.1461 g and BTV 500 mL.**
10. A 0.1 mM solution by definition contains 0.1 mmole of solute/L. How much is present in 150 mL?
    $$\frac{0.1\text{ mmole}}{1\text{ L}} = \frac{?}{0.150\text{ L}} \qquad ? = \mathbf{0.015\ mmole}$$
11. There is 150 µg of dissolved enzyme in a total volume of 1 mL. To express as a percent (w/v) solution, convert this to g/100 mL:
    $$\frac{150\ \mu\text{g}}{1\text{ mL}} = \frac{15{,}000\ \mu\text{g}}{100\text{ mL}} = \frac{15\text{ mg}}{100\text{ mL}} = \frac{0.015\text{ g}}{100\text{ mL}}$$
    so this is a **0.015% w/v solution**
12. Determine the molar concentration of 100 g of NaCl per liter of solution.
    $$\frac{58.44\text{ g}/1{,}000\text{ mL}}{1\text{ M}} = \frac{100\text{ g}/1{,}000\text{ mL}}{?} \qquad ? \approx \mathbf{1.711\ M}$$

13. The recipe as written requires 100 g of $CuSO_4$ because:

$$\frac{20\text{ g}}{100\text{ mL}} = \frac{?}{500\text{ mL}} \qquad ? = 100\text{ g}$$

Set up a proportion to compensate for the different forms of copper sulfate:

$$\frac{100\text{ g}}{?} = \frac{160}{178} \qquad \mathbf{? = 111.25\,g}$$

so this is the amount needed of the hydrated form

14. To use the anhydrous form you will need to add <25 g. The MW of the hydrated form is 270.3 g and the MW of the anhydrous form is 162.2 g. To calculate how much of the anhydrous form to use, set up a proportion:

$$\frac{25\text{ g}}{?} = \frac{270.3}{162.2} \qquad ? \approx 15.0\text{ g}$$

Use **15.0** g of the anhydrous form instead of 25 g of the hydrated form.

15. Convert 3 M NaCl to a percent (w/v).
3 M NaCl contains 3×58.44 g per liter = 175.32 g/L

$$\frac{175.32\text{ g}}{1{,}000\text{ mL}} = \frac{?}{100\text{ mL}}$$ ? = 17.532 g per 100 mL, so this is a **17.532%** solution of NaCl.

16. Convert 10 mg/mL to units of g/L. Multiply the numerator and denominator by 1,000:

$$\frac{10\text{ mg}}{\text{mL}} = \frac{10\text{ g}}{\text{L}}$$

A 1 M solution of glucose contains 180.16 g per liter

$$\frac{180.16\text{ g/L}}{1\text{ M}} = \frac{10\text{ g/L}}{?} \qquad ? \approx \mathbf{0.0555\,M}$$

17. 25% = 25 g/100 mL of NaCl = 250 g/1,000 mL
1 M NaCl = 58.44 g/1,000 mL
Using a proportion, if 58.4 g/L is 1 M, then 250 g/L is 4.28 M.

$$\frac{58.44\text{ g/L}}{1\text{ M}} = \frac{250\text{ g/L}}{?} \qquad ? \approx \mathbf{4.28\ M}$$

Or, by unit canceling:

$$\left(\frac{250\ \cancel{\text{g}}}{1\text{ L}}\right)\left(\frac{1\text{ mole}}{58.44\ \cancel{\text{g}}}\right) \approx \frac{4.28\text{ mole}}{1\text{ L}} = \mathbf{4.28\ M}$$

18. For 500 mL, you need 100 µg antibiotic/mL×500 mL = 50,000 µg of antibiotic.
The product is not pure; use a proportion equation to calculate how much to add:

$$\frac{891\ \mu\text{g antibiotic}}{1\text{ mg powder}} = \frac{50{,}000\ \mu\text{g antibiotic}}{?}$$

? ≈ **56.12 mg** of impure form of antibiotic powder

# Preparing Laboratory Solutions That Contain More Than One Solute

13



## 13.1 THE $C_1V_1 = C_2V_2$ EQUATION

This chapter will be about preparing solutions with more than one component, but first, it is necessary to introduce the topic of dilutions. A **dilution** *is when one substance (often but not always water) is added to another to reduce the concentration of the first substance. The original substance being diluted may be called the* **stock solution**. *The diluting substance is called the* **diluent.** In a biotechnology setting, the diluent is almost always water or an aqueous solution (e.g., buffer). As a familiar example, to make orange juice from concentrate, you pour the concentrated orange juice into a pitcher and add three cans of cold water to it. The concentrated stock solution is the orange juice concentrate, the diluent is water, and the orange juice is the diluted material.

There are many times that dilutions are prepared in the laboratory. Of particular importance in this chapter, buffers for molecular biology are often made in a concentrated form and diluted. Another common example is antibiotics that are prepared and sterilized in a concentrated form and then are diluted when added to nutrient media (solutions in which cells are grown). Drugs are also often diluted to a proper dose before administration.

In this chapter, we primarily consider cases where the concentration of the stock solution and the desired concentration of the final solution are both known. The question is how much of the stock solution is required and how much diluent must be added to it. For example, suppose you have a liter of a 2 M stock solution of Tris buffer and you want to dilute some of it so that you have 100 mL of 1 M Tris. How much of the stock solution should you remove and how much diluent should you add? There is a very convenient formula, Equation 13.1, to do this calculation. It is:

DOI: 10.1201/9780429282744-15

**EQUATION 13.1: The $C_1V_1 = C_2V_2$ Equation**

**HOW TO MAKE A LESS CONCENTRATED SOLUTION FROM A MORE CONCENTRATED SOLUTION**

$$(\text{Concentration}_{\text{stock}})(\text{Volume}_{\text{stock}}) = (\text{Concentration}_{\text{final}})(\text{Volume}_{\text{final}})$$

This equation can be abbreviated:

$$C_1V_1 = C_2V_2$$

Box 13.1 outlines the procedure to use the $C_1V_1 = C_2V_2$ equation and the example problems below illustrate its application.

**BOX 13.1: Using the $C_1V_1 = C_2V_2$ Equation**

Step 1. Determine the concentration of the stock solution; this is $C_1$.

Step 2. Determine the volume of stock solution required. This is usually the unknown.

Step 3. Determine the final concentration required; this is $C_2$.

Step 4. Determine the final volume required; this is $V_2$.

Step 5. Insert the values determined in steps 1-4 into the formula and solve for the unknown.

Notes:

- Any unit can be used for volume, as long as the same units are used for $V_1$ and $V_2$. Any unit can be used for concentration, as long as the same units are used for $C_1$ and $C_2$.
- The $C_1V_1 = C_2V_2$ equation is used when calculating how to prepare a LESS CONCENTRATED SOLUTION FROM A MORE CONCENTRATED SOLUTION. Do not use this equation when dilutions are not involved.

**Example Problem:**

How would you prepare 100 mL of a 1 M solution of Tris buffer from a 2 M stock of Tris buffer?

***Answer:***

Consider first, is this a situation where a less concentrated solution is being made from a more concentrated solution? Yes. Therefore, it is appropriate to apply the $C_1V_1 = C_2V_2$ equation:

Step 1: Concentrated solution = 2 M = $C_1$
Step 2: The volume of concentrated stock necessary is ? (the unknown)
Step 3: The concentration you want to prepare is 1 M = $C_2$
Step 4: The volume you want to prepare is 100 mL = $V_2$
Step 5: Substituting into Equation 13.1:

$$C_1V_1 = C_2V_2$$

$$2\,\text{M}(?) = 1\,\text{M}(100\,\text{mL})$$

$$2\,\text{M}(?) = 100\,\text{M}(\text{mL})$$

$$? = \frac{100\,\cancel{\text{M}}\,(\text{mL})}{2\,\cancel{\text{M}}}$$

$$? = \mathbf{50\ mL}$$

Take **50 mL** of the concentrated stock solution and **bring to volume (BTV) 100 mL**.

Observe that the units of concentration match (M) and the units of volume match (mL).

**Example Problem:**

The technician in Figure 13.1 has a stock solution of a buffer that is labeled "50X." This is an expression that we have not encountered previously. In this expression, the "**X**" means "*times.*" In this picture, the stock solution is 50 times more concentrated than the usual concentration for this buffer. (One reason that stock solutions are made is that some solutions are very stable when stored in a concentrated form. Also, concentrated solutions are convenient because they take up less room on the shelf than diluted ones.) In this problem, the technician needs 3 L of the buffer at a concentration of "1X." 1X is the normal concentration for this buffer. How should she prepare it?

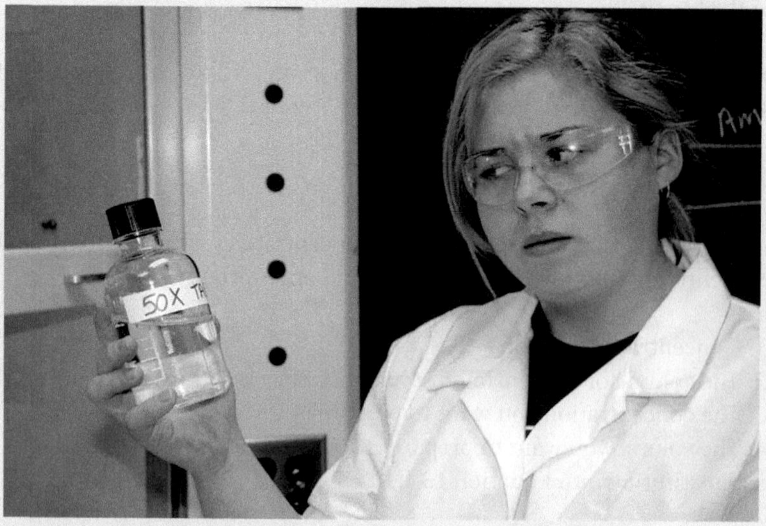


**FIGURE 13.1** Sometimes solutions are prepared in a concentrated form.

*Answer:*

This is a dilution problem. Decide volume needed, 3 L.

$$\text{Use } C_1V_1 = C_2\,V_2 \text{ equation}$$

$$(50X)(?) = (1X)(3{,}000\text{ mL})$$

$$? = \mathbf{60\text{ mL}}$$

Take **60 mL** of the concentrated stock and **bring to a final volume of 3,000 mL**.

**Example Problem:**

Promega Corporation (a company that sells products for molecular biology) provides a particular reagent, STR buffer, as part of a kit that is used to produce a "DNA Fingerprint" of DNA from a crime scene. The reagent is supplied as 10X, meaning that it is a stock that is 10 times more concentrated than it will be when used in the laboratory. Based on the information in the following table, what is the concentration of STR buffer in the final reaction mixture? (Observe that in this situation we know the initial and final volumes and the final concentration is the unknown.)

| PCR Master Mix Component | Volume per Sample (μL) | Number of Reactions | Final Volume (μL) |
|---|---|---|---|
| Sterile water | 17.30 | | |
| STR 10X buffer | 2.50 | | |
| Multiplex 10X primer pair mix | 2.50 | | |
| Taq DNA polymerase (at 5 U/μL) | 0.20 (1 U) | | |
| Total volume | 22.50 | | |

*Answer:*

The initial concentration is 10X; this is $C_1$. The total volume is 22.50 µL; this is $V_2$. 2.50 µL of stock is used for each reaction; this is $V_1$. The unknown is $C_2$. Substituting into the equation:

$$C_1V_1 = C_2V_2$$

$$(10X)(2.50\,\mu L) = ?(22.50\,\mu L)$$

$$? \approx \mathbf{1.11X}$$

**Practice Problems**

1. ***Suppose you start with 5X solution A and you want a final volume of 10 µL of 1X solution A. How much solution A do you need?***
2. ***How would you mix 75 mL of 95% ethanol if you have 250 mL of 100% ethanol?***
3. ***How would you mix 25 mL of 35% acetic acid from 25% acetic acid?***
4. ***If you have only 65 mL of 0.3 M $Na_2SO_4$, how much 0.1 mM solution can you make?***
5. ***If you have a liter of 75% ethanol, how much will you need to use to make 300 mL of 20% ethanol?***
6. ***If you have 65 µL of 0.3 M sodium sulfate, how much 0.1 mM solution can you make?***
7. ***If you have 100 mL of 10X buffer A, how could you prepare 450 mL of 1X buffer A?***
8. a. ***How would you prepare a 2 M stock solution of NaCl? FW is 58.44.***
   b. ***How would you use this NaCl stock to prepare a 100 mM solution of NaCl?***
9. ***You are going to make a series of standard solutions, each of which contains a specific amount of the protein, bovine serum albumin, BSA. (BSA is often used as a standard in protein assays.) To do this, you begin with a stock solution of BSA at a concentration of 2 mg/mL. Use the $C_1V_1 = C_2V_2$ equation to calculate how to dilute this stock solution to make 400 µL of each of the following standards.***
   a. ***50 µg/mL*** b. ***100 µg/mL*** c. ***200 µg/mL*** d. ***300 µg/mL***
10. ***You are going to make a series of standard solutions of reagent A. The stock solution has a concentration of 1 mg/mL. The total volume needed is 1 mL. Fill in the table below to show how the stock will be diluted to make the various standards.***

| Standard Number | Concentration of Standard (µg/mL) | Amount of Stock Solution Required | Amount of Diluent Required |
|---|---|---|---|
| 1 | 30 | | |
| 2 | 50 | | |
| 3 | 60 | | |
| 4 | 80 | | |

*Answers*

1. $C_1 V_1 = C_2 V_2$

$$(5X)(?) = (1X)(10\,\mu L)$$

$$? = \frac{(1X)(10\,\mu L)}{5X}$$

$$? = \mathbf{2\,\mu L}$$

So you need 2 μL of compound A.

2. $C_1 V_1 = C_2 V_2$

$$(100\%)(?) = (95\%)(75\,mL)$$

$$? = \mathbf{71.25\,mL}$$

Take **71.25 mL** of 100% ethanol **and BTV 75 mL**. (The number 250 in the problem is extraneous.)

3. You cannot make a more concentrated solution from a less concentrated one.

4. $C_1 V_1 = C_2 V_2$

$$(0.3\,M)(65\,mL) = (0.0001\,M)(?)$$

$$? = 195{,}000\,mL = 195\,L$$

You can make quite a lot – **195 L!**

5. $C_1 V_1 = C_2 V_2$

$$(75\%)(?) = (20\%)(300\,mL)$$

$$? = \mathbf{80\,mL}$$

6. $C_1 V_1 = C_2 V_2$

$$(0.3\,M)(65\,\mu L) = (0.0001\,M)(?)$$

$$? = 195{,}000\,\mu L = \mathbf{195\,mL}$$

7. $C_1 V_1 = C_2 V_2$

$$(10X)(?) = (1X)(450\,mL)$$

$$? = \mathbf{45\,mL}$$

**Use 45 mL of the 10× stock and BTV 450 mL**

8. a. How would you prepare a 2 M stock solution of NaCl? FW is 58.44.
   Decide how much to make, for example, 100 mL.
   Using Formula 12.1 from Section 12.5:
   (2 moles/L) (58.44 g/mole) (0.1 L) = **11.688 g**
   **Dissolve 11.688 g of NaCl and BTV 100 mL**

   b. How would you use this NaCl stock to prepare a 100 mM solution of NaCl?
   Decide how much to make, for example, 100 mL.

$$C_1 V_1 = C_2 V_2$$

$$(2\,M)(?) = (0.1\,M)(100\ mL)$$

$$? = \mathbf{5\,mL}$$

**Take 5 mL of the stock and BTV 100 mL**

9. a. $C_1 V_1 = C_2 V_2$

$$(2{,}000\ \mu g/mL)(?) = (50\ \mu g/mL)(400\ \mu L)$$

$$? = \mathbf{10\ \mu L}$$

So combine **10 µL** of BSA stock with **390 µL of diluent**. (It would be difficult to bring these to volume because of the small volumes required, rather, the required amount of diluent is calculated.)

b. Use **20 µL** of BSA stock and **380 µL of diluent.**

c. Use **40 µL** of BSA stock and **360 µL of diluent.**

d. Use **60 µL** of BSA stock and **340 µL of diluent.**

10. $C_1 V_1 = C_2 V_2$

$$(1{,}000\ \mu g/mL)(?) = (30\ \mu g/mL)(1{,}000\ \mu L)$$

$$? = \mathbf{30\ \mu L}$$

| Standard Number | Concentration of Standard (µg/mL) | Amount of Stock Solution Required (µL) | Amount of Diluent Required (µL) |
|---|---|---|---|
| 1 | 30 | **30** | **970** |
| 2 | 50 | **50** | **950** |
| 3 | 60 | **60** | **940** |
| 4 | 80 | **80** | **920** |

## 13.2 INTRODUCTION TO SOLUTIONS WITH MORE THAN ONE COMPONENT

Chapter 12 discussed how to prepare a solution containing a single solute. Now we extend the discussion to solutions with more than one solute. Table 13.1 shows three examples of recipes for solutions with more than one solute.

- Recipe I is relatively simple to interpret. It states the *amounts* of four solutes to weigh out and combine in water. The final volume of the solution is specified.
- Recipe II also states how much of each solute is required; however, the solutes are prepared as individual solutions before being combined. To prepare Recipe II, first make a 1 M solution of $MgCl_2$, a 0.4% solution of thymidine, and a 20% solution of glucose. Then, mix 5 mL of the $MgCl_2$ solution, 10 mL of the thymidine solution, and 25 mL of the glucose solution. Additional water is not added to the mixture of the three solutes in this example.
- Recipe III is different in that it does not state the *amount* of each solute required. Rather, the recipe states the *final concentration* of each solute. If the recipe or procedure gives only the final concentration(s) needed for the solute(s), you will have to

**TABLE 13.1 Examples of Three Laboratory Solutions That Contain More than One Solute**

| Recipe I | | Recipe II | | Recipe III |
|---|---|---|---|---|
| $Na_2HPO_4$ | 6 g | 1 M $MgCl_2$ | 5 mL | 0.1 M Tris |
| $KH_2PO_4$ | 3 g | 0.4% thymidine | 10 mL | 0.01 M EDTA |
| NaCl | 0.5 g | 20% glucose | 25 mL | 1% SDS |
| $NH_4Cl$ | 1 g | | | |
| Dissolve in purified water and BTV 1 L | | | | |

*calculate the amount(s)* you need of each. The reason authors often record concentrations instead of amounts is they do not know what volume you will need. Recipes like Recipe III are discussed in this chapter.

## 13.3 EXAMPLE 1: SM BUFFER

Consider the following recipe for SM buffer, which is used in various molecular biology procedures:

***SM Buffer***

**0.2 M Tris, pH 7.5**
**1 mM $MgSO_4$**
**0.1 M NaCl**
**0.01% gelatin**

This is the entire recipe as it might appear in a manual. It contains four solutes. The recipe lists the final concentration of each solute; Tris is present in the final solution at a concentration of 0.2 M, $MgSO_4$ at a final concentration of 1 mM, and so on. The final volume of the solution is not given because the author does not know how much you need. Water is not listed as a component, but it is assumed that the solution will be prepared in water. The first instinct people sometimes have when looking at a recipe like this is to prepare four separate solutions of 0.2 M Tris, 1 mM magnesium sulfate, 0.1 M NaCl, and 0.01% gelatin and then to mix them together; however, this instinct is wrong. If you combine any volume of 0.2 M Tris with any volume of 1 mM $MgSO_4$ or any of the other solutes, they will dilute one another, giving the wrong final concentrations.

Consider two correct strategies to prepare this solution.

### 13.3.1 STRATEGY 1: PREPARING SM BUFFER WITHOUT STOCK SOLUTIONS

In overview, decide what volume you want to make. Prepare 0.2 M Tris, but do not bring it to the final volume. You will need to adjust the pH of the Tris solution to 7.5, since that is specified in the recipe. Then, calculate how many grams of each of the other solutes are required to make the desired volume at the desired concentration. These solutes are weighed out and dissolved directly in the Tris buffer. The steps are:

**Step 1: Decide how much volume to prepare, for example, 1 L.**

**Step 2: Weigh out the Tris. One liter of 0.2 M Tris requires 24.22 g of Tris base (FW = 121.1).** Dissolve the Tris in about 700 mL of water and bring the pH to 7.5. Do not bring the Tris to volume yet.

**Step 3: Weigh out the NaCl. One liter of 0.1 M NaCl requires 5.844 g of NaCl** (FW = 58.44). Add this amount to the Tris buffer.

**Step 4: Weigh out the magnesium sulfate.** One liter of 1 mM $MgSO_4$ requires 1/1,000 of its FW. (Magnesium sulfate comes in more than one hydrated form. Read the label on the chemical's container to determine the correct molecular weight.) Weigh out the correct amount; add it to the Tris buffer. (For example, $MgSO_4 \cdot 7H_2O$ has a FW of 246.5. Add 0.2465 g of this form of $MgSO_4$.)

**Step 5: Weigh out the gelatin.** 0.01% gelatin is 0.1 g in 1 L. Weigh out 0.1 g of gelatin and add to the Tris buffer.

**Step 6: Stir the mixture until all the components are dissolved, then BTV of 1 L with water.**

**Step 7: Check the pH.** It is good practice to check the pH at the end; it should be close to 7.5 because the pH of Tris is fairly stable with dilution. Record the final pH, but do not readjust it, unless directed to do so by a procedure you are following.

Box 13.2 summarizes and generalizes this strategy for making a multicomponent solution without stocks. Box 13.3 shows a standard method of bringing a solution to the proper pH.

**BOX 13.2: General Procedure to Prepare a Multicomponent Solution without Stocks**

Step 1. Decide what volume to make.

Step 2. Weigh out and dissolve first component. Do not bring to volume yet.

Step 3. Adjust pH if necessary.

Step 4. Weigh out and dissolve the rest of components. Mix.

Step 5. Bring to volume.

Step 6. Check pH.

**BOX 13.3: General Procedure to Bring a Solution to the Correct pH Using a Strong Acid or a Strong Base**

Step 1. Determine the amount(s) of solute(s) required to get the correct concentration.

Step 2. Mix the solute(s) with most, but not all the solvent required. Do not bring the solution to volume yet.

Step 3. Place the solution on a magnetic stir plate, add a clean stir bar, stir, Figure 13.2

Step 4. Check the pH.

Step 5. Add a small amount of acid or base, whichever is needed to bring the solution to the desired pH. If the recipe does not specify which acid or base to use, it is usually acceptable to add HCl or NaOH. (Handle both with safety precautions.)

Step 6. Stir and recheck pH.

Step 7. Repeat steps 5 and 6 until the pH is correct.

Step 8. Bring the solution to the proper volume, recheck and record the pH.

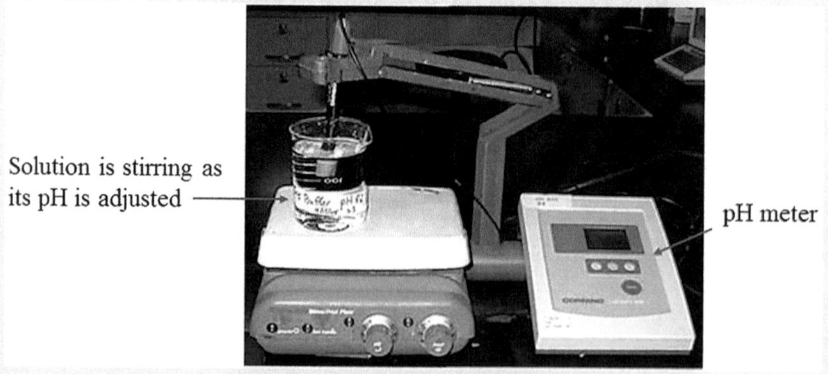


**FIGURE 13.2** Bringing a solution to the required pH.

**NOTES ABOUT ADJUSTING THE PH OF A SOLUTION**

- **Temperature:** pH the solution when it is at the temperature at which you plan to use it. Note also that some solutions change temperature during mixing. Restore the buffer to the correct temperature before making the final adjustment of its pH.
- **Overshooting the pH or the volume:** If you accidentally overshoot the pH or the volume, it is generally best to discard the solution and begin again to avoid inconsistencies in your solutions. For example, if you are adding HCl (an acid) to bring down the pH to 7.0 and you accidentally add too much HCl resulting in a pH below 7.0, then, discard the solution and begin again. Do not add base to bring the pH back up to 7.0. If you add base, you are changing the composition of the solution.

### 13.3.2 STRATEGY 2: PREPARING SM BUFFER WITH STOCK SOLUTIONS

In this strategy, the four solutes are each prepared separately as concentrated stock solutions. Then, when the four stocks are combined, they dilute one another to the proper final concentrations.

**Step 1: Prepare a stock solution of Tris buffer at pH 7.5.** There is no set rule as to what concentration a stock solution should be, other than it should be significantly higher than the concentration of the diluted solution. Also note that if you try to make a stock solution that is too concentrated, the solute will not totally dissolve. For the present problem, a useful concentrated stock solution might be 1 M (i.e., 5X, that is, 5 times more concentrated than needed). To make 1 L of 1 M stock, dissolve 121.1 g of Tris base in about 900 mL of water. Bring the solution to pH 7.5 and then to a volume of 1 L.

**Step 2: Prepare a stock solution of magnesium sulfate, for example, 1 M.** To make 100 mL of this stock, dissolve 0.1 FW of $MgSO_4$ in water and bring to a volume of 100 mL. (For example, $MgSO_4 \cdot 7H_2O$ has a FW of 246.5. Use 24.65 g of this form of $MgSO_4$.)

**Step 3: Prepare a stock solution of NaCl, for example, 1 M.** To make 100 mL of stock, dissolve 5.844 g in water and bring to a volume of 100 mL.

**Step 4: Prepare a stock solution of gelatin, for example, 1%,** by dissolving 1 g in a final volume of 100 mL of water.

**Step 5: Combine the right amounts of each stock to make the final solution.** Decide how much volume to make. Because this is a situation where concentrated solutions are being diluted, use the $C_1V_1 = C_2V_2$ equation four times, once for each solute. For example, to figure out how much Tris stock is required to make 1 L:

$$C_1V_1 = C_2V_2$$

$$(1\text{ M})(?) = (0.2\text{ M})(1{,}000\text{ mL})$$

$$? = \mathbf{200\text{ mL}}$$

Therefore, to make 1,000 mL of SM buffer, combine:

| Components | Final Concentration |
|---|---|
| **200 mL** of the 1 M Tris stock, pH 7.5 | 0.2 M Tris |
| **1 mL** of the 1 M magnesium sulfate stock | 1 mM $MgSO_4$ |
| **100 mL** of the 1 M NaCl stock | 0.1 M NaCl |
| **10 mL** of the 1% gelatin stock | 0.01% gelatin |

Sep 6: Place in a graduated cylinder or volumetric flask and bring to the final volume with purified water. Check the pH; it should be close to 7.5.

Box 13.4 summarizes and generalizes this procedure.

Both strategy 1 and 2 are correct. It is generally efficient to make stock solutions of solutes that are used often because weighing out chemicals is time consuming. For example, many solutions require NaCl; therefore, it might be useful to keep a 1 M stock solution of NaCl on hand. Chemicals that are infrequently used should not be kept as stock solutions because microorganisms can grow in them and they may slowly degrade. (Sterilizing solutions can sometimes extend their shelf life.)

**BOX 13.4: General Procedure to Prepare a Multicomponent Solution with Stocks**

Step 1. Decide what volume to make.

Step 2. Prepare concentrated stocks of each component.

Step 3. Use $C_1V_1 = C_2V_2$ equation to determine how much of each stock is required.

Step 4. Measure out the volumes of each component required, as determined in Step 3.

Step 5. Mix and bring to volume.

Step 6. Check pH.

## 13.4 EXAMPLE 2: TE BUFFER

Consider another example of a common biological solution:

*TE Buffer*

**Tris, pH 7.6 10 mM**
**$Na_2$-EDTA 1 mM**

This buffer contains Tris at a pH of 7.6 and a final concentration of 10 mM and $Na_2$-EDTA at a final concentration of 1 mM. As for SM buffer, it is incorrect to prepare 10 mM Tris buffer and 1 mM $Na_2$-EDTA and then to mix them together because they will dilute one another. It is conventional to prepare TE buffer by combining stock solutions of Tris, at the desired final pH, and $Na_2$-EDTA. (For example, this strategy is outlined in: Sambrook, et al. *Molecular Cloning: A Laboratory Manual,* 2nd ed. Cold Spring Harbor Laboratory Pr, 1989.)

To make TE buffer:

**Step 1: Decide how much volume of TE to prepare, for example, 100 mL.**

**Step 2: Prepare stock solution of sodium-EDTA**. $Na_2$-EDTA does not go into solution easily and is relatively insoluble in water if the pH is <8.0. Therefore, $Na_2$-EDTA is commonly prepared as a concentrated stock solution with a pH of 8.0. To make 100 mL of a 0.5 M stock of $Na_2$-EDTA, add 18.61 g of EDTA, disodium salt, dihydrate (FW = 372.2) to 70 mL of water. Adjust the pH to 8.0 slowly with stirring by adding pellets of NaOH or concentrated NaOH solution. When the $Na_2$-EDTA is dissolved, bring the solution to volume.

**Step 3: Prepare stock solution of Tris buffer**. The Tris buffer needs to be dissolved and brought to the proper pH before it is combined with the $Na_2$-EDTA. Like the $Na_2$-EDTA, the Tris should also be prepared as a concentrated stock solution (e.g., 0.1 M). To make 100 mL of 0.1 M Tris stock (FW = 121.1), dissolve 1.211 g of Tris base in about 70 mL of water, adjust it to pH to 7.6 with HCl, and then bring it to 100 mL final volume.

**Step 4: Use the $C_1V_1 = C_2V_2$ equation twice, once for each solute, to calculate how much of each stock will be required to make a solution of TE with the proper concentration of both solutes**. The desired volume of TE in this example is 100 mL.

To calculate how much 0.1 M stock of Tris is required:

$$C_1 \quad V_1 = C_2 \qquad V_2$$

$$(0.1\ \text{M})\,(?) = (0.001\ \text{M})\,(100\ \text{mL})$$

$$? = \mathbf{10\ mL}$$

(Note that the units must be consistent on both sides of the equation, so 10 mM was converted to 0.010 M.)

To calculate how much 0.5 M $Na_2$-EDTA stock is required:

$$C_1 \quad V_1 = C_2 \qquad V_2$$

$$(0.5\ \text{M})(?) = (0.001\ \text{M})\,(100\ \text{mL})$$

$$? = 0.2\ \text{mL} = \mathbf{200\ \mu L}$$

**Step 5:** Combine 10 mL of Tris stock and 200 µL of $Na_2$-EDTA stock and bring the solution to the final volume, 100 mL, with water.

**Step 6. Check the pH.**

## Practice Problems

1. *Suppose you have the following "recipe":*

| | |
|---|---|
| *5X buffer A* | *2 μL* |
| *Enzyme mix* | *2 μL* |
| *Reagent B* | *2 μL* |
| *Reagent C* | *3 μL* |
| *Water* | *1 μL* |

*What is the concentration of buffer A in this solution after it is mixed?*

2. a. *How would you prepare a stock solution of 2.0 M Tris buffer in water? (MW = 121.1) (Since the volume is unspecified, you can choose the volume.)*
   b. *How would you prepare a stock solution of 30% sodium dodecyl sulfate (SDS) in water (w/v)? (Again, since the volume is unspecified, you can choose a volume.)*
   c. *How would you use these stock solutions (as prepared in parts a and b) to prepare 100 mL of a solution containing:*

| *COMPONENT* | *FINAL CONCENTRATION* |
|---|---|
| *Tris buffer* | *1 M* |
| *SDS* | *10%* |

3. *Write a procedure to:*
   a. *First prepare stock solutions.*
   b. *Use these stock solutions to prepare 200 mL of breaking buffer.*

| *STOCK SOLUTIONS* | *BREAKING BUFFER* |
|---|---|
| *1 M Tris, pH 7.6* | *0.2 M Tris* |
| *1 M Mg acetate* | *0.2 M NaCl* |
| *1 M NaCl* | *0.01 M Mg acetate* |
| | *0.01 M β-mercaptoethanol* |
| | *5% (v/v) Glycerol* |

*Tris FW = 121.1*
*NaCl FW = 58.44*
*Magnesium acetate·4H$_2$O FW = 214.40*
*β-mercaptoethanol FW = 78.13, comes as a liquid, density = 1.1 g/mL*

*Notes:*

- **β-mercaptoethanol comes as a liquid. It can be weighed out in grams, but it is much easier to measure β-mercaptoethanol with a pipette. The density of β-mercaptoethanol is 1.1 g/mL. This means that 1 mL of β-mercaptoethanol weighs 1.1 g.**
- **Magnesium acetate comes as a tetrahydrate with four bound waters. The molecular weight given in the problem is for the tetrahydrate form**
- **Glycerol is a liquid. Assume the stock solution is 100%.**

4. *Write a procedure to prepare 100 mL of the following solution. Do not use stock solutions.*

*SOLUTION Q*
*100 mM Tris buffer, pH 7.5 (FW = 121.1)*
*2% NaCl*
*10 μg/mL Proteinase K*

5. *The following table shows the components that are combined when PCR is performed. (PCR, polymerase chain reaction, is a method of amplifying the amount of a specific sequence of DNA. PCR is described in more detail in*

***Chapter 24, so at this point, do not worry about the purpose of the components of this reaction.)***

| COMPONENT | VOLUME |
|---|---|
| 5X PCR reaction buffer | 10 μL |
| Nucleotide mixture, 10 mM each | 1 μL |
| Upstream primer | 1 μL |
| Downstream primer | 1 μL |
| PCR enzyme, 5 units/μL | 0.25 μL |
| DNA | 7 μL |
| Water | 29.75 μL |

a. ***What is the final concentration of reaction buffer in the reaction mixture?***

b. ***The nucleotide mixture consists of four nucleotides, each present in a stock solution at a concentration of 10 mM. What is the final concentration of each nucleotide in the reaction mixture?***

c. ***How many units of PCR enzyme are present in the reaction mixture? Note that this question does not ask for the final concentration of the enzyme.***

6. ***You have the following stock solutions:***

   ***1 M Tris buffer, pH 7.6***
   ***1 M $MgCl_2$***
   ***1 M DTT***

   ***How would you use these stock solutions to make 1 mL of 10X ligation buffer? The recipe for 10X ligation buffer is:***

   ***600 mM Tris, pH 7.6***
   ***100 mM $MgCl_2$***
   ***70 mM DTT***

7. ***Phosphate-buffered saline (PBS) is a commonly used reagent in many biotechnology applications. A recipe for its production is shown here. How would you make 1 L of this solution (without using stock solutions)?***

   ***PBS 1X pH 7.4***

| Component | Concentration | FW |
|---|---|---|
| NaCl | 0.137 M | 58.44 |
| KCl | 2.7 mM | 74.55 |
| $Na_2HPO_4$ | 0.01 M | 141.96 |
| $KH_2PO_4$ | 1.8 mM | 136.09 |

8. ***Finding the math. You are following a procedure from a manual. There is a list of materials required for the procedure, part of which is shown here:***

   ***Materials List***

   ***PBS:***

   ***137 mM NaCl***
   ***2.7 mM KCl***
   ***10 mM $Na_2HPO_4$***
   ***1.8 mM $KH_2PO_4$***

   ***ROCK inhibitor Y27632 (ROCK inhibitor is used to enhance the survival of cultured stem cells) Prepare a 10 mM stock solution by adding 3 mL sterile PBS to a 10 mg vial of ROCK inhibitor Y27632. Mix thoroughly.***

a. ***Based on this materials list, what solution(s) must you prepare?***

b. ***What solution(s) is (are) being prepared as a concentrated stock solution?***

c. ***Will you need to know the formula weights for any compounds? If so, which ones?***

d. ***A step in the procedure reads:***

   ***To a 15 mL conical tube, add 2 mL of culture medium with 10 μM ROCK Inhibitor Y27632.***

   ***Explain what you will need to do to complete this step.***

9. ***Solution recipes are sometimes written in sentence form, like this:***
***Reaction mix dye (10% glycerol, 0.5% SDS, 0.025% xylene cyanol, 0.025% bromophenol blue).***
***How would you prepare reaction mix dye? (Note that glycerol comes as a liquid, the other ingredients come as powders.)***

## *Answers*

1. What is the concentration of buffer A in this solution after it is mixed?
The total volume is 10 µL.

$$C_1 V_1 = C_2 V_2$$

$$(5X)(2\,\mu L) = (?)(10\,\mu L)$$

$$? = \mathbf{1X}$$

2. a. How would you prepare a stock solution of 2.0 M Tris buffer in water? (MW=121.1) For example, for 1 L, weigh out **242.2 g Tris, BTV 1 L.**
b. How would you prepare a stock solution of 30% SDS in water (w/v)?
For example, for 100 mL weigh out **30 g SDS, BTV 100 mL.**
c. To use these stock solutions (as prepared in parts a and b) to prepare 100 mL of solution containing the proper final concentration, use the $C_1V_1 = C_2V_2$ equation twice, once for each solute:

**Tris**

$$C_1 V_1 = C_2 V_2$$

$$(2\,M)(?) = (1\,M)(100\,mL)$$

$$? = \mathbf{50\,mL}$$

**SDS**

$$C_1 V_1 = C_2 V_2$$

$$(30\%)(?) = (10\%)(100\,mL)$$

$$? = \mathbf{33.33\,mL}$$

| COMPONENT | FINAL CONCENTRATION | STOCK TO USE |
|---|---|---|
| Tris buffer | 1 M | 50 mL |
| SDS | 10% | 33.33 mL |

**Combine 50 mL of the Tris stock solution and 33.33 mL of the SDS stock and BTV 100 mL.**

3. STOCKS
1 M Tris (pH 7.6).
To make 1 L of stock, dissolve 121.1 g of Tris base in about 700 mL water. After the Tris is dissolved, bring it to pH 7.6 and then BTV 1 L.
1 M Mg acetate. To make 1 L of stock, dissolve 214.40 g of magnesium acetate (tetrahydrate) in water. Bring it to volume.
1 M NaCl. To make 1 L of stock, dissolve 58.44 g in water. BTV.

BREAKING BUFFER

| | To make 200 mL: |
|---|---|
| 0.2 M Tris | **40 mL of 1 M Tris pH 7.6** |
| 0.2 M NaCl | **40 mL of 1 M NaCl** |
| 0.01 M Mg acetate | **2 mL of 1 M Mg acetate** |
| 0.01 M β-mercaptoethanol | **142 μL** (see note below) |
| 5% Glycerol | **10 mL glycerol** |

BTV of 200 mL with purified water

You want 200 mL of a 0.01 M solution of β-mercaptoethanol, so you need 0.15626 g. You can use a proportion to figure out how many mL will contain 0.15626 g:

$$\frac{1.100\text{ g}}{1\text{ mL}} = \frac{0.15626\text{ g}}{?}$$

$? \approx 0.142$ mL = 142 μL Therefore, you need **142 μL** of β-Mercaptoethanol.

4. Write a procedure to prepare 100 mL of the following solution without using stock solutions.

   SOLUTION Q
   100 mM Tris buffer, pH 7.5
   2% NaCl
   10 μg/mL Proteinase K

   For 100 mL of 100 mM Tris solution (FW 121.1), weigh out 1.211 g of Tris base. Dissolve in about 60 mL of water and adjust the pH to 7.5. Do not BTV yet.
   100 mL of 2% NaCl requires 2 g, add to the Tris solution.
   10 μg Proteinase K/mL × 100 mL = 1,000 μg = 1 mg, weigh and add to the Tris solution.
   Dissolve all the components and BTV 100 mL. Check pH.

5. a. What is the final concentration of reaction buffer in the reaction mixture?

$$C_1 V_1 = C_2 V_2$$

$$(5\text{X})(10\,\mu\text{L}) = (?)(50\,\mu\text{L})$$

$$? = \mathbf{1X}$$

   b. What is the final concentration of each nucleotide in the reaction mixture?

$$C_1 V_1 = C_2 V_2$$

$$(10\text{ mM})(1\,\mu\text{L}) = ?(50\,\mu\text{L})$$

$$? = \mathbf{0.2\text{ mM}}$$

   c. How many units of PCR enzyme are present in the reaction mixture

$$(5\text{ units}/\mu\text{L})\ (0.25\,\mu\text{L}) = \mathbf{1.25\text{ units}}$$

6. Use the $C_1V_1 = C_2V_2$ equation three times, once for each solute:

| Use | |
|---|---|
| 1 M Tris stock 0.600 mL | = **600 µL** |
| 1 M $MgCl_2$ stock 0.100 mL | = **100 µL** |
| 1 M DTT stock 0.070 mL | = **70 µL** |
| water | **230 µL** |
| | **1,000 µL** |

(A solution with such a low volume is usually not "brought to volume," rather the right amount of water is calculated to reach the correct volume.)

7. The amounts of each component are shown here:

| Component | Concentration | FW | Amount Required |
|---|---|---|---|
| NaCl | 0.137 M | 58.44 | **8.0063 g** |
| KCl | 2.7 mM | 74.55 | **0.2013 g** |
| $Na_2HPO_4$ | 0.01 M | 141.96 | **1.4196 g** |
| $KH_2PO_4$ | 1.8 mM | 136.09 | **0.2450 g** |

To prepare the solution:

Step 1: Add the required amount of each chemical to about 800 mL of purified water in a suitable container.

Step 2: Mix well.

Step 3: Adjust the solution to pH 7.4.

Step 4: Bring the solution to 1,000 mL with purified water.

8. a. Based on this materials list, you must prepare two solutions: PBS and ROCK inhibitor.

   b. ROCK inhibitor is prepared as a concentrated stock solution at a concentration of 10 mM. The directions say to prepare this by combining a 10 mg vial of ROCK inhibitor with 3 mL of sterile PBS.

   c. You will need formula weights for all four components of PBS.

   d. A step in the procedure reads:

   "To a 15 mL conical tube, add 2 mL of culture medium with 10 µM ROCK Inhibitor Y27632."

   To complete this step, you need to add the right amount of the ROCK inhibitor stock solution to 2 mL of culture medium. This is a $C_1V_1 = C_2V_2$ problem:

$$10 \text{ mM} = 10{,}000 \ \mu\text{M}$$

$$C_1 \ V_1 = C_2 \ V_2$$

$$(10{,}000 \ \mu\text{M ROCK Inhibitor})(?) = (2 \text{ mL})(10 \ \mu\text{M ROCK Inhibitor})$$

$$? = 0.002 \text{ mL} = \mathbf{2 \ \mu L}$$

**So, combine 2 µL of ROCK Inhibitor with 2 mL of culture medium (technically, 1,998 µL of culture medium, but in practice this would be rounded to 2 mL) and put it into a 15 mL conical tube.**

9. Reaction mix dye (10% glycerol, 0.5% SDS, 0.025% xylene cyanol, 0.025% bromophenol blue).

   The first step in preparing reaction mix dye is to decide on a volume. Suppose you decide to make 100 mL. Then, you need **10 mL of glycerol, 0.5 g of SDS, 0.025 g of xylene cyanol, and 0.025 g of bromophenol blue**. These ingredients would be mixed into purified water and then the solution would be brought to 100 mL.

# Dilutions

# 14



## 14.1 INTRODUCTION

In Chapter 13, we introduced the $C_1V_1 = C_2V_2$ equation and showed how it is often used when preparing various buffers and other laboratory solutions. The $C_1V_1 = C_2V_2$ equation is a valuable calculation tool when performing dilutions, but there are situations where you will need additional ways to think about dilutions. This is partly because you will encounter varied terminology and varied strategies to describe and deal with dilutions in the scientific literature. It is important to understand what various authors mean when they discuss dilutions.

There are also times when the $C_1V_1 = C_2V_2$ equation provides an answer that is mathematically correct but is not practical. For example, suppose you have a suspension of bacterial cells at a concentration of $10^6$ cells/mL and you want to dilute them so that you have 5 mL of cells with a concentration of $10^1$ cells/mL. Substituting into the $C_1V_1 = C_2V_2$ equation:

$$C_1 \quad V_1 = C_2 \qquad\qquad V_2$$

$$(10^6 \text{ cells/mL})(?) = (10^1 \text{ cells/mL})(5\text{ mL})$$

$$? = 0.00005\text{ mL} = \mathbf{0.05\ \mu L}$$

This volume, 0.05 μL, is too low to accurately measure with normal measuring devices. It is therefore necessary to dilute this cell suspension using more than one step, as we will

DOI: 10.1201/9780429282744-16

demonstrate later in this chapter. In this situation, and in other situations as well, it is useful to have strategies in addition to the $C_1V_1 = C_2V_2$ equation to handle dilution calculations. This chapter therefore broadens our strategies for dealing with dilutions in a variety of situations.

## 14.2 INTRODUCTION TO DILUTION TERMINOLOGY

There are various ways to speak about dilutions; unfortunately, this variation in terminology can (and does) lead to confusion. Let us illustrate dilution terminology with an example. A baker buys a bottle of food coloring and dilutes it to decorate cookies. The baker takes 1 mL of the concentrated food coloring and adds 9 mL of water so that the total volume of the diluted food coloring solution is 10 mL, Figure 14.1a. Various people might refer to this same dilution using different terminology, Figure 14.1b.

Observe that the word **"to"** and the symbol **":"** are used inconsistently. Sometimes the word **"to"** or the symbol **":"** is used before the volume of the *diluting substance*, the **diluent**. (In this example, the diluent is 9 mL of water.) Other times, the word **"to"** or the symbol **":"** is used before the total volume of the final mixture. (In this example, the total volume of the final mixture is 10 mL.) The key to avoiding confusion is to keep track of whether you are talking about the *total volume of the final mixture* or about the *amount of diluting substance*. When reading what other people have written, try to determine what they mean.

In this book, the dilution terminology conforms to that suggested by the American Society for Microbiology (ASM). (*ASM Style Manual for Journals and Books*. American Society for Microbiology, 1991.) This terminology is logical and consistent, even when three or more substances are combined. This terminology is summarized in Box 14.1.

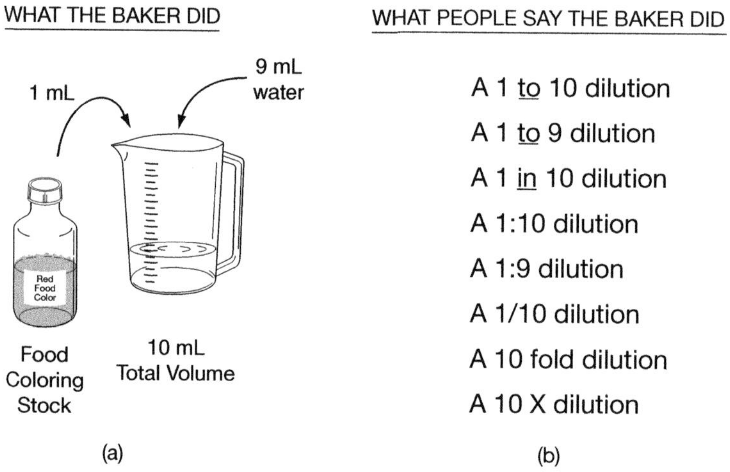


**FIGURE 14.1** Dilutions and terminology. (a) What the baker did. (b) What people say the baker did – using varied terminology.

**BOX 14.1: Dilution Terminology Based on ASM Recommendations**

1. **One part food coloring combined with nine parts water means the food coloring is one part in 10 mL total volume or 1/10 food coloring.** The denominator in an expression with a slash (/) is the total volume of the solution, never the amount of the diluting substance.
2. **An undiluted substance, by definition, is called 1/1.**
3. **When talking about dilutions, the symbol ":" means parts. If 1 mL of food coloring is combined with 9 mL of water,** that is one part food coloring plus nine parts water or 1:9 food coloring to water. In this text, a dilution of one part plus nine parts diluent is not referred to as a 1:10 dilution (unless we are demonstrating how other people describe dilutions).

For example,

A **1:2 dilution** *means there are THREE parts total volume.*

A $\frac{1}{2}$ **dilution** *means there are TWO parts total volume.*

**Therefore,**

**½ is the same as 1:1.**

**1:2 is the same as 1/3.**

**1:3:5 A:B:C means that one part A, three parts B, and five parts C are combined for a total of nine parts.**

*(The parts can be any unit as long as they are all the same. For example, the last expression might mean 1 mL of A, 3 mL of B, and 5 mL of C. Or, it might mean 1 g of A, 3 g of B, and 5 g of C, and so on.)*

**Practice Problems**

*(Follow ASM recommendations.)*

1. ***Suppose you dilute 1 oz of orange juice concentrate with 3 oz of water.***
   a. ***Express this dilution using the word "in."***
   b. ***Express this dilution using the word "to."***
   c. ***Express this dilution with a ":" and then with a "/."***
2. ***Express each of the following as a dilution (using a /).***
   a. ***1 mL of original sample + 9 mL of water***
   b. ***1 mL sample + 10 mL water***
   c. ***3 mL sample in a total volume of 30 mL***
   d. ***3 mL sample + 27 mL water***
   e. ***0.5 mL sample + 11.0 mL water***
3. ***Express each of the following as a dilution (using a /).***
   a. ***one part sample: nine part diluent***
   b. ***one part sample: ten parts diluent***
   c. ***1:3*** d. ***1:1*** e. ***1:4***
4. ***Express each of the dilutions in problem 2 as a 1:____.***

*Answers*

1. a. One part orange juice in four parts total
   b. One part orange juice to three parts water  c. **1:3 or ¼**
2. a. 1 mL/10 mL = **1/10**  b. 1 mL/11 mL = **1/11**
   c. 3 mL/30 mL = **1/10**  d. 3 mL/30 mL = **1/10**
   e. 0.5 mL/11.5 mL = 0.5/11.5 = **1/23**
3. a. **1/10**  b. **1/11**  c. **1/4**  d. **1/2**  e. **1/5**
4. a. **1:9**  b. **1:10**  c. 3:27 or **1:9**
   d. 3:27 or **1:9**  e. 0.5:11 or **1:22**

## 14.3 DILUTION EXPRESSED AS A FRACTION

Suppose that 1 mL of a stock solution is removed and is diluted with 9 mL of buffer. This is a 1 mL/10 mL dilution, which equals a 1/10 dilution (the units cancel). We will refer to "1/10" as the **dilution,** expressed as a fraction. Dilutions have no units because the units in the numerator and the denominator are the same and cancel. Figure 14.2 shows a series of dilutions. What is the dilution, expressed as a fraction, for each?

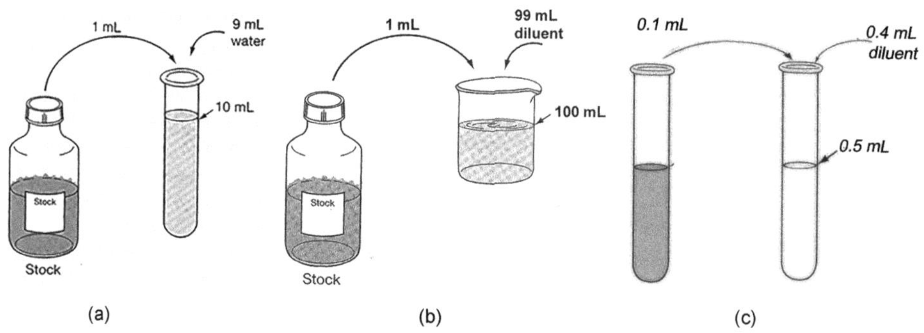


**FIGURE 14.2** Dilutions. (a) A 1/10 dilution. (b) A 1/100 dilution. (c) A 1/5 dilution.

**Practice Problems**

***What is the dilution, expressed as a fraction, for each of these dilutions?***

1. ***1 mL of stock is removed and combined with 4 mL of water.***
2. ***1 mL of stock is removed and combined with 9 mL of buffer.***
3. ***2 mL of stock is removed and combined with 8 mL of buffer.***
4. ***35 mL of stock is removed and combined with 65 mL of buffer.***
5. ***You take 1 mL of a solution and add 99 mL of diluent.***
6. ***0.1 mL of stock is removed and combined with 9.9 mL of water.***
7. ***1 mL of stock is removed and combined with 10 mL of buffer.***
8. ***250 mL of stock is combined with buffer to give a total volume of 1,000 mL.***
9. ***You take 0.5 mL of a solution and add 4.5 mL of diluent.***
10. ***You take 1 mL of a solution and add 8 mL of diluent.***

*Answers*

| | | |
|---|---|---|
| 1. 1 mL/5 mL = **1/5** | 2. **1/10** | 3. 2/10 = **1/5** |
| 4. 35/100 = **7/20** | 5. **1/100** | 6. 0.1/10 = **1/100** |
| 7. **1/11** | 8. 250/1,000 = **1/4** | 9. 0.5/5 = **1/10** |
| 10. **1/9** | | |

## 14.4 DILUTIONS AND PROPORTIONAL RELATIONSHIPS

The concepts of dilution and proportion are related. For example,

**1 mL of food coloring mixed with 9 mL of water is equivalent to a dilution of 10 mL of food coloring mixed with 90 mL of water.**

$$\frac{\textbf{1 mL}}{\textbf{10 mL}} = \frac{\textbf{10 mL}}{\textbf{100 mL}} = \frac{\textbf{1}}{\textbf{10}}$$

$$\textbf{1 mL in 10 mL total} = \textbf{10 mL in 100 mL total} = \textbf{1 / 10 dilution}$$

Similarly, all the following are equivalent to 1/10 dilutions:

| | | |
|---|---|---|
| **2 mL food coloring** | **100 μL enzyme solution** | **17 fluid ounces juice** |
| **+ 18 mL water** | **+ 900 μL buffer solution** | **+ 153 fluid ounces water** |
| **20 mL total volume** | **1000 μL total volume** | **170 fluid ounces total** |
| $\frac{\textbf{2 mL}}{\textbf{20 mL}} = \frac{\textbf{1}}{\textbf{10}}$ | $\frac{\textbf{100 μL}}{\textbf{1,000 μL}} = \frac{\textbf{1}}{\textbf{10}}$ | $\frac{\textbf{17 oz}}{\textbf{170 oz}} = \frac{\textbf{1}}{\textbf{10}}$ |

### DILUTION PRACTICALITIES

There are often multiple strategies for diluting substances all of which are equivalent mathematically, but some of which are impractical in the laboratory. For example, removing 1 μL of stock solution and adding 9 μL of diluent is numerically equivalent to diluting 1 L of stock solution with 9 L of diluent. Both are 1/10 dilutions. But the two dilutions are not the same from a practical perspective. Keep in mind these considerations:

- **Measuring very small volumes:** Micropipettes are used to measure very small volumes. The finest of these devices will measure volumes down to 0.5 μL, but larger volumes, say, 5 μL, are easier to measure accurately. A dilution strategy that requires measuring <1 μL of solution is seldom practical.
- **Total volume of the dilution:** The final volume after dilution may be constrained by laboratory glassware, cost, or by storage considerations. A typical laboratory will have glassware for volumes up to 1 or 2 L, and buffers and other commonly used reagents are often diluted to these volumes; dilution volumes greater than a liter may be impractical. Antibodies and other expensive reagents

are often purchased, stored, and used in volumes in the order of microliters or a few milliliters. When the final volume must be low and a substance must be diluted by many orders of magnitude, use a dilution series (Section 14.8) rather than diluting a substance in one step with a large volume of diluent.

- There are times when the original stock is limited in quantity, which means that the first dilution is constrained. For example, if you have only 500 µL of a valuable antibody, your first dilution cannot be 1 mL of antibody + 9 mL of diluent.
- There are times that a certain volume of diluted substance is required. For example, if you need 3 mL of diluted material in each of five tubes to run a test, you need at least 15 mL of diluted material. In this case, a 1/10 dilution that is 1 mL stock + 9 mL of diluent will not provide enough material for all five tubes.
- **Mixing:** Thorough mixing of dilutions is critical. It requires care to ensure that a very small volume, for example, 1 µL, is entirely mixed into a much larger volume, say, 1 L.
- **Bringing to volume:** When aqueous solutions or suspensions are diluted with water, it is common practice to calculate the amount of diluent needed rather than bringing the solution to volume in a volumetric flask or graduated cylinder.

**Practice Problems**

1. ***Express each of the following dilutions as two equivalent fractions:***
   a. ***2 mL/10 mL***
   b. ***10 mL of stock solution and 90 mL of buffer***
   c. ***0.1 mL of stock and 9.9 mL of buffer***
   d. ***One pint of stock and nine pints of water***
   e. ***25 mL of stock and 225 mL of buffer***
   f. ***0.5 mL of stock and 9.5 mL of water***
2. ***If you take a 0.5 mL sample of blood and add 1.0 mL of water and 3.0 mL of reagents, what is the final dilution of the blood?***

*ANSWERS*

1. a. **2/10 or 1/5** b. **10/100 or 1/10** c. **0.1/10 or 1/100**
   d. **1/10 or 10/100** e. **25/250 or 1/10** f. **0.5/10 or 1/20**
2. Total volume: 0.5 mL blood + 1.0 mL water + 3 mL reagent = 4.5 mL. So dilution expressed as a fraction is **0.5/4.5 or 1/9**

## 14.5 CALCULATIONS FOR PREPARING A DILUTION WITH A PARTICULAR DILUTION AND A PARTICULAR VOLUME

### EXAMPLE 1: HOW COULD YOU PREPARE 10 ML OF A 1/10 DILUTION OF FOOD COLORING?

Proportions can be used to determine how to make this dilution. The desired dilution is 1/10 and the total volume is 10 mL. Using a proportion equation:

$$\frac{1}{10} = \frac{?}{10\text{ mL}}$$

$$? = \mathbf{1\ mL}$$

This means that you need 1 mL of food coloring, the stock. Then, to get the desired volume, you will need to add 9 mL of water, as illustrated in Figure 14.3.

## EXAMPLE 2: HOW COULD YOU MAKE 10 ML OF A 1/5 DILUTION OF FOOD COLORING?

Using a proportion equation:

$$\frac{1}{5} = \frac{?}{10\ \text{mL}}$$

$$? = \mathbf{2\ mL}$$

This means you would combine 2 mL of food coloring stock with 8 mL of water. The total volume will be 10 mL. Thus, the dilution will be 2/10 = 1/5. This is illustrated in Figure 14.4.

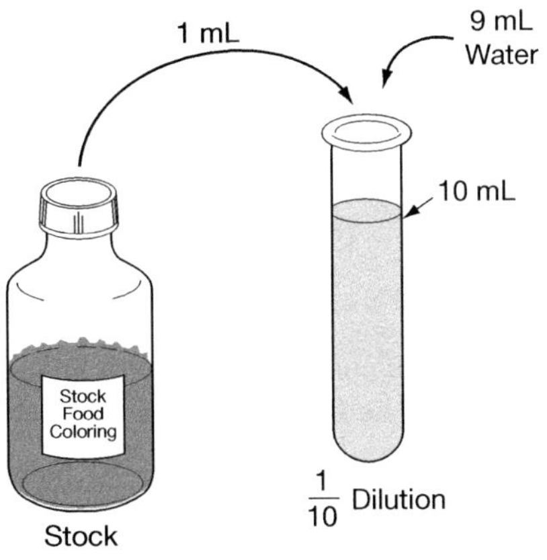


**FIGURE 14.3** Preparing 10 mL of a 1/10 dilution. Combine 1 mL of the food coloring with 9 mL of water. Observe that the total volume will be 10 mL and the dilution, expressed as a fraction, will be 1/10.

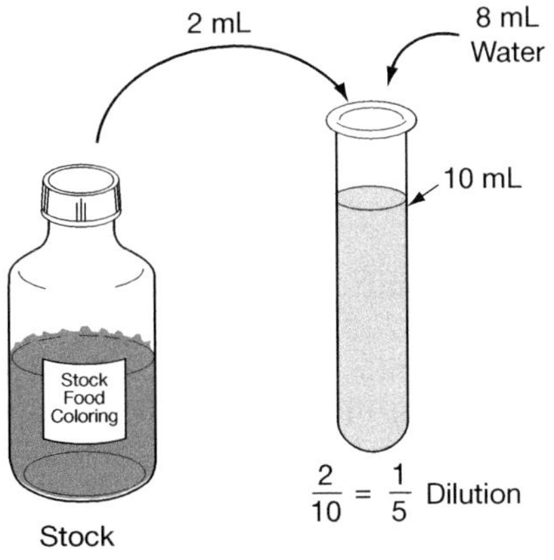


**FIGURE 14.4** Preparing 10 mL of a 1/5 dilution. Combine 2 mL of food coloring with 8 mL of water. The total volume will be 10 mL. Thus, the dilution, expressed as a fraction, will be 2/10 = 1/5.

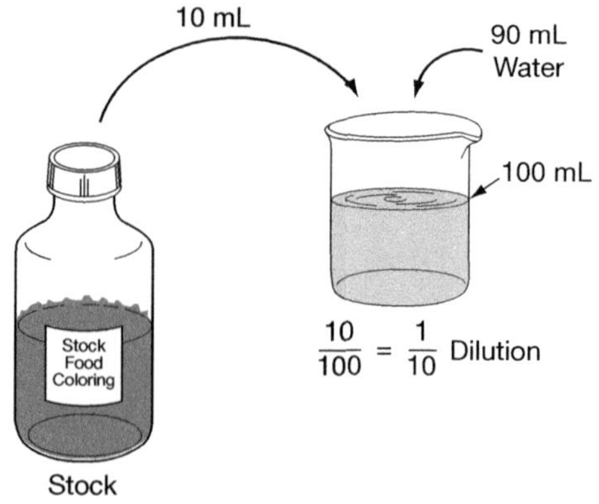


**FIGURE 14.5** Preparing 100 mL of a 1/10 dilution. Combine 10 mL of food coloring stock with 90 mL of water. The total volume will be 100 mL. Thus, the dilution, expressed as a fraction, will be 10/100, which is equivalent to 1/10.

## EXAMPLE 3: HOW COULD YOU MAKE 100 ML OF A 1/10 DILUTION OF FOOD COLORING?

$$\frac{1}{10} = \frac{?}{100\,\text{mL}}$$

$$? = \mathbf{10\ mL}$$

This means you combine 10 mL of food coloring stock with 90 mL of water. The total volume will be 100 mL. Thus, the dilution will be 10/100 = 1/10. This is illustrated in Figure 14.5.

## EXAMPLE 4: HOW COULD YOU MAKE 250 ML OF A 1/4 DILUTION OF FOOD COLORING?

This may be less obvious than the three examples above, but it can be easily solved using the logic of proportions:

$$\frac{1}{4} = \frac{?}{250\,\text{mL}}$$

$$? = \mathbf{62.5\ mL}$$

This means you need 62.5 mL of the food coloring stock. You will also need water. How much? The total volume required is 250 mL of which 62.5 mL will be food coloring stock. So the amount of water required is:

$$250\,\text{mL} - 62.5\,\text{mL} = 187.5\,\text{mL}$$

This is illustrated in Figure 14.6.

Proportions can thus be used to calculate how to make a particular volume of a specific dilution. We can summarize this procedure in Equation 14.1.

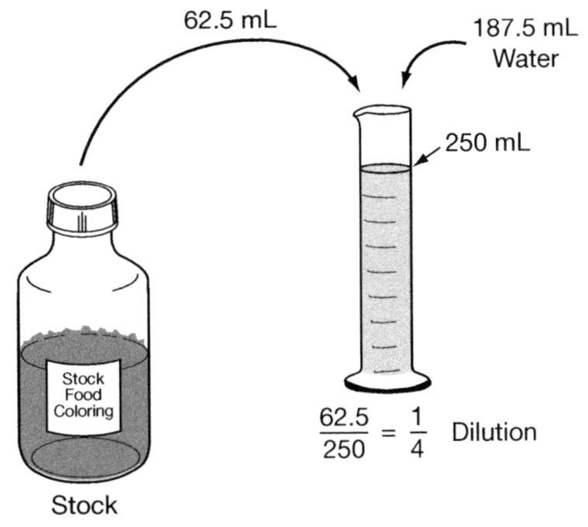


**FIGURE 14.6** Preparing 250 mL of a 1/5 dilution. Take 62.5 mL of food coloring and add enough water to get 250 mL total volume (187.5 mL). The food coloring dilution, expressed as a fraction, will be: $\frac{62.5\ \cancel{\text{mL}}}{250\ \cancel{\text{mL}}} = \frac{1}{4}$.

**EQUATION 14.1: Calculating How to Make a Particular Volume of a Specific Dilution**

Use a proportion equation to determine how much stock to use: Put the desired dilution, expressed as a fraction, on one side. On the other side, put the unknown in the numerator and the desired final (total) volume in the denominator. The unknown is the amount of stock required. Generally, determine by subtraction how much diluent is required, although there are times when it is practical to bring the solution to volume using a graduated cylinder or volumetric flask.

$$\textbf{Dilution expressed as a fraction} = \frac{\textbf{volume of stock}}{\textbf{desired final volume}}$$

or

$$\textbf{Dilution expressed as a fraction} = \frac{\textbf{volume of stock}}{(\textbf{volume of stock}) + (\textbf{volume of diluent})}$$

**Practice Problems**

1. ***How would you prepare 10 mL of a 1/10 dilution of buffer?***
2. ***How would you prepare 250 mL of a 1/300 dilution of a cell suspension?***
3. ***How would you prepare 1 mL of a 1/50 dilution of an enzyme?***
4. ***How would you prepare 1,000 µL of a 1/100 dilution of food coloring?***
5. ***How would you prepare 23 mL of a 3/5 dilution of solution Q?***
6. ***Suppose you have a stock of a buffer solution that is used in experiments. The stock is ten times more concentrated than it is used (like frozen orange juice that is sold in a concentrated form). How would you prepare 10 mL of the buffer solution at the right concentration?***
7. ***Suppose you have a stock of buffer that is five times more concentrated than it is used. How would you prepare 15 mL at the correct concentration?***
8. ***Suppose you need $10^3$ µL of a solution. The solution is stored at a concentration that is 100 times the concentration at which it is normally used. How would you dilute the solution?***
9. ***How would you prepare 50 mL of a 0.01 dilution of buffer?***

*Answers*

1. $\frac{?}{10\text{ mL}} = \frac{1}{10}$ $\quad ? = \frac{(1)10\text{ mL}}{10}$ $\quad ? = 1\text{ mL}$ buffer

**1 mL + 9 mL diluent** will give 1/10 dilution

2. $\frac{?}{250\text{ mL}} = \frac{1}{300}$ $\quad ? = \frac{1(250\text{ mL})}{300}$ $\quad ? \approx 0.833\text{ mL}$ cell suspension

**0.833 mL + 249.167 mL of diluent** = 250 mL

3. $\frac{?}{1\text{ mL}} = \frac{1}{50}$ $\quad ? = \frac{1(1\text{ mL})}{50}$ $\quad ? = 0.02\text{ mL}$ enzyme

**0.02 mL + 0.98 mL of diluent** = 1 mL

4. $\frac{?}{1{,}000\ \mu\text{L}} = \frac{1}{100}$ $\quad ? = \frac{1(1{,}000\ \mu\text{L})}{100}$ $\quad ? = 10\ \mu\text{L}$ food coloring

**10 μL + 990 μL of diluent** = 1,000 μL

5. $\frac{?}{23\text{ mL}} = \frac{3}{5}$ $\quad ? = \frac{3(23\text{ mL})}{5}$ $\quad ? = 13.8\text{ mL}$ of Q

**13.8 mL + 9.2 mL of diluent** = 23 mL

6. Since the stock is ten times more concentrated than it is used, it must be diluted 1/10.

$\frac{?}{10\text{ mL}} = \frac{1}{10}$ $\quad ? = \frac{1(10\text{ mL})}{10}$ $\quad ? = 1\text{ mL}$ stock

**1 mL + 9 mL of diluent** = 10 mL

7. Since the stock is five times more concentrated than it is used, it must be diluted 1/5.

$\frac{?}{15\text{ mL}} = \frac{1}{5}$ $\quad ? = \frac{1(15\text{ mL})}{5}$ $\quad ? = 3\text{ mL}$ stock

**3 mL + 12 mL of diluent** = 15 mL

8. Since the stock is 100 times more concentrated than it is used, it must be diluted 1/100.

$\frac{?}{10^3\ \mu\text{L}} = \frac{1}{100}$ $\quad ? = \frac{1(10^3\ \mu\text{L})}{100}$ $\quad ? = 10\ \mu\text{L}$ stock

**10 μL + 990 μL of diluent** = 1,000 μl

9. Express the dilution in fraction form: 0.01 = 1/100

$\frac{?}{50\text{ mL}} = \frac{1}{100}$ $\quad ? = 0.5\text{ mL}$ buffer

**0.5 mL + 49.5 mL of diluent** = 50 mL

## 14.6 CALCULATING THE CONCENTRATION OF SOLUTE AFTER DILUTING A STOCK SOLUTION

Suppose you prepare a dilution of a stock solution by removing some of the stock and adding diluent. There are now two solutions. The stock solution contains the solute(s) at its original concentration. The dilution contains the solute at a lower concentration. For example, suppose the original stock solution contains 10 mg/mL of a solute. You remove 1 mL of this stock and add 9 mL of buffer. The dilution, expressed as a fraction, is 1/10 mL or 1/10. The concentration of solute in the original stock solution, of course, is still 10 mg/mL. What is the concentration of the solute in the diluted sample? To calculate the concentration of solute in the dilution, multiply the original concentration times 1/10, the dilution expressed as a fraction:

$$(\text{Original concentration})(\text{dilution}) = \text{concentration in the diluted sample}$$

$$\left(\frac{10\text{ mg}}{1\text{ mL}}\right)\left(\frac{1}{10}\right) = \frac{\mathbf{1\ mg}}{\mathbf{1\ mL}}$$

This is another way to think about the same problem: when you removed 1 mL from the stock solution, you removed 10 mg of solute. This is because the concentration of the stock is 10 mg/mL – in every mL of stock there are 10 mg of solute. You took this 10 mg of solute and added to it 9 mL of buffer. The total volume in the diluted solution is 10 mL. In that 10 mL are 10 mg of solute. The concentration of solute in the diluted sample is 10 mg per 10 mL or 10 mg/10 mL or 1 mg/mL. It may be simplest to remember this rule:

**EQUATION 14.2: To Calculate the Concentration of Substance in a Dilution**

To calculate the concentration of a substance in a diluted sample, multiply the original concentration of the substance times the dilution:

$$(\text{Original concentration})(\text{dilution}) = \text{concentration in the diluted sample}$$

**Example Problem:**

A solution of 100% ethanol is diluted 1/10. What is the concentration of ethanol in the diluted solution?

***Answer:***

Using Equation 14.2 to calculate the concentration in the diluted sample:

$$(\text{Concentration of substance in original solution})(\text{dilution})$$
$$= \text{concentration in diluted sample}$$

$$(100\%\ \text{ethanol})\left(\frac{1}{10}\right) = \mathbf{10\%\ ethanol}$$

The diluted solution has a concentration of 10% ethanol.

**Example Problem:**

This example is illustrated in Figure 14.7.

A stock solution contains 10 mg/mL of a particular enzyme. The stock solution is diluted by taking 1 mL of the solution (which contains 10 mg of enzyme) and mixing it with 4 mL of water. What is the concentration of enzyme in the diluted solution?

***Answer:***

Using Equation 14.2:

$$(\text{Concentration of substance in original solution})(\text{dilution})$$
$$= \text{concentration in diluted sample}$$

$$\left(\frac{10\ \text{mg}}{1\ \text{mL}}\right)\left(\frac{1}{5}\right) = \frac{\mathbf{2\ mg}}{\mathbf{1\ mL}}$$

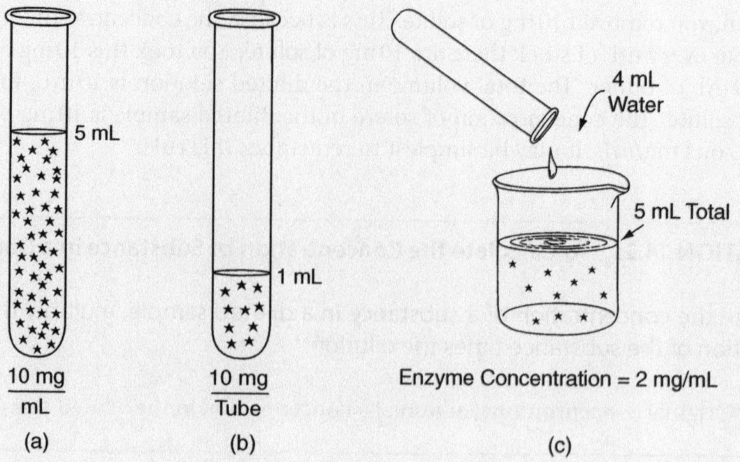


**FIGURE 14.7** Dilution of an enzyme solution. (a) The original solution has a concentration of 10 mg enzyme/mL. Each * represents an mg of enzyme. (b) 1 mL of solution is removed containing 10 mg of enzyme. (c) The 1 mL of solution is diluted with 4 mL of water. The resulting diluted solution contains 10 mg of enzyme in 5 mL. The concentration of enzyme is therefore 10 mg/5 mL = 2 mg/mL.

A second way to understand this problem:

The diluted solution has a total volume of 5 mL and it contains 10 mg of enzyme. The concentration of enzyme in the dilution therefore is:

$$\frac{10\text{ mg enzyme}}{5\text{ mL}} = \frac{\mathbf{2\ mg\ enzyme}}{\mathbf{1\ mL}}$$

This is the same answer as Equation 14.2 provided.

Yet another way to understand this problem is to use the $C_1V_1 = C_2V_2$ equation. Observe that the unknown is $C_2$ (unlike many of the problems we saw in Chapter 13 where the unknown was $V_1$).

$$C_1V_1 = C_2V_2$$

$$(10\text{ mg/mL})(1\text{ mL}) = (?)(5\text{ mL})$$

$$? = \mathbf{2\ mg / mL}$$

**Example Problem:**

A stock solution initially has a concentration of 20 mg of solute per liter.

A diluted solution is prepared by removing 1 mL of stock solution and adding 14 mL of water.

a. What is the concentration of solute in the diluted solution?
b. How much solute is present in 1 mL of the diluted solution?

*Answer:*

a. The concentration in the stock solution is 20 mg/L. The solution was diluted 1/15. Using Equation 14.2, the concentration in the diluted solution is:

$$\left(\frac{20\text{ mg}}{1\text{ L}}\right)\left(\frac{1}{15}\right)\approx\frac{\mathbf{1.3\ mg}}{\mathbf{1\ L}}$$

b. This part can be solved using proportions:

$$\frac{1.3\text{ mg}}{1{,}000\text{ mL}}=\frac{?}{1\text{ mL}}\qquad ?\approx\mathbf{0.0013\ mg}$$

This can also be solved using the unit canceling method:

$$\frac{1.3\text{ mg}}{1{,}000\text{ mL}}(1\text{ mL})=\mathbf{0.0013\ mg}$$

0.0013 mg is the amount of solute present in 1 mL of the diluted solution.

**Practice Problems**

1. ***If you prepare a 1/40 dilution of a 50% solution, what is the final concentration of the solution?***
2. ***If you prepare a 1/10 dilution of a 10 mg/mL solution, what is the final concentration of the solution?***
3. ***If you prepare a 1:1 dilution of a 10 mg/mL solution, what is the final concentration of the solution?***
4. ***How much 1/5 diluted solution can be made if you have 1 mL of original solution?***
5. ***A stock solution of enzyme contains 10 mg/mL of enzyme. You remove 100 mL of this stock and dilute it with 400 mL of buffer.***
   a. ***What is the concentration of enzyme in the resulting diluted solution?***
   b. ***How much enzyme will be present in 300 μL of the resulting dilution?***

*Answers*

1. $(50\%)\left(\frac{1}{40}\right)=\mathbf{1.25\%}$

2. $\left(\frac{10\text{ mg}}{1\text{ mL}}\right)\left(\frac{1}{10}\right)=\frac{\mathbf{1\ mg}}{\mathbf{1\ mL}}$

3. $1{:}1=\frac{1}{2}$ so $\left(\frac{10\text{ mg}}{1\text{ mL}}\right)\left(\frac{1}{2}\right)=\frac{10\text{ mg}}{2\text{ mL}}=\frac{\mathbf{5\ mg}}{\mathbf{1\ mL}}$

4. 1 mL+4 mL = 1/5 dilution. With 1 mL, you can make **5 mL** diluted solution.
5. a. When 100 mL of stock solution is mixed with 400 mL of buffer, the dilution can be expressed as:

$$\frac{100\text{ mL}}{500\text{ mL}} = \frac{1}{5}$$

Using Equation 14.2, the concentration of enzyme in the resulting dilution is:

$$\left(\frac{10\text{ mg}}{1\text{ mL}}\right)\left(\frac{1}{5}\right) = \frac{\mathbf{2\ mg}}{\mathbf{1\ mL}}$$

b. 300 µL = 0.3 mL. There are 2 mg/mL enzyme in the diluted solution, and we need to know how much enzyme is in 0.3 mL. By the unit canceling method:

$$\left(\frac{2\text{ mg}}{1\text{ mL}}\right)(0.3\text{ mL}) = \mathbf{0.6\ mg}$$

or

$$\left(\frac{300\ \mu\text{L}}{1}\right)\left(\frac{1\text{ mL}}{1{,}000\ \mu\text{L}}\right)\left(\frac{2\text{ mg}}{\text{mL}}\right) = \mathbf{0.6\ mg}$$

By proportions:

$$\frac{2\text{ mg}}{1\text{ mL}} = \frac{?}{0.3\text{ mL}} \qquad ? = \mathbf{0.6\ mg}$$

## 14.7 CALCULATING THE CONCENTRATION IN A STOCK SOLUTION IF YOU KNOW THE CONCENTRATION IN THE DILUTED SOLUTION

Suppose you have a concentrated solution and a dilution made from the concentrated stock and suppose you know the concentration of solute in the ***diluted solution*** but not in the original stock. This is the inverse of the situation discussed in Section 14.6. To calculate the concentration of material in the original stock solution, apply Equation 14.3:

**EQUATION 14.3: Calculating the Concentration of a Substance in an Original Stock Solution, Given the Concentration in the Dilution**

Multiply the concentration of the substance in the diluted solution times the reciprocal of the dilution (expressed as a fraction):

$$(\textbf{Concentration of substance in diluted solution})(\textbf{reciprocal of dilution})$$
$$= \textbf{concentration of substance in original stock}$$

**Example Problem:**

A solution of ethanol is diluted 1/10. The concentration of ethanol in the diluted solution is 10%. What was the concentration in the original stock solution?

***Answer:***

Using Equation 14.3, the concentration of solute in the original solution is:
(Concentration of substance in diluted solution) (reciprocal of dilution) = concentration of substance in original stock

$$(10\%)\left(\frac{10}{1}\right) = \mathbf{100\%}$$

The original solution had a concentration of 100% ethanol.

**Example Problem:**

A stock solution has a total volume of 100 mL. It is diluted by removing 1 mL of stock solution and adding 24 mL of water. The concentration of solute in the dilution is 1.5 g/L.

a. What is the concentration of solute in the stock solution?
b. How much solute is present in the total 100 mL of stock?

***Answer:***

a.
(Concentration of substance in diluted solution) (reciprocal of dilution) = concentration of substance in original stock

$$\left(\frac{1.5\text{ g}}{1\text{ L}}\right)\left(\frac{25}{1}\right) = \frac{\mathbf{37.5\ g}}{\mathbf{1\ L}}$$

b. This can be solved using the logic of proportions:

$$\frac{37.5\text{ g}}{1{,}000\text{ mL}} = \frac{?}{100\text{ mL}}$$

$$? = \mathbf{3.75\ g}$$

This is the amount of solute present in 100 mL of the original solution.

Note also that the $C_1V_1 = C_2V_2$ equation will work to perform a part of this problem, that is, calculating the concentration of solute in the stock solution. Now, the unknown is $C_1$.

$$C_1V_1 = C_2V_2$$

$$(?)(1\text{ mL}) = (1.5\text{ g/L})(25\text{ mL})$$

$$? = \mathbf{37.5\ g/L}$$

**A NOTE ABOUT TERMINOLOGY:**

You may come across the term "dilution factor." Sometimes this term is used to mean a dilution, expressed as a fraction, but other times this term is used to refer to the *reciprocal* of the dilution. For example, if 1 mL of stock is diluted with 9 mL of diluent, some people might say the "dilution factor is 1/10" but other people might say the "dilution factor is 10." We avoid the term "dilution factor" in this book because it is not used consistently in the literature.

**Practice Problems**

1. ***A diluted solution has a concentration of 15 mg/L. It was diluted 1/100. What was the concentration of solute in the original, undiluted stock solution?***
2. ***A diluted solution has a concentration of 1 mg/mL. It was diluted 1/20. What is the concentration of solute in the original stock?***
3. ***A diluted solution has a concentration of 1 mM. It was diluted 1/250. What is the concentration in the original stock solution?***
4. ***You are performing a test to determine the concentration of protein in a sample. The sample is first diluted 1/100. The protein concentration is 0.15 mg/L in the diluted sample. What was the concentration of protein in the original stock solution?***
5. ***In a protein assay, the amount of protein in 1 mL of diluted sample is 8.7 mg. If the original sample was diluted 1/50, what was the concentration of protein in the original sample?***
6. ***A suspension of bacterial cells is diluted by removing 1 mL of cells and adding 9 mL of sterile medium. The concentration of cells in the diluted solution is $1 \times 10^8$ cells/mL. What is the concentration of bacterial cells in the original solution?***
7. ***You have 100 µL of a protein sample. The sample is diluted by taking 5 µL of the sample and adding 20 µL of buffer. A protein assay is performed on the diluted sample. The concentration of protein in the diluted sample is 40 mg/mL.***
   a. ***Draw a sketch of this.***
   b. ***What was the concentration of protein in the original, undiluted sample?***
   c. ***How much protein was present altogether in the original, undiluted sample?***
8. ***You have 50 µL of a protein sample. The sample is diluted by taking 1 µL of the sample and adding 19 µL of buffer. A protein assay is performed on the diluted sample. The concentration of protein in the diluted sample is 0.20 mg/mL.***
   a. ***Draw a sketch of this.***
   b. ***What was the concentration of protein in the original, undiluted sample?***
   c. ***How much protein was present altogether in the original, undiluted sample?***
9. ***Suppose you do an assay to determine how much protein is present in a sample. To perform the assay, it is necessary to dilute the original sample 1/100. The assay shows that the concentration of protein in the diluted sample was 0.5 mg/mL.***
   a. ***What was the concentration of protein in the undiluted sample?***
   b. ***How much protein was present in 100 mL of the original, undiluted sample?***
10. ***You grow 10 L of bacterial cells in a fermenter. You plan to harvest a valuable enzyme product. You take a 100 mL sample of this bacterial cell suspension from the fermenter. (This 100 mL is intended to be used for various tests, either***

***now or stored for later.) You remove 1 mL of cells from the 100 mL sample and grind them up to form a viscous cell paste. You dissolve the cell paste in 9 mL of buffer to give you 10 mL of diluted cell paste. You remove 5 mL from the cell paste suspension and assay it to see how much protein it contains. You remove the other 5 mL and assay it for enzyme. The results are as follows:***

***5 mL contains 50 mg of protein.***

***5 mL contains 100 units of enzyme.***

a. ***Draw this situation. (It is important to sketch problems like this that involve multiple steps.)***

b. ***What is the concentration of enzyme in the sample that was assayed? Express your answer as Units enzyme/mg protein. (Hint: look at the units.) (Note that the units used to talk about enzymes are simply called "Units.")***

c. ***How many units of enzyme are present in the entire 10 L of bacterial cells? Express your answer as Units of enzyme. (Hint, remember that amount and concentration are not synonyms. The question asks for the amount of enzyme. Watch the units. Refer to your sketch!)***

## *Answers*

1. Applying Equation 2:

(Concentration in diluted sample)(reciprocal of dilution) = concentration in original stock

$$(15\ \text{mg/L})(100/1) = \mathbf{1{,}500\ mg\ /\ L}$$

2. (1 mg/mL) (20/1) = **20 mg/mL**
3. (1 mM) (250/1) = **250 mM**
4. (0.15 mg/L) (100/1) = **15 mg/L**
5. $\frac{1}{50}$ dilution had $\frac{8.7\ \text{mg}}{\text{mL}}$

$$\left(\frac{8.7\ \text{mg}}{1\ \text{mL}}\right)(50) = \frac{435\ \text{mg}}{1\ \text{mL}} = \frac{\mathbf{0.435\ g}}{\mathbf{1\ mL}} = \text{concentration protein in undiluted sample}$$

6. $\left(1 \times 10^8\ \frac{\text{cells}}{\text{mL}}\right)\left(\frac{10}{1}\right) = \mathbf{1 \times 10^9\ cells\ /\ mL}$

7. a.

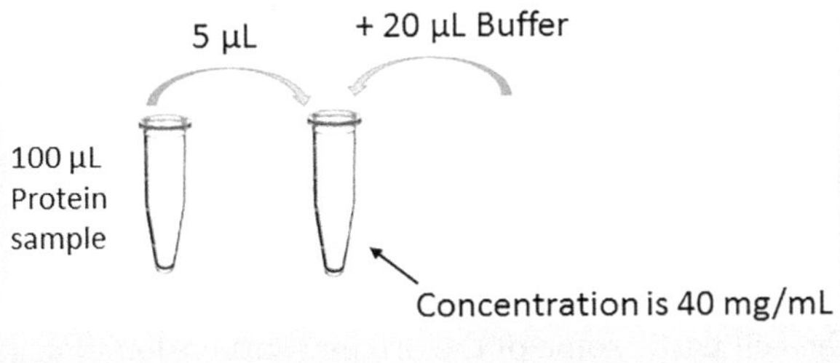


b. Dilution is 5/25 = 1/5.

$$(40\ \text{mg/mL})(5/1) = \mathbf{200\ mg\ /\ mL}$$

c. $(200\ \text{mg/mL})(0.100\ \text{mL}) = \mathbf{20\ mg}$

8. a.

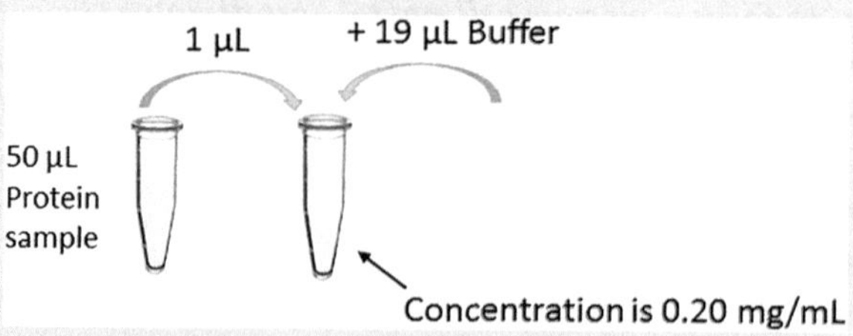


b. Dilution is **1/20**.

c. $(4\ \text{mg/mL})(0.050\ \text{mL}) = \mathbf{0.20\ mg}$

$(0.20\ \text{mg/mL})(20/1) = \mathbf{4\ mg/mL}$

9. a. $\left(\frac{0.5\ \text{mg}}{\text{mL}}\right)(100) = \frac{\mathbf{50\ mg}}{\mathbf{1\ mL}} = \text{Concentration protein in undiluted sample}$

b. $\frac{50\ \text{mg}}{\text{mL}} = \frac{?}{100\ \text{mL}}$

$? = \mathbf{5{,}000\ mg}$

10. a.

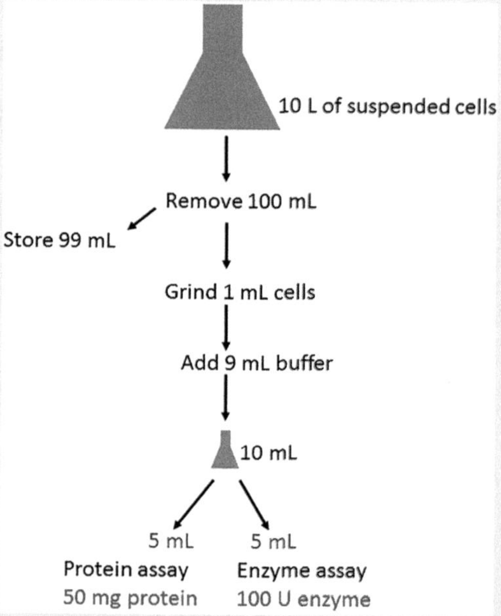


b. 100 Units/50 mg = **2 Units/mg**

c. There were 100 Units in 5 mL of cell paste. So the concentration of enzyme in the cell paste was

$$100\ \text{Units}/5\ \text{mL} = 20\ \text{Units/mL}.$$

To make the cell paste, some of the original suspension of cells was diluted by taking 1 mL of cells and adding 9 mL of buffer. So the dilution was 1/10.

By Equation 14.3, the concentration of enzyme in the original cells was:

$$(20\ \text{units/mL})(10/1) = 200\ \text{units/mL}.$$

The amount of enzyme in the original cells was:

$$\left(\frac{200\ \text{units}}{1\ \text{mL}}\right)(10{,}000\ \text{mL}) = \mathbf{2 \times 10^6\ units\ total}$$

## 14.8 DILUTION SERIES

Cell culturists often need to know the concentration of cells in their cultures. Imagine a suspension containing a great many bacterial cells, perhaps $10^7$ cells/mL. Now imagine trying to count so many cells – in each mL there would be about ten million cells! It is necessary to dilute this suspension by many orders of magnitude before it is possible to count the cells. Let us consider how such a dilution might be accomplished.

Suppose you decide that you want to dilute the original stock solution of bacteria 1/100,000 and that you want 10 mL final volume. Set this up as a proportion, as we did in Section 14.5:

$$\frac{1\text{ mL}}{100{,}000\text{ mL}} = \frac{?}{10\text{ mL}} \qquad ? = \mathbf{0.0001\ mL}$$

This means that to dilute the bacterial broth by a dilution of 1/100,000 in one step, with a final volume of 10 mL, would require removing 0.0001 mL of bacterial broth. This is not a practical strategy for preparing a dilution because it is extremely difficult to accurately measure a volume of only 0.0001 mL. A better strategy is to dilute the original solution of cells using two or more steps. Figure 14.8 shows how one might prepare 10 mL of a 1/100,000 dilution of bacterial cells in three steps.

Here are the steps that are being performed in Figure 14.8.

### A DILUTION SERIES

1. 0.1 mL of the original bacterial broth is mixed with 9.9 mL of diluent.
   **This is a dilution of 0.1/10 mL = 1/100 dilution.**
2. 0.1 mL of the diluted bacterial broth prepared in step 1 is mixed with 9.9 mL of diluent.
   **This is a dilution of 1/100.**
3. 1 mL of the diluted bacterial broth prepared in step 2 is mixed with 9 mL of diluent.
   **This is a dilution of 1/10.**

   The bacteria were therefore diluted 1/100 in the first tube, 1/100 in the second tube, and 1/10 in the third tube. The final, total dilution is:

$$\left(\frac{1}{100}\right)\left(\frac{1}{100}\right)\left(\frac{1}{10}\right) = \frac{1}{100{,}000}$$

**The third tube has the desired dilution and the desired volume.**

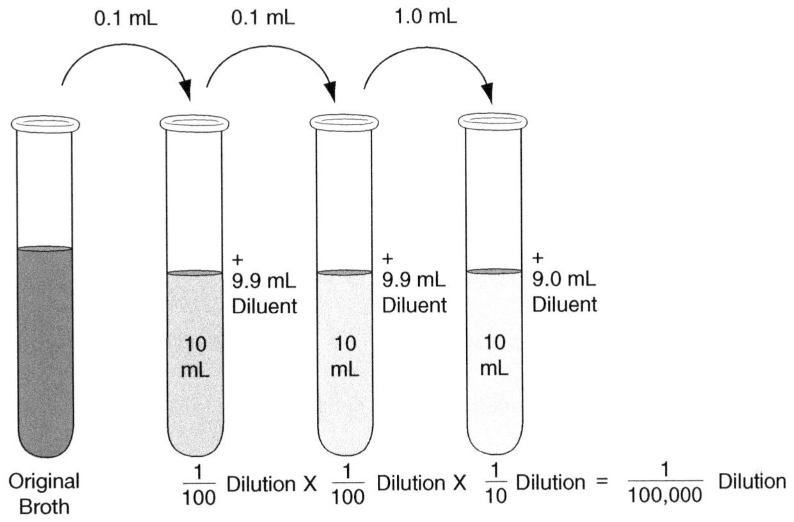


**FIGURE 14.8** A dilution series used to dilute a bacterial stock solution 1/100,000.

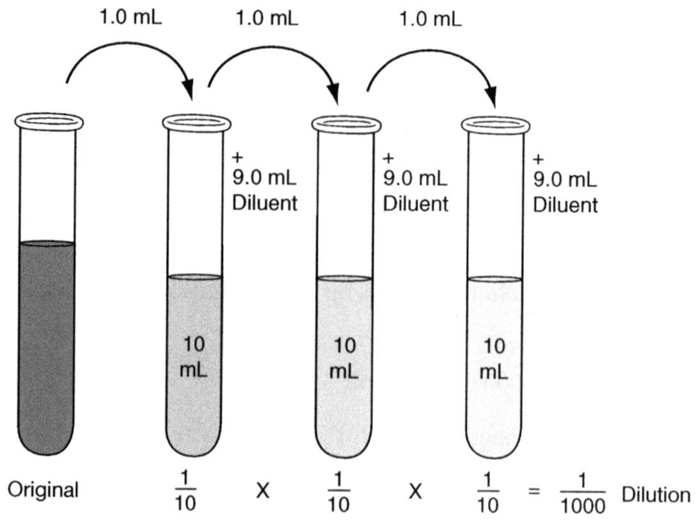


**FIGURE 14.9** A serial dilution.

This procedure, involving a series of connected dilutions, is called a **dilution series.** Sometimes people refer to a **serial dilution** to mean a series of dilutions that all have the same dilution (for example, all are 1/10 dilutions or all are 1/2 dilutions). Note, however, that the terms "dilution series" and "serial dilutions" are sometimes used interchangeably, without regard for whether the dilutions are all the same. Figure 14.9 shows an example of a 1/10 serial dilution, where each dilution is the same (1/10).

Observe in Figures 14.8 and 14.9 that to determine the final, total dilution, expressed as a fraction, in a dilution series, the dilutions in each intermediate tube are multiplied by one another. This is summarized in Equation 14.4.

**EQUATION 14.4: Calculating the Final Dilution in a Dilution Series**

The dilution in the final tube in a dilution series is determined by multiplying the dilution in the first tube, times the dilution in the second tube, and so on until reaching the last tube.

$$\textbf{Dilution in final tube} = (\textbf{dilution in first diluted tube})$$
$$(\textbf{dilution in second diluted tube})$$
$$\ldots(\textbf{dilution in last diluted tube})$$

Continuing with the bacteria example, as shown in Figure 14.8, suppose that the original bacterial broth contained $1 \times 10^7$ bacteria per mL. What is the concentration of bacteria in each of the three dilution tubes?

In the **first** dilution tube, the concentration of cells is:

$$1 \times 10^7 \text{ bacteria per mL} \times 1/100 = 1 \times 10^5 \text{ bacteria per mL}$$

In the **second** dilution tube, the concentration of cells is:

$$1 \times 10^5 \text{ bacteria per mL} \times 1/100 = 1 \times 10^3 \text{ bacteria per mL}$$

In the **third (final)** dilution tube, the concentration of cells is:

$$1 \times 10^3 \text{ bacteria per mL} \times 1/10 = 1 \times 10^2 \text{ bacteria per mL}$$

Another way to think about this is: The final, total dilution is 1/100,000. Therefore, the concentration of bacterial cells in the **final** diluted solution must be:

$$\left(\frac{1 \times 10^7 \text{ bacteria}}{\text{mL}}\right)\left(\frac{1}{100{,}000}\right) = \frac{\mathbf{1 \times 10^2 \text{ bacteria}}}{\mathbf{1 \text{ mL}}}$$

The procedure to find the concentration of solute (or cells) in the final tube in a dilution series can be generalized into Equation 14.5.

**EQUATION 14.5: Calculating the Concentration of a Substance in the Final Tube in a Dilution Series**

The concentration of a substance in the final tube in a dilution series is determined by multiplying the concentration of substance in the original solution times the dilution in the first tube, times the dilution in the second tube, and so on until reaching the last tube.

$$\textbf{Concentration in final tube} = (\textbf{concentration in original tube})$$
$$(\textbf{dilution in first diluted tube})$$
$$(\textbf{dilution in second diluted tube})$$
$$\ldots(\textbf{dilution in last diluted tube})$$

**Example Problem:**

As shown in Figure 14.10, a broth contains bacterial cells at a concentration of $10^5$ cells/mL. You dilute this broth by removing 1 mL of it and adding 9 mL of sterile medium. This gives you dilution tube 1 of bacterial cells. You remove 0.1 mL from this diluted tube and add 9.9 mL of sterile medium to give you dilution tube 2. What is the concentration of bacterial cells in each of the two diluted tubes?

***Answer:***

The first dilution is 1/10, so the concentration of cells in dilution tube #1 is:

$$\left(10^5 \text{ cells/mL}\right)(1/10) = \mathbf{10^4 \text{ cells / mL}}$$

The second dilution is 0.1/10 or 1/100. Therefore, the concentration in dilution tube #2 is:

$$\left(10^4 \text{ cells/mL}\right)(1/100) = \mathbf{10^2 \text{ cells / mL}}$$

You can also apply Equation 14.5 to calculate the concentration of cells in the second (final) tube:

Applying Equation 14.5:

$$\left(10^5 \text{ cells/mL}\right)(1/10)(1/100) = \mathbf{10^2 \text{ cells / mL}}$$

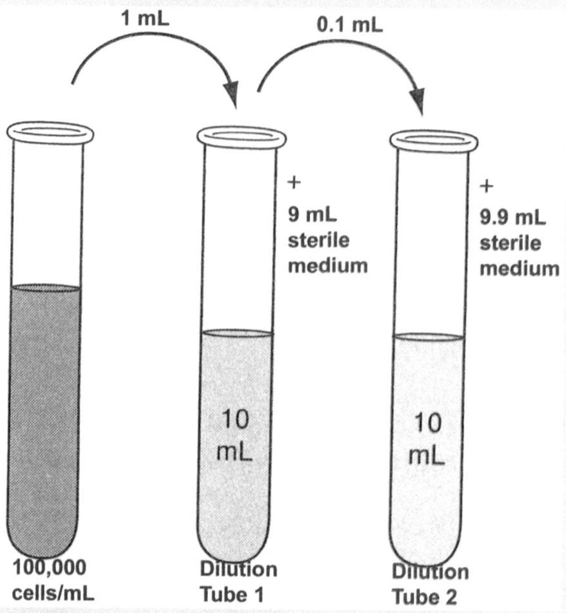

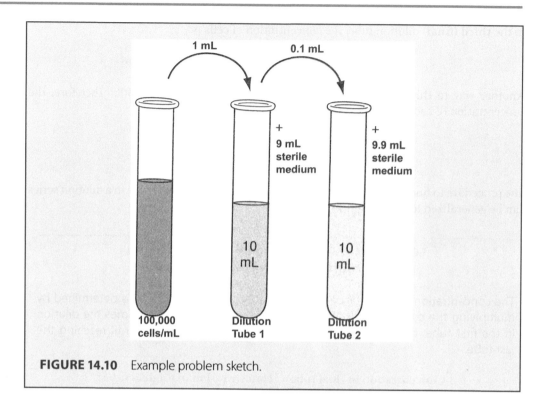

**FIGURE 14.10** Example problem sketch.

## Practice Problems

1. ***As shown in Figure 14.11, you begin with a broth containing bacterial cells at a concentration of $2 \times 10^7$ cells/mL. You dilute the broth by removing 1 mL and adding 9 mL of sterile medium to give you dilution tube 1 of bacterial cells. You remove 0.1 mL from this first dilution tube and add 9.9 mL of sterile medium to***

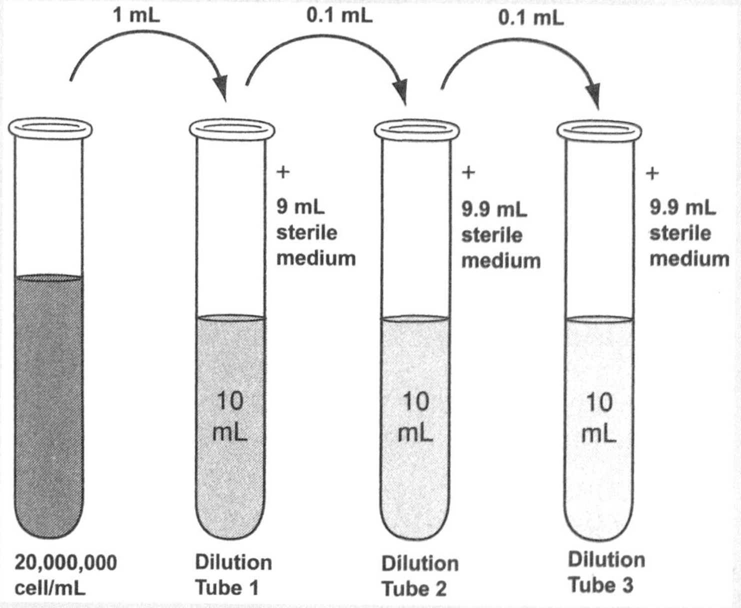


**FIGURE 14.11** Practice Problem 1.

*give dilution tube 2. You remove 0.1 mL from this second dilution tube and add 9.9 mL of sterile medium to give dilution tube #3. What is the concentration of bacterial cells in each of the three dilution tubes?*

2. ***Explain how a dilution series could be used to prepare a*** $1 \times 10^6$ ***dilution of bacterial cells.***
3. ***As shown in Figure 14.12 (on page 228), an original stock solution contains*** $2 \times 10^5$ ***mammalian cells/mL. A dilution series is prepared where the stock solution is first diluted 1/10, then this first dilution is used to make a 1/100 dilution. What is the concentration of cells after the second dilution?***
4. ***An original stock solution contains*** $2.5 \times 10^6$ ***bacterial cells/mL. A dilution series is prepared where the stock solution is first diluted 1/10, then 0.1 mL of this first dilution is removed and diluted with 9.9 mL sterile medium to make a 1/100 dilution. A third dilution is made by taking 0.5 mL from the second dilution tube and adding 4.5 mL of sterile medium.***
   a. ***Sketch this.***
   b. ***Calculate the concentration of cells in the third, final dilution tube.***

*Answers*

1. The first dilution is 1/10, so the concentration of cells in dilution tube 1 is:

$$\left(2\times10^{7}\text{ cells/mL}\right)(1/10)=\mathbf{2\times10^{6}\text{ cells / mL}}$$

The next dilution is 0.1/10 or 1/100. Therefore, the concentration in dilution tube 2 is:

$$\left(2\times10^{6}\text{ cells/mL}\right)(1/100)=\mathbf{2\times10^{4}\text{ cells / mL}}$$

The next dilution is 0.1/10 or 1/100. Therefore, the concentration in dilution tube 3 is:

$$\left(2\times10^{4}\text{ cells/mL}\right)(1/100)=\mathbf{2\times10^{2}\text{ cells / mL}}$$

2. There are many ways to do this. For example:
   A $1/10^6$ dilution could be obtained with three $1/10^2$ dilutions.
   0.1 mL of culture + 9.9 mL of diluent = 1/100
   Take 0.1 mL of above + 9.9 mL of diluent = (1/100) (1/100) = $1/10^4$
   Take 0.1 mL of above + 9.9 mL of diluent = (1/100) ($1/10^4$) = $1/10^6$
3. Applying Equation 14.5:

$$\left(2\times10^{5}\text{ mammalian cells/mL}\right)(1/10)(1/100)=\mathbf{2\times10^{2}\text{ cells / mL}}$$

4. a. (Figure 14.13)
   b. Applying Equation 14.5:

$$\left(2.5\times10^{6}\text{ bacterial cells/mL}\right)(1/10)(1/100)(0.5/5)=\mathbf{250\text{ cells / mL}}$$

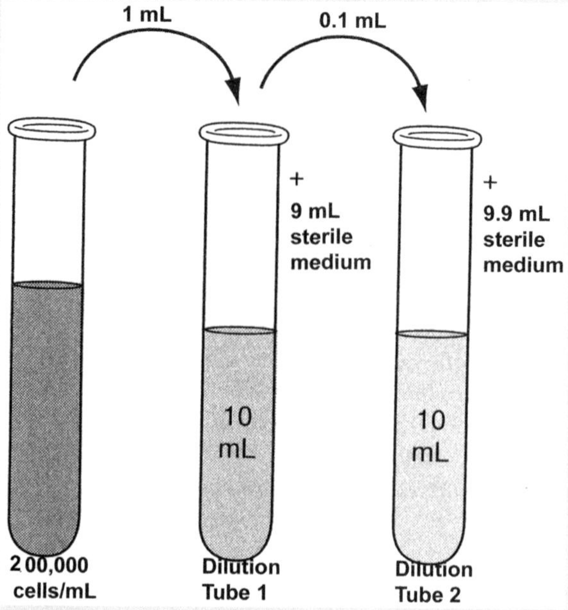

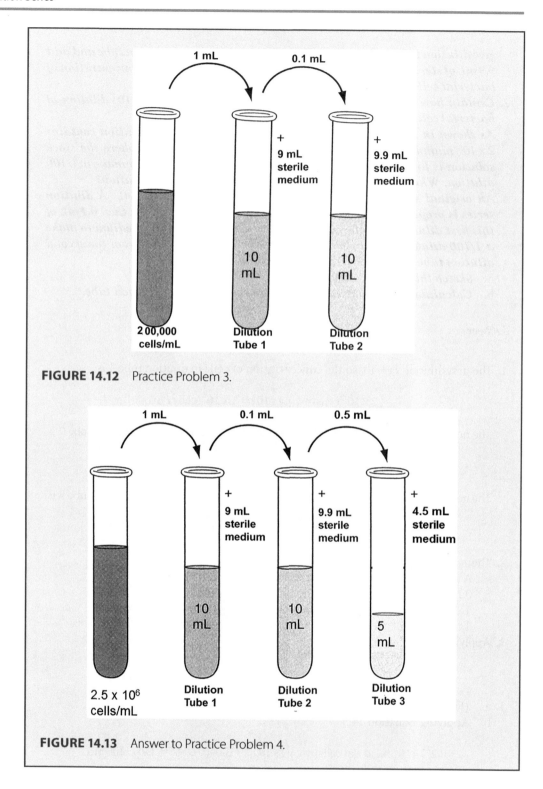

**FIGURE 14.12** Practice Problem 3.

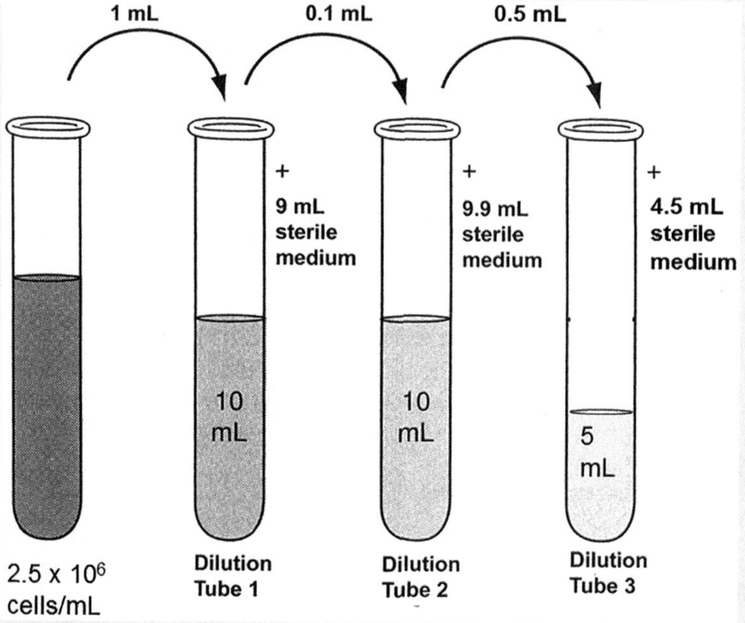


**FIGURE 14.13** Answer to Practice Problem 4.

## 14.9 PLANNING A DILUTION SERIES

In practice, there are many situations where you are not given a dilution strategy and more than one strategy may be correct to solve a problem. Box 14.2 outlines a general strategy you can use to devise a dilution series.

**BOX 14.2: A General Strategy for Planning a Dilution Series**

Step 1. Determine how much the stock needs to be diluted overall.

Step 2. Determine what volume (if any) is needed of each intermediate dilution.

Step 3. Determine what volume of stock solution is available.

Step 4. Devise a dilution series. Generally, dilutions that are a multiple of 1/10 (such as 1/10 or 1/100) are multiples of 1/5 (such as 1/5 or 1/50) or are multiples of ½ (such as ½ or ¼) are preferred.

The example problems below illustrate this general strategy.

**Example Problem:**

A solution contains 10 g KCl/L. How could this solution be diluted to obtain 1 mL of solution with a KCl concentration of 0.100 mg/L?

**Answer:** ***(Refer to Figure 14.14.)***

Step 1: The KCl concentration in the original solution is 10 g/L = 10,000 mg/L.
The desired concentration is 0.100 mg/L.
Therefore, the initial solution has 100,000 times more KCl per liter than the desired dilution.
Observe that to prepare the desired dilution in one step requires 0.00001 mL of the original stock:

$$\frac{1}{100{,}000} = \frac{?}{1\ \text{mL}}$$

$$? = 0.00001\ \text{mL} = \text{amount of original stock solution required.}$$

(Note that if this is not clear, you could get the same answer for ? using the $C_1V_1 = C_2V_2$ equation.)

It is not possible to accurately measure 0.00001 mL with normal equipment. Therefore, it is best to dilute the KCl solution in steps.

Step 2: In this situation, the intermediate dilutions will not be used. (A later example problem will illustrate a situation where the intermediate dilutions are used.)

Step 3: The volume of stock solution is not specified so we will assume it is unlimited. (A later example problem will illustrate a situation where the stock solution is limited.)

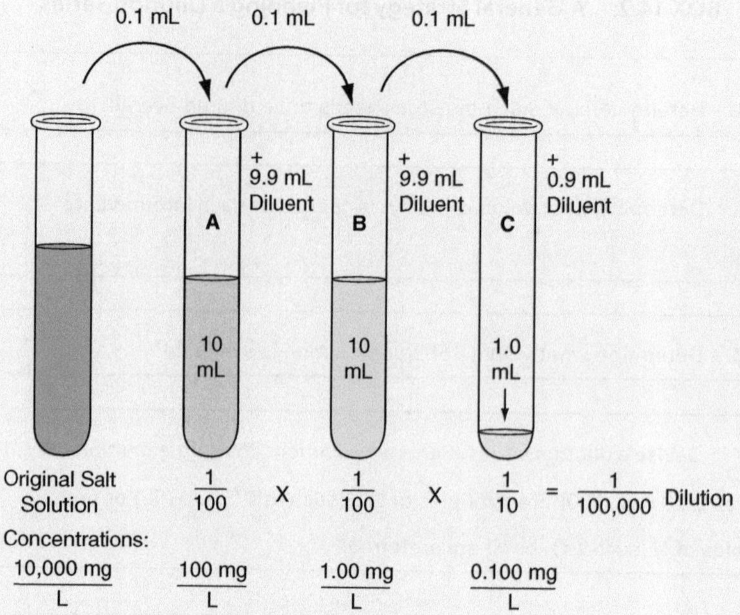


**FIGURE 14.14** Diluting a potassium chloride solution.

Step 4: Devise a series of dilutions that will work. In this case, dilutions that are multiples of 1/10 are straightforward:

Tube A: Remove 0.1 mL of the original KCl solution and add 9.9 mL of water. This is a 1/100 dilution. The concentration of KCl in this dilution is 100 mg/L because:

$$(\text{Original concentration})(\text{dilution}) = (\text{concentration after first dilution})$$

$$\left(\frac{10{,}000 \text{ mg}}{1 \text{ L}}\right)\left(\frac{1}{100}\right) = \frac{\mathbf{100\ mg}}{\mathbf{1\ L}}$$

Tube B: Remove 0.1 mL from tube A and add 9.9 mL of water. This is also a 1/100 dilution. The concentration of KCl in this dilution tube is 1.00 mg/L because:

$$(\text{Concentration after first dilution})(\text{dilution}) = (\text{concentration after second dilution})$$

$$\left(\frac{100 \text{ mg}}{1 \text{ L}}\right)\left(\frac{1}{100}\right) = \frac{\mathbf{1.00\ mg}}{\mathbf{1\ L}}$$

Tube C: Remove 0.1 mL from the tube B and add 0.9 mL of water. This is a 1/10 dilution. The volume in this tube is 1 mL, as desired and the concentration of KCl is 0.100 mg KCl/L because:

$$(\text{Concentration after 2nd dilution})(\text{dilution}) = (\text{concentration after final dilution})$$

$$\left(\frac{1.00 \text{ mg}}{1 \text{ L}}\right)\left(\frac{1}{10}\right) = \frac{\mathbf{0.100\ mg}}{\mathbf{1\ L}}$$

You can also apply Equation 14.5 to calculate the concentration of KCl in the (final) tube:

$$(10{,}000 \text{ mg/L})(1/100)(1/100)(1/10) = \mathbf{0.100\ mg/L}$$

**Example Problem:**

Plasmids are circular DNA molecules that can transport a gene from one bacterium into another. In nature, plasmids may carry genes that make a bacterium resistant to an antibiotic; as bacteria exchange plasmids carrying resistance genes, resistance to antibiotics spreads among bacterial populations. In the laboratory, plasmids can be used to transport useful genes into bacteria. Suppose that in an experiment, it is necessary to add 0.01 µg of plasmid to a tube and suppose that 1 mL of plasmid in solution at a concentration of 1 mg plasmid/mL is available. Suggest a strategy by which the addition of 0.01 µg of plasmid might be accomplished. Assume that it is not possible to measure a volume <1 µL.

***Answer:***

Step 1: The concentration of plasmid in the stock solution is 1 mg/mL = 1 µg/µL. If the plasmid is drawn directly from the stock tube, only 0.01 µL is needed, which is a volume too small to accurately measure. The stock must be diluted.

For example, if the stock is diluted 1,000X, or we can also say it is diluted 1/1,000, its concentration will be:

$$\left(\frac{1\,\mu g}{1\,\mu L}\right)\left(\frac{1}{1{,}000}\right)=\frac{0.001\,\mu g}{1\,\mu L}$$

Then, 10 µL of the diluted plasmid solution will contain 0.01 µg of plasmid.

There are micropipettes available that can accurately measure 10 µL volumes. Therefore, in this situation, an overall dilution of 1/1,000, is reasonable. Let us assume that we decide to dilute the stock 1/1,000.

Step 2: The intermediate dilutions will not be used.

Step 3: 1 mL of stock solution is available. You might or might not want to use all of it at once. Generally, diluted biological materials are less stable than concentrated ones. Therefore, it is common to discard the intermediate dilutions (assuming they are not used in a procedure). Therefore, it is good practice not to use more of the stock than necessary.

Step 4: There are various strategies to dilute the stock plasmid solution 1,000 times. As in the previous example, dilutions that are a multiple of 1/10 are straightforward:

Tube A: Remove 10 µL of the original plasmid stock and add 990 µL of buffer or water for a 1/100 dilution.

Tube B: Remove 10 µL from the dilution in tube A and add 90 µL of buffer or water resulting in a 1/10 dilution. The total dilution in tube B is therefore:

$$(\mathbf{1/100})(\mathbf{1/10})=\mathbf{1/1{,}000}$$

**The concentration of plasmid in this tube is 0.001 µg/µL, the desired concentration, so 10 µL at this concentration will contain the desired 0.01 µg of plasmid.**

This two dilution strategy involves volumes that can be measured with reasonable accuracy. (There are other strategies that will also work. For example, three 1/10 dilutions is a reasonable strategy.)

**Example Problem:**

Antibodies are often used in research studies to locate and tag biological molecules, such as specific cellular proteins. Antibodies are purchased as concentrated stock solutions that are diluted right before use. The optimal dilutions of antibodies are best determined by experimentation. For example, an antibody manufacturer might suggest a 1/1,000 dilution as a starting point for a particular application. But you need to experiment to see if this is the best dilution. Suppose you decide to try dilutions of 1/500, 1/1,000, 1/2,000, and 1/4,000 to see which dilution best works for your application. Suggest a strategy to use a dilution series to prepare all four of these dilutions. Assume you will need at least **2 mL** of each of these dilutions for your assay. Antibodies are expensive, so suggest a strategy that minimizes, or close to minimizes, the use of stock.

Step 1: The final dilution is 1/4,000, so this is the overall dilution required.

Step 2: You need 2 mL of each intermediate dilution.

Step 3: Use the minimum amount of stock to provide sufficient material in each dilution tube.

Step 4: In this case, dilutions that are all multiples of 1/10 will not work. (Why not?) Dilutions of ½ will work. Let us start by considering the first dilution. The first dilution is 1/500. We need at least 2 mL of it plus however much is removed to make the second dilution. You might think about making 3, 4, and 5 mL and seeing if these amounts will work. Let us try making 4 mL. By Equation 14.1:

*Use a proportion expression to determine how much stock to use: put the desired dilution, expressed as a fraction, on one side. On the other side, put the unknown in the numerator and the desired final (total) volume in the denominator. Determine by subtraction how much diluent is required.*

$$\frac{1}{500} = \frac{?}{4\text{ mL}}$$

$$? = \mathbf{0.008\text{ mL} = 8\text{ µL}}$$

Thus,

Tube A: (**8 µL stock + 4 mL diluent**, technically 3,992 µL, but that is close enough to 4 mL that most people would not measure 3,992 µL.) This tube is a 1/500 dilution, and it uses relatively little of the valuable antibody stock.

Tube B: A ½ dilution of tube A will work to obtain a 1/1,000 dilution. **Remove 2,000 µL from tube A and add 2,000 µL of diluent.**

Tube C: A ½ dilution of tube B will work to obtain a 1/2,000 dilution. **Remove 2,000 µL from tube B and add 2,000 µL of diluent.** This will give you a 1/2,000 dilution.

Tube D: This is another ½ dilution. It might be accomplished by removing **1,500 µL from tube C and adding 1,500 µL of diluent.** (You could also use 1,000 µL from tube C and add 1,000 µL of diluent, but it is useful to have a bit extra, when possible.)

This procedure is sketched in Figure 14.15.

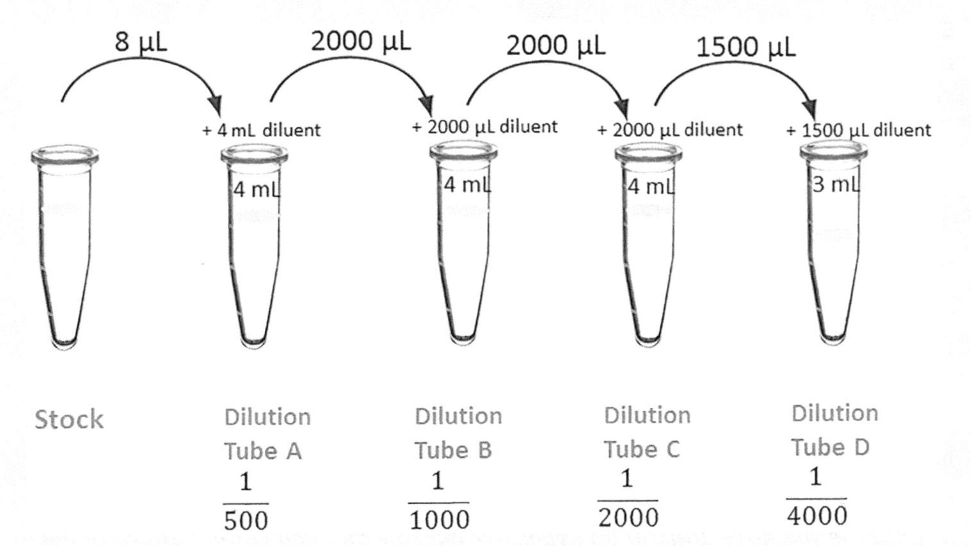


**FIGURE 14.15** Antibody example.

## 14.10 SUMMARY

This chapter includes a series of equations that relate to working with dilutions expressed as fractions. These equations are summarized in Box 14.3.

**BOX 14.3: Summary of the Equations in This Chapter**

**Equation 14.1: Calculating How to Make a Particular Volume of a Specific Dilution**

$$\text{Dilution expressed as a fraction} = \frac{\text{volume of stock}}{\text{desired final volume}}$$

**Equation 14.2: The Concentration of Substance in a Dilution**

$$(\text{Original concentration})(\text{dilution}) = \text{concentration in the diluted sample}$$

**Equation 14.3: Calculating the Concentration of a Substance in an Original Stock Solution, Given the Concentration in the Dilution**

$$(\text{Concentration of substance in diluted solution})(\text{reciprocal of dilution})$$
$$= \text{concentration of substance in original stock}$$

**Equation 14.4: Calculating the Final Dilution in a Dilution Series**

$$\text{Dilution in final tube} = (\text{Dilution in first tube})(\text{dilution in second tube})$$
$$\ldots(\text{dilution in last tube})$$

**Equation 14.5: Calculating the Concentration of a Substance in the Final Tube in a Dilution Series**

$$\text{Concentration in final tube} = (\text{concentration in original tube})$$
$$(\text{Dilution in first diluted tube})$$
$$(\text{dilution in second diluted tube})$$
$$\ldots(\text{dilution in last diluted tube})$$

### More Practice Problems

1. ***Suppose you have 20 µL of an expensive enzyme and you cannot afford to purchase more. The enzyme has a concentration of 1,000 Units/mL. You are going to do an experiment that requires tubes with a concentration of 1 Unit/mL of enzyme and each tube will have 5 mL total volume. (The enzyme is diluted in buffer.) How much enzyme does each tube require? ________ How many tubes can you prepare before you run out of enzyme? ____________***
2. ***Suppose you have 20 µL of an expensive enzyme that has 1,000 Units/mL. You are going to use the enzyme in an experiment that requires tubes with 0.01 Units/mL of enzyme and each tube will have 5 mL total volume. (The enzyme is diluted in buffer.) How much enzyme will each tube require? _______ Will you be able to accurately measure this amount of enzyme? ____ Show how you can dilute 10 µL of the original 20 µL of enzyme so that you can use it in your experiment. Use a diagram and words to demonstrate your strategy for preparing the enzyme.***
3. ***Antibodies are frequently shipped and stored very concentrated relative to how much is necessary in an experiment. Show how you would use a dilution series to dilute an antibody solution 500,000X. Assume you have 1 mL of antibody to begin, but you want to save at least 0.5 mL of the antibody for future experiments.***
4. ***Counting seems like a simple mathematical process. However, counting microorganisms is not so simple. For one thing, microorganisms, such as bacteria, are not visible to the eye. Another problem is that bacteria may be present in extremely large numbers in a sample. For example, in nutrient broth, there might be $1 \times 10^9$ bacterial cells per mL. Therefore, microbiologists have devised various methods to count bacterial cells. One such method is called viable cell counting. To perform a viable cell count, a sample of bacterial cells is first serially diluted. Then, 0.1 mL of diluted cells are spread on a petri dish that contains nutrient agar. It is assumed that every living cell in the 0.1 mL placed on the agar divides to form a colony of bacterial cells. A colony contains so many individual cells that it is visible to the eye. It is also assumed that each colony originates from a single cell. It is possible to count the colonies and therefore to estimate the number of bacteria in the 0.1 mL of broth.***

   ***Assume you begin with a culture of bacteria that contains $1 \times 10^9$ bacteria/mL. Show how you could dilute the culture so that the final tube has a concentration of 200 bacteria/0.1 mL.***
5. ***As shown in Figure 14.16, you are performing a viable cell count of bacteria. The original broth has an unknown concentration of bacteria. You dilute the culture as shown in the diagram and plate 0.1 mL of the last three dilutions onto three Petri dishes with nutrient agar. The following day you count the number of colonies on the plates with the results shown in the illustration. What was the concentration of bacteria in the original tube?***

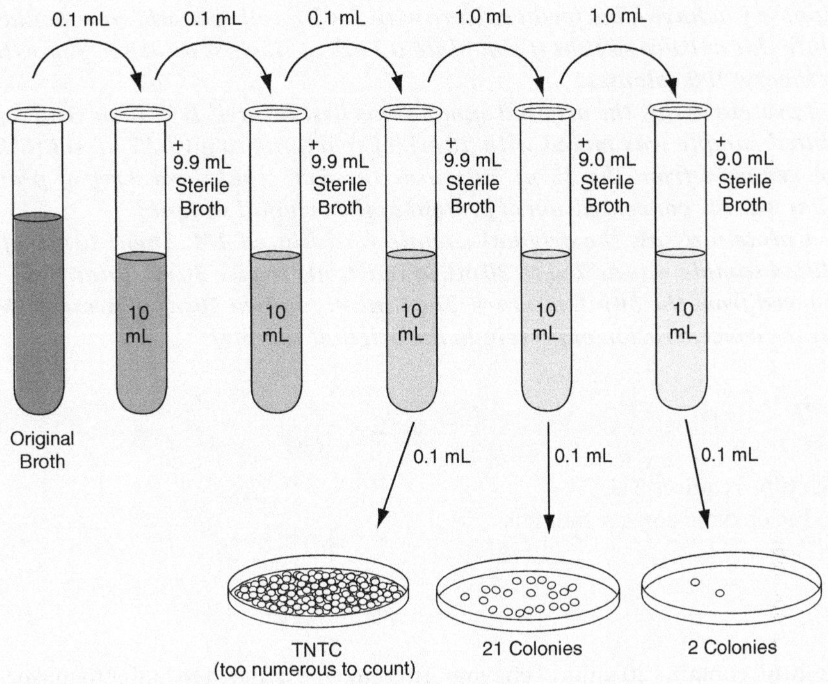


**FIGURE 14.16** Viable cell count Problem 5.

6. ***As shown in Figure 14.17, you are performing a viable cell count of bacteria. The original broth has an unknown concentration of bacteria. You dilute the culture as shown in the diagram and plate 0.1 mL of the last three dilutions on three nutrient agar plates. The following day you count the number of colonies on the plates with the results shown in the illustration. What was the concentration of bacteria in the original tube?***

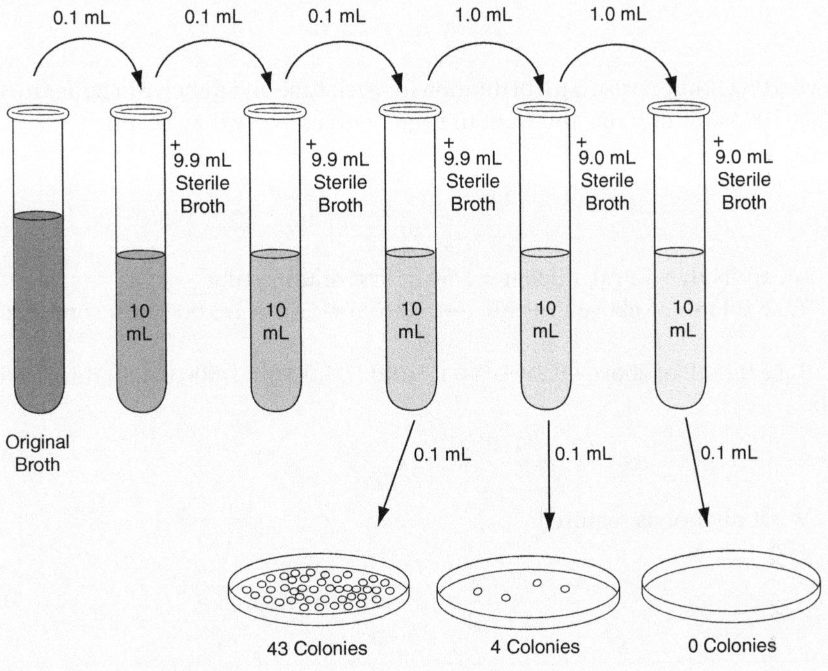


**FIGURE 14.17** Viable cell count Problem 6.

7. ***Suppose you have a bacterial culture with $1 \times 10^7$ cells per mL. How would you dilute this culture so that if you plate 0.1 mL of the last dilution, you will get (in theory) 100 colonies?***
8. ***In a protein assay, the original sample was first diluted 1/5. Then, 5 mL of the diluted sample was mixed with 20 mL of reactants to give 25 mL total. 5 mL was removed from the 25 mL mixture. The 5 mL contained 3 mg of protein. What was the concentration of protein in the original sample?***
9. ***In a protein assay, the original sample was diluted 1/4. Then, 10 mL of the diluted sample was added to 20 mL of reactants to give 30 mL total. 5 mL was removed from the 30 mL mixture. The 5 mL contained 10 mg of protein. What was the concentration of protein in the original sample?***

*Answers*

1. Each tube requires 5 U.

   The enzyme concentration is:

$$\frac{1{,}000\ \text{U}}{1\ \text{mL}} = \frac{1{,}000\ \text{U}}{1{,}000\ \mu\text{L}} = \frac{1\ \text{U}}{1\ \mu\text{L}}$$

   The 20 µL contains 20 units of enzyme. This enzyme is added to buffer to make 5 mL total volume. Therefore, you can make **four tubes** with **5 U** per tube.
2. Each tube requires (5) (0.01 U) = **0.05 U**. The enzyme concentration is 1 U/µL.

$$\frac{?}{0.05\ \text{U}} = \frac{1\ \mu\text{L}}{1\ \text{U}}$$

$$? = 0.05\ \mu\text{L} = \text{amount needed, but this volume is too low to measure.}$$

   Therefore, make 1/100 dilution, **10 µL enzyme + 990 µL = 1/100**. After dilution, there are:

$$\left(\frac{1\ \text{U}}{1\ \mu\text{L}}\right)\left(\frac{1}{100}\right) = \frac{1\ \text{U}}{100\ \mu\text{L}} = \frac{10^{-2}\ \text{U}}{1\ \mu\text{L}}$$

   Need 0.05 U/tube so use **5 µL** of dilution for each tube and dissolve in buffer to 5 mL.
3. Want 500,000X dilution and want to begin with no more than 0.5 mL.

$$\text{Here is one possibility: dilute: } \frac{1}{500{,}000} = \left(\frac{1}{50}\right)\left(\frac{1}{100}\right)\left(\frac{1}{100}\right)$$

   0.1 mL antibody + 4.9 mL diluent = 1/50 in first dilution tube

   Take 0.1 mL of above + 9.9 mL → (1/100) (1/50) = 1/5,000 in second dilution tube

   Take 0.1 mL of above + 9.9 mL → (1/100) (1/5,000) = 1/500,000 in third dilution tube
4. Have $\frac{1\times 10^9\ \text{cells}}{1\ \text{mL}}$ want $\frac{2\times 10^3\ \text{cells}}{1\ \text{mL}} = \frac{2\times 10^2\ \text{cells}}{0.1\ \text{mL}}$

   What dilution is required?

$$\frac{1\times 10^9}{2\times 10^3} = \frac{1}{2}\times 10^6 \text{ or } 5\times 10^5 \text{ dilution}$$

There are various strategies. It would be common practice to begin with 1/10 or 1/100 dilutions. The final dilution would then need to have a five in the denominator:

$$\left(\frac{1}{100}\right)\left(\frac{1}{100}\right)\left(\frac{1}{50}\right) = \frac{1}{5\times10^5} = \text{dilution needed}$$

0.1 mL culture + 9.9 mL diluent = (1/100) → (1/100) ($1\times10^9$) = $10^7$ cells/mL
0.1 mL of above + 9.9 mL diluent = (1/100) → (1/100) ($1\times10^7$) = $10^5$ cells/mL
0.1 mL of above + 4.9 mL diluent = (1/50) → (1/50) ($1\times10^5$) = 2 $\times10^3$ cells/mL = 200 cells/0.1 mL

5. The first plate has too many colonies to count and the third plate has fewer colonies than are desirable for a plate count. The middle plate has 21 colonies, so it is the one we will use for calculations. The concentration of cells added to this plate was about 21 cells/0.1 mL = 210 cells/mL. The dilution tube from which these cells were drawn had been diluted $1\times10^7$. So there were originally about $210\times10^7 = 2.10\times10^9$ bacterial cells/mL in the original broth.
6. The first plate can be used for calculations. There are about 43 colonies on the first plate, so the concentration of bacteria applied to that plate was about 430 cells/mL. The dilution tube from which these cells were drawn had been diluted $1/10^6$. Therefore, there were about $430\times10^6$ = **$4.30\times10^8$ cells/mL** in the original broth.
7.

$$10^7\ \text{cells/mL, dilute to}\ \frac{100\ \text{cells}}{0.1\ \text{mL}} = 1{,}000\ \text{cells/mL}$$

$$\frac{10^7}{10^3} = 1\times10^4 = \ \text{dilution needed}$$

$$0.1\ \text{mL culture} + 9.9\ \text{diluent} = \frac{1}{100}\ \text{dilution} = \frac{1}{10^2}\ \text{dilution} \rightarrow 10^5\ \frac{\text{cells}}{\text{mL}}$$

$$0.1\ \text{mL of above} + 9.9\ \text{mL diluent} = \frac{1}{100}\ \text{dilution}$$

$$= \frac{1}{10^2}\ \text{dilution} \rightarrow 10^3\ \frac{\text{cells}}{\text{mL}}\ \text{will form}\ 10^2\ \text{colonies / 0.1 mL}$$

8. The sample was diluted 1/5 and then 5/25 → (1/5) (5/25) = 5/125 total dilution. There were 3 mg protein in 5 mL = 0.6 mg protein/mL. Multiplying times the dilution: (0.6 mg/mL) (125/5) = **15 mg/mL**.
9. The sample was diluted 1/4 and then 10/30 → 10/120 total dilution.

   There were 10 mg protein/5 mL = 2 mg/mL protein in the solution. Multiplying times the dilution:

   (2 mg/mL) (120/10) = **24 mg/mL** in the original sample.

# III

# Describing Relationships with Equations and Graphs

**Chapters in This Unit**



## INTRODUCTION

At the time of writing, it is fall 2020, one week before Thanksgiving. The United States has now recorded more than 12 million cases of COVID-19; one million new cases were added in the last week alone. Daily case numbers are approaching 200,000. More than 255,000 people in the United States have died of the virus. With the epidemic raging, people are trying to decide what to do about Thanksgiving. Public health officials are pleading with the public to forego travel and attending large family gatherings. A team of scientists created the graph below to summarize the risks of gatherings. The graph is used to determine the probability that at a given event – such

DOI: 10.1201/9780429282744-17

as a Thanksgiving dinner – at least one person will be infected. This probability depends largely on two factors: the number of cases of illness circulating in the given population at the moment and the number of people at the event. If one person is infected, it does not necessarily mean that others will catch the virus, but it does mean that others are at risk. The risk is particularly high if the event is inside and people are not wearing masks. Thanksgiving dinner is a classic example of a gathering that is normally held inside, in close quarters, and where people are eating and cannot be masked. The X-axis on the graph is the size of the gathering and the Y-axis is the number of cases circulating in the population of interest. In this particular graph, the population is all people in the United States. Reading this graph, we can see that if ten people gather on 11/22/2020, there is a 4.35% chance that one of them will be infected with the virus causing COVID-19. This is based on the estimation, from recent data, that about 1.5 million people in the United States are infected at this moment. This graph can similarly be used to determine the probability that one person will be infected at larger gatherings.

The point of interest to us at the moment is not what to do about Thanksgiving dinner in 2020, rather, that graphs, such as this one, are an important way to depict data. Graphs are used to summarize data and show ***relationships***: in this situation, the relationship between cases of illness, size of gathering, and probability one person is infected. It is important for every biotechnologist to be able to prepare graphs and to interpret graphs others have created. This unit introduces these skills.

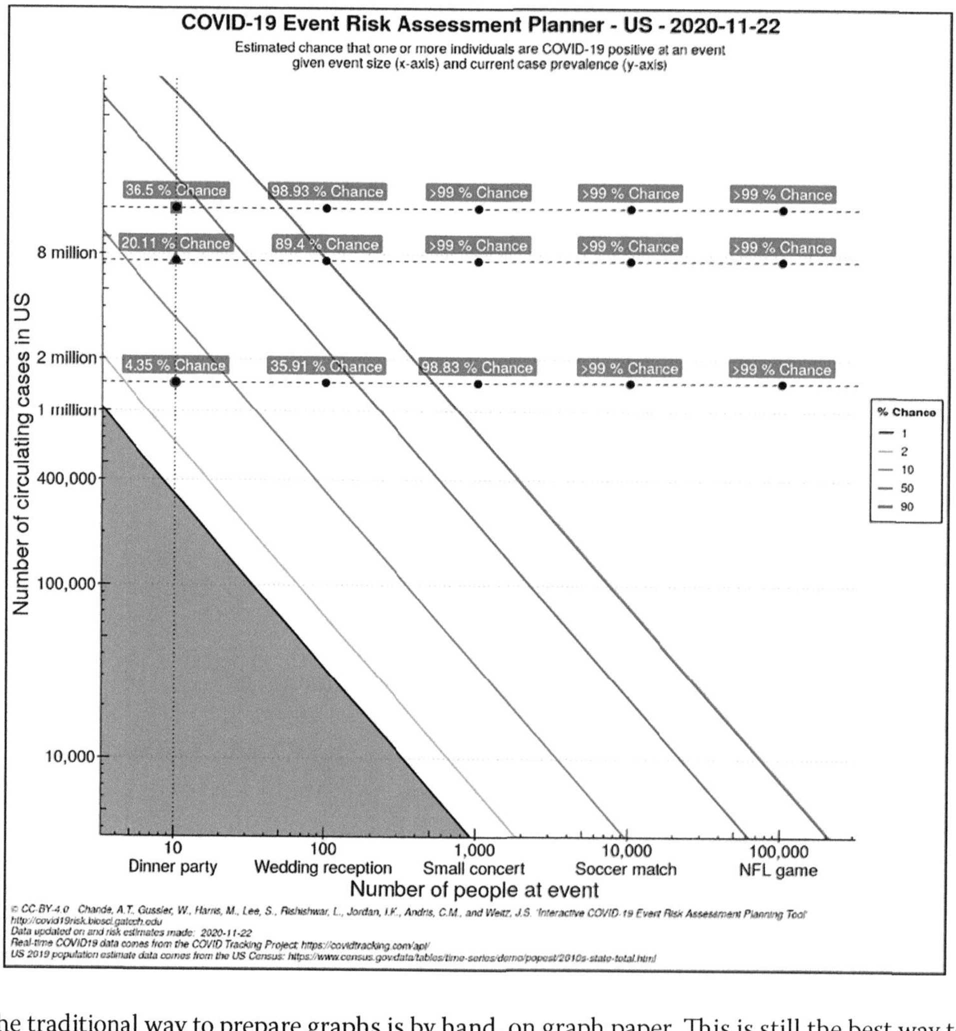


The traditional way to prepare graphs is by hand, on graph paper. This is still the best way to learn about graphing. However, in the workplace, graphs are normally computer generated, and employers are likely to assume you can prepare graphs with a computer. Also, some of the interesting problems in this text are time consuming to plot by hand and can be more readily and more accurately plotted by a computer program. Therefore, it is a good idea to practice preparing graphs both by hand and using a computer software program. Graph paper templates are readily available online, so you practice graphing by hand. At the time of writing, Excel is the most common computer software program used for graphing. Tutorials for using Excel are available on-line; use a web browser to find them. Note, however, that Excel has periodically changed its format, and therefore any specific directions are likely to become outdated. Usually, once you understand Excel's basic commands, some experimentation will allow you to create the graph you want, regardless of the version of the program.

In addition to graphs, biotechnologists use equations to depict relationships. Like graphs, all biotechnologists must have some facility with equations, although we do not need to go as far into algebraic manipulations as you would in a typical algebra class. This unit discusses the use of graphs and equations to summarize data and show relationships between different factors. We focus on the most common ways in which these mathematical tools are applied in biotechnology settings.

# Graphing Linear Equations

15



## 15.1 BRIEF REVIEW OF THE BASIC TECHNIQUES OF GRAPHING

Graphs and equations are tools for working with relationships between two (or sometimes more) variables. The general rules regarding graphing will be briefly reviewed in the first part of this chapter. The use of graphing as a tool to perform various tasks in a laboratory will be demonstrated in later sections.

A basic two-dimensional graph, Figure 15.1, consists of a vertical and a horizontal line that intersect at a point called the **origin**. *The horizontal line is the* **X-axis**, and *the vertical line is the* **Y-axis**. The X- and Y-axes are each divided into evenly spaced subdivisions that are assigned numerical values. To the right of the origin on the X-axis the values are positive numbers, and to the left of the origin the values are negative. On the Y-axis values above the origin are positive; below the origin, they are negative.

A basic two-dimensional graph shows the relationship between two variables: one that is assigned to the X-axis and the other to the Y-axis. *At any given point on the graph, the value of the variable on the X-axis is paired with a corresponding value of the variable on the Y-axis.* The two values are called **coordinates** because they are coordinated, or associated,

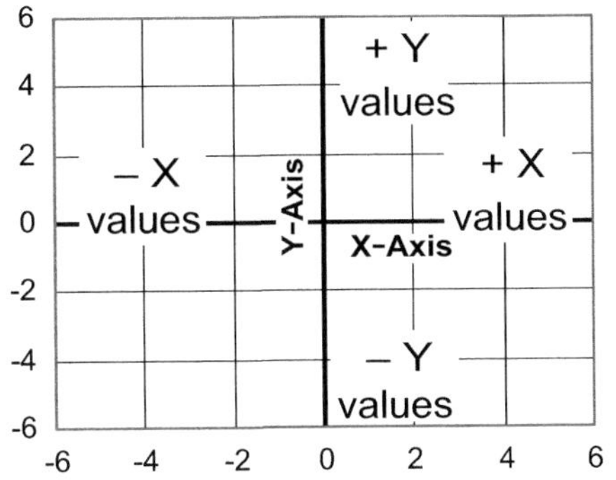


**FIGURE 15.1** A two-dimensional graph.

DOI: 10.1201/9780429282744-18

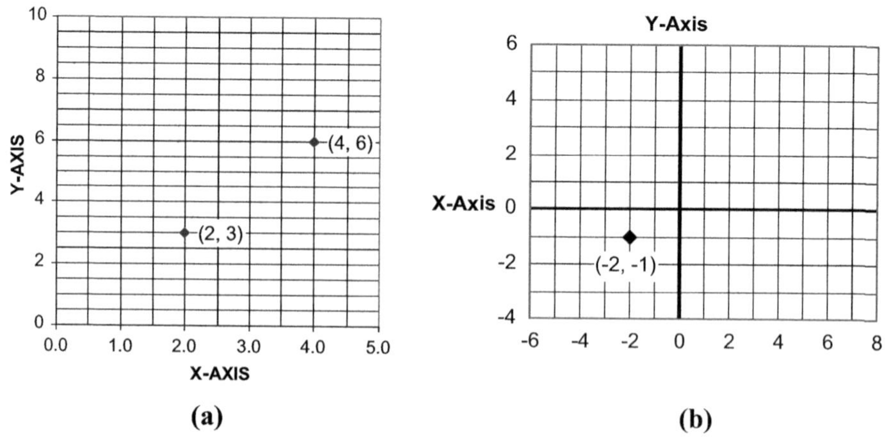


**FIGURE 15.2** Coordinates and graphs. (a) The points (2,3) and (4,6). (b) The point (–2, –1).

with one another. A pair of coordinates can be plotted on the graph as shown in Figure 15.2a. The first point shown on the graph has an X-coordinate of 2 because it is a distance of 2 to the right of the origin and a Y-coordinate of 3, because it is a distance of 3 above the origin. This point can be written as $X = 2$, $Y = 3$, or as (2, 3). The second point on this graph has the coordinates (4, 6). Similarly, the point in Figure 15.2b has coordinates $X = -2$, $Y = -1$. To prepare a graph, one marks the locations of a series of points by using their coordinates.

## 15.2 GRAPHING STRAIGHT LINES

Two variables may be related to one another in such a way that when their data points are plotted on a graph, the points form a straight line. The two variables are then said to have a **linear relationship**. There are many applications in the laboratory that involve linear relationships.

Consider the simple equation:

$$Y = 2X$$

It is possible to find many combinations of values for X and Y that are solutions to this equation. For example:

If $X = 3$, then $Y = 6$

If $X = 4$, then $Y = 8$

and so on

These solutions and more are represented in both tabular and graphical form in Figure 15.3. Each pair of X- and Y-values are the coordinates of a point on the graph. The points form a straight line when connected.

In the linear equation $Y = 2X$, the value 2 is called the **slope**. In the equation $Y = 3X$ the slope is 3, and in the equation $Y = 4X$ the slope is 4. The equations $Y = 2X$, $Y = 3X$, and $Y = 4X$ are plotted on the same graph in Figure 15.4. Each equation is linear; the difference between the three lines is their steepness. Just as a hill may be more or less steep, so a line has a slope

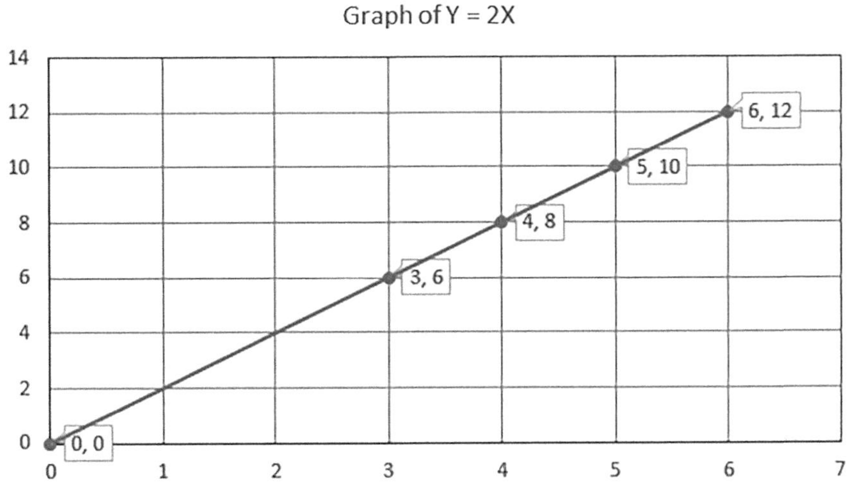


| Examples of Solutions for the Equation Y = 2X | |
|---|---|
| **X** | **Y** |
| *0* | *0* |
| *3* | *6* |
| *4* | *8* |
| *5* | *10* |
| *6* | *12* |

**FIGURE 15.3** Graph of the equation Y = 2X.

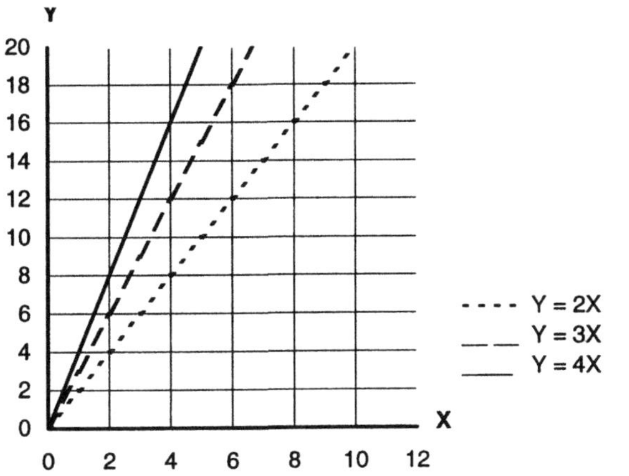


| Y = 3X | | Y = 4X | |
|---|---|---|---|
| X | Y | X | Y |
| *0* | *0* | *0* | *0* |
| *1* | *3* | *1* | *4* |
| *2* | *6* | *2* | *8* |
| *3* | *9* | *3* | *12* |
| *4* | *12* | *4* | *16* |
| *5* | *15* | *5* | *20* |

**FIGURE 15.4** Slope. The greater the absolute value of the slope of a straight line, the steeper the line. (The absolute value is the magnitude of a number without regard to whether it is + or –.)

that is more or less steep. The equation Y = 4X defines a steeper line than the other two equations because its slope, 4, is the largest.

Given a straight line plotted on a graph, the slope of the line is calculated by determining how steeply the line rises or falls. For example, consider the line for Y = 2X in Figure 15.5. From point **a** to point **b**, X increases from 2 to 3, a change of +1. Y increases from 4 to 6, a change of +2. *The amount by which the X-coordinate changes is called the* **run**; *the amount by which the Y-coordinate changes is called the* **rise**. The rise divided by the run is a numerical measure of the steepness of the slope. To calculate the slope of any straight line, choose any two points on the line. The coordinates for the first point are $(X_1, Y_1)$ and for the second point are $(X_2, Y_2)$. Then,

$$\textbf{Slope} = \frac{\textbf{Rise}}{\textbf{Run}} = \frac{\textbf{Change in Y}}{\textbf{Change in X}} = \frac{Y_2 - Y_1}{X_2 - X_1}$$

We can also say:

$$\textbf{Slope} = \frac{\textbf{Vertical change}}{\textbf{Horizontal change}}$$

For the line Y = 2X:

$$\textbf{Slope} = \frac{\textbf{Rise}}{\textbf{Run}} = \frac{2}{1} = 2$$

Any two points on the line Y = 2X will give a slope of 2. Similarly, any two points on the line Y = 3X will give a slope of 3 and any two points on the line Y = 4X will yield a slope of 4. This is because straight lines have a constant "steepness." In contrast, in Chapter 17, we will look at the graphs of exponential equations where the graph changes in steepness; therefore the value for the slope varies depending on where you are on the graph.

Figure 15.6 shows the graph of a line that goes "downhill" from left to right. For this line, as the X-values increase, the Y-values decrease. The slope is therefore negative.

Figure 15.7 shows the plot for the equation **A = 2C + 4**. (Substitution of other symbols for X and Y does not change the basic meaning of the equation.) The difference between the plot of **Y = 2X** and **A = 2C + 4** is that the latter line crosses the vertical axis higher than the origin. The line A = 2C+4 intercepts, or passes through, the Y-axis at (0, 4). *The point at which a line passes through the Y-axis, that is, where X = 0, is termed the* **Y-intercept.** If the line passes through the Y-axis at the point where both X and Y are zero, the intercept is often not written. Thus, the Y-intercept of the line Y = 2X is (0,0).

If an equation gives a straight line when it is graphed, it can be expressed in the form:

$$\textbf{Y} = \textbf{Slope}(\textbf{X}) + \textbf{Y-intercept}$$

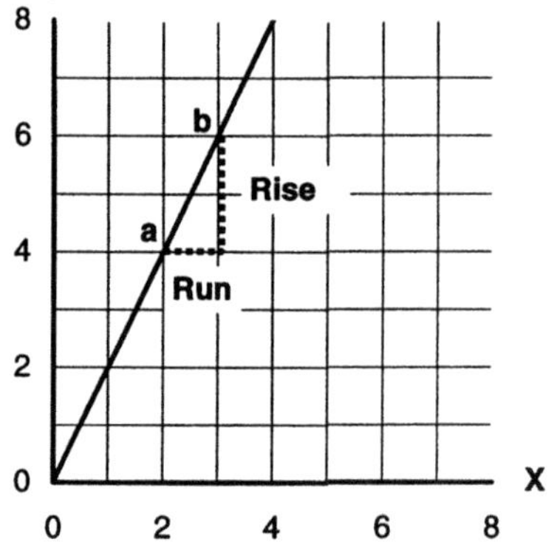


**FIGURE 15.5** Determining the slope of a line. The slope can be calculated based on the coordinates of any two points on the line. Slope = rise/run, which in this case = 2/1 = 2.

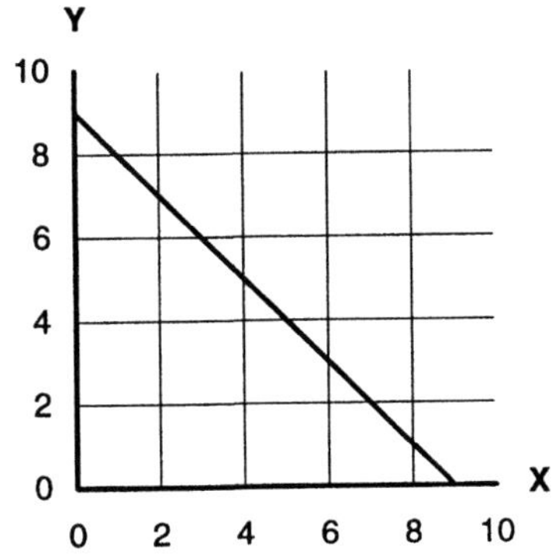


**FIGURE 15.6** A line with a negative slope. All lines that go "downhill" from left to right have a negative slope.

**Examples of Solutions for the Equation A = 2C + 4**

| C | A |
|---|---|
| 0 | 4 |
| 1 | 6 |
| 2 | 8 |
| 3 | 10 |
| 4 | 12 |
| 5 | 14 |

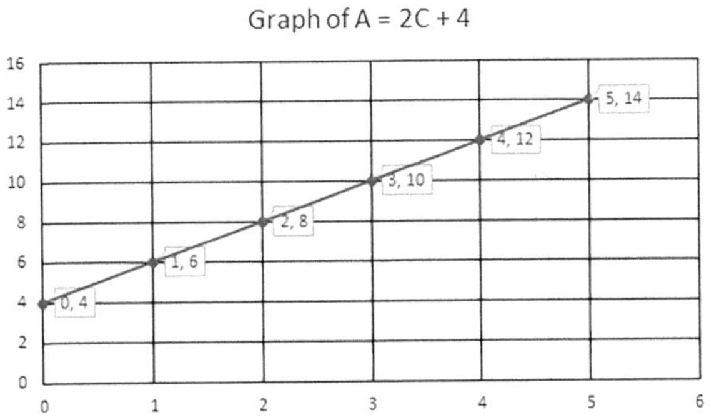


**FIGURE 15.7** A graph with a non-zero Y-intercept.

This general equation for a straight line is sometimes written as Equation 15.1. This is known as the slope-intercept form.

**EQUATION 15.1: The Equation for a Straight Line**

$$Y = mX + a$$

where m is the slope
a is the Y-intercept

Note: There are other common ways to write the general equation for a straight line that use different symbols to represent the slope or the Y-intercept. For example, the Y-intercept is often called "b." However, "b" has another meaning in spectrophotometry, as you will see in Chapter 16, so we use "a" to represent the Y-intercept in this text.

It is possible to determine the equation for a straight line from its graph. For example, the line drawn in Figure 15.8 has a Y-intercept of (0, 4) and a slope of 0.5. Therefore, the equation for this line is:

$$\mathbf{Y = 0.5X + 4.}$$

The general procedure to find the equation for any graphed straight line is shown in Box 15.1.

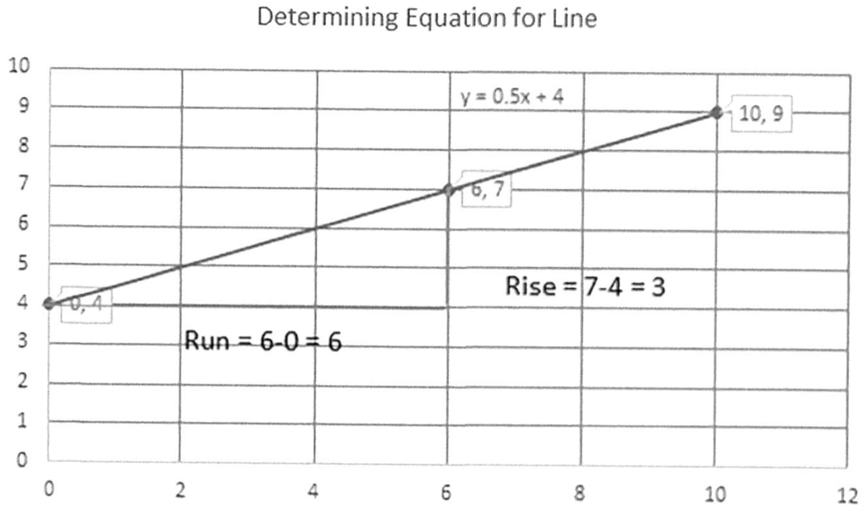


**FIGURE 15.8** Determining the equation for a line. Slope = (7−4)/(6−0) = 0.5. Y-intercept = (0, 4). Equation is Y = 0.5X + 4.

**BOX 15.1: Procedure to Find the Equation for a Straight Line on a Graph**

We can generally describe a straight line with an equation in the form:

$$Y = mX + a$$

where:
m is the slope
a is the Y-intercept

Step 1. Find the Y-intercept, that is, the value of Y when X = 0. The intercept may be positive, negative, or zero.

Step 2. Find the slope by picking any two points for which you can find the coordinates and calculating

$$(Y_2 - Y_1)/(X_2 - X_1).$$

The slope may be positive, negative, or zero. (A horizontal line has a slope of zero.)

Step 3. Write the equation for the line by filling in the values for the slope and Y intercept:

Y = *slope* (X) + *Y-intercept*

Notes:

- The axes of a graph can have units in which case the slope and the intercept will also have units. Include the units, if present, when writing the equation for a line.
- The equation for a horizontal line is Y = 0 (X) + Y-intercept, or just Y = Y-intercept.
- For example, Y = 3 is the equation for a horizontal line.
- This pattern does not fit vertical lines, such as X = 2.

**Example Problem:**

Which of the following equations describe a straight line?

**a.** $C = 2B$ **b.** $Q = 25.4T - 5$ **c.** $Y = X^2 + 3$ **d.** $C = -V - 34$

***Answer:***

All except **c** are equations for a straight line. The exponent in equation **c** means that it does not describe a straight line. The rest of the equations have 2 variables, a slope, and a Y-intercept, which may or may not be zero. Equation **b** fits the form of a linear equation as shown here:

$$\mathbf{Y = mX + a}$$

$$\mathbf{Q = 25.4T + (-5)}$$

Equation **d** also fits the slope-intercept form of:

$$\mathbf{Y = mX + a}$$

$$\mathbf{C = (-1)V + (-34)}$$

**Example Problem:**

The graph below shows the ideal response of a pH meter relative to the pH of a solution. The meter's response is measured in units of mV, as shown on the Y-axis. Observe that the response of the pH meter varies depending on the temperature of the solution.

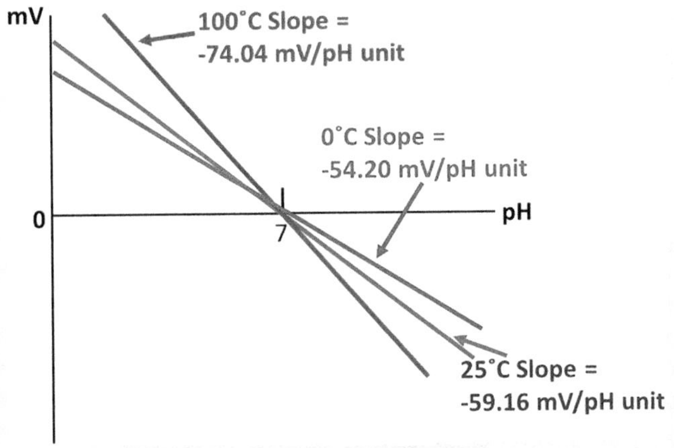


**a.** The response of the pH meter was measured at three temperatures: 0°C, 25°C, and 100°C. At which temperature does the relationship have the steepest slope?

**b.** What is the change in mV per pH unit at each temperature? Describe how temperature affects the response of the pH meter.

**c.** Predict the response in mV of a pH meter in a solution at pH 3 at 25°C.

*Answer:*

a, b. **The slope is steepest at 100°C**, where there is an increase of +74.04 mV for each pH *decrease* of one (the slope is negative). At 25°C, there is a change of +59.16 mV for each pH *decrease* of one. At 0°C, there is a change of +54.20 mV for each pH *decrease* of one. This means that the pH meter is more responsive to a change in pH when it is warmer than when it is colder. Typically, we work at 25°C and so an ideal pH metering system is expected to have a response of 59.16 mV for each change in one pH unit, i.e., when the pH increases by one, the response decreases by 59.16 mV, and vice versa.

c. Note that at pH 7, the pH meter response is 0 mV. pH 3 is four units *lower* than pH 7, so the mV response should be:

$$0 \text{ mV} + 4 \text{pH units } (59.16 \text{ mV/pH unit}) = 236.64 \text{ mV} \approx \mathbf{237\ mV.}$$

**Practice Problems**

1. ***For each of the following graphs, describe in words the relationship that is displayed.***

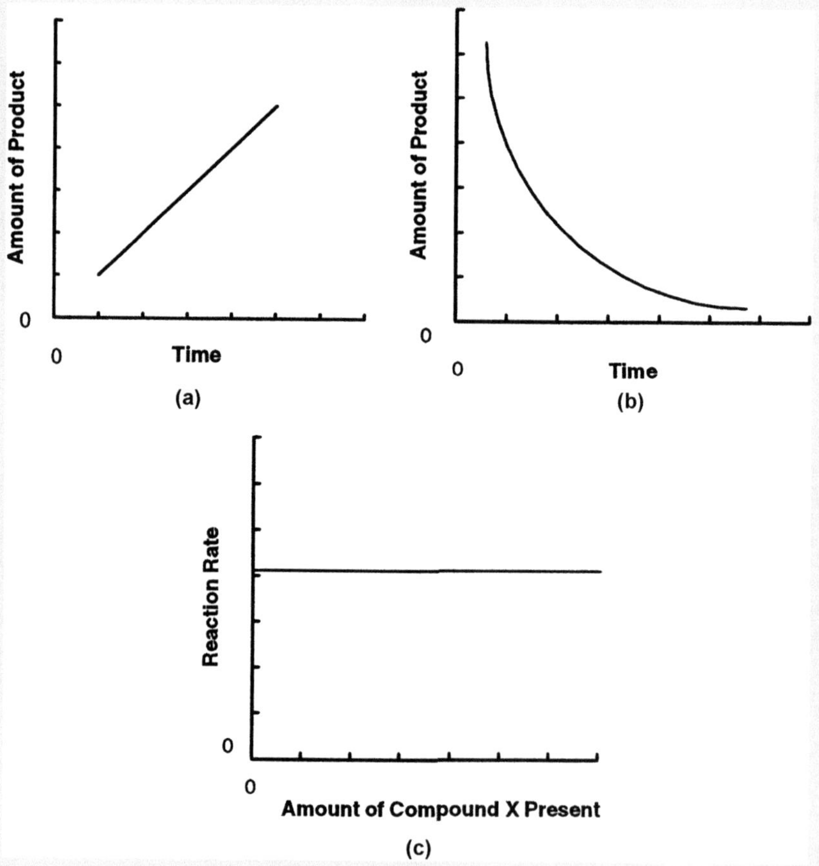

2. ***This figure shows a graph with 4 points, labeled a, b, c, and d. Write the coordinates for each of the four points.***

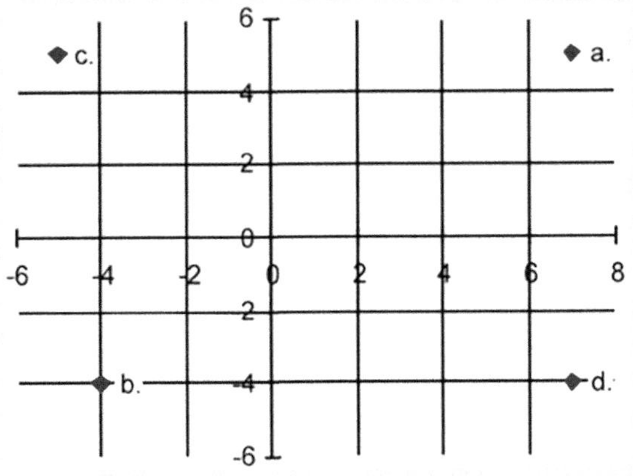


3. ***In the graph in problem 2, as you move from point a to point b, by how much does the value of X change?___ By how much does the value of Y change?______. As you go from point b to point c, how much does the value of X change?____ How much does the value of Y change?___________***

4. ***Draw a graph and plot each of these points on the graph:***

   $X = 4, Y = 6$

   $X = 5,\ Y = -2$

   $(-4,3)$

   $(1,1)$

5. ***A table showing solutions for the equation $Y = 5X + 1$ is shown below. Fill in the blanks in the table, and then plot the line.***

| *X* | *Y* |
|---|---|
| *1* | *6* |
| *5* | *26* |
| *10* | *51* |
| *12* | __ |
| __ | *76* |
| __ | *101* |

6. ***Suppose two variables, A and Q, are related by the equation $A = 3Q - 4$. Prepare a table showing at least five solutions for this equation and then graph the equation.***

7. ***What is the slope and the Y-intercept for each of these equations?***
   ***a.*** $Y = 3X + 2$ ***b.*** $C = 0.2X - 1$ ***c.*** $Y = 0.005X$

8. ***What is the slope and Y-intercept for each of these lines?***

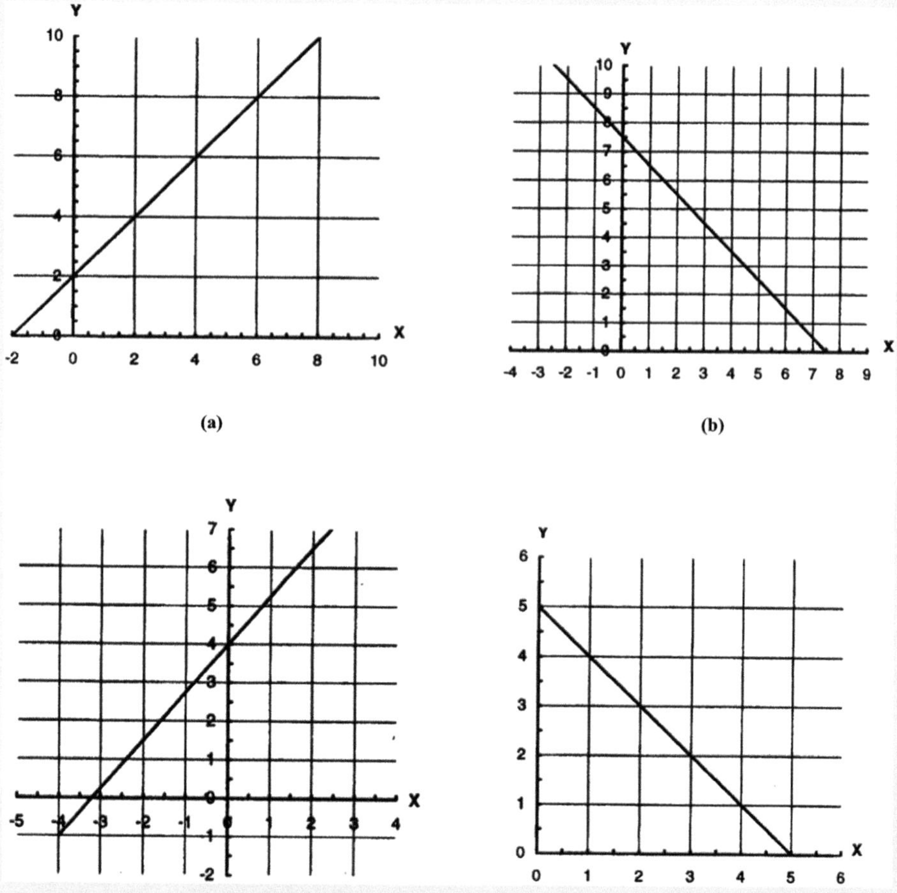

(a) (b) (c) (d)

9. ***Which of these graphs shows a linear relationship between two variables?***

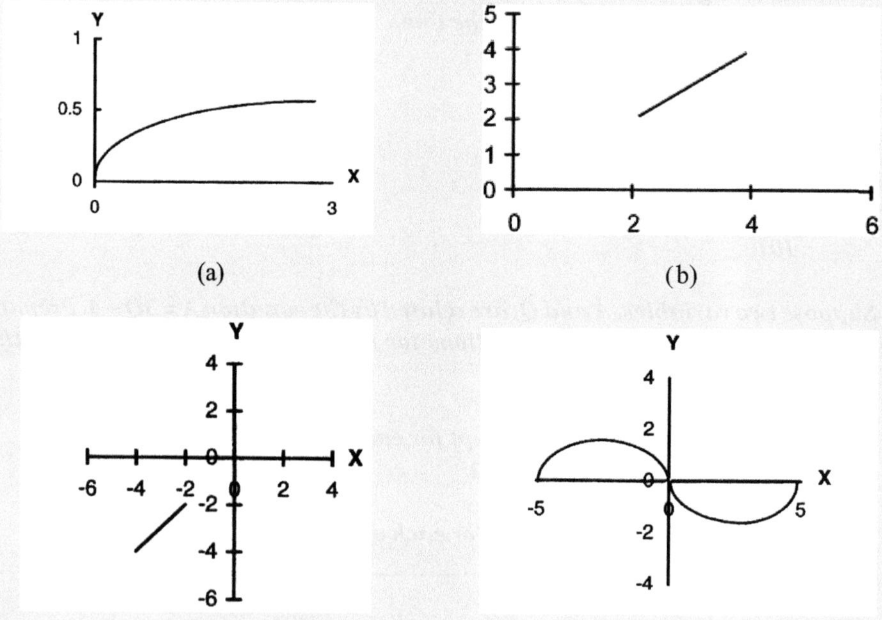

(a) (b) (c) (d)

10. ***Which of these equations will form a straight line when plotted on a graph?***
    - *a.* $Y = 45X - 1$ *b.* $C = 34D + 17$ *c.* $34 + 2 - 4D = E$ *d.* $Q = R$

11. ***For each linear equation below, give the slope, the Y-intercept, and sketch the graph:***
    - *a.* $Y = (10\ \text{cm/min})\,X + 1\ \text{cm}$
    - *b.* $3 - X = Y$
    - *c.* $12\ (\text{mg}) + 7\ (\text{mg/cm})\,X = Y$

12. ***Find the equations for the lines graphed in each of the following examples.***

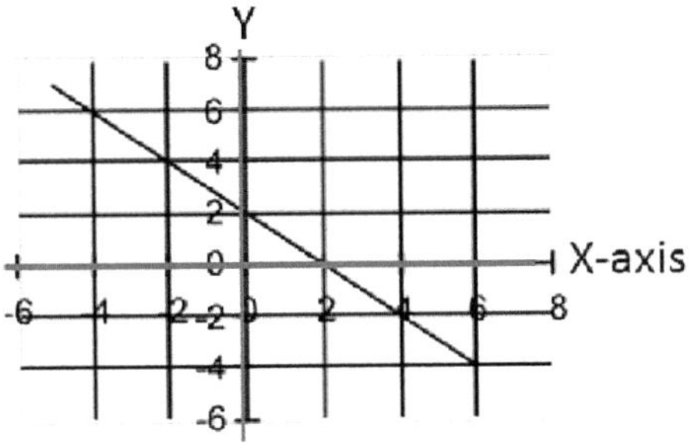


(a)

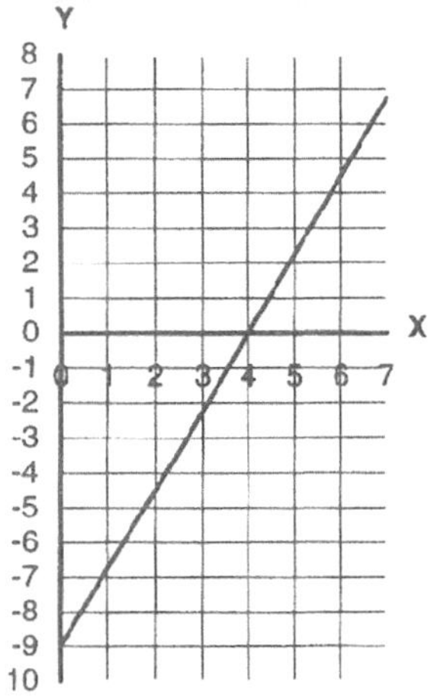


(b)

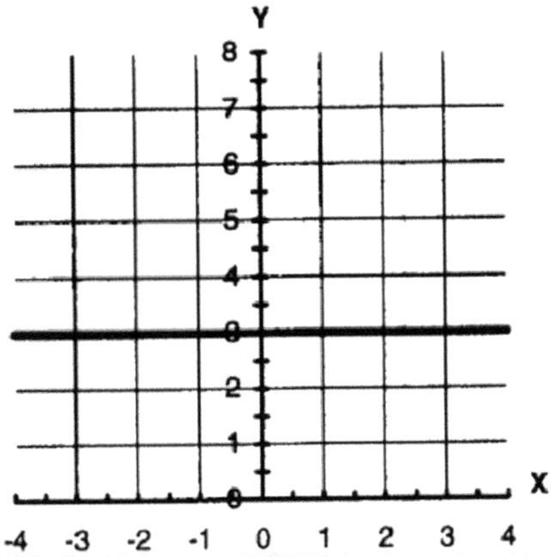


(c)

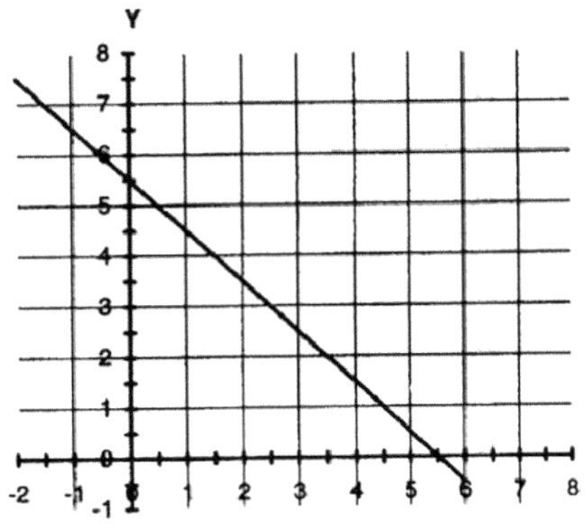


(d)

13. ***Graph the line that contains the following points: (1, 1), (6, 6), (9, 9). What is the equation for this line?***

14. ***The relationship between the temperature in degrees Fahrenheit and degrees Celsius is given by the equation:*** $°F = 9/5\ (°C) + 32°$.
    - *a.* ***There are two constants in this equation. What are they?***
    - *b.* ***Which of the two constants is the Y-intercept?***
    - *c.* ***Which of the two constants is the slope of the line?***
    - *d.* ***Graph this relationship.***

### Answers

1. a. The amount of product increases in a linear fashion over time.
   b. The amount of product decreases in a nonlinear fashion over time.
   c. The reaction rate is constant, regardless of the amount of compound X present.

2. a. **(7, 5)** b. **(−4, −4)** c. **(−5, 5)** d. **(7, −4)**

3. Change in X = **−11**, change in Y = **−9**,
   Change in X = **−1**, change in Y = **9**

4.
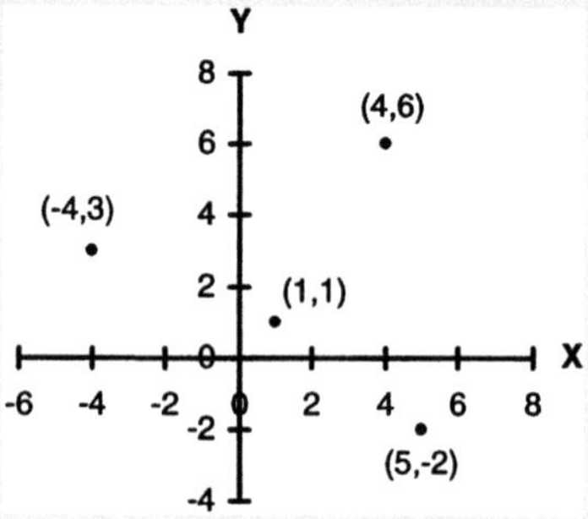


5.

| X | Y |
|---|---|
| 1 | 6 |
| 5 | 26 |
| 10 | 51 |
| 12 | 61 |
| 15 | 76 |
| 20 | 101 |

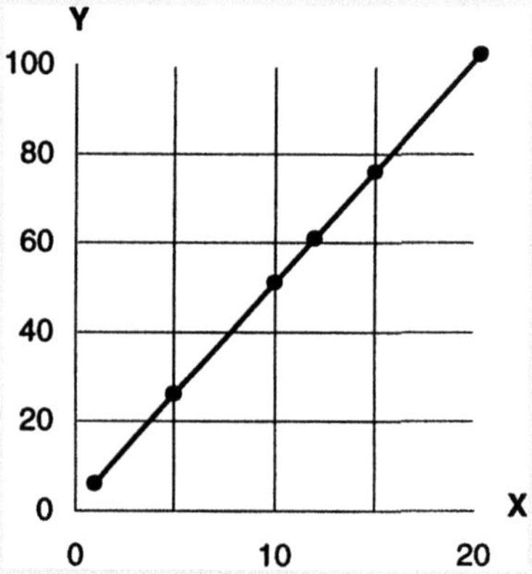


6.

A = 3Q–4

| Q | A |
|---|---|
| −1 | −7 |
| 0 | −4 |
| 1 | −1 |
| 2 | 2 |
| 3 | 5 |

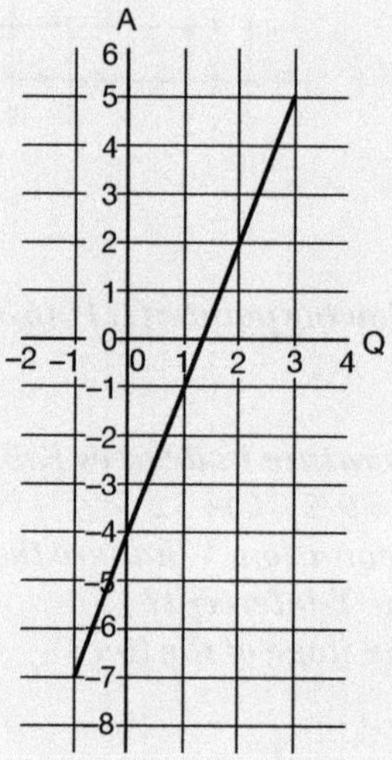

7. a. Slope **3**, Y-intercept **(0, 2)** b. Slope **0.2**, Y-intercept **(0, –1)**
   c. Slope **0.005**, Y-intercept **(0, 0)**

8. a. Slope **1**, Y-intercept **(0, 2)** b. Slope **–1**, Y-intercept **(0, 7.5)**
   c. Slope **1.25**, Y-intercept **(0, 4)** d. Slope **–1**, Y-intercept **(0, 5)**

9. a. Not linear b. Linear c. Linear d. Not linear

10. All will form a line.

11. a. Slope = **10 cm/min**, Y-intercept = **(0 min, 1 cm)**
    b. Slope = **–1**, Y-intercept = **(0, 3)**
    c. Slope = **7 mg/cm**, Y-intercept = **(0 cm, 12 mg)**

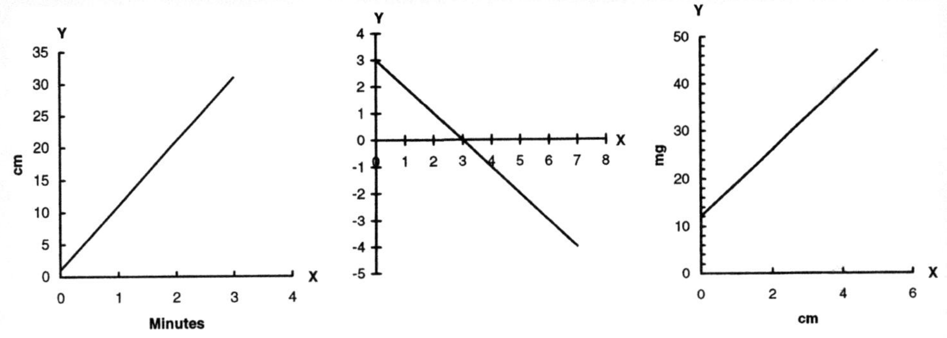

(a) (b) (c)

12. a. $Y = -1X + 2$ b. $Y = 2.25X - 9$ c. $Y = 3$ d. $Y = -1X + 5.5$

13. $Y = 1X + 0$

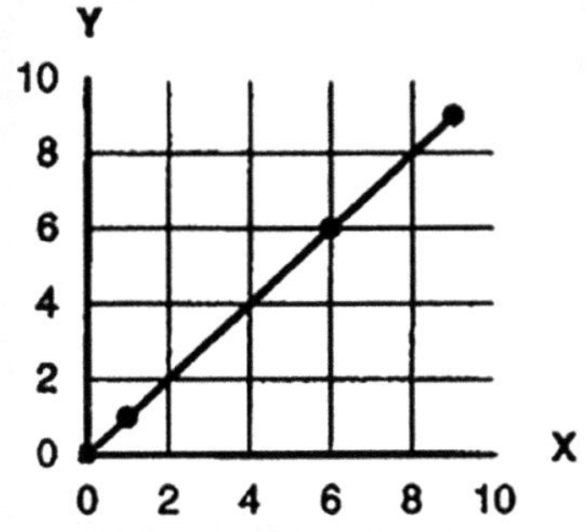


14. a. **9/5** and **32**
    b. **32**
    c. **9/5**
    d.

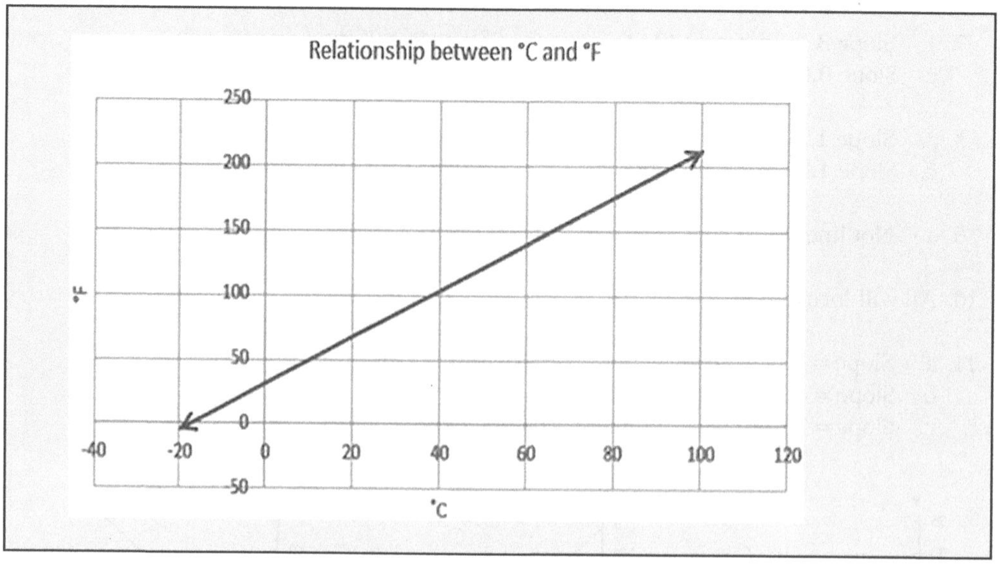


## 15.3 AN APPLICATION OF GRAPHING: STANDARD CURVES AND QUANTITATIVE ANALYSIS

This section discusses an important laboratory application of graphs of linear relationships, that is, in quantitative analysis. **Quantitative analysis** *is the determination of how much of a particular material is present in a sample. The substance of interest is called the* **analyte**. To make such determinations, a standard curve is often used. A **standard curve** *is a graph of the relationship between the concentration or amount of a material of interest and the response of a particular instrument.* Note that the term standard "curve" is used for this sort of graph; however, the desired relationship between concentration (or amount) and instrument response is typically linear.

A standard curve is constructed as follows: a series of standards containing known concentrations of the material of interest are prepared. The response of an instrument to each standard is measured. A standard curve is plotted with the response of the instrument on the Y-axis and the concentration of standard on the X-axis. Once graphed, the standard curve is used to determine the concentration of the material of interest in the samples. This process is summarized in Box 15.2 and is illustrated with an example.

**EXAMPLE:**

Step 1: Standards are prepared containing 1.0, 2.0, 3.0, 5.0, 6.0, and 7.0 mg/mL of a compound of interest.

Step 2: An instrument's response to each standard is measured, Table 15.1.

Step 3: The resulting data are plotted as points on a graph with the concentration of standard on the X-axis and the instrument response on the Y-axis, Figure 15.9a.

Step 4: If the data reasonably fit a line, they are connected into a line, Figure 15.9b and 15.9c.

Step 5: The standard curve is used to determine the concentration of the material of interest in samples, Figure 15.10.

Observe in Figure 15.9a that the points approximate a line, but they do not all fall exactly on the line. This is what we would expect due to small errors in measurement and natural variability in instrument response. In a situation like this, where it is reasonable to assume that the relationship is linear, we connect the points into a straight line. The points are not connected "dot to dot" as illustrated in Figure 15.9b, because this would suggest that the slight

**BOX 15.2: Preparing a Standard Curve for Quantitative Analysis**

Step 1. Make a series of standards that contain a known concentration of the analyte. At least 5 standards are recommended. The standard concentrations should span the range of concentrations expected in samples.

Step 2. Determine instrument's response to each standard.

Step 3. Graph the data with concentration (or amount) of analyte on the X-axis and instrument response on the Y-axis.

Step 4. Assuming data reasonably fit a line, connect the points into a straight line.

Step 5. Test the instrument's response to the sample(s). Use the standard curve to determine the concentration (or amount) of analyte in the sample(s).

Notes:

- Be aware of thresholds in the relationship between instrument response and standard concentration. Do not connect points into the standard curve line that exceed a threshold. (Thresholds are discussed in the text below.)
- Samples that have an instrument response higher than any standard should be diluted first.

**TABLE 15.1 Instrument Response Versus Concentration of Standards**

| Concentration of Standard (mg/mL) | Instrument Response |
|---|---|
| 1 | 0.24 |
| 2 | 0.53 |
| 3 | 0.72 |
| 5 | 1.28 |
| 6 | 1.51 |
| 7 | 1.79 |

variations from the line are meaningful. Rather, the points are connected into a single line that "best fits," or best averages all the points, as shown in Figure 15.9c.

There are two ways to get a "best fit" line for the points on a graph. One method is to place a ruler over the graph and draw a straight line that appears "by eye" to be closest to all the points. Most people are able to draw a reasonable "best fit" line "by eye," but two people will seldom draw a line with exactly the same slope and Y-intercept. *A more accurate method to draw a line of best fit is the statistical technique,* **the least squares method.** This statistical method is explained in Section 15.15. Computer graphing programs, such as Excel, are able to automatically compute and display the line of best fit.

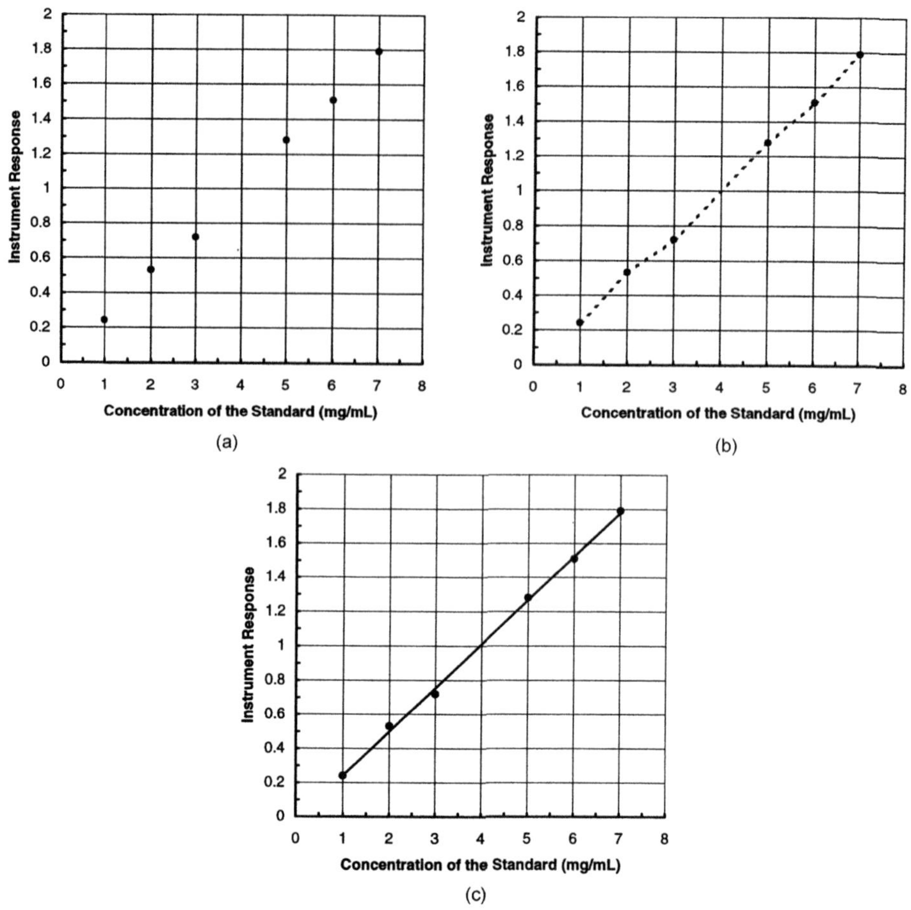


**FIGURE 15.9** A standard curve. (a) Data from Table 15.1 are graphed. The concentration of compound in the standards is on the X-axis, instrument response is on the Y-axis. (b) The points are not connected "dot to dot," as shown here, because this would suggest that slight variations from a straight line are meaningful. (c) The points are connected into a "best fit line" that best averages all the points.

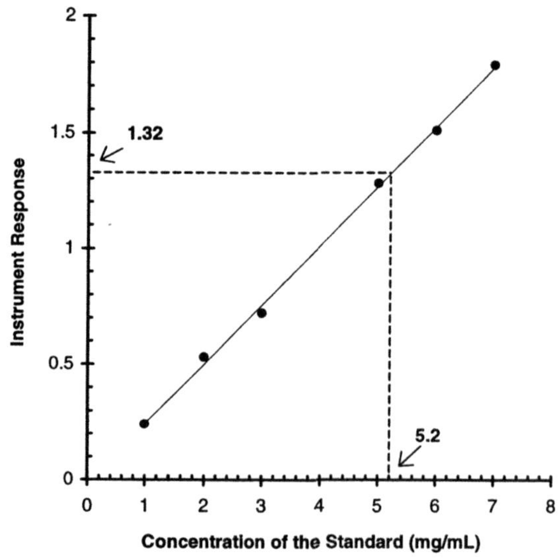


**FIGURE 15.10** Using a standard curve to determine the concentration of a material in a sample. In this example, a sample gives an instrument reading of 1.32 that corresponds to a concentration of 5.2 mg/mL.

Regardless of whether the points are connected into a line "by eye" or using the method of least squares, the standard curve can be used to determine the level of compound in each unknown sample. In the example illustrated in Figure 15.10, a sample gives an instrument reading of 1.32. From the standard curve, one can see that a reading of 1.32 corresponds to a concentration of 5.2 mg/mL.

**Example Problem:**

Biologists commonly use a protein assay to determine the concentration of protein in a solution. (An **assay** *is a test of a sample.*) Various protein assays are available, many of which measure the color change in a protein solution when it reacts with various dyes. The amount of color appearing is generally proportional to the amount of protein present within a given range of protein concentration.

The graph below shows the relationship between the concentration of protein in a series of standards and the amount of color after the standards are reacted with dye. The amount of color is measured in terms of the *amount of light absorbed by the dye*; this measurement is called **absorbance**.

a. In what range of protein concentration does the assay give useful results? What happens at higher concentrations of protein and very low concentrations of protein?
b. Suppose you have a sample containing an unknown amount of protein. The sample reacted with the dye and has an absorbance of 0.70. Based on the standard curve, what is the concentration of protein in the unknown?

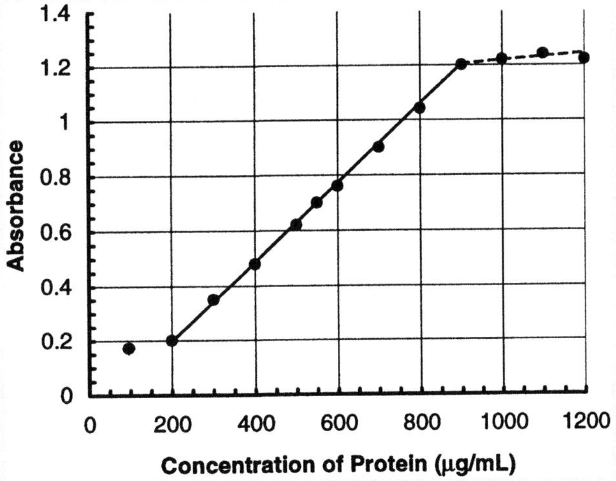


***Answer:***

a. The assay is useful in the middle range of protein concentrations. The data points and graph above 900 μg/mL and below 200 μg/mL are not useful because the absorbance plateaus. You can see this on the graph where the points do not follow the linear relationship that fits the other points.
b. You can see from the dashed lines on the graph below that the unknown's absorbance of 0.70 corresponds to a concentration of about 550 μg/mL.

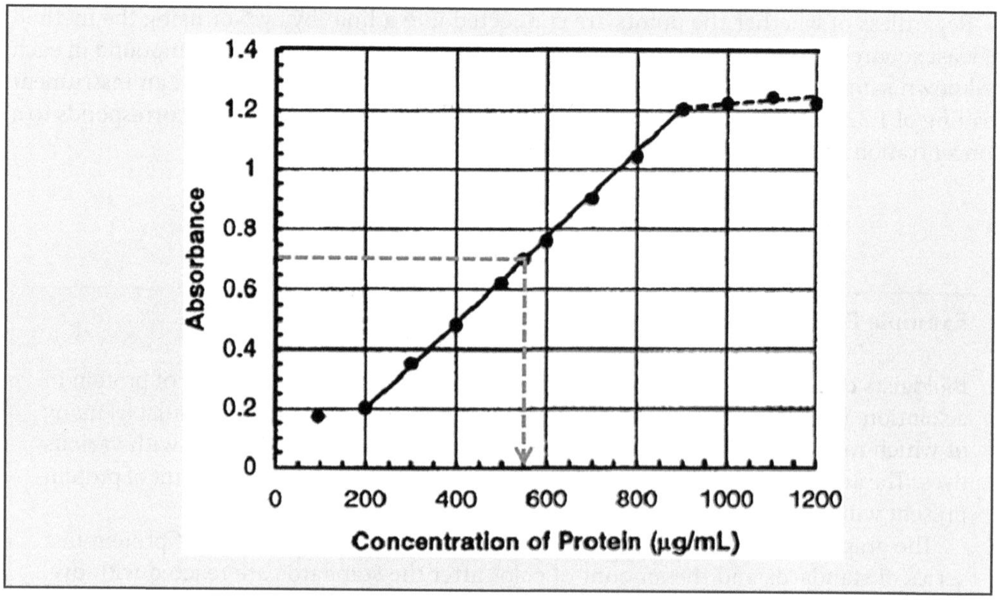


**Example Problem:**

The concentration of compound Z in samples needs to be determined. The response of an instrument to compound Z is linear with respect to its concentration. A series of standards are prepared, and the instrument's response is measured. The resulting data are shown below.

**a.** Plot a standard curve for compound Z based on the data provided. Draw the line that best fits the points.
**b.** A sample with an unknown concentration of compound Z gives an instrument response of 1.35. Based on the standard curve, what is the concentration of compound Z in the sample?
**c.** Suppose that the response of the instrument used in this example is known to be inaccurate at readings above 2.2. If a sample has a reading of 2.67, how can you determine its concentration of compound Z?
**d.** If a sample is diluted 1/20 and has an instrument reading of 0.45, what was the concentration of compound Z in the original sample?

| Concentration of Compound Z in Standard (mg/mL) | Instrument Response |
|---|---|
| 100 | 0.30 |
| 150 | 0.44 |
| 250 | 0.68 |
| 400 | 1.13 |
| 550 | 1.48 |
| 650 | 1.82 |
| 850 | 2.10 |

*Answer:*

a.

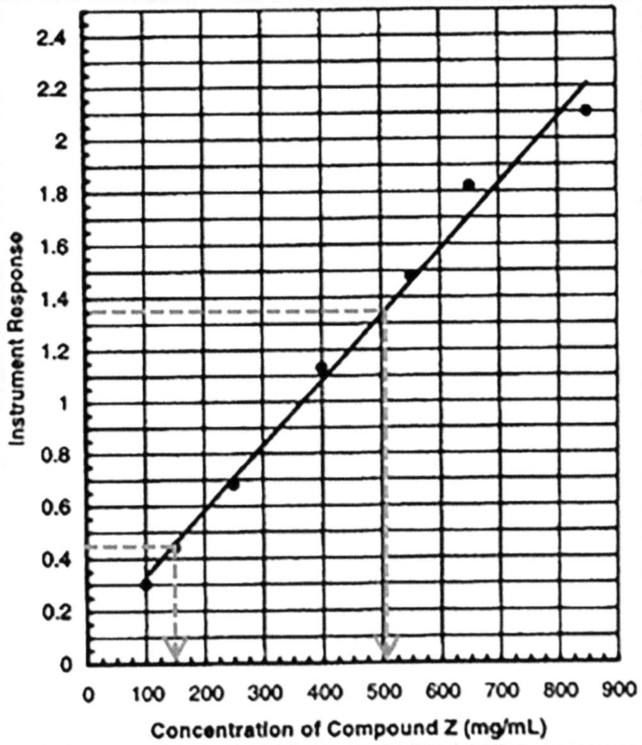


b. You can see from the dashed lines on the standard curve that the concentration of compound Z in the sample is about **500 mg/mL**.
c. It is necessary to dilute the sample before reading its absorbance.
d. As shown by the dashed lines on the standard curve, a value of 0.45 corresponds to a concentration of about 150 mg/mL. However, the sample was diluted, and this dilution needs to be taken into consideration. Therefore, we multiply 150 mg/mL times the reciprocal of the dilution:

$$(150\ \text{mg/mL})(20/1) = \mathbf{3{,}000\ mg\ /\ mL}$$

The concentration of compound Z in the original undiluted sample was **3,000 mg/mL**.

**Practice Problem**

a. ***Plot a standard curve based on the data below. Draw the line that best fits the values.***
b. ***Suppose you have a sample that gives an instrument response of 2.35. This value is higher than the reading of the highest standard. Therefore, you dilute the sample 1/100. The instrument reading of the diluted sample is 0.78. What was the amount of the material of interest in the original solution?***

| Amount of Standard (g) | Instrument Response |
|---|---|
| 0 | 0.00 |
| 10 | 0.14 |
| 20 | 0.28 |
| 30 | 0.41 |
| 40 | 0.52 |
| 50 | 0.71 |
| 65 | 0.84 |
| 75 | 1.04 |
| 80 | 1.15 |

*Answer*

a.

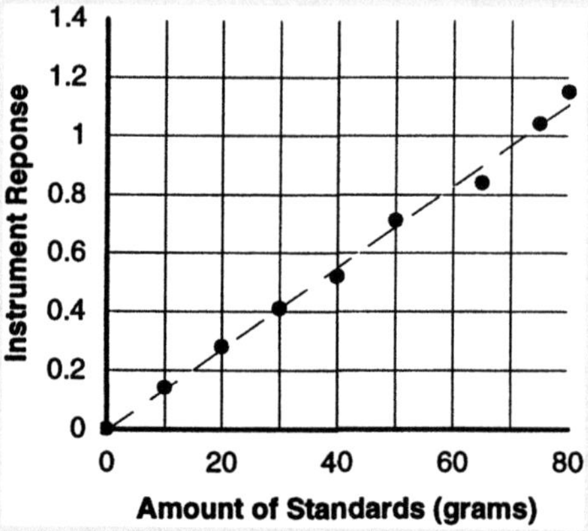

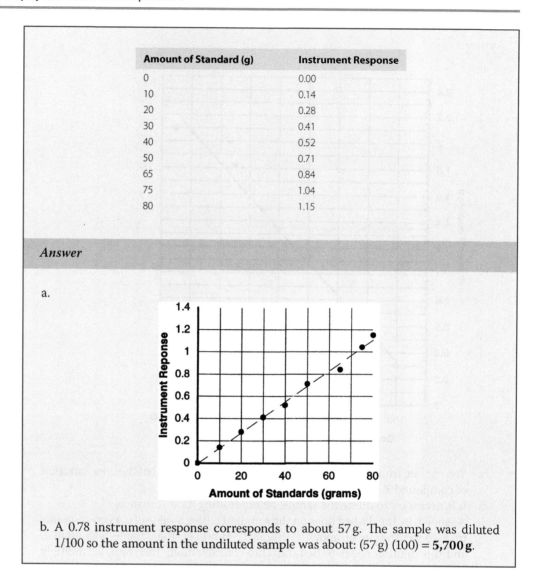

b. A 0.78 instrument response corresponds to about 57 g. The sample was diluted 1/100 so the amount in the undiluted sample was about: (57 g) (100) = **5,700 g**.

## 15.4 USING GRAPHS TO DISPLAY THE RESULTS OF AN EXPERIMENT

Many experiments involve manipulating one variable and measuring the result of that manipulation on a second variable. For example, an investigator interested in the effect of light intensity on the rate of seedling growth could expose different groups of seedlings to different light intensities and measure their growth rates. The two experimental variables, light intensity and seedling growth rate, can be plotted on a two-dimensional graph.

When plotting data from experiments, one distinguishes between the **dependent variable** and the **independent variable**. In the example above, the investigator is looking at whether seedling growth rate is dependent on the light intensity. Growth rate is therefore called the dependent variable. *A variable the investigator controls is an* **independent variable**. *A variable that changes in response to the independent variable is called a* **dependent variable**. It is conventional to plot the dependent variable on the Y-axis and the independent variable on the X-axis. In this example, light intensity is plotted on the X-axis and seedling growth rate on the Y-axis.

Let us consider how the results of another hypothetical experiment might be displayed graphically. Suppose investigators are interested in the effects of a plant hormone on the number of fruits produced by a certain plant. Investigators perform an experiment to determine the relationship, if any, between this hormone and fruit production. The investigators divide plants into twelve groups, each of which is treated identically except for the application of differing levels of the hormone. The investigators count the fruits produced by each plant. The results of this hypothetical experiment are shown in tabular form in Table 15.2 and graphically in Figure 15.11. Fruit production is the dependent variable and is plotted on the Y-axis; applied hormone concentration is on the X-axis. These data strongly suggest that the hormone boosts fruit production.

There are several important concepts illustrated by this graph:

1. ***Thresholds:*** In the central portion of the graph the points appear to form a straight line, that is, there appears to be a linear relationship between hormone level and fruit production. Below about 4.0 mg/L of hormone and above about 35.0 mg/L of hormone, the relationship changes, that is, the data points are no longer approximated by the best fit line for the points from 4 to 35 mg/mL. The values 4.0 and 35 mg/L are threshold values. A **threshold** *is a point on a graph where there is a change in the relationship.* Thresholds at low and high values, as illustrated in Figure 15.11a, are common when working with biological data. Above 35.0 mg/mL and below 4.0 mg/mL the line is "flat," which means that there is no relationship between fruit production and hormone level.

**TABLE 15.2 Experimental Data**

| Hormone Level (mg/L)-Independent Variable | Average Fruit Production per Plant-Dependent Variable |
|---|---|
| 0.0 | 3.2 |
| 3.0 | 3.7 |
| 5.0 | 3.8 |
| 10.0 | 6.5 |
| 15.0 | 12.7 |
| 20.0 | 15.2 |
| 25.0 | 17.0 |
| 30.0 | 24.8 |
| 40.0 | 32.3 |
| 50.0 | 36.0 |
| 55.0 | 36.2 |
| 60.0 | 36.5 |

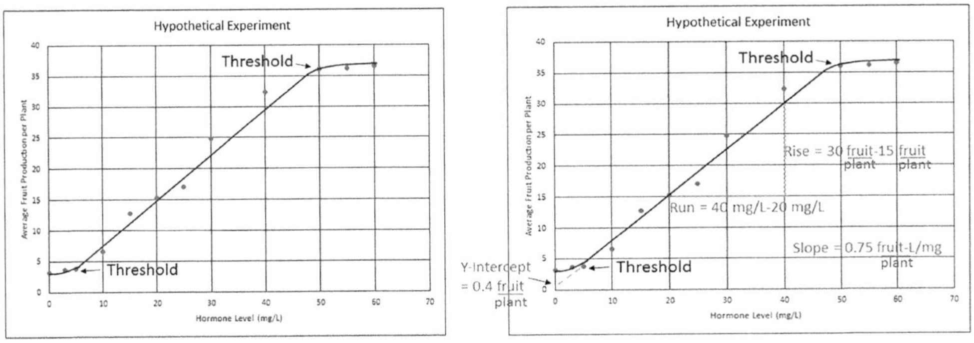


(a) (b)

**FIGURE 15.11** Hypothetical experiment. (a) The effect of hormone application on fruit production. (b) Determining the equation for the line.

2. ***Best Fit Line:*** The middle points on the graph (those between the threshold points) are close to forming a line and it is reasonable to conclude that the relationship between fruit production and hormone level is linear between 4.0 and 35.0 mg/L of applied hormone. Therefore, it is acceptable to represent these middle points with a straight line. A line may be drawn either "by eye" or using the statistical method of least squares.

   Once the points between the threshold points are represented by a line, it is possible to determine the equation for the best fit line. The slope has units since both the X- and Y-axes have units. The Y-axis has units of "average fruit production per plant," or, more simply, "fruit/plant;" the X-axis has units of mg/L. The slope of the line, Figure 15.11b, is:

   $$\frac{0.75(\text{fruit})(\text{L})}{(\text{plant})(\text{mg})}$$

   To determine the Y-intercept of the line, it is necessary to determine where the intercept would be <u>if</u> there were no lower threshold. By using a ruler to extend the line to the Y-axis, the Y-intercept can be determined to be 0.4 fruit, Figure 15.11b. The equation for this line in Figure 15.11 is therefore:

   $$Y = \frac{0.75(\text{fruit})(\text{L})}{(\text{plant})(\text{mg})} X + 0.40 \text{ fruit / plant}$$

   The slope is the amount by which average production of fruit per plant increases with 1 mg/L of increased hormone. The Y-intercept is the amount of fruit production per plant expected if there were no hormone added and if the relationship was linear for all values of hormone (which is not the case).
3. ***Prediction:*** Equations and graphs are tools that can be used to make predictions. For example, the experiment did not involve testing the effect of 13.0 mg/L of hormone on fruit production. Yet, we can infer from the graph that if 13.0 mg/L of hormone were to be applied, the average fruit production per plant would be about 10. It is also possible to use the equation to predict the amount of fruit with 13.0 mg/L of hormone:

   $$Y = \frac{0.75(\text{fruit})(\text{L})}{(\text{plant})(\text{mg})}\left(\frac{13 \text{ mg}}{\text{L}}\right) + \frac{0.40 \text{ fruit}}{\text{plant}} \approx \mathbf{10.2 \text{ fruit / plant}}$$

   The use of equations and graphs for prediction is powerful. However, when studying natural systems there are often thresholds, we cannot predict how much fruit production there will be with 100 mg/L of hormone because this is outside the linear range of our data. Even if there were no threshold at 35 mg/L, we still could not predict fruit production with 100 mg/L of hormone because we would not know if there was a threshold before reaching 100 mg/L.
4. ***Using Graphs to Summarize Data:*** The graph of the hypothetical experiment contains the same information as Table 15.2. However, it is usually easier to see a relationship between two variables when the data are displayed on a graph than when they are listed in a table.

So far, we have looked at data where two variables are indeed related to one another. What would a graph look like if the two variables studied are not related to one another? One possibility is shown in Figure 15.12a where the points appear to be scattered without pattern on the graph. Another possibility is shown in Figure 15.12b where the graph is "flat." The value

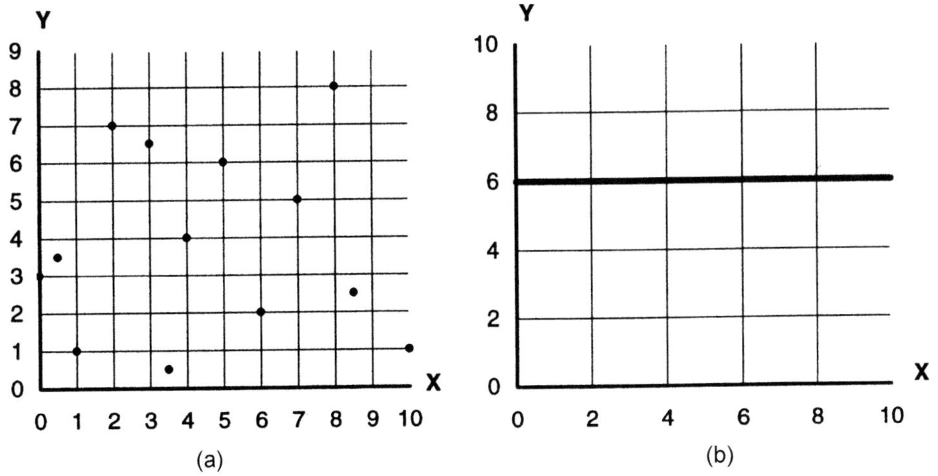


**FIGURE 15.12** Graphs of variables that are not related. (a) The points are scattered without pattern on the graph. (b) The value of the Y variable is constant regardless of the value of the X variable.

of the Y-variable is constant regardless of the value for the variable on the X-axis. Observe in the hypothetical fruit and hormone experiment, Figure 15.11, the graph of the data is "flat" at high and low hormone levels. Therefore, we can reasonably conclude that at low and high levels of hormone, the production of fruit is controlled by factors other than the level of this hormone.

Figure 15.10 illustrates a situation where the variable on the Y-axis clearly appears to be related to the variable on the X-axis. The graphs in Figure 15.12 illustrate situations where two variables clearly appear to be unrelated to one another. In practice, it is sometimes ambiguous whether there is a relationship between two variables. For example, in Figure 15.13, there appears to be a faint relationship between the adult height of a daughter and the height of her mother. But the relationship is inconsistent because maternal height is not the only factor affecting a woman's adult height. Paternal genes and nutrition also affect height. Therefore, the plot of daughter versus mother's height does not form a very "good" line.

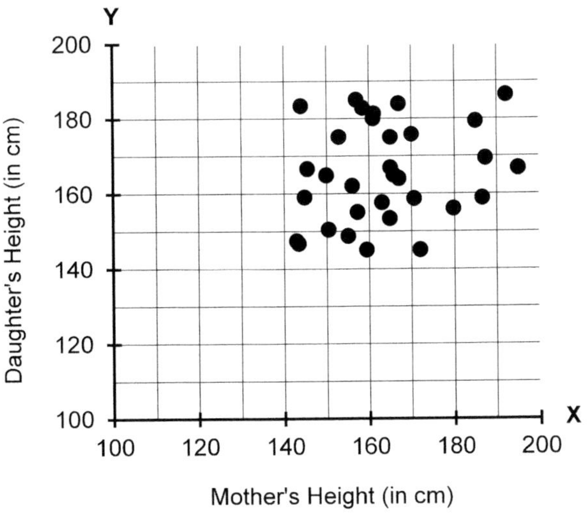


**FIGURE 15.13** Two variables whose relationship to one another is ambiguous.

**Practice Problems**

1. ***It is important to know whether exposure to agents such as low level radiation, pesticides, or asbestos is likely to cause cancer. Two different predictions of cancer risk due to exposure to small concentrations of cancer-causing materials are shown in the graphs below.***

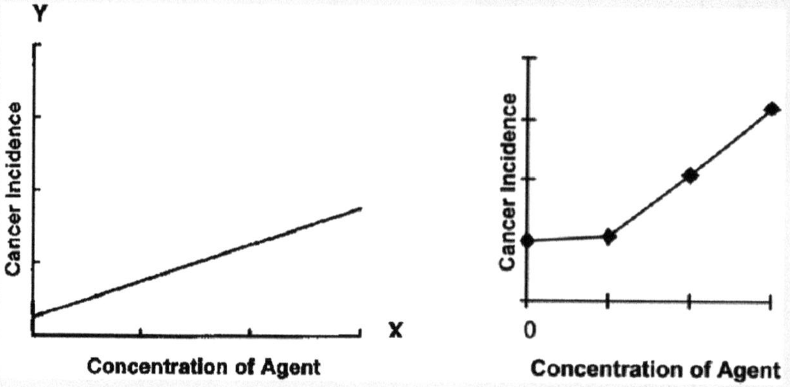


(a) (b)

   a. ***If graph (a) is correct (no threshold) and a population of humans is exposed to small amounts of potentially carcinogenic materials, will the incidence of cancer in the population increase? Explain.***
   b. ***If graph (b) is correct, will exposure to small amounts of potentially carcinogenic materials result in an increase in the incidence of cancer?***
   c. ***Speculate as to why exposures to small amounts of carcinogenic materials may not increase the likelihood of cancer while exposure to large amounts does increase the probability of cancer.***
   d. ***Explain why neither graph (a) nor (b) intersect the Y-axis at zero.***
   e. ***Why is it important to know whether graph (a) or (b) more accurately reflects the truth about a given material? (To learn more about this issue, see, for example, Goldman, M. "Cancer Risk of Low-Level Exposure." Science, vol. 271, no. 5257, 1996, pp. 1821–22. doi:10.1126/science.271.5257.1821. More recently, Nohmi, Takehiko. "Thresholds of Genotoxic and Non-Genotoxic Carcinogens." Toxicological Research, vol. 34, no. 4, 2018, pp. 281–90. doi:10.5487/tr.2018.34.4.281.)***

2. ***Suppose an investigator is studying the genetics of plant productivity. The investigator determines the mass of 500 parent plants and 1,000 of their offspring plants. The investigator plots offspring plant mass versus parent masses.***
   a. ***Which of the graphs below (a) or (b) would indicate that there is a roughly linear relationship between the mass of the parent plant and the mass of the offspring? (Assume the scales and units are the same on both graphs.) Explain.***
   b. ***Suppose the data suggest that there is no relationship between the mass of the parent plant and the mass of its offspring. Suggest a hypothesis to explain that observation and suggest an experiment to test your hypothesis.***

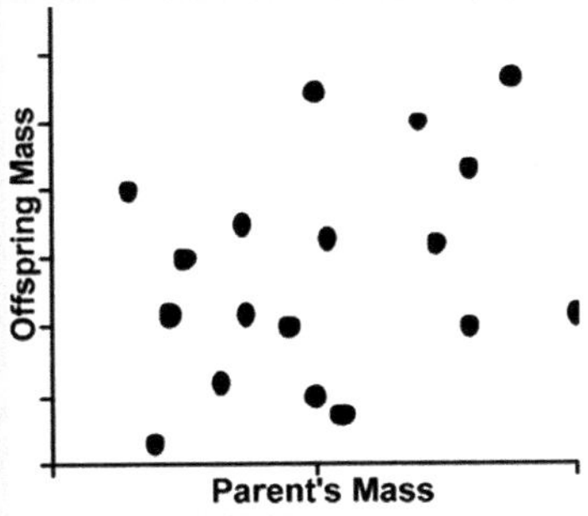


(a)

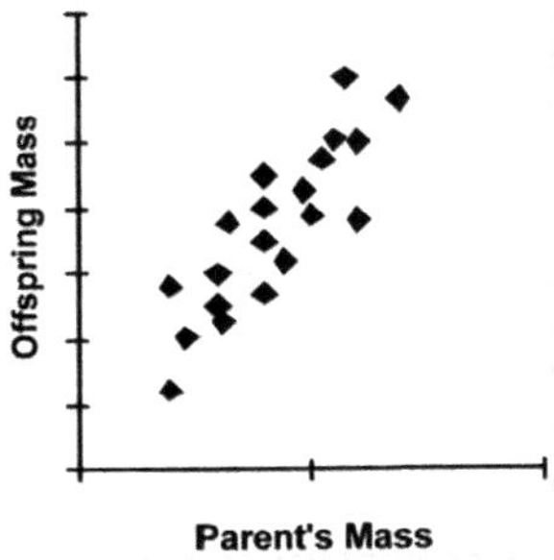


(b)

3. a. ***Draw the best fit line "by eye" for each of the graphs below. Be careful not to extrapolate (extend the line) past the data, except to find the Y-intercept.***
   b. ***Calculate the slope for each of the lines – do not forget the units.***
   c. ***What is the Y-intercept for each line?***
   d. ***What is the equation for each of these lines? Include the units.***
   e. ***Examine graph (a) to approximate the mosquito density if there are 5 in. of rain.***
   f. ***Use the equation for the line in graph (a) to predict mosquito density if there are 5 in. of rain. (The answers for 3e and 3f should be about the same.)***
   g. ***From graph (b) determine the average shrub's height at 20 months of age. Confirm your determination using the equation for the line in graph (b).***
   h. ***From graph (c) determine average seedling height with 50 mg of nutrient. Confirm your determination using the equation for the line in graph (c).***

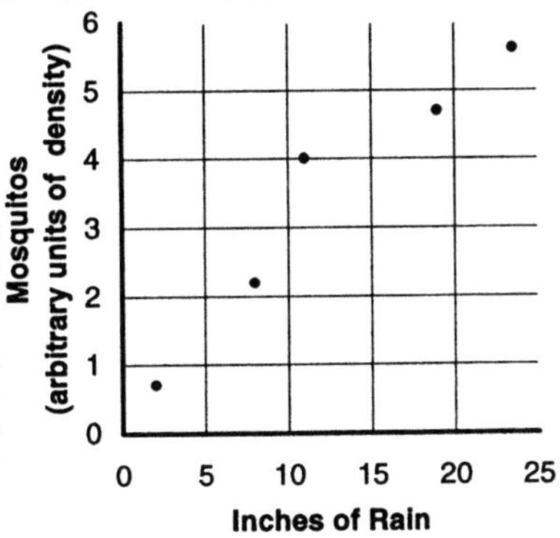


(a)

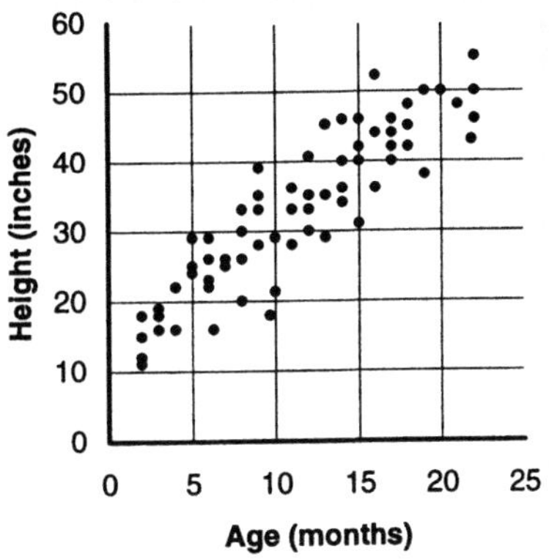


(b)

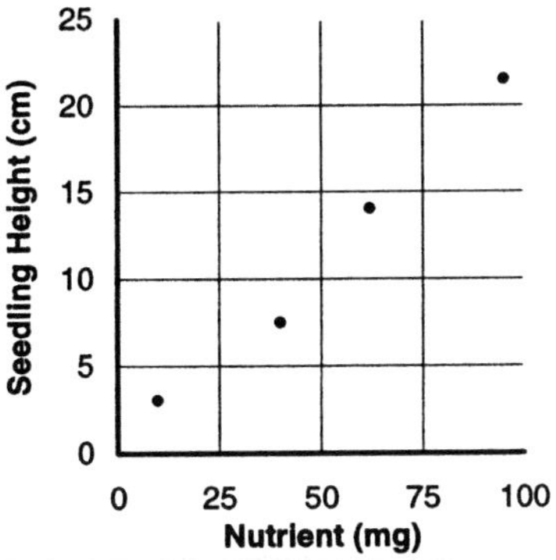


(c)

4. ***Ten students took a course midterm and final. The scores for each student are plotted below.***
   a. ***What was the approximate average score for the midterm, 20, 40, 60, or 80?***
   b. ***What was the approximate average score for the final, 20, 40, 60, or 80?***
   c. ***Which exam had lower scores?***
   d. ***Was there a clear relationship between a student's midterm grade and their final grade? If the same class and the same exams were given the following year, could the teacher predict the final score of a student based on their midterm? Explain.***

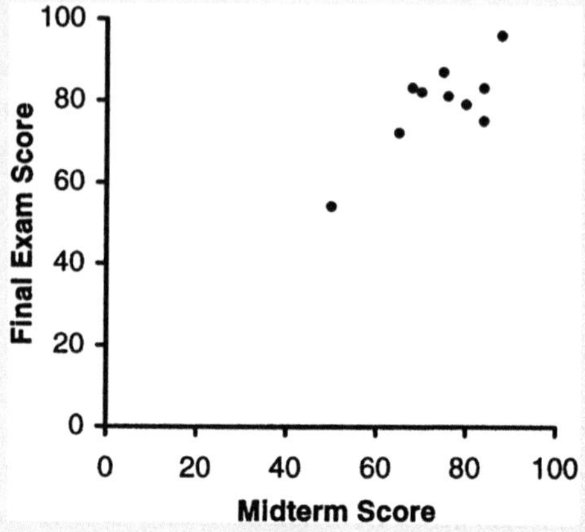


*Answers*

1. a. Yes. The graph shows a linear relationship between cancer incidence and exposure level, even with the lowest exposures to the agent.
   b. No, the graph has a threshold. At low levels of exposure, below the threshold, no change in cancer incidence occurs.
   c. Possible explanations include: (1) individuals are able to detoxify and handle low levels of the agent and (2) multiple receptors must be activated before an effect occurs.
   d. A background level of cancer is found in the population even in the absence of exposure to the agent.
   e. Regulatory agencies need to know whether low level exposure is safe to decide what levels (if any) of compound can be allowed. For example, this is important to know when deciding whether a particular pesticide can be used on crops, and if so, what levels are "safe."

2. a. Graph (b) indicates a roughly linear relationship between the mass of the parent and the offspring where a higher parental mass is associated with a higher offspring mass.
   b. Environmental factors may play a major role in determining mass. One experiment would be to take genetically identical clones of the plant and measure their mass under different, controlled environmental conditions. There are other experiments you might devise as well.

3. a.

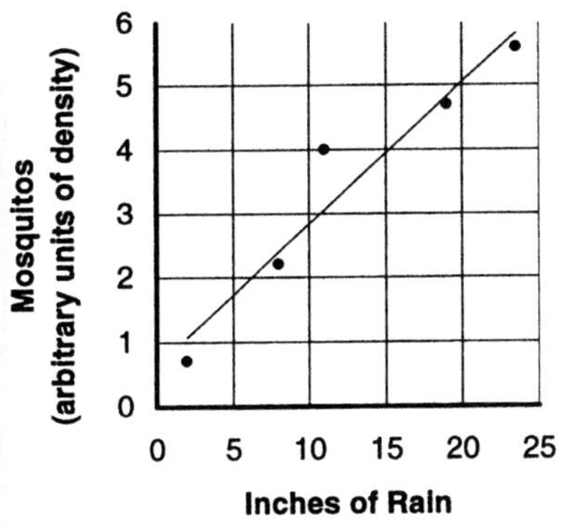


(a)

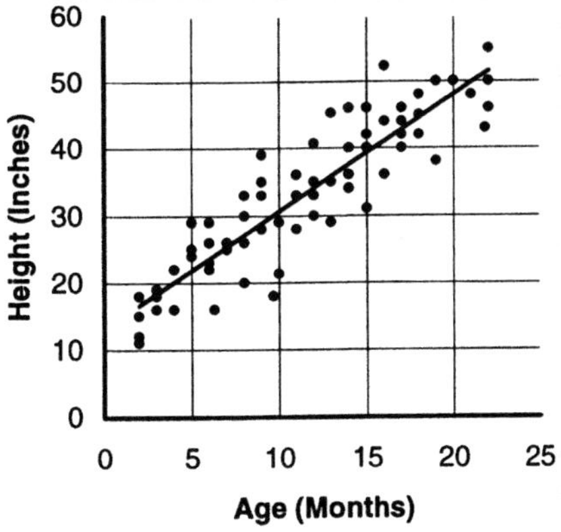


(b)

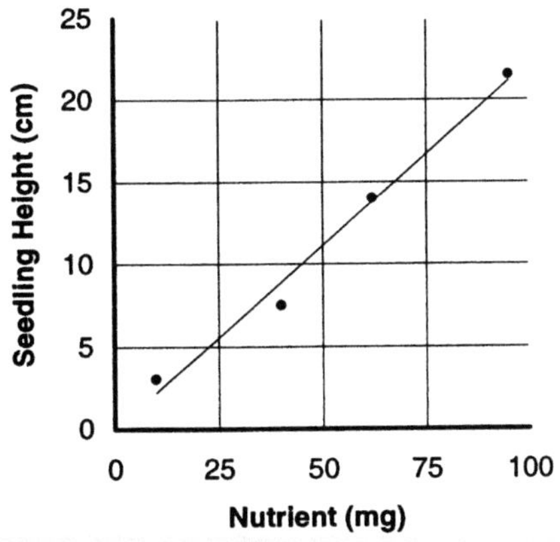


(c)

(Your answers may vary slightly from these.)

b. (a) Slope = **0.22 mosquitos/in. rain** (b) Slope = **1.8 in./month**
(c) Slope = **0.24 cm/mg**

c. (a) Y-intercept = **0.6 mosquitos** (b) Y-intercept = **13 in.**
(c) Y-intercept = **0 cm**

d. (a) **Y = (0.22 mosquitos/in. rain) (X) + 0.6 mosquitos**
(b) **Y = (1.8 in./month) (X) + 13 in.**
(c) **Y = (0.24 cm/mg) (X) + 0 cm**

e. **1.7 mosquitos**

f. Y = (0.22 mosquitos/in.) (5 in.) + 0.6 mosquitos = **1.7 mosquitos**

g. Y = (1.8 in./month) (20 months) + 13 in. = **49 in.**

h. Y = (0.24 cm/mg) (50 mg) + 0 cm = **12 cm**

4. a. **80** b. **80**

c. The slope is close to 1, so the test scores were roughly equal.

d. The relationship is roughly linear which means there is a general relationship between the two scores. Midterm scores are therefore fairly predictive, although other classes might differ.

## 15.5 A STATISTICAL METHOD TO CALCULATE THE LINE OF BEST FIT

Consider a standard curve, as shown in Figure 15.9. Recall that the variable that is controlled by the investigator (in this example the concentration of compound) is termed the "independent variable" and is plotted on the X-axis. The variable that varies in response to the independent variable (in this example, the instrument's response to the standards) is the "dependent variable" and is plotted on the Y-axis. When a standard curve is prepared, we expect that the response of the instrument will be entirely determined by the concentration of compound in the standard. If this expectation is met (and if the relationship between concentration and instrument response is linear), then all the points will lie exactly on a line. However, there are sometimes slight errors or inconsistencies when a standard curve is constructed. These small errors cause the points to not lie exactly on the line, as shown in Figure 15.14.

As is shown in Figure 15.14, the points can easily be represented with a line, although the points do not all fall exactly on the line. Some of the points are a little above the line, others a little below. In a situation like this, where a series of points approximate a line, we can use a ruler to draw "by eye," a line that seems to best describe the points. However, drawing a line "by eye" is not the most accurate method nor does it give consistent results, Figure 15.15. It is more accurate to use a statistical method to calculate the equation for the line that best describes the relationship between the two variables. *The statistical linear regression method used to determine the equation for a line is called* **the method of least squares**. The least squares method calculates the equation for a line such that the total squared deviation of the

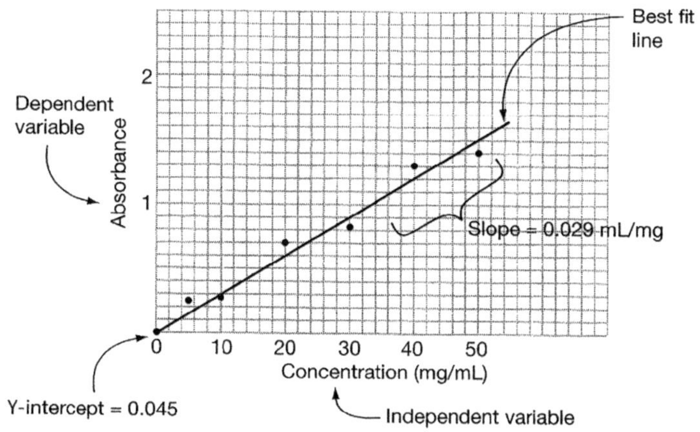


**FIGURE 15.14** The relationship between the concentration of compound and the response of an instrument; a standard curve. In this case there were slight inconsistencies in the standards and so the points do not lie exactly on a line.

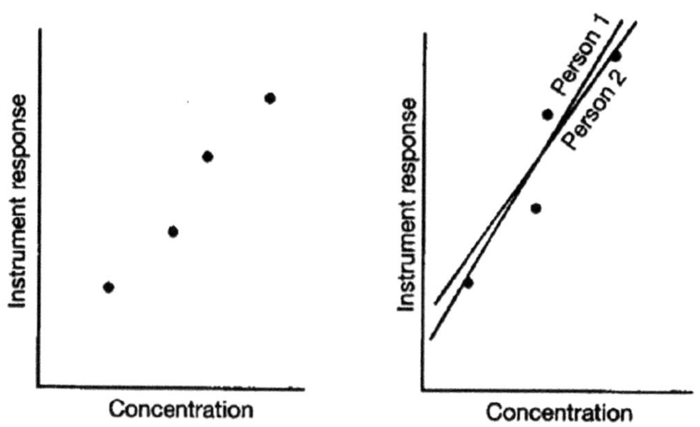


**FIGURE 15.15** Drawing a best fit line "by eye." Two people connect the points into a best fit line by eye with slightly different results.

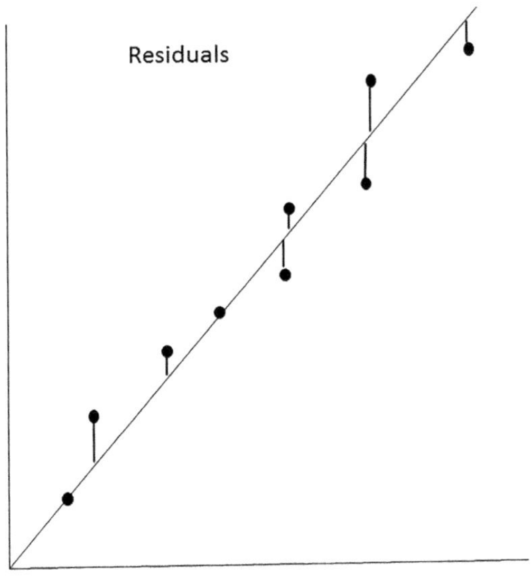


**FIGURE 15.16** The basis of a best fit line. ***The distance of a given point to the best fit line*** is called its "residual." In this example, there are nine points, each with a residual distance to the line. The best fit line minimizes the sum of the residuals of all the points. (Actually, the method minimizes the sum of the ***squared*** residuals, which makes sense given that the method is called the "least squared" method.)

points from the line is minimized, Figure 15.16. *The equation for the line calculated using the method of least squares is called the* **regression equation**. *The line itself is called the* **best fit line.**

Recall that the equation for a line can be written as:

$$\mathbf{Y = Slope(X) + Y\text{-}intercept}$$

or

$$\mathbf{Y = mX + a}$$

where:
m is the slope
a is the Y-intercept
X is the independent variable
and Y is the dependent variable

The least squares method is used to calculate: (1) the slope and (2) the Y-intercept of the line that best fits the points. (The equations to perform these calculations are shown later.)

When the linear regression equations are applied to the data graphed in Figure 15.14, the slope for the linear regression line is calculated to be **0.0285 mL/mg**. The Y-intercept is calculated to be **0.045**. Therefore, the linear regression equation for the line in Figure 15.14 is:

$$\mathbf{Y = \frac{(0.0285\ mL)}{mg} X + 0.045}$$

Note that the slope and the Y-intercept can have units. (In this example, the instrument response, absorbance, has no units; therefore, the Y-intercept has no units.)

Some calculators are able to facilitate the calculation of the equation for the line of best fit; computers are also used for this. Many modern laboratory instruments calculate the best fit line automatically, so this calculation is rarely done "by hand" anymore. An example of a standard curve graphed with Excel (a commonly used software program) is shown in Figure 15.17. In Excel, the best fit line is termed a "trend line."

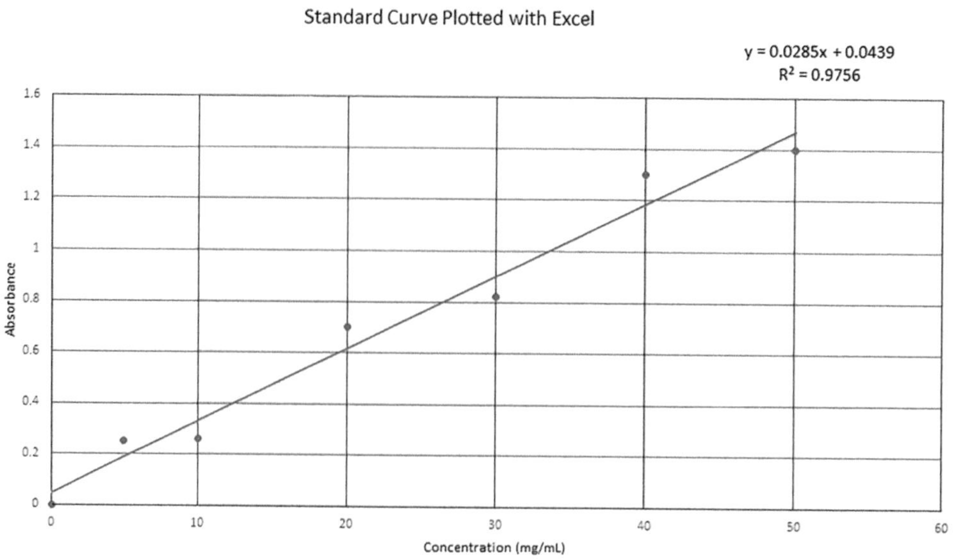


**FIGURE 15.17** Standard curve plotted with Excel that shows the equation for the line (the trend line) and the $R^2$ value.

Note in Figure 15.17 that Excel also provided a value called $R^2$, "R-squared." R-squared is a statistical measure of how closely the data fit the calculated best fit line. (It is also known as the coefficient of determination.) The $R^2$ value is defined as the percentage of the response of the Y-variable that is explained by the linear model. Since it is a percentage, $R^2$ can vary between 0 and 1 or between 0% and 100%. The closer $R^2$ is to 1 (or 100%), the better. In our example, the change in absorbance, that is, the Y-value, is almost entirely explained by changes in analyte concentration, the X-value. Hence, the data fit the linear model quite well and there is a high value for $R^2$, which is 0.9756. But $R^2$ is not exactly 1, so there is some variation in the Y-values that is explained by other factors. Perhaps there was a small amount of pipetting error, or some fluctuation within the spectrophotometer, or some random error. The closer $R^2$ is to 1, the more confident we can be that our linear plot correctly explains the variation in absorbance values.

Although calculating best fit lines "by hand" is seldom done anymore, the method for doing these calculations manually is shown below so that you can see how it is done.

### 15.5.1 CALCULATING THE LINE OF BEST FIT

This section describes the method of least squares that is used to calculate the linear regression equation. It is based on the following assumptions:

- The values of the independent variable, X, are controlled by the investigator.
- The dependent variable, Y, must be approximately normally distributed.

  (For example, if the same standard is measured in the same instrument many times, the instrument response values will vary slightly from reading to reading due to random error. These various measurements are expected to be normally distributed. See Section 20.2 for a discussion of the normal distribution.)
- If there is a relationship between the two variables, it is linear.

(1) To calculate the slope of the linear regression line, the equation is:

$$m = \frac{n\sum xy - \sum x \sum y}{n\sum x^2 - \left(\sum x\right)^2}$$

The symbol "$\Sigma$" means to add up.

(2) To calculate the Y-intercept, the equation is:

$$a = \bar{y} - m\bar{x}$$

where:

$$\bar{x} = \frac{\sum x}{n}$$

$$\bar{y} = \frac{\sum y}{n}$$

n = sample size

These calculations are summarized in Box 15.3.

**BOX 15.3: Calculation of the Linear Regression Equation**

Step 1. Arrange the data into a table of X and Y pairs.

Step 2. Calculate the sum of the X values, $\Sigma X$

Step 3. Calculate the mean of the X values, $\bar{X}$

Step 4. Calculate $\Sigma X^2$ by squaring each X value and adding the results together.

Step 5. Calculate $(\Sigma X)^2$ by squaring the sum of the X values.

Step 6. Calculate the sum of the Y values, $\Sigma Y$

Step 7. Calculate the mean of the Y values, $\bar{Y}$

Step 8. Calculate the $\Sigma X\ \Sigma Y$

Step 9. Multiply each X by its corresponding Y value and add the products to get $\Sigma XY$.

Step 10. Calculate the slope, m, as: $m = \dfrac{n\sum xy - \sum x \sum y}{n\sum x^2 - \left(\sum x\right)^2}$

Step 11. Calculate the Y intercept as: $a = \bar{Y} - m\bar{X}$

Step 12. Place the values calculated for the slope and Y intercept into the equation $Y = mX + a$

Note: Keep track of the units when calculating and expressing the equation of a line.

**TABLE 15.3 Calculating the Line of Best Fit**

| Concentration of Analyte X (mg/mL) | Instrument Response Y (In This Case, Y Has No Units) | XY (mg/mL) | $X^2$ $(mg^2/mL^2)$ |
|---|---|---|---|
| 0 | 0 | 0 | 0 |
| 5 | 0.25 | 1.25 | 25 |
| 10 | 0.26 | 2.60 | 100 |
| 20 | 0.70 | 14.00 | 400 |
| 30 | 0.82 | 24.60 | 900 |
| 40 | 1.30 | 52.00 | 1,600 |
| 50 | 1.40 | 70.00 | 2,500 |
| $\Sigma X = 155$ mg / mL | $\Sigma Y = 4.73$ | $\Sigma XY = 164.45$ mg / mL | $\Sigma X^2 = 5{,}525$ mg$^2$/mL$^2$ |
| $\bar{X} \approx 22.14$ mg / mL | $\bar{Y} \approx 0.676$<br>N = 7 | $(\Sigma X)(\Sigma Y) = 733.15$ mg / mL | $(\Sigma X)^2 = 24{,}025$ mg$^2$/mL$^2$ |

As an example, we show how the linear regression equation is calculated for the data graphed in Figures 15.14 and 15.17. Table 15.3 shows the data for this example along with preliminary calculations.

The values from Table 15.3 can be "plugged into" the equations for the best fit line.

The slope of the regression line is:

$$m = \frac{n\sum xy - \sum x \sum y}{n\sum x^2 - \left(\sum x\right)^2}$$

$$m = \frac{7(164.45\text{ mg/mL}) - 733.15\text{ mg/mL}}{7(5{,}525\text{ mg}^2/\text{mL}^2) - (24{,}025\text{ mg}^2/\text{mL}^2)} = \frac{418\text{ mg/mL}}{14{,}650\text{ mg}^2/\text{mL}^2} \approx \mathbf{0.0285\ mL/mg}$$

The Y-intercept is:

$$a = 0.676 - (0.0285\text{ mL/mg})(22.14\text{ mg/mL}) \approx \mathbf{0.044}$$

Therefore, the regression equation for this line is:

$$\hat{Y} \approx \frac{(0.0285\text{ mL})}{1\text{ mg}} X + 0.044$$

By convention, the symbol $\hat{Y}$ is used to distinguish a regression equation.

# Spectrophotometry

16



## 16.1 INTRODUCTION

Section 15.3 introduced the concept of standard curves, which are of fundamental importance in quantitative analysis. Observe that in the standard curves in Chapter 15, the Y-axis is sometimes termed "instrument response." There are various kinds of instruments (detectors) that can be used in differing situations, but detectors that measure the absorbance of light are common in biotechnology settings. **Spectrophotometers** *are laboratory instruments that measure how much light is absorbed as it passes through a liquid sample.* This chapter delves more deeply into the calculations involved in standard curves, particularly those involving spectrophotometers that detect the absorption of light.

Biologists often work with aqueous solutions (or suspensions) that contain a substance of interest, for example, a protein, DNA, RNA, cells, or an inorganic compound. *The substance of interest in a sample is called the* **analyte**. The job of a spectrophotometer is to measure how the analyte affects a beam of light that is shined through the sample. As the light passes through the sample, some, all, or none of the light's energy may be **absorbed** by the analyte. Light energy that is not absorbed is **transmitted** unchanged through the sample. A spectrophotometer can be used for quantitative analysis because, under certain conditions, the amount of light that is absorbed by the sample is proportional to the amount of analyte in the sample. The more analyte that is present in the sample, the more light energy that is absorbed.

DNA, RNA, proteins, and other molecules of importance to biologists frequently absorb a particular kind of light, that is, ultraviolet (UV) light. Our eyes cannot detect ultraviolet light, but some types of spectrophotometers have detectors that can "see" UV light. Therefore, some types of spectrophotometers can detect whether a sample contains an analyte that absorbs UV light. It is also possible to add reagents to samples that cause an analyte of interest to become colored:

$$\text{Analyte without color} \xrightarrow{\text{reagent}} \text{colored product}$$

DOI: 10.1201/9780429282744-19

Light that our eyes can see and that has color is called visible (vis) light. Thus, sometimes assays using spectrophotometers require the addition of reagents that produce a colored product. Other times, analytes absorb UV light, and the absorbance of UV light can be directly detected by the spectrophotometer.

## 16.2 TRANSMITTANCE AND ABSORBANCE MEASUREMENTS IN A SPECTROPHOTOMETER

To understand quantitative analysis with a spectrophotometer, it is necessary to know a little about how these instruments work. Remember that the job of a spectrophotometer is to determine how an analyte in a liquid sample affects a beam of light passing through it. But an analyte is seldom alone in a sample solution, rather, it is dissolved in a solvent and sometimes various reagents are added to the sample as well. When the sample is placed in the spectrophotometer, not only the analyte may absorb light but the solvent and added reagents may absorb light as well. Moreover, the sample is contained in a *holder, called a* **cuvette**. Although cuvettes appear transparent, a small amount of light is absorbed by their walls. Therefore, a beam of light passing through a sample is affected not only by the analyte but also by the solvent, added reagents, and the walls of the cuvette. The absorbance that is not due to the analyte must be distinguished from the total absorbance to determine the absorbance of the analyte. The way this is accomplished is to prepare a **blank** *that contains no analyte but does contain the solvent and any reagents that are intentionally added to the sample.* The interaction of light with the sample is compared to its interaction with the blank. For example, if a sample consists of a protein of interest dissolved in a buffer, then the analyte is the protein, and the blank would consist of just the buffer.

Within a spectrophotometer a beam of light, **incident light**, is directed first at the blank and then at the sample. As the light beam passes through the material in the sample or blank, some or all of its energy may be absorbed; the remainder of the light is transmitted, Figure 16.1. Note in Figure 16.1 that the incident light has a particular color. In practice, only a small portion of the light emitted by a light bulb in a spectrophotometer is directed at the sample. The spectrophotometer allows the user to select light of a specific wavelength. Thus, when working with a spectrophotometer, the wavelength of light involved in the analysis is always specified.

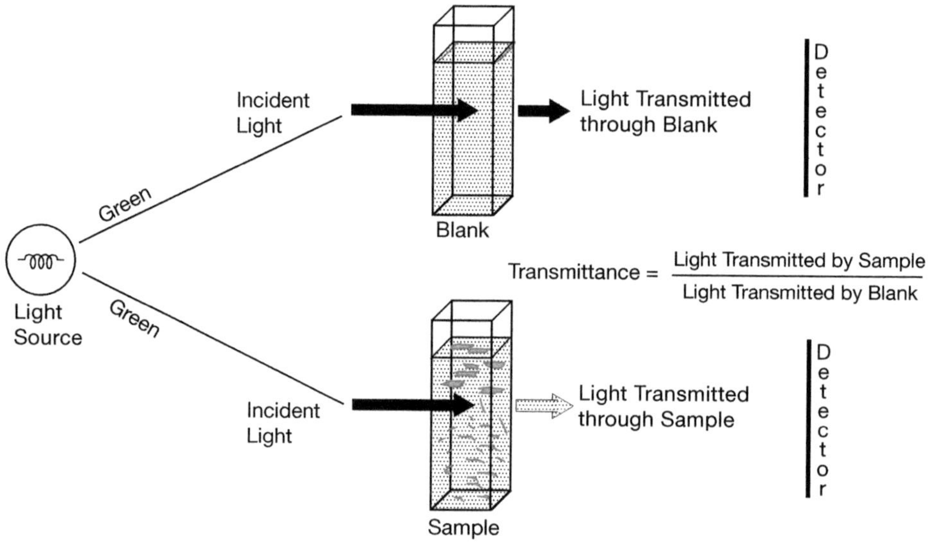


**FIGURE 16.1** A spectrophotometer measures the interaction of light with the sample and with the blank to determine the transmittance. The blank contains the solvent in which the sample is dissolved and any reagents that are added to the sample but does not contain the analyte. Light that is not absorbed as it passes through the sample or the blank is detected.

The light that is transmitted through the sample or blank strikes a **detector** *that measures the amount of light arriving at its surface.* The spectrophotometer compares the amount of light that was transmitted through the sample with the amount of light transmitted through the blank. *The ratio of the light transmitted through the sample to that transmitted through the blank is called the* **transmittance,** abbreviated **t**:

$$\frac{\text{light transmitted through the sample}}{\text{light transmitted through the blank}} = \text{transmittance} = \text{t}$$

It is also common to speak of **percent transmittance,** *the transmittance times 100%*:

$$\%\text{T} = (\text{t})(100\%)$$

Percent transmittance ranges from 0% (no light passed through the sample, relative to the blank) to 100% (all light was transmitted through the sample, relative to the blank).

Thus, observe in Figure 16.1 that the property a spectrophotometer actually detects is transmitted light. However, analysts are generally interested in the amount of light *absorbed* by the analyte. Therefore, it is customary to convert transmittance to **absorbance**. **Absorbance** *is defined as the negative log of the transmittance (see Chapter 2 for a discussion of logs)*:

$$\text{A} = -\log_{10}(\text{transmittance})$$

$$\text{A} = -\log \text{t}$$

Transmittance and absorbance do not have units.

It makes sense that as the concentration of analyte in a sample increases, the transmittance of light through the sample decreases. Observe in Figure 16.2a that this is the case, but the decline in transmittance is not linear with respect to concentration of analyte. In contrast, there is a linear relationship between the absorbance of light by a sample and the concentration of analyte, Figure 16.2b. As the concentration of analyte increases, so does the absorbance of light; and this increase is linear with respect to concentration. Because the relationship between absorbance and concentration is linear, absorbance is a convenient measure to use for quantitative analysis of the concentration of analyte in a sample.

A sample that absorbs a great deal of light transmits very little light and *vice versa,* Table 16.1. For example, if the percent transmittance is 100%, then there is no light absorbance by the sample relative to the blank; the incident light passes through the analyte without being absorbed. Suppose in another case that an analyte absorbs so much light that the percent transmittance is only 0.1%. In this example, the transmittance (t) is 0.001 and the absorbance is 3:

$$\text{A} = -\log(0.001) = -\log(10^{-3}) = -(-3) = 3$$

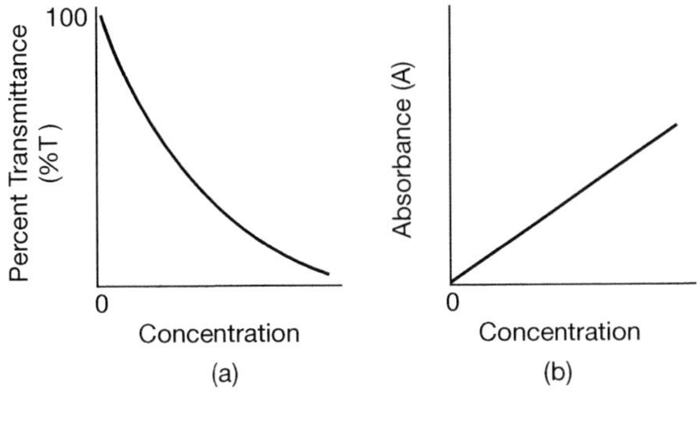


**FIGURE 16.2** The relationship between transmittance and absorbance of light and the concentration of analyte. (a) Transmittance versus concentration of analyte in a sample is not linear. (b) The relationship between absorbance and analyte concentration is linear.

**TABLE 16.1 The Relationship between Absorbance and Transmittance**

| t | %T | A |
|---|---|---|
| | $A = -\log_{10}(t)$ | |
| 0.000 | 0.00 | ∞ |
| 0.001 | 0.10% | 3 |
| 0.010 | 1.00% | 2 |
| 0.100 | 10.0% | 1 |
| 1.000 | 100% | 0 |

An absorbance of 3 is very high and the measurements from most spectrophotometers are generally not useful when there is so little transmitted light. The practical range of absorbance is conventionally considered to be from about 0.1 to 2 although modern spectrophotometers usually have a wider range in which they are accurate.

All but the oldest spectrophotometers automatically convert transmittance values to absorbances and so can display a measurement either in terms of absorbance or transmittance. It is also possible to use a calculator to convert transmittance to absorbance, and *vice versa*, as illustrated in these examples:

**Example Problem:**

Convert a transmittance value of 0.63 to absorbance.

***Answer:***

$$A = -\log(t)$$

$$A = -\log(0.63)$$

$$\mathbf{A \approx -(-0.20) = 0.20}$$

**Example Problem:**

Convert an absorbance value of 0.380 to transmittance and % transmittance.

***Answer:***

$$0.380 = -\log(t)$$

$$-0.380 = \log(t)$$

$$10^{-0.380} = t$$

$$\mathbf{0.417 \approx t}$$

or

$$\mathbf{41.7\% \approx \%T}$$

Alternatively, we can say:

$$\text{antilog}(-0.380) = t$$

$$\mathbf{0.417 \approx t}$$

**or 41.7% ≈ %T**

**Example Problem:**

A solution contains 2 mg/mL of a light absorbing substance. Using a particular wavelength of incident light, the solution transmits 50% of incident light relative to a blank.

a. What is the absorbance in this case?
b. What is the predicted absorbance of a solution containing 8 mg/mL of the same substance?
c. What is the predicted transmittance of a solution containing 8 mg/mL of the same substance?

***Answer:***

a. The absorbance of 2 mg/mL of this substance is equal to –log (0.50) ≈ **0.30**.
b. The relationship between absorbance and concentration is linear (within a certain range, as discussed later). Also, if there is no analyte in a sample, the concentration is zero, then the absorbance (in principle) must also be zero. Assuming linearity and assuming that both the X and Y-intercepts are zero, this can be solved as a proportion problem:

$$\frac{2\text{ mg/mL}}{0.30} = \frac{8\text{ mg/mL}}{?} \quad \mathbf{? = 1.20}$$

c. Observe in Figure 16.2 that the relationship between transmittance and concentration is not linear. Therefore, it is not possible to simply use a proportion based on the transmittance to solve the problem. (Many math problems in the laboratory can be solved with proportions – but not all of them!) Rather, calculate that if the absorbance of 8 mg/mL solute is 1.20 (from part b) then:

$$A = -\log(t)$$

$$1.2 = -\log(t)$$

$$-1.2 = \log(t)$$

$$10^{-1.2} = t$$

$$\mathbf{0.063 \approx t}$$

$$\text{or } \mathbf{\%\,T \approx 6.3\%}$$

Alternatively, we can say:

$$\text{Antilog}(-1.20) = t$$

$$\mathbf{0.063 \approx t}$$

$$\text{or } \mathbf{\%\,T \approx 6.3\%}$$

### Practice Problems

1. ***Convert the following transmittance values to % T.***
   a. ***0.876*** b. ***0.776*** c. ***0.45*** d. ***1.00***

2. ***Convert the following values to absorbance values.***

| | |
|---|---|
| a. ***t = 0.876*** | e. ***T = 25%*** |
| b. ***t = 0.776*** | f. ***T = 15%*** |
| c. ***t = 0.45*** | g. ***T = 95%*** |
| d. ***t = 1.00*** | h. ***T = 45%*** |

3. ***Fill in the following table:***

| ***Absorbance*** | ***transmittance (t)*** | ***% Transmittance (T)*** |
|---|---|---|
| ***0.01*** | ____ | ____ |
| ____ | ***0.56*** | ____ |
| ____ | ____ | ***1.0%*** |

4. ***Convert the following absorbance values to transmittance.***
   a. ***1.24*** b. ***0.95*** c. ***1.10*** d. ***2.25***

5. ***A solution contains 2 mM of a light absorbing substance. Using a particular wavelength of incident light, the solution transmits 34% of incident light relative to a blank.***
   a. ***What is the absorbance in this case?***
   b. ***What is the predicted absorbance of a solution containing 7 mM of the same substance?***
   c. ***What is the predicted transmittance of a solution containing 7 mM of the same substance?***

### *Answers*

1. a. 0.876 = **87.6% T** b. 0.776 = **77.6% T**
   c. 0.45 = **45% T** d. 1.00 = **100% T**

2.

| | A | | A |
|---|---|---|---|
| a. t = 0.876 | ≈ **0.057** | e. T = 25% | ≈ **0.60** |
| b. t = 0.776 | ≈ **0.110** | f. T = 15% | ≈ **0.82** |
| c. t = 0.45 | ≈ **0.35** | g. T = 95% | ≈ **0.022** |
| d. t = 1.00 | ≈ **0.00** | h. T = 45% | ≈ **0.35** |

3.

| Absorbance | transmittance (t) | % Transmittance (T) |
|---|---|---|
| 0.01 | **0.98** | **98%** |
| **0.25** | 0.56 | **56%** |
| **2.0** | **0.01** | 1.0% |

4. a. **0.0575** b. **0.11** c. **0.0794** d. **0.00562**

5. a. The absorbance of 2 mM of this substance is equal to –log (0.34) ≈ **0.47**.
   b. The relationship between absorbance and concentration is usually proportional (within a certain range, as discussed later).

$$\frac{2\text{ mM}}{0.469} = \frac{7\text{ mM}}{?} \qquad ? \approx \mathbf{1.640}$$

   c. Transmittance = antilog (–1.640) ≈ **0.0229** = **2.29% T**

## 16.3 STANDARD CURVES AND SPECTROPHOTOMETRY

Quantitative applications of spectrophotometry have the purpose of determining the concentration (or amount) of an analyte in a sample. Quantitative analysis with a spectrophotometer typically involves a "standard curve," that is, *a graph of absorbance (Y-axis) versus analyte concentration (X-axis).* To construct a calibration curve, standards are prepared with known concentrations of analyte. The absorbances of the standards are determined at a specified wavelength and the results are graphed. Given a standard curve, it is possible to determine the concentration of an analyte in a sample based on the sample's absorbance. This process is summarized in Box 16.1 and illustrated in an example problem.

**BOX 16.1 Preparing a Standard Curve for Quantitative Analysis**

Step 1. Make a series of standards that contain a known concentration of the analyte. At least 5 standards are recommended. The standard concentrations should span the range of concentrations expected in samples.

Step 2. Determine instrument's response to each standard.

Step 3. Graph the data with concentration (or amount) of analyte on the X-axis and instrument response on the Y-axis.

Step 4. Assuming data reasonably fit a line, connect the points into a straight line.

Step 5. Test the instrument's response to the sample(s). Use the standard curve to determine the concentration (or amount) of analyte in the sample(s).

**Example Problem:**

a. Construct a standard curve for red food coloring.
b. Determine the concentration of red food coloring in a sample with an absorbance of 0.50.

***Answer:***

a.

Step 1. Prepare a series of standards of known concentration by diluting a stock solution with distilled water.
Prepare the blank; in this case, the blank is simply distilled water.

Step 2."Blank" the spectrophotometer, that is, place the blank in the spectrophotometer and adjust the spectrophotometer to read 0 absorbance or 100% transmittance (at the proper wavelength for red food coloring.)
Read the absorbance of each standard at the specified wavelength. Example results are shown below.
Step 3. Plot the data on a graph with standard concentration on the X-axis and absorbance on the Y-axis, as shown below.
Step 4. Draw a best fit line to connect the points.
Step 5. Read the absorbance of the unknown at the specified wavelength.

| **Concentration of Standard** | **Absorbance** |
|---|---|
| 0.0 ppm | 0.00 |
| 2.0 ppm | 0.14 |
| 4.0 ppm | 0.26 |
| 6.0 ppm | 0.45 |
| 8.0 ppm | 0.59 |
| 10.0 ppm | 0.75 |
| 12.0 ppm | 0.91 |
| *Unknown* | *0.50* |

Determine the concentration of the unknown based on the standard curve.

**Example Data**

**a.** The standard curve is:

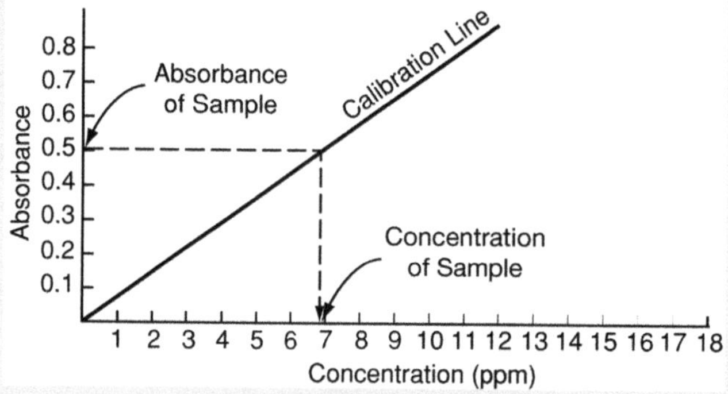


b. Based on the standard curve, the unknown's concentration is about **6.7 ppm.**

Observe that the graph in Figure 16.3 has two thresholds. At very low absorbance levels, the spectrophotometer is not able to detect the difference between a tiny amount of absorbance and no absorbance at all. At high absorbance levels, the instrument is not able to accurately measure the small amount of light passing through the sample. (As noted above, many spectrophotometers are not accurate at absorbances much higher than 2, although some spectrophotometers can be used at higher absorbances.) All quantitative spectrophotometric assays have a range of concentration within which the values obtained are reliable. Above this concentration range, the absorbances are too high to be useful and below this range the absorbance values are too low. It is essential that the standards and samples all have concentrations such that their absorbance falls in the range where the values are accurate.

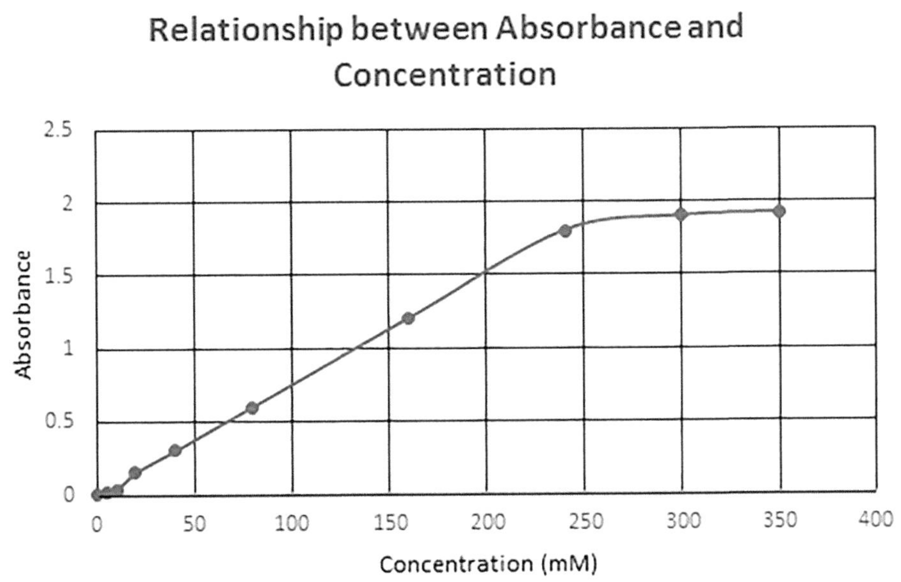


**FIGURE 16.3** The relationship between absorbance and concentration is linear at intermediate concentrations of analyte but not at high or very low concentrations.

## 16.4 THE EQUATION FOR THE CALIBRATION LINE: BEER'S LAW

Within a certain range, the relationship between concentration of the analyte and its absorbance is linear. The line on a standard curve has an equation, as does every line. Recall that the general equation for a line is:

$$Y = mX + a$$

where:

m is the slope
a is the Y-intercept

For the line on any calibration plot (standard curve), the Y-axis is absorbance, and the X-axis is concentration (or amount). Therefore, in the equation for the line on any spectrophotometry calibration curve, we can substitute A (for absorbance) and C (for concentration) as follows:

$$A = mC + a$$

For a calibration line, the Y-intercept is normally zero since, when the concentration of the analyte is zero (as it is in the blank), the absorbance is set to zero. Thus, the equation for the line on a calibration curve is:

$$A = mC + 0$$

or simply

$$A = mC$$

in words:

$$\text{Absorbance} = (\text{slope of calibration line})(\text{concentration of analyte})$$

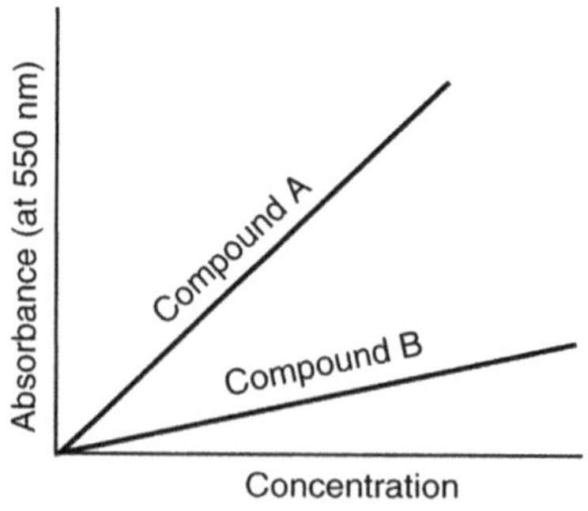


**FIGURE 16.4** The slope of the calibration line. The calibration line for compound A is steeper than for compound B under the conditions of the measurement.

Consider the slope of a calibration line. If the slope is relatively steep, it means that there is a dramatic change in absorbance as the concentration of analyte increases. Conversely, if the slope is not very steep, then as the concentration of analyte increases, the absorbance does not increase dramatically.

What determines the steepness of the slope of a standard curve (at a specified wavelength)? One factor is the nature of the analyte. Different compounds have differing patterns of absorbance of light. In Figure 16.4, for example, compound A absorbs more light under the conditions of the measurement than does compound B. (Assume that the concentrations of both compounds are equal and that the conditions were identical when the data were taken.) The line for compound A has a steeper slope than that for compound B because compound A has a greater inherent tendency to absorb light under these conditions than compound B. Thus, given a particular set of conditions, the slope of a calibration line will vary from one compound to another.

*The inherent tendency of a material to absorb light under specific conditions and at a specified wavelength is called its* **absorptivity** (abbreviated in this text with the Greek letter alpha, $\alpha$). The greater the absorptivity of a material, the more it absorbs light under those conditions. The absorptivity of a specific compound under particular conditions is constant. The value of the absorptivity constant of a particular compound has units that vary depending on the units in which the concentration of the analyte is expressed (such as moles/L, mg/mL, and ppm). It is essential to note the units if you calculate an absorptivity constant and to be aware of the units when you use a published absorptivity constant. (As was noted in Chapter 5, a constant value that is used in an equation depends on the units. If the units change, so does the value for the constant.)

A second factor that affects the slope of the calibration line is the path length, which is the width of the cuvette holding the sample, and it is usually abbreviated "b." If the light has to pass through a longer path, then there is more absorbing material present and more of the light will be absorbed. Thus, the two main factors that affect the slope are:

1. The inherent tendency of the analyte to absorb light under the conditions used
2. The path length

Returning to the equation for the calibration line, we can rewrite the equation to include the path length and the analyte's absorptivity, both of which contribute to the slope. The equation thus becomes:

$$A = mC$$

$$A = (\alpha b)C$$

where:

A = the absorbance
$\alpha$ = the absorptivity constant for that compound at that wavelength

b = the pathlength
C = the concentration
(α b) = m = the slope

This equation, which shows the relationship between absorbance, concentration, absorptivity, and path length, is famous. It forms the basis for quantitative analysis by absorption spectrophotometry. Its discovery is variously attributed to Beer, Lambert, and Bouguer, but it is generally referred to simply as "**Beer's law**." **Beer's law** *states that the amount of light emerging from a sample is reduced by three things*:

1. The concentration of absorbing substance in the sample (C in the equation).
2. The distance the light travels through the sample (pathlength or b).
3. The probability that a photon of a particular wavelength will be absorbed by the specific material in the sample (the absorptivity or α).

**Example Problem:**

a. Using Beer's law, what is the concentration of analyte in a sample where the absorptivity constant is 15,000 L/mole · cm and the absorbance is 1.30 in a 1 cm cuvette?
b. Suppose that the absorbance of the analyte above is measured in a 1.25 cm cuvette. Will its absorbance be less than, more than, or equal to 1.30?
c. Will changing to a 1.25 cuvette affect the absorptivity constant?

***Answer:***

a. Substituting into the equation for Beer's law:

$$A = \alpha \quad b \quad C$$

$$1.30 = \frac{(15{,}000\ \text{L})(1\ \cancel{\text{cm}})\ \text{C}}{\text{mole} \cdot \cancel{\text{cm}}}$$

The cm cancel:

$$1.30 = \frac{(15{,}000\ \text{L})\,\text{C}}{1\ \text{mole}}$$

Solving for the concentration:

$$C = \frac{1.30}{\dfrac{(15{,}000\ \text{L})}{1\ \text{mole}}}$$

$$C = \frac{1.30\ \text{mole}}{15{,}000\ \text{L}}$$

$$\approx \mathbf{8.67 \times 10^{-5}\ \frac{mole}{L}}$$

b. This change in cuvette will affect the path length. Since the path length is longer, the absorbance will be greater than 1.30.
c. The absorptivity constant is unchanged by using a different cuvette since it is an intrinsic property of this analyte.

**Example Problem:**

DNA polymerase is an enzyme that participates in the assembly of DNA strands from building blocks of nucleotides. The absorptivity constant of this enzyme (at a certain wavelength) is 0.85 mL/mg·cm. (*Worthington Enzyme Manual: Enzymes and Related Biochemicals*, edited by Von Worthington, Worthington Biochemical Corp., 1993.) If a solution of DNA polymerase has an absorbance of 0.60, what is its concentration? Observe that the pathlength is not specified in this problem, so assume that it is 1 cm, which is most common.

***Answer:***

Substituting into the equation for Beer's law:

$$A = \alpha \ b C$$

$$0.60 = \frac{0.85 \text{ mL}}{\text{mg} \cdot \cancel{\text{cm}}}(1 \ \cancel{\text{cm}})(C)$$

$$C = \frac{0.60}{\frac{0.85 \text{ mL}}{1 \text{ mg}}}$$

$$\approx \frac{\mathbf{0.71 \ mg}}{\mathbf{1 \ mL}}$$

Although there is a lower limit of concentration below which an analyte cannot be detected, spectrophotometry is generally a method used to evaluate analytes that are present at very low levels in a sample. You can easily demonstrate that this is so by taking food coloring and trying to measure its absorbance or transmittance. You will find that the absorbance of undiluted food coloring is far too intense to measure in a spectrophotometer. In fact, food coloring must be diluted a great deal before its absorbance falls into the linear range of a spectrophotometer. Samples often must be diluted before they can be analyzed spectrophotometrically.

**Example Problem:**

Assume that a spectrophotometer is able to read accurately in the absorbance range from 0.1 to 1.8. The molar absorptivity constant for NADH (an important molecule involved in energy production in cells) is 15,000 L/mole·cm, at a specified wavelength. Using Beer's law, calculate the concentration range of NADH that can be accurately quantified under these conditions based on the limits of the spectrophotometer.

***Answer:***

This involves calculation of the molar concentrations that will produce absorbances of 0.1 and 1.8. From Beer's law:

$$C = \frac{A}{\alpha \, b}$$

Substituting 0.1 and 1.8 into the equation and assuming a customary pathlength of 1 cm:

$$C = \frac{0.1}{\frac{(15{,}000\ \text{L})(1\ \cancel{\text{cm}})}{\text{mole}\cdot\cancel{\text{cm}}}} \approx \mathbf{6.7 \times 10^{-6}\ mole/L}$$

$$C = \frac{1.8}{\frac{(15{,}000\ \text{L})(1\ \cancel{\text{cm}})}{\text{mole}\cdot\cancel{\text{cm}}}} = \mathbf{120 \times 10^{-6}\ mole/L}$$

Thus, the range of NADH concentrations that can be detected under these conditions with this spectrophotometer is from $6.7 \times 10^{-6}$ to $120 \times 10^{-6}$ mole/L. These are dilute solutions of NADH.

## 16.5 CALCULATING THE ABSORPTIVITY CONSTANT

There are situations where it is desirable to know the absorptivity constant for a given compound under specific conditions based on data from your own spectrophotometer in your own laboratory. This section shows two strategies to determine the absorptivity constant. The first strategy is based on the absorbance of a single standard. The second strategy is more reliable because it involves constructing a standard curve with more than one standard and calculating the absorptivity constant from the slope of the calibration line.

### Strategy 1: Calculating an Absorptivity Constant Based on One Standard

Beer's equation can be rearranged as follows:

$$\text{Absorptivity constant} = \frac{\text{absorbance}}{(\text{pathlength})(\text{concentration})}$$

$$\text{or} \quad \alpha = \frac{A}{bC}$$

If the pathlength, absorbance, and concentration of a single standard is known, these values can be plugged into the equation above to determine the absorptivity constant as is illustrated in the example below.

**Example:**

A standard containing 75 ppm of compound Y is placed in a 1 cm cuvette. The absorbance of this standard is 1.20 under specified conditions. Assuming that there is a linear relationship between the concentration of compound Y and the absorbance and assuming that the standard was prepared properly, what is the absorptivity constant for this compound under these conditions?

***Answer:***

Substituting into the equation for Beer's law:

$$\text{Absorptivity constant} = \frac{\text{absorbance}}{(\text{concentration})(\text{pathlength})}$$

$$\alpha = \frac{1.20}{(75\ \text{ppm})(1\ \text{cm})} = \mathbf{0.016/ppm \cdot cm}$$

This first strategy will give a value for the absorptivity constant. However, it is usually not the best method to use because it is based on only one standard. If that single standard is diluted incorrectly or if for some reason the absorbance value is slightly off what it should be, then the absorptivity constant calculated will also be inaccurate.

## Strategy 2: Calculating an Absorptivity Constant from a Standard Curve

A better way to calculate the absorptivity constant for a particular compound at a specified wavelength is to base it on the absorbance of a series of standards. This is readily accomplished using a standard curve. Recall that the slope of the calibration line is ***the absorptivity constant (α)*** multiplied by ***the path length***. Determining the absorptivity constant based on the slope of a standard curve is illustrated in the example below and is summarized in Box 16.2.

**Example Problem:**

The calibration curve for compound Q is shown below. What is the absorptivity constant for this compound under these conditions? (Assume the path length is 1 cm.)

***Answer:***

Step 1. Calculate the slope of the calibration line. In this case, the slope is 0.014 mL/mg. Note that there are units to the slope because the concentration has units.

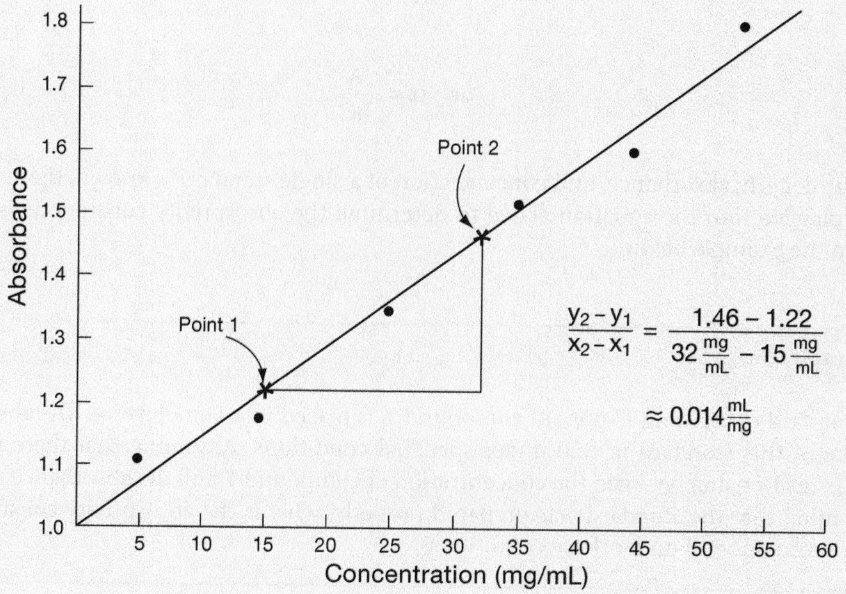

Step 2. The path length is 1 cm.

Step 3. From Beer's law, the slope of the calibration line is:

$$\text{Slope} = (\text{pathlength})(\text{absorptivity constant})$$

$$\text{or} \quad m = (b)(\alpha)$$

$$\text{so the absorptivity constant} = \frac{\text{slope}}{\text{pathlength}}$$

$$\text{or} \quad \alpha = \frac{m}{b}$$

In this example, under the conditions used:

$$\alpha = \frac{m}{b}$$

$$\alpha = \frac{\frac{0.014 \text{ mL}}{1 \text{ mg}}}{1 \text{ cm}}$$

$$\alpha = \left(\frac{0.014 \text{ mL}}{1 \text{ mg}}\right)\left(\frac{1}{1 \text{ cm}}\right)$$

$$\alpha = \frac{\mathbf{0.014\ mL}}{\mathbf{1\ cm \cdot mg}}$$

**BOX 16.2 Determination of the Absorptivity Constant from a Calibration Curve**

Step 1. Prepare a calibration curve with concentration on the X-axis and absorbance on the Y-axis.

Step 2. Calculate the slope of the calibration line using the equation:

$$m = \frac{Y_2 - Y_1}{X_2 - X_1}$$

Step 3. Determine the path length, b. It is generally 1 cm assuming a standard cuvette and holder are used.

Step 4. Use this equation to solve for the absorptivity constant:

$$\alpha = \frac{m}{b}$$

Notes:

- When calculating slope, pick two points that are actually on the best fit line. Remember that the data used to make your graph may include points that do not actually sit right on the best fit line. Do not use those points that do not sit on the line to calculate slope.
- Graphing software programs will conveniently and accurately provide the slope, m, of the best fit line based on the least squared method.

## 16.6 QUANTITATIVE ANALYSIS OF A SAMPLE

Generally, the best way to determine the concentration of an analyte in a sample is to always construct a calibration curve based on a series of standards. The standards should be treated alongside the samples so that all conditions and preparation steps are identical for the standards and the samples. Sometimes analysts rely on calibration curves from previous runs, or on single standards, or on published absorptivity constants. These are situations where the use of these "shortcuts" is appropriate, but a standard curve is usually the preferred method. The next example problem illustrates the use of a "shortcut."

**Example Problem:**

In a clinical laboratory, a validated standard is purchased with a concentration of 10 mg/mL of analyte.

The absorbance of this standard (at a specified wavelength) = 1.6

The absorbance of a patient's sample is 0.8.

What is the concentration of analyte in the patient sample, assuming that all parts of the assay were done correctly?

***Answer:***

$$\frac{10\text{ mg/mL}}{1.6} = \frac{?}{0.8} \quad ? = \mathbf{5\ mg/mL}$$

In this case, analysts relied on a single standard rather than preparing a calibration curve with multiple standards. This may be appropriate where the valid range of the assay is known, the single standard is known to be properly diluted, and the instruments used are properly calibrated and maintained.

**Practice Problems**

1. a. ***Prepare a standard curve from the data below.***
   b. ***Does this data show a linear relationship where absorbance increases as standard concentration increases? If so, what is the equation for the line?***
   c. ***If all or part of the graph shows a linear relationship, where absorbance increases with standard concentration, determine the value of the absorptivity constant based on the line. Remember to include the units. (Assume the path length is 1 cm.)***

d. ***Does this graph show a threshold? If so, where? If so, why is there a threshold?***

| *Standard #* | *Concentration in mg/L* | *Absorbance* |
|---|---|---|
| *1* | *2* | *0.22* |
| *2* | *4* | *0.45* |
| *3* | *10* | *1.11* |
| *4* | *12* | *1.34* |
| *5* | *20* | *2.23* |
| *6* | *30* | *2.21* |
| *7* | *40* | *2.22* |
| *8* | *50* | *2.21* |

2. a. ***Prepare a standard curve from the data below.***
   b. ***Calculate the absorptivity constant based on the slope of the line. (Assume a path length of 1 cm.)***
   c. ***Determine the concentration of compound in the samples based on the standard curve.***

| *Standard #* | *Concentration in mM* | *Absorbance* |
|---|---|---|
| *1* | *0* | *0.0* |
| *2* | *80* | *0.2* |
| *3* | *160* | *0.4* |
| *4* | *240* | *0.8* |
| *5* | *320* | *1.0* |

| *Sample* | *Absorbance* |
|---|---|
| *A* | *0.18* |
| *B* | *0.31* |
| *C* | *0.96* |
| *D* | *1.0* |

3. a. ***Prepare a standard curve from the data below.***
   b. ***Determine the absorptivity constant. (Assume the path length is 1 cm.)***
   c. ***What is the concentration of an unknown that is diluted 5 fold and has an absorbance of 0.30?***

| *Standard #* | *Concentration in mM* | *Absorbance* |
|---|---|---|
| *1* | *1* | *0.22* |
| *2* | *2* | *0.46* |
| *3* | *5* | *1.08* |
| *4* | *6* | *1.34* |
| *5* | *10* | *2.18* |

***For problems 4–11, assume Beer's law applies.***

4. ***A certain sample has an absorbance of 1.6 when measured in a 1 cm cuvette.***
   a. ***If the same sample's absorbance is measured in a 0.5 cm cuvette, will its absorbance be greater than, less than, or equal to 1.6?***
   b. ***Based on Beer's law, what is the absorbance of this sample in the 0.5 cm cuvette?***

5. ***A 25 ppm solution of a certain compound has an absorbance of 0.87. What do we expect will be the absorbance of a 40 ppm solution? Explain.***

6. ***A 10 mg/mL solution of a compound has a transmittance of 0.680.***
   a. ***What is the absorbance of this solution?***
   b. ***What will be the absorbance of a 16 mg/mL solution of this compound?***
   c. ***What will be the transmittance of a 16 mg/mL solution of this compound?***

7. ***A solution contains 30 mg/mL of a light absorbing substance. In a 1 cm cuvette it transmits 75% of the incident light.***
   a. ***What will be the transmittance of 60 mg/mL of the same substance?***
   b. ***What will be the absorbance of 60 mg/mL of the same substance?***
   c. ***What will be the transmittance of 90 mg/mL of the same substance?***
   d. ***What will be the absorbance of 90 mg/mL of the same substance?***

8. ***A standard solution of bovine serum albumin (a protein that is commonly used as a standard) containing 1.0 mg/mL had an absorbance of 0.65 under specified conditions.***
   a. ***Based on Beer's law, what is the protein concentration in a partially purified protein preparation if the absorbance of the preparation is 0.15 under these conditions?***
   b. ***Give two possible sources of error in this analysis.***

9. ***The absorptivity constant of ATP (a molecule involved in many cellular activities, including energy transfer) is 15,400 L/mole · cm under specified conditions. (Value from Segel, I.H. Biochemical Calculations. 2nd ed. John Wiley and Sons, 1976.) A solution of purified ATP has an absorbance of 1.6 in a 1 cm cuvette. What is its concentration?***

10. ***The molar absorptivity constant for NADH (a molecule important in the production of energy in cells) is 15,000 L/mole · cm under specified conditions. (Value from Segel, I.H. Biochemical Calculations. 2nd ed. John Wiley and Sons, 1976.) A sample of purified NADH has an absorbance of 0.98 in a 1.2 cm cuvette. What is its concentration?***

11. ***Calculate the range of molar concentrations that can be used to produce absorbance readings between 0.1 and 1.8 if a 1 cm cuvette is used and the compound has a molar absorptivity of 10,000 L/mole · cm.***

12. ***Try this as a challenge: Suppose a 15 ppm solution of a sulfanilamide drug (an antibiotic) has a transmittance of 0.60 at 270 nm in a 1.00 cm cuvette. The solvent is water and the molecular weight of the drug is 245. What is the <u>molar absorptivity constant</u> at this wavelength? (This means the absorptivity constant has units of L/mole · cm.)***

## *Answers*

1. a.

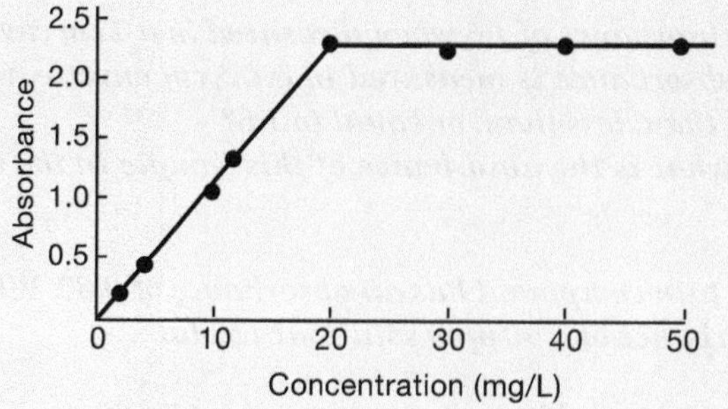

b. The graph is linear from 2 to about 20 mg/L concentrations.

$$\text{Slope} = m = \frac{Y_2 - Y_1}{X_2 - X_1} = 1.1 / 10 \text{ mg/L}$$

$$= \frac{0.11 \text{ L}}{\text{mg}}$$

**Absorbance = (0.11 L/mg) C + 0**

c. $\textbf{Absorptivity constant} = \alpha = \dfrac{\textbf{slope}}{\textbf{path length}} = \textbf{0.11 L/mg} \cdot \textbf{cm}$

d. This graph has an upper threshold at concentrations above about 20 mg/L where the graph plateaus. This is an indication of the limitation of the spectrophotometer at low light transmittances.

2. a.

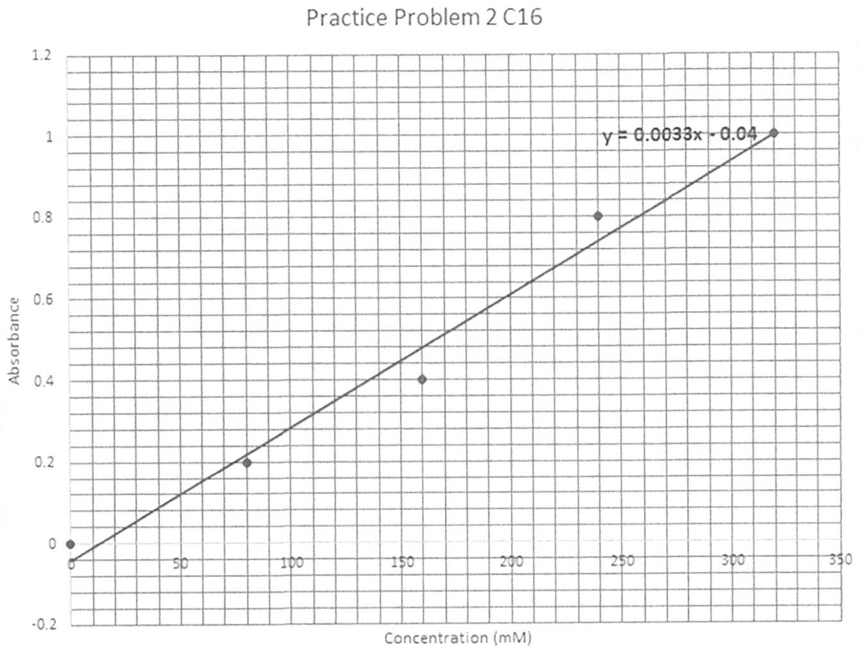


b.

$$\alpha = \frac{\text{slope}}{\text{pathlength}}$$

Slope = 0.0033/mM

$$\alpha = \frac{\textbf{0.0033}}{\textbf{mM cm}}$$

c. To find the concentration in the samples, we can use the equation for the line on the standard curve. (Here we have used the equation provided by graphing software. If you calculate the equation for the line "by hand," you may have slightly different answers.)

$$Y = m \qquad X + a$$

$$A = (0.0033/\text{mM})\ C - 0.04$$

For example, for sample A:

$0.18 = (0.0033/\text{mM})\ C - 0.04$

$0.22 = (0.0033/\text{mM})\ C$

$$C = \frac{0.22}{0.0033/\text{mM}} \approx 66.7\ \text{mM}$$

Thus:

| | Absorbance | Concentration (in mM) |
|---|---|---|
| Sample A | 0.18 | **≈ 66.7** |
| Sample B | 0.31 | **≈ 106.1** |
| Sample C | 0.96 | **≈ 303.0** |
| Sample D | 1.0 | **≈ 315.2** |

3. a.

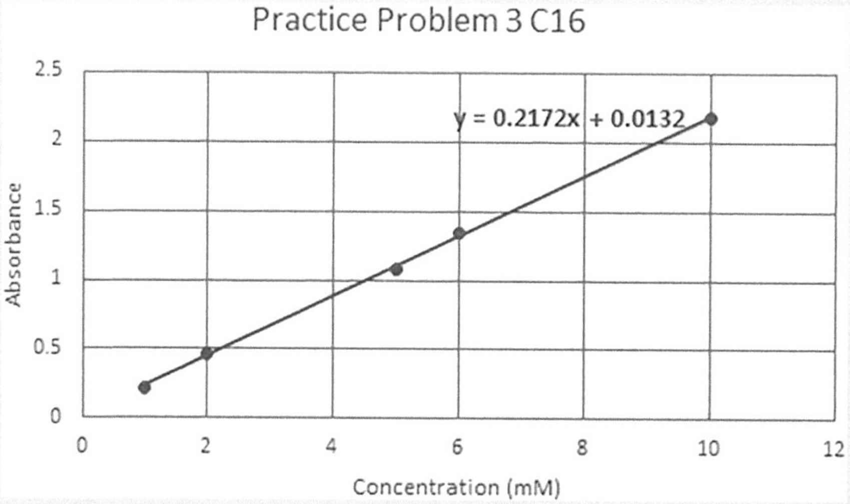


b. $\alpha = \dfrac{\text{slope}}{\text{pathlength}}$

Slope ≈ 0.2172/mM

$$\alpha = \frac{\mathbf{0.2172}}{\mathbf{cm \cdot mM}}$$

c. C ≈ 1.320 mM (diluted) C = (1.320 mM) (5) ≈ **6.60 mM undiluted**

4. a. When the pathlength decreases the absorbance decreases b. **0.8**

5. $\dfrac{?}{40\ \text{ppm}} = \dfrac{0.87}{25\ \text{ppm}}$ ? ≈ **1.39** Absorbance

Absorbance is a linear function of concentration, and the Y-intercept is reasonably assumed to be zero (or to be very close to zero), so this is a proportion problem.

6. t = 0.680 A = −log (t)
 a. A = −log (0.680) ≈ **0.167**
 b. Because there is a proportional relationship between absorbance and concentration:

$\dfrac{?}{16\ \text{mg/mL}} = \dfrac{0.167}{10\ \text{mg/mL}}$ A ≈ **0.267**

c. $A = -\log(t)$

$0.267 = -\log(t)$

$t = 10^{-0.267}$

$t \approx \mathbf{0.540}$

7. $A = -\log(0.75) \approx 0.12494$

a, b. $\frac{A}{60\ \text{mg/mL}} = \frac{0.12494}{30\ \text{mg/mL}}$ The absorbance of 60 mg/mL ≈ **0.250**

$t = 10^{-A}$

$t = 10^{-0.250}$

Transmittance ≈ **0.562**

c, d. $\frac{A}{90\ \text{mg/mL}} = \frac{0.12494}{30\ \text{mg/mL}}$ Absorbance ≈ **0.375**

$t = 10^{-A}$

$t = 10^{-0.375}$

Transmittance ≈ **0.422**

8. $A = 0.65$ of 1 mg/mL

a. $\frac{?}{0.15} = \frac{1\ \text{mg/mL}}{0.65}$ C ≈ **0.231 mg/mL**

b. The proteins in the preparation may not have the same amino acid composition as the BSA. There might be impurities in the partially purified preparation that interfere with the analysis. The standard solution may not have been prepared correctly.

9. $\alpha_{ATP} = 15{,}400\ \text{L/mole}\cdot\text{cm}$

$A = \alpha\ \ b\ \ C$

$$1.6 = \frac{15{,}400\ \text{L}(1\ \not{\text{cm}})}{(\text{mole}\cdot\not{\text{cm}})}C$$

$$C = \frac{1.6\ \text{mole}}{15{,}400\ \text{L}} \approx \mathbf{1.04 \times 10^{-4}\ mole/L}$$

10. $\alpha_{NADH} = 15{,}000\ \text{L/mole}\cdot\text{cm}$

$A = \ \alpha\ \ b\ \ C$

$$0.98 = \frac{15{,}000\ \text{L}}{\text{mole}\cdot\text{cm}}(1.2\ \text{cm})(C)$$

$$C = \frac{0.98\ \text{mole}\cdot\not{\text{cm}}}{15{,}000\,(1.2)\ \not{\text{cm}}\cdot\text{L}}$$ C ≈ $\mathbf{5.44 \times 10^{-5}\ mole/L}$

11. $A = \alpha\, b\, C$

or $C = \frac{A}{\alpha\, b}$

For lower limit: $0.1 = \frac{10{,}000\ \text{L}\,(1\ \not{\text{cm}})\,C}{\text{mole}\cdot\not{\text{cm}}}$

$$C = \frac{0.1\text{ mole}}{10{,}000\text{ L}} \qquad \mathbf{C = 1 \times 10^{-5}\ mole/L}$$

For upper limit:

$$1.8 = \frac{10{,}000\text{ L}\,(1\ \cancel{\text{cm}})\,C}{\text{mole}\ \cancel{\text{cm}}}$$

$$C = \frac{1.8\text{ mole}}{10{,}000\text{ L}} \qquad \mathbf{C = 1.8 \times 10^{-4}\ mole/L}$$

Therefore, the range of concentration that can be measured for this compound is from $\mathbf{1.8 \times 10^{-4}}$ **mole/L to** $\mathbf{1 \times 10^{-5}}$ **mole/L**.

12. First, convert 15 ppm to units of molarity. 15 ppm = 15 g/$10^6$ mL = 0.015 g/$10^3$ mL = 0.015 g/L

1 M = 245 g/L, so what molarity is 0.015 g/L?

$$\frac{245\text{ g/L}}{1\text{ M}} = \frac{0.015\text{ g/L}}{?} \qquad ? \approx 6.12244898 \times 10^{-5}\text{ M}$$

Convert transmittance to absorbance: t = 0.60 A ≈ 0.22185
Substitute into Beer's equation:

$$\begin{matrix} A & \alpha & b & C \end{matrix}$$

$$0.22185 = \alpha(1\text{ cm})\left(6.1224489 \times 10^{-5}\text{ moles/L}\right)$$

$$\alpha = \frac{0.22185}{(1\text{ cm})\left(6.1224489 \times 10^{-5}\text{ moles/L}\right)}$$

$$\boldsymbol{\alpha \approx 3{,}624\ \text{L/mole} \cdot \text{cm}}$$

## 16.7 INTRODUCTION TO ELISAs

This section introduces an important *method of quantitative analysis* called **ELISA** (enzyme-linked immunosorbent assay). ELISAs rely on antibodies and their affinity for (attraction to) antigens. **Antibodies** *are proteins that circulate in the body and help protect us from pathogenic invaders (like bacteria or viruses).* An **antigen** *is the agent to which the antibody responds.* For example, an antigen might be a protein on the surface of a viral or bacterial invader. Each kind of antibody only recognizes and binds its own antigen. **ELISAs** *are tests based on the fact that antibodies find and bind specifically to their target antigen.*

ELISAs have many applications. For example, they can be used in research to look for proteins produced by experimentally treated cells. They are commonly used in medicine to look for substances in blood, or other body fluids, for the purpose of diagnosing disorders. They can be used to test food samples for unwanted substances. They can be used to see if a person has been infected by a particular pathogen and therefore has developed antibodies against that pathogen. ELISAs are of particular importance during the COVID-19 pandemic because they can be used to test whether people have antibodies against the virus that causes the disease.

We introduce ELISAs in this chapter because ELISAs involve standard curves and a *type of spectrophotometer* called a **plate reader**. The difference between a plate reader and the conventional spectrophotometers we have discussed so far is that a plate reader can read and print out at once the absorbances of multiple samples contained in the wells of a 96-well plate.

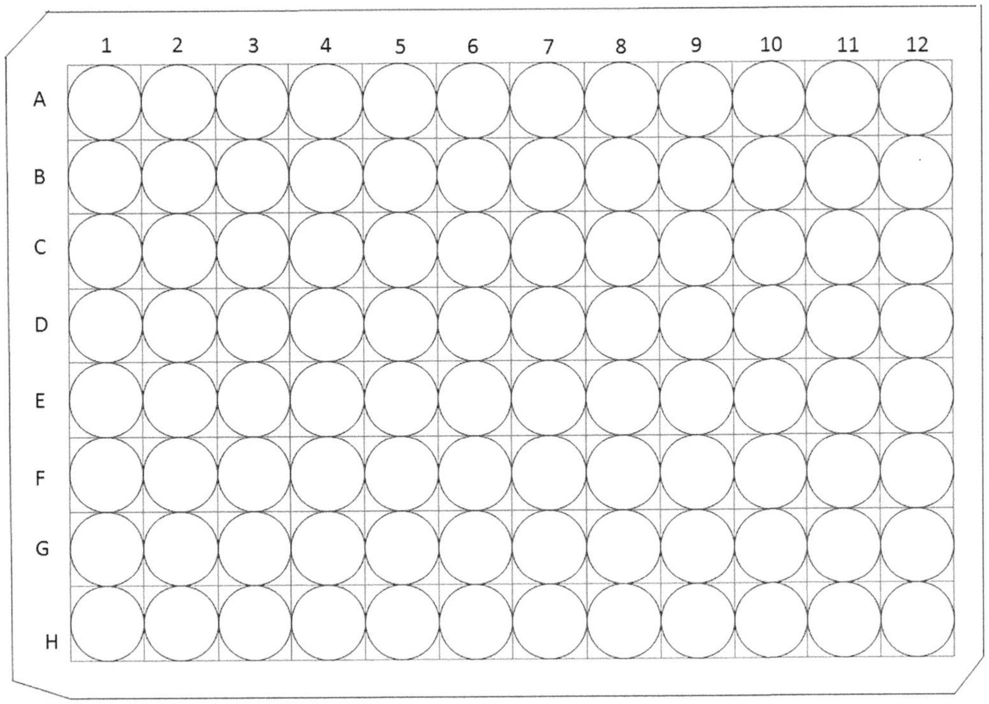


**FIGURE 16.5** Top view of a 96-well plate. 96 wells, each of which is a tiny test tube, are present. The first well, at the upper left corner, is labeled A1. The first row is labeled A1–A12. The second row is labeled B1–B12, and so on.

A *96-well plate is a plastic holder that contains 96 tiny test tubes called "wells,"* Figure 16.5. The plastic used to manufacture the plate is designed so that antibodies and other proteins stick to it tightly. From a mathematical point of view, the calculations involved in performing quantitative ELISAs are the same as we have already discussed in this chapter. Standards are diluted, assayed, and used to prepare a standard curve. The concentration (or amount) of analyte in test samples can then be determined based on the standard curve.

As an example, suppose we are interested in detecting and quantifying the bacterial pathogen *Salmonella* to see if it is present in food samples. A protein that is part of this pathogen is the target ***antigen*** of interest. *Salmonella* is also the ***analyte*** of interest or the target of the assay. It is possible to purchase a 96-well plate in which the bottom surface of each well is coated with tightly adhered antibodies that recognize and bind to a *Salmonella* protein and (ideally) nothing else, Figure 16.6a. When an assay is performed, standards containing known amounts of the *Salmonella* protein are introduced into some of the wells. The antibodies coating the bottoms of these wells will recognize, bind to, and anchor the *Salmonella* protein inside the wells. These standards will be used to create the standard curve. Other wells are filled with test samples from foods that might or might not contain the *Salmonella* pathogen. If *Salmonella* is present in any of the food samples, the *Salmonella* protein will be recognized by, and will bind to, the antibodies in the well. If there is no *Salmonella* protein in a test sample, then nothing will stick to the antibodies coating the wells. After introducing the standards and test samples into the wells of the 96-well plate, the plate is washed to remove anything that did not stick. *Salmonella* proteins that were recognized and bound by the antibodies will remain anchored to the bottom of the wells, Figure 16.6b. At this point the *Salmonella* protein–antibody complex is invisible, so steps are performed that cause the complex to become colored. The more *Salmonella* protein in a well, the more intense the color that develops, Figure 16.6c. Finally, the plate is put into the plate reader that detects and quantifies how much color (if any) is present in each well. The more color, the more *Salmonella* protein present in that well.

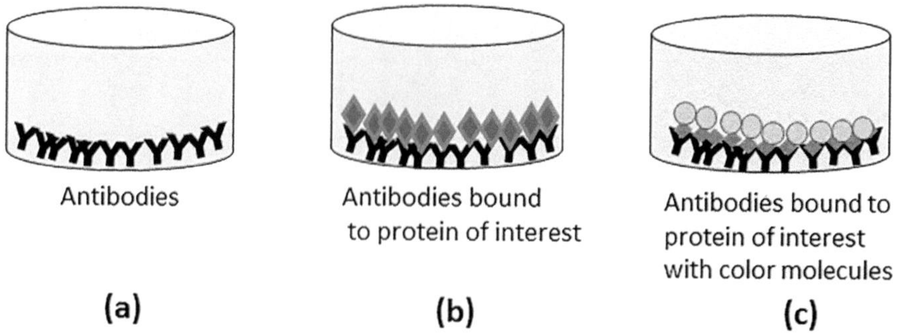


**FIGURE 16.6** ELISA testing for the presence and quantity of a protein of interest. (a) Closer view of a single well from a 96-well plate that has been coated with antibody against the protein of interest. For example, if the protein of interest is a *Salmonella* protein, then the bottoms of the wells are coated with antibody against that protein. (b) The protein of interest, the antigen, which was present in a standard or in a sample has bound specifically to the antibodies coating the well. (c) A series of steps were performed resulting in a colored deposit in any well where the antibody is bound to the protein of interest. The more protein of interest that was present in the well, the more color that appears.

**Example Problem:**

An outbreak of *Salmonella* has occurred causing severe illness in a number of people. A testing laboratory has been hired to test a variety of food samples to determine which food is causing the outbreak. ELISA is a method of choice for a study such as this. Analysts purchase 96-well plates that have been coated with antibody that recognizes the *Salmonella* protein. The steps that are performed by analysts in the laboratory are as follows:

**Step 1**: A series of standards with known levels of *Salmonella* protein are prepared by dissolving the protein in an aqueous buffer.

**Step 2**: Analysts create a chart, shown in Table 16.2, that indicates which wells will contain the standards and which wells will contain the food samples being tested. (Note that not every well on the 96-well plate is used in this assay.)

**Step 3**: A specific volume of each standard is added to its own well of the 96-well plate. The *Salmonella* protein in each standard binds tightly to the antibody that coats the bottom of the well.

**Step 4**: Three food samples are prepared, and the proper volume of each food sample is added to its own well. If the *Salmonella* pathogen is present in a food sample, its protein will bind to the antibody that coats the bottom of the well.

**Step 5**: Procedural steps are performed to make the antibody–protein complex colored in any well that contained the *Salmonella* protein. The more *Salmonella* protein present, the more color that appears. The resulting plate is shown in Figure 16.7.

**Step 6**: The 96-well plate is put into the plate reader which provides an absorbance reading for each well. The absorbance is proportional to the amount of color in that well. The more *Salmonella* protein present, the more intense the color, and the higher the absorbance reading. Table 16.3a shows these readings.

Based on the results in Table 16.3a, prepare a standard curve and determine the amount of *Salmonella* (if any) present in each of the three food samples. Observe that each standard and each test sample is assayed twice. These two assays of the same thing are called "replicates." For your analysis, average the two results. (Note that if there is a dramatic difference between replicates, it alerts the analyst that there is a problem, and troubleshooting would have to be performed.)

***Answer:***

The averaged values for the replicate standards and samples are shown in Table 16.3b.

The standard curve for these data is shown in Figure 16.8.

Using the equation for the line in Figure 16.8, the values for the samples are:

Food sample 1:

$$0.334 = 0.011(?) + 0.0004$$

$$? \approx \mathbf{30.327\ pg/mL}$$

Food sample 2:

$$\approx \mathbf{100.600\ pg/mL}$$

Food sample 3:
No detectable *Salmonella* contamination

Based on these results, foods 1 and 2 are contaminated and may be associated with the *Salmonella* outbreak.

**TABLE 16.2 Layout for *Salmonella* ELISA Showing Which Wells of a 96-Well Plate Will Contain Which Standards and Which Samples**

| | 1 | 2 | 3 | 4 | 5 | 6 | 7 | 8 | 9 | 10 | 11 | 12 |
|---|---|---|---|---|---|---|---|---|---|---|---|---|
| A | Standard 0 pg/mL | Standard 0 pg/mL | Food 1 | Food 1 Replicate | | | | | | | | |
| B | Standard 10 pg/mL | Standard 10 pg/mL | Food 2 | Food 2 Replicate | | | | | | | | |
| C | Standard 20 pg/mL | Standard 20 pg/mL | Food 3 | Food 3 Replicate | | | | | | | | |
| D | Standard 50 pg/mL | Standard 50 pg/mL | | | | | | | | | | |
| E | Standard 75 pg/mL | Standard 75 pg/mL | | | | | | | | | | |
| F | Standard 150 pg/mL | Standard 150 pg/mL | | | | | | | | | | |
| G | | | | | | | | | | | | |
| H | | | | | | | | | | | | |

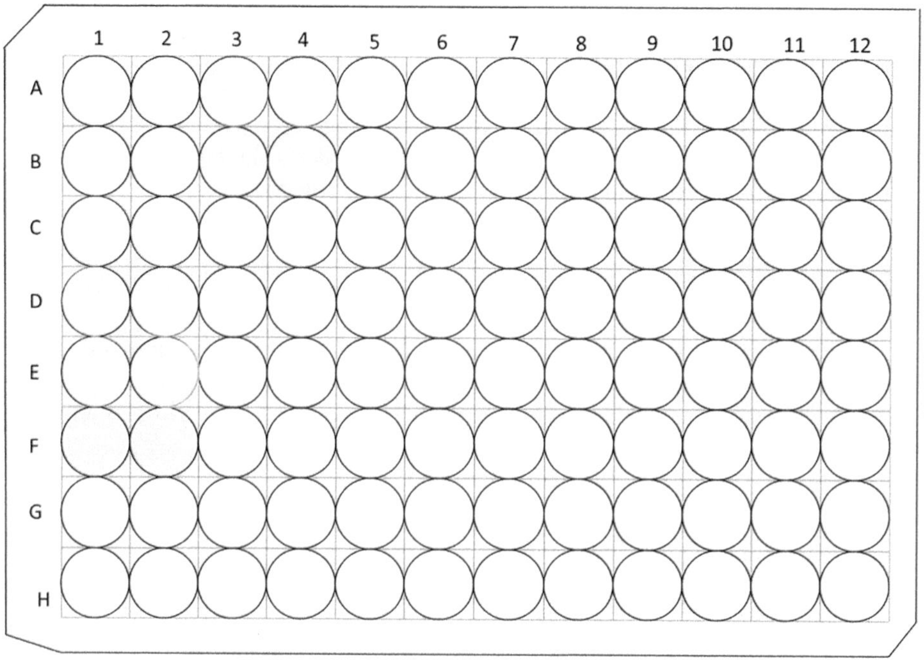


**FIGURE 16.7** ELISA testing for the presence and quantity of ***Salmonella*** in foods. The standards are present in columns 1 and 2, rows A–F. Observe that as the standard concentration increases, the color intensity in the wells also increases. Columns 3 and 4, rows A–C, contain the three test samples. Each standard and each sample is tested in replicate (twice).

**TABLE 16.3A Plate Reader Absorbance Values for *Salmonella* Assay**

| | 1 | 2 | 3 | 4 | 5 | 6 | 7 | 8 | 9 | 10 | 11 | 12 |
|---|---|---|---|---|---|---|---|---|---|---|---|---|
| A | 0.001 | 0.002 | 0.331 | 0.337 | | | | | | | | |
| B | 0.110 | 0.112 | 1.101 | 1.113 | | | | | | | | |
| C | 0.221 | 0.219 | 0.002 | 0.000 | | | | | | | | |
| D | 0.556 | 0.553 | | | | | | | | | | |
| E | 0.824 | 0.821 | | | | | | | | | | |
| F | 1.655 | 1.660 | | | | | | | | | | |
| G | | | | | | | | | | | | |
| H | | | | | | | | | | | | |

**TABLE 16.3B Plate Reader Absorbance Values for *Salmonella* Assay with Replicates Averaged**

| | 1 | 2 | Replicate averages | 3 | 4 | Replicate averages | 5 | 6 | 7 | 8 | 9 | 10 | 11 | 12 |
|---|---|---|---|---|---|---|---|---|---|---|---|---|---|---|
| A | 0.001 | 0.002 | **0.002** | 0.331 | 0.337 | **0.334** | | | | | | | | |
| B | 0.110 | 0.112 | **0.111** | 1.101 | 1.113 | **1.107** | | | | | | | | |
| C | 0.221 | 0.219 | **0.220** | 0.002 | 0.000 | **0.001** | | | | | | | | |
| D | 0.556 | 0.553 | **0.555** | | | | | | | | | | | |
| E | 0.824 | 0.821 | **0.823** | | | | | | | | | | | |
| F | 1.655 | 1.660 | **1.658** | | | | | | | | | | | |
| G | | | | | | | | | | | | | | |
| H | | | | | | | | | | | | | | |

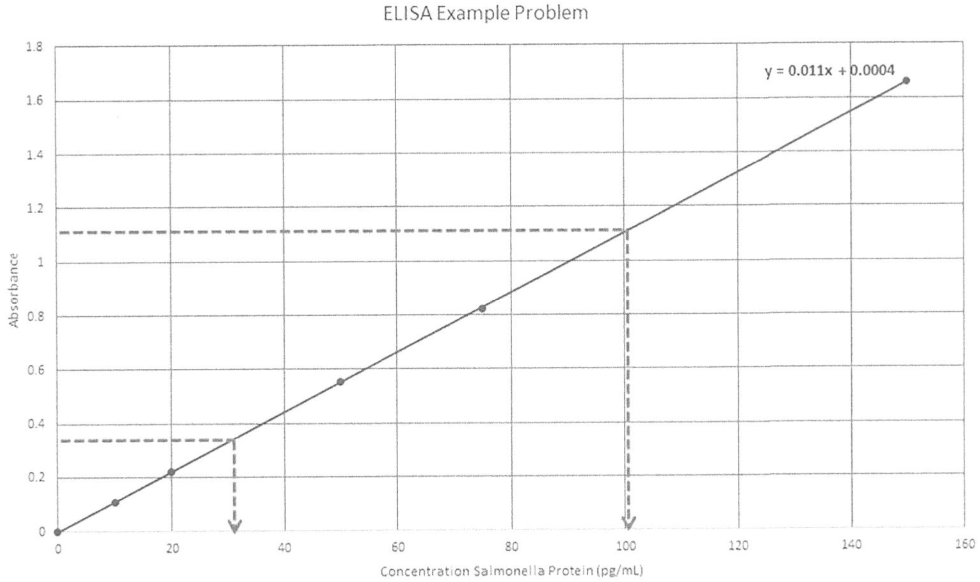


**FIGURE 16.8** Standard curve results of an ELISA for ***Salmonella*** contaminants in foods. Observe that it is possible to "read off" the values for concentration of Salmonella protein in the samples, based on this curve, as shown with the dashed lines. However, it is more accurate to calculate the values based on the equation for the best fit line provided by the software program.

### 16.7.1 FINDING THE MATH

**Case Study: An ELISA for Egg White Proteins**

**BACKGROUND**

This case study relates to a commercial test kit used to test food samples for low levels of egg white protein contamination. Why test foods for egg white protein contaminants? Egg white protein, unlike the pathogenic bacterium, *Salmonella*, seems like it should be an ordinary and harmless substance in foods. The answer is that some people are allergic to egg white proteins; for these people, eating processed food with even tiny amounts of egg white proteins can cause a life-threatening reaction. In a food processing facility, it is possible for egg white proteins to accidentally move from one processed food into another food that is not supposed to have any egg products. This is a particular problem in bakeries where eggs are a common ingredient. For this reason, it is important to have a test that can determine the presence of egg white protein contaminants.

It is possible to purchase ELISA kits that detect and quantify egg white protein contamination. These kits contain coated plates, reagents, and instructions. However, even when using convenient test kits, there are usually a few preparations that analysts must perform. Also, analysts must be able to interpret the instructions that come with the kit. This case study examines some of the preparations that are required when using an ELISA test kit. This case study also involves the analysis of example test results.

Figure 16.9 shows the information and instructions that come with an ELISA test kit for egg white protein detection. Read the information and instructions carefully and answer the questions below. Assume that you are testing **five food samples** for the presence of egg white protein. Observe that the procedure recommends testing duplicates of each standard and each sample. Assume that you will do so.

Note that for our purposes in this text, we are interested in finding the math required, and it is not important that you understand every step in the procedure. Of course, if you were doing this procedure in a real-life situation, it would be essential to understand each step.

**Questions:**

1. Highlight each place in Figure 16.9 where you will need to perform a math calculation to carry out the assay.
2. For each place you marked in Question 1, explain the calculation required. Perform the calculations. (If you are not sure how to proceed, see the hint below.)
3. Assume you have now carried out the assay procedure and the data you obtain are shown in Table 16.4. Analyze these results.

**Hint: Here are some hints to guide your analysis:**

a. What reagents need to be prepared in advance?
b. How many samples are being tested?
c. How many standards are being tested?
d. Given the number of samples and/or standards involved, how much reagent(s) should you prepare?

**DIRECTIONS ELISA TEST KIT FOR EGG WHITE PROTEIN**

| COMPONENTS SUPPLIED WITH KIT | |
|---|---|
| **Component** | **Amount Supplied** |
| 96-well plate coated with antibodies to recognize egg white protein | One 96-well plate |
| Egg white protein standards (0; 0.4; 1; 4; 10 ppm egg white protein) | One vial each standard; 1.0 mL/vial |
| Conjugate: ready to use | 15 mL |
| Substrate solution: ready to use | 15 mL |
| Stop solution: ready to use | 15 mL |
| Extraction and Sample Dilution Buffer (Tris): 10X concentrate. Dilute 1+9 with purified water. Stored at 4 °C the diluted buffer is stable for at least one week. If during the cold storage crystals precipitate, the concentrate should be warmed at 37 °C for 15 minutes. | 2 times 120 mL |
| Washing Solution (PBS + SDS): 10X concentrate. Dilute 1 + 9 with purified water. Stored at 4 °C the diluted buffer is stable for at least 4 weeks. If during the cold storage crystals precipitate, the concentrate should be warmed at 37 °C for 15 minutes. | 60 mL |

**ASSAY PROCEDURE**

**PART I: PREPARATION OF FOOD SAMPLES**

1. Remove at least 5 grams of each food sample.

2. Pulverize completely with mortar and pestle or other method.

**FIGURE 16.9** Instructions that accompany ELISA test kit for egg white protein.

(*Continued*)

3. Suspend 1 g of the pulverized sample in 20 mL of pre-diluted Extraction and Sample Dilution Buffer.

4. Incubate for 15 minutes in a water bath at 60 °C with shaking every 2 minutes.

5. Centrifuge 10 minutes at 2000 × g.

6. Apply 100 μL of each particle-free food solution to a well. If the results of a sample are out of the measuring range, further dilution with pre-diluted Extraction and Sample Dilution Buffer is necessary. The additional dilution has to be considered when calculating the concentration.

**PART II: ASSAY PROCEDURE**

The washing solution is supplied as a 10X concentrate and must be diluted 1 + 9 with purified water before use.

The ready-to-use standards should be assayed twice.

A duplicate measurement of each sample is also recommended.

1. Prepare samples as described above.

2. Pipette 100 μL of ready to use standards and of prepared samples in duplicate into the appropriate wells of the 96-well plate.

3. Incubate for 20 minutes at room temperature.

4. Wash the plate three times as follows: Discard the contents of the wells. Pipette 300 μL of diluted washing solution into each well. After the third repetition empty the wells again and remove residual liquid by striking the plate against a paper towel. The wash procedure is critical to ensure good results.

5. Pipette 100 μL of conjugate into each well.

6. Incubate for 20 minutes at room temperature.

7. Wash the plate as outlined in step 4.

8. Pipette 100 μL of substrate solution into each well.

9. Allow the reaction to develop for 20 minutes at room temperature.

10. Stop the reaction by adding 100 μL of stop solution into each well. The wells with positive results will turn yellow.

11. Measure the absorbance in each well using a plate reader.

**PART III: ANALYSIS OF DATA**

12. Construct a standard curve by plotting the average absorbance reading for each standard against its concentration, with absorbance on the Y-axis and concentration on the X-axis.

13. Calculate the average absorbance for each sample and determine its concentration of egg white protein in ppm based on the standard curve.

**FIGURE 16.9 (*CONTINUED*)** Instructions that accompany ELISA test kit for egg white protein.

**TABLE 16.4 Results of ELISA for Egg White Protein**

| Sample or Standard | Absorbance |
|---|---|
| 0 ppm egg white protein standard | 0.001 |
| 0 ppm egg white protein standard | 0.000 |
| 0.4 ppm egg white protein standard | 0.076 |
| 0.4 ppm egg white protein standard | 0.072 |
| 1 ppm egg white protein standard | 0.181 |
| 1 ppm egg white protein standard | 0.191 |
| 4 ppm egg white protein standard | 0.751 |
| 4 ppm egg white protein standard | 0.744 |
| 10 ppm egg white protein standard | 1.891 |
| 10 ppm egg white protein standard | 1.923 |
| Food sample 1 | 0.561 |
| Food sample 1 | 0.651 |
| Food sample 2 | 0.123 |
| Food sample 2 | 0.134 |
| Food sample 3 | 1.724 |
| Food sample 3 | 1.689 |
| Food sample 4 | 2.340 |
| Food sample 4 | 2.351 |
| Food sample 5 | 0.002 |
| Food sample 5 | 0.001 |

**Answers:**

1. The places where a math calculation is required are highlighted in yellow and underlined in Figure 16.10.
2. Calculations Required:

Two of the reagents that come with this kit are supplied as concentrated stock solutions. This is probably because they are more stable when concentrated than when diluted. Therefore, these two solutions must be diluted before use.

(Note that Chapters 13 and 14 discussed the dilution of concentrated stock solutions.)

The directions say to dilute each of the two reagents 1+9. This means you want one part of the concentrated stock solution plus 9 parts purified water for a total of 10 parts.

But first, it is necessary to decide what volume of each solution to prepare.

Let us begin with the extraction and sample dilution buffer. From the directions, we see that this buffer is used for the food samples that are being tested but is not required for the standards.

We are testing **5** food samples each in duplicate = **10** food samples.

According to the directions, each food sample is suspended in 20 mL of extraction buffer, so the total volume of extraction and sample dilution buffer required is **200 mL**.

How much concentrated stock solution is required and how much purified water? We can do this calculation by proportions:

$$\frac{1 \text{ part}}{10 \text{ part}} = \frac{?}{200 \text{ mL}}$$

$$? = \mathbf{20\ mL}$$

So **20 mL** of extraction and sample dilution buffer concentrate would be brought to **200 mL** with purified water.

| COMPONENTS SUPPLIED WITH KIT | |
|---|---|
| **Component** | **Amount Supplied** |
| 96-well plate coated with antibodies to recognize egg white protein | 1 96-well plate |
| Egg white protein standards (0; 0.4; 1; 4; 10 ppm egg white protein) | 1 vial each standard; 1.0 mL/vial |
| Conjugate: ready to use | 15 mL |
| Substrate solution: ready to use | 15 mL |
| Stop solution: ready to use | 15 mL |
| Extraction and Sample Dilution Buffer (Tris): 10X concentrate. Dilute 1+9 with purified water. Stored at 4 °C the diluted buffer is stable for at least one week. If during the cold storage crystals precipitate, the concentrate should be warmed at 37 °C for 15 minutes. | 2 times 120 mL |
| Washing Solution (PBS + SDS): 10X concentrate. Dilute 1 + 9 with purified water. Stored at 4 °C the diluted buffer is stable for at least 4 weeks. If during the cold storage crystals precipitate, the concentrate should be warmed at 37 °C for 15 minutes. | 60 mL |

**ASSAY PROCEDURE**

**PART I: PREPARATION OF FOOD SAMPLES**

1. Remove at least 5 grams of food sample.
2. Pulverize completely with mortar and pestle or other method.
3. Suspend 1 g of the pulverized sample in 20 mL of Extraction and Sample Dilution Buffer.
4. Incubate for 15 minutes in a water bath at 60 °C with shaking every 2 minutes.
5. Centrifuge 10 minutes at 2000 X.
6. Apply 100 µL of each particle-free food solution to a well. If the results of a sample are out of the measuring range, further dilution with pre-diluted Extraction and Sample Dilution Buffer is necessary. The additional dilution has to be considered when calculating the concentration.

**PART II: ASSAY PROCEDURE**

The washing solution is supplied as a 10X concentrate and has to be diluted 1 + 9 with purified water before use. The ready-to-use standards should be assayed twice. A duplicate measurement of each sample is also recommended.

1. Prepare samples as described above.
2. Pipette 100 µL of ready to use standards or prepared samples in duplicate into the appropriate wells of the 96-well plate.
3. Incubate for 20 minutes at room temperature.
4. Wash the plate three times as follows: Discard the contents of the wells. Pipette 300 µL of diluted washing solution into each well. After the third repetition empty the wells again and remove residual liquid by striking the plate against a paper towel. The wash procedure is critical to ensure good results.
5. Pipette 100 µL of conjugate into each well.
6. Incubate for 20 minutes at room temperature.
7. Wash the plate as outlined in step 4.
8. Pipette 100 µL of substrate solution into each well.
9. Allow the reaction to develop for 20 minutes at room temperature.
10. Stop the reaction by adding 100 µL of stop solution into each well. The wells with positive results will turn yellow.
11. Measure the absorbance in each well using a plate reader.

**PART III: ANALYSIS OF DATA**

12. Construct a standard curve by plotting the average absorbance reading for each standard against its concentration with absorbance on the Y- and concentration on the X-axis.
13. Calculate the average absorbance for each sample and determine its concentration of egg white protein in ppm from the standard curve.

**FIGURE 16.10** Highlighting calculations required.

Alternatively, as discussed in Chapter 12, the $C_1V_1 = C_2V_2$ equation can be used to readily perform the required calculation:

$$C_1V_1 = C_2V_2$$

$$(10X)(?) = (1X)(200 \text{ mL})$$

$$? = \mathbf{20\ mL}$$

So **20 mL** of extraction buffer concentrate would be brought to **200 mL** with purified water.

Next, consider the washing solution. How much concentrated stock solution is required and how much purified water?

There are 10 food samples. There are also 5 standards, each of which is tested in duplicate. So there are **20** standards and samples in total.

In steps 4 and 7, each well is washed 3 times. So there are 6 washes.

There will be 20 wells, each washed 6 times for a total of **120** washes.

Each wash requires **300 µL** of diluted washing solution for a total of **36,000 µL** of diluted washing solution = **36 mL**.

The same dilution calculation strategies as previously described can be applied here. Let us use the $C_1V_1 = C_2V_2$ equation:

$$C_1V_1 = C_2V_2$$

$$(10X)(?) = (1X)(36 \text{ mL})$$

$$? = \mathbf{3.6\ mL}$$

**So remove 3.6 mL of the concentrated washing solution and bring to a volume of 36 mL with purified water.**

So now we know how to prepare the extraction and sample dilution buffer and washing buffer.

A chart showing the positions of these samples and standards (like the chart shown in Figure 16.2) would also need to be prepared. The required equipment and supplies would be assembled, much as one might do when preparing to follow a recipe to prepare something in the kitchen.

3. The results of the replicates for each sample and standard are inspected to be sure that none of the replicates are far apart in absorbance value. They are reasonable, and so the replicate values are averaged as shown in Table 16.5.

   Before proceeding with the analysis, it is important to note that food sample 4 provided an absorbance value outside the range of the standards. This value cannot be used. Food sample 4 must therefore be diluted *before* it is assayed. It is likely that another complete run of the ELISA test would need to be performed with this

**TABLE 16.5 Results of ELISA for Egg White Protein with Replicates Averaged**

| Sample or Standard | Absorbance | Average of Replicates |
|---|---|---|
| 0 ppm egg white protein standard | 0.001 | 0.001 |
| 0 ppm egg white protein standard | 0.000 | |
| 0.4 ppm egg white protein standard | 0.076 | 0.074 |
| 0.4 ppm egg white protein standard | 0.072 | |
| 1 ppm egg white protein standard | 0.181 | 0.186 |
| 1 ppm egg white protein standard | 0.191 | |
| 4 ppm egg white protein standard | 0.751 | 0.748 |
| 4 ppm egg white protein standard | 0.744 | |
| 10 ppm egg white protein standard | 1.891 | 1.907 |
| 10 ppm egg white protein standard | 1.923 | |
| Food sample 1 | 0.561 | 0.606 |
| Food sample 1 | 0.651 | |
| Food sample 2 | 0.123 | 0.129 |
| Food sample 2 | 0.134 | |
| Food sample 3 | 1.724 | 1.707 |
| Food sample 3 | 1.689 | |
| Food sample 4 | 2.340 | ! |
| Food sample 4 | 2.351 | |
| Food sample 5 | 0.002 | 0.002 |
| Food sample 5 | 0.001 | |

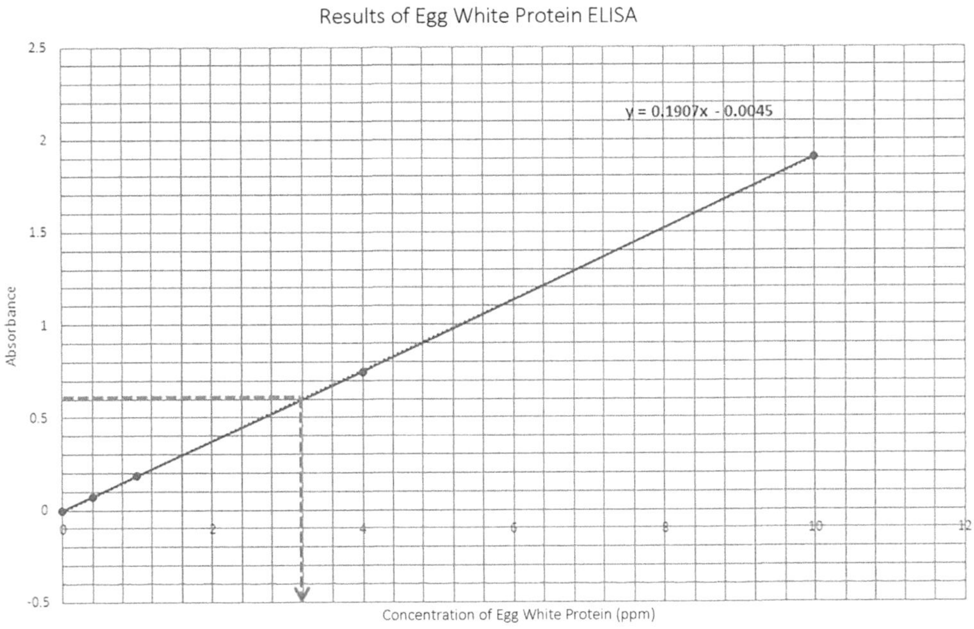


**FIGURE 16.11** Standard curve for egg white protein ELISA. The dashed lines show how it is possible to "read off" the concentration of egg white protein in food sample 1 using the standard curve graph.

sample and more reagents would be needed. For our purposes, we will go ahead and analyze the results of the rest of the samples and ignore the out-of-range sample.

The standard curve is plotted in Figure 16.11.

Using the equation for the line on Figure 16.11, the values for the samples are:

Food sample 1:
$0.606 = 0.1907\,(?) - 0.0045$
**? ≈ 3.201 ppm**

Food sample 2:
**≈ 0.700 ppm**

Food sample 3:
**≈ 8.975 ppm**

Food sample 4:
Must be diluted and assay repeated

Food sample 5:
No detectable egg white protein

These results indicate that egg white protein has contaminated some of the food samples and further investigation would likely be required to assess and fix the problem.

# Graphing Exponential Equations

17



## 17.1 EXPONENTIAL RELATIONSHIPS: GROWTH OF CELL POPULATIONS

Chapters 15 and 16 focused primarily on relationships that form a straight line when graphed. Although linear relationships are extremely important, not all relationships that biotechnologists encounter are linear. This chapter discusses two important examples of nonlinear relationships: (1) the relationship between the number of cultured cells present and time elapsed and (2) the relationship between the amount of radioactivity present and time elapsed. A third example is found in Chapter 23 where electrophoresis of DNA fragments is discussed. Yet another example is discussed in Chapters 24 and 25, where we look at the exponential amplification of DNA using a method called polymerase chain reaction.

Biotechnologists frequently work with cultured cells, both microbial cells and eukaryotic cells (a term that includes insect, yeast, and animal cells). Cultured cells are those grown in flasks, dishes, tubes, vats, or other vessels. Cultured cells are used in research laboratories to probe biological processes and to test the effects of treatments (such as drugs) on cells. Cells are also used as "factories" to manufacture products, the commercial basis of the enterprise we call "biotechnology." In all these cases, it is important to monitor the growth of the cells. For example, it is important that cells are at a certain stage of growth before introducing a gene of interest into them. It is necessary to have a certain number of cells before beginning an experiment. Understanding patterns of cell growth is thus important.

New cells form by **cell division**. In cell division, *a single cell divides to form two daughter cells*. Suppose we begin with a single bacterial cell that divides to form two cells. The two cells each split to form four cells, which divide into eight cells and so on. Suppose that the cells divide every hour and therefore every hour the number of bacterial cells doubles. We say that these cells have a **generation time** of 1 hour, Figure 17.1. (Note that the terms "doubling time" and "generation time" are used interchangeably.) The relationship between time elapsed and number of bacteria in this example is summarized in Table 17.1 and graphed in Figure 17.2. Observe that this relationship does not form a straight line when graphed.

DOI: 10.1201/9780429282744-20

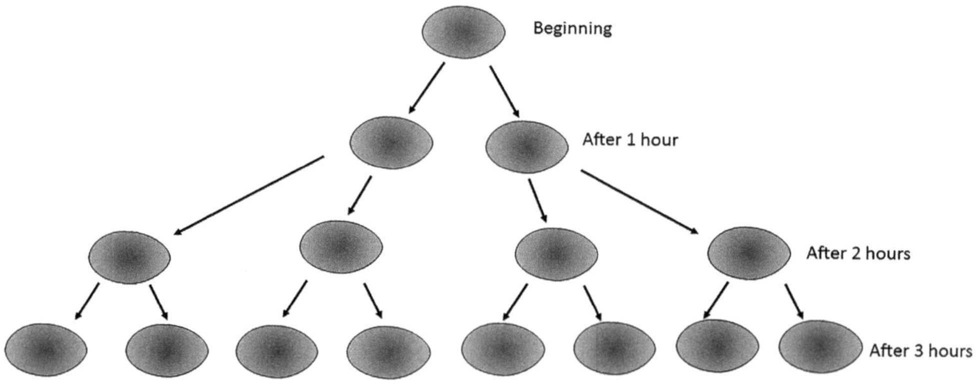


**FIGURE 17.1** Cell division. These cells have a generation time of 1 hour.

**TABLE 17.1 Population Growth Where the Generation Time Is 1 hour**

| Time Elapsed (hours) | Number of Cells Present |
|---|---|
| 0 | 1 |
| 1 | 2 |
| 2 | 4 |
| 3 | 8 |
| 4 | 16 |
| 5 | 32 |
| 6 | 64 |
| 7 | 128 |

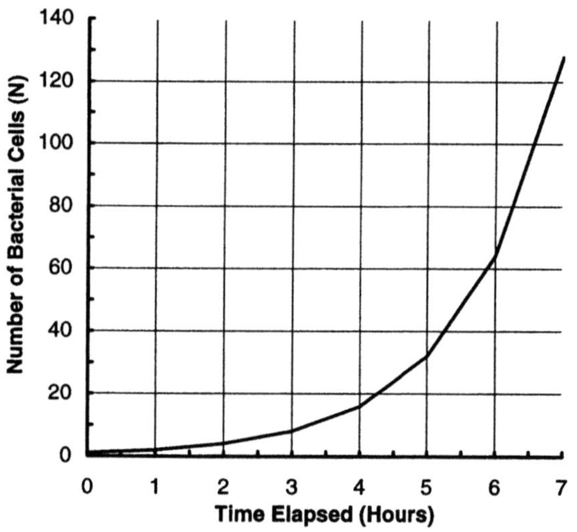


**FIGURE 17.2** Cell growth. A plot where there is initially only one cell present and the population doubles every hour.

How could we write an equation that describes the relationship graphed in Figure 17.2? There are two variables: the number of generations that have occurred and the number of bacteria. The equation needs to include both variables to show that the population doubles at a regular interval. The equation that describes this relationship is:

$$\mathbf{Y = 2^t}$$

where:

t is the number of generations that have elapsed
Y is the number of bacterial cells present

For example:

When t=2, two generations have elapsed

$$Y = 2^2 = 4$$

the number of cells present is 4

When t=4, four generations have elapsed

$$Y = 2^4 = 16$$

the number of cells present is 16

Now, suppose that we begin with a population of 100 bacterial cells that double as before. The equation that describes these data is:

$$\mathbf{Y = 2^t(100)}$$

This example is illustrated in tabular form in Table 17.2 and graphically in Figure 17.3. The graph where there are initially 100 cells present is much like the graph where there is initially only one bacterium, but with a Y-intercept of 100.

**TABLE 17.2 Bacterial Population Growth Beginning with 100 Cells and a Generation Time of 1 hour**

| Time Elapsed (hours) | Number of Bacterial Cells Present |
|---|---|
| 0 | 100 |
| 1 | 200 |
| 2 | 400 |
| 3 | 800 |
| 4 | 1,600 |
| 5 | 3,200 |
| 6 | 6,400 |
| 7 | 12,800 |

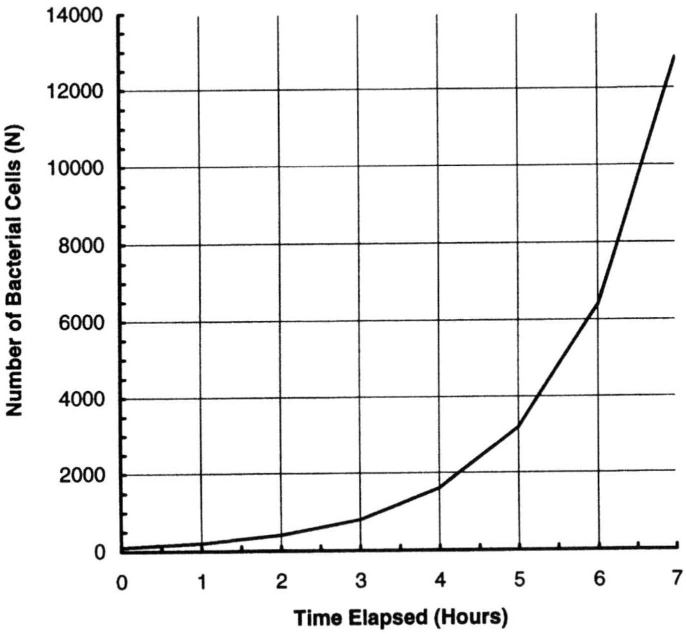


**FIGURE 17.3** Bacterial growth. A plot where there are initially 100 bacterial cells present and the bacteria population doubles every hour.

Being able to calculate cultured cell numbers is important in the laboratory in situations where we want to predict approximately how many cells will be present in a culture after a certain time or want to know how long a culture must be incubated to get a certain number of cells. It is possible to write a general growth equation, Equation 17.1, that applies to any doubling cell population, regardless of how many cells there are initially and regardless of how long it takes the population to double:

**EQUATION 17.1: General Equation for Cell Population Growth**

$$N = 2^t (N_0)$$

where:
$N_0$ is the number of bacteria initially
N is the number of cells after t generations
t is the number of generations elapsed (observe that t in this equation is not time) (for example, if the cells double every 2 hours, then after 6 hours three generations have elapsed).

**Example Problem:**

A type of bacterium has a doubling time of 20 minutes. There are initially 10,000 bacteria present in a flask. How many bacteria will there be in 1 hour?

*Answer:*

**Strategy 1: Intuitive, Using a Table:**

| Time Elapsed (minutes) | Number of Generations Elapsed | Number of Bacteria Present |
|---|---|---|
| 0 | 0 | 10,000 |
| 20 | 1 | 20,000 |
| 40 | 2 | 40,000 |
| 60 | 3 | 80,000 |

Thus, after 60 minutes we predict there will be 80,000 bacteria in the flask.

**Strategy 2: Using Equation 17.1**

Three generations have elapsed (the first at 20 minutes, the second at 40 minutes, and the third at 60 minutes). Substituting the number of generations elapsed and the number of cells originally present into the equation gives:

$$N = 2^t (N_0)$$

$$N = 2^3 (10{,}000)$$

$$N = 8(10{,}000)$$

$$\mathbf{N = 80{,}000}$$

The equation for population growth and the "intuitive" approach both give the same answer.

**Example Problem:**

*Lactococcus lactis* is a type of bacterium used extensively in the production of cheese and buttermilk. Under optimal conditions, it has a generation time of 26 minutes. There are initially 10,000 bacteria present in a flask. How many bacteria will there be in 1 hour?

*Answer:*

The first step in answering this question is to calculate how many generations have elapsed in 1 hour:

$$\frac{1\text{ generation}}{26\text{ minutes}} = \frac{?}{60\text{ minutes}}$$

$$? \approx 2.31\text{ generations}$$

Use Equation 17.1:

$$N = 2^t(N_0)$$

$$N = 2^{2.31}(10{,}000)$$

$$\mathbf{N \approx 4.96 \times 10^4\ bacteria}$$

**Practice Problems**

1. ***A population of bacteria begins with 1,000 individuals. How many doubling times (generations) have elapsed when there are:***
   a. ***2,000 bacteria present?***
   b. ***16,000 bacteria present?***
   c. ***32,000 bacteria present?***

2. ***If the doubling time of a population of bacteria cells is 45 minutes, how many generations have elapsed after:***
   a. ***1 hour*** b. ***2 days*** c. ***2 weeks***

3. ***Chinese hamster ovary (CHO) cells are a type of eukaryotic cell that is widely used in biotechnology as a factory to manufacture pharmaceutical products. CHO cell generation time under normal conditions is about 15 hours. Suppose a culture begins with $10^4$ cells. About how many cells will be present after 3 days?***
4. ***A type of bacterium has a generation time of 40 minutes. If the population initially has 25,000 cells, about how many will be present after 10 hours?***
5. ***HeLa cells are a type of eukaryotic cell that is important in research laboratories. Its generation time is about 25 hours. If a culture begins with 500 HeLa cells, about how many will be present in 2 days?***
6. ***True or false: A type of bacterium has a doubling time of 20 minutes. There are initially 10,000 bacteria present. Therefore, after 10 minutes there will be 15,000 bacteria. Explain your reasoning.***

*Answer:*

1. a. There are initially 1,000 bacteria present so **1 generation** or doubling time elapsed when there are 2,000 bacteria present.
   b. **4 generations** have elapsed when 16,000 bacteria are present.
   c. **5 generations** have elapsed when 32,000 bacteria are present.

2. Doubling time=45 minutes.
   a. After 1 hour: 60 minutes/45 minutes≈**1.333 generations**
   b. 2 days=2,880 minutes. 2880 minutes/45 minutes=**64 generations**
   c. 2 weeks=20,160 minutes. 20,160 minutes/45 minutes=**448 generations**

3. 3 days=72 hours. $\frac{72\text{ hours}}{15\text{ hours}} = 4.8$ this means that 4.8 generations elapsed

$$N = 2^t (N_0)$$

$$N = 2^{4.8}(10{,}000)$$

$$\mathbf{N \approx 2.79 \times 10^5\ CHO\ cells}$$

4. 10 hours = 600 minutes. $\frac{600\text{ minutes}}{40\text{ minutes}} = 15$

$$N = 2^t (N_0)$$

$$N = 2^{15}(25{,}000)$$

$$\mathbf{N \approx 8.19 \times 10^8\ cells}$$

5. 2 days = 48 hours. $\frac{48\text{ hours}}{25\text{ hours}} = 1.92$

$$N = 2^t (N_0)$$

$$N = 2^{1.92}(500)$$

$$\mathbf{N \approx 1{,}892\ HeLa\ cells}$$

6. **False**. If one generation is 20 minutes, then 10 minutes is 0.5 generations. Substituting into the equation:

$$N = 2^{0.5}\,(10{,}000) \approx 14{,}142$$

Observe that when relationships are exponential, we cannot apply the same logic as we do for linear relationships.

The relationship between the number of cells present and the time (or number of generations) elapsed is called **exponential** *because the independent variable is in the exponent.* As you can see in Figures 17.2 and 17.3, an exponential relationship is not linear if it is plotted on a regular two-dimensional graph.

It is more convenient to work with graphs that are linear in form than with those that are not. Therefore, it is often desirable to convert an exponential relationship to a form that is linear when plotted. The way this is accomplished involves logarithms. If, instead of plotting the number of bacterial cells on the Y-axis, we plot the *log* of the number of bacterial cells, the plot is linear. This approach is illustrated in tabular form in Table 17.3 and graphically in Figure 17.4.

**TABLE 17.3 Cell Growth Log of the Number of Cells (Generation Time = 1 hour)**

| Time Elapsed (hours) | Number of Cells Present of Number of Cells | Log |
|---|---|---|
| 0 | 100 | 2.00 |
| 1 | 200 | ≈ 2.30 |
| 2 | 400 | ≈ 2.60 |
| 3 | 800 | ≈ 2.90 |
| 4 | 1,600 | ≈ 3.20 |
| 5 | 3,200 | ≈ 3.51 |
| 6 | 6,400 | ≈ 3.81 |
| 7 | 12,800 | ≈ 4.11 |

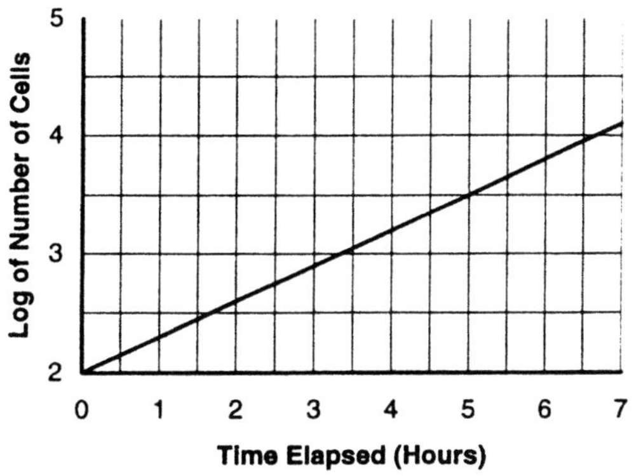


**FIGURE 17.4** When the log of cell number is plotted versus time, a straight line is formed. this population doubles every hour.

## 17.2 SEMILOGARITHMIC PLOTS

There is an alternative method to graph bacterial growth so that the plot is linear in form. This method involves the use of a **semilogarithmic plot**, *a type of graph "paper" that substitutes for calculating logs.* Semilogarithmic graph "paper" has normal, linear subdivisions on the X-axis, Figure 17.5. (We use the term semilogarithmic "paper" to describe this type of plot, whether it is actually prepared on paper or on a computer.) However, the divisions on the Y-axis are not even, rather, they are initially widely spaced and then become narrower as one moves toward powers of 10. This spacing takes the place of calculating logs. The graph paper shown in Figure 17.5 is called "semilogarithmic" paper because only the Y-axis has logarithmic spacing. (It is also possible to create a "log–log" plot where both axes are logarithmic.)

Observe in Figure 17.5a that the Y-axis has ten major divisions. These ten divisions together are called a "cycle." The first division in a cycle never begins with 0 because there is no log of 0. Rather, the first division is a power of 10, for example, 0.1, 1, 10, or 100. The second division in each cycle is twice the first, the third division is three times the first, and so on. For example, the Y-axis in Figure 17.5a begins at the bottom with 1. Therefore, the next division is 2, the next 3, and so on to 10. The Y-axis in Figure 17.5b begins with 10. Therefore, the next division is 20, then 30, and so on to 100. The Y-axis in Figure 17.5c begins with 0.1. Therefore, the next division is 0.2, then 0.3, and so on to 1.0.

Figure 17.5 illustrates one cycle semilogarithmic paper. The graph paper in Figure 17.6a is called "two-cycle semilogarithmic paper" because it repeats the same pattern twice. Three-cycle semilogarithmic paper, Figure 17.6b, repeats the pattern three times. The beginning of each new cycle is ten times greater than the beginning of the previous cycle. For example, if the first cycle goes from 1 to 10, then the second cycle must range from 10 to 100, the third cycle from 100 to 1000, and so on. Thus, a cycle begins on a power of ten and ends on the next, consecutive power of ten.

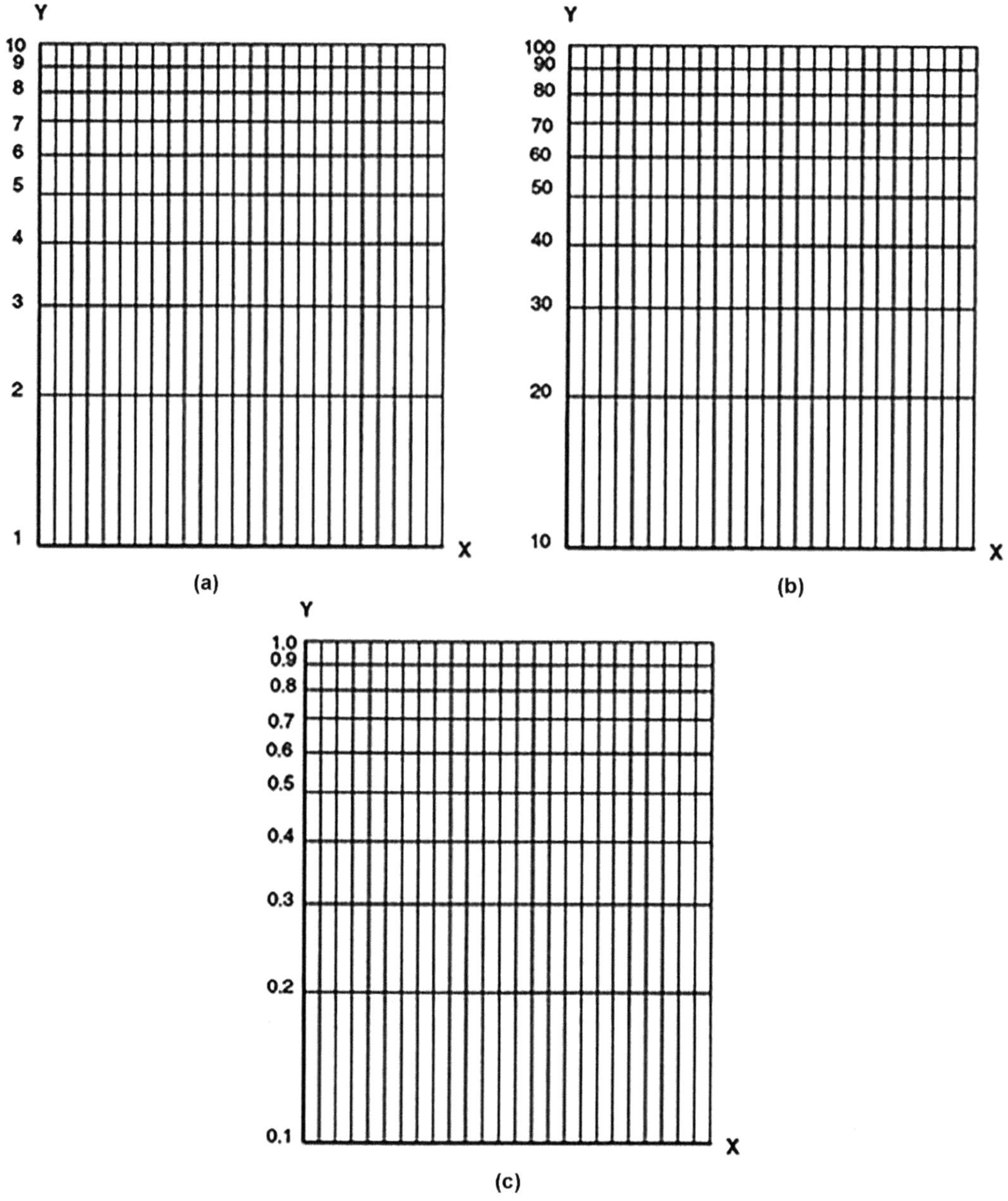


**FIGURE 17.5** Labeling semilogarithmic paper. (a) Labeling the Y-axis when the first division is 1. (b) Labeling the Y-axis when the first division is 10. (c) Labeling the Y-axis when the first division is 0.1.

It is possible to purchase, or generate on a computer, semilogarithmic paper with various numbers of cycles. To determine how many cycles you need, examine the data to be plotted. For example, in Tables 17.2 and 17.3, the Y-values vary between 100 and 12,800. In this case there is no need for a cycle from 1 to 10 or 10 to 100 so the bottom cycle can begin at 100. The first cycle required to plot these data runs from 100 to 1,000. The second cycle ranges from 1,000 to 10,000, and a third cycle, from 10,000 to 100,000, is needed to plot the value "12,800." Thus, three-cycle semilog paper is required to plot these data. Figure 17.7 shows the semilogarithmic plot of the data from Table 17.2. Observe how the Y-axis is labeled in this figure. Also, compare the plots in Figures 17.4 and 17.7. Both graphs are linear in form and either is an acceptable way to plot these data. Note also that it is important to distinguish the two types of graphs and read/interpret values from them correctly.

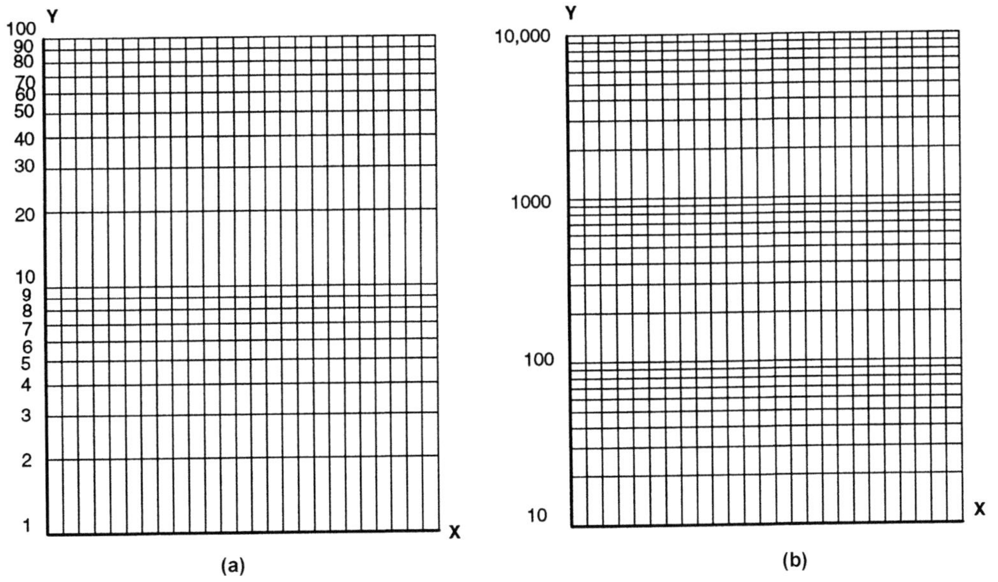


**FIGURE 17.6** Cycles on semilogarithmic paper. (a) Two-cycle semilogarithmic paper. (b) Three-cycle semilogarithmic paper.

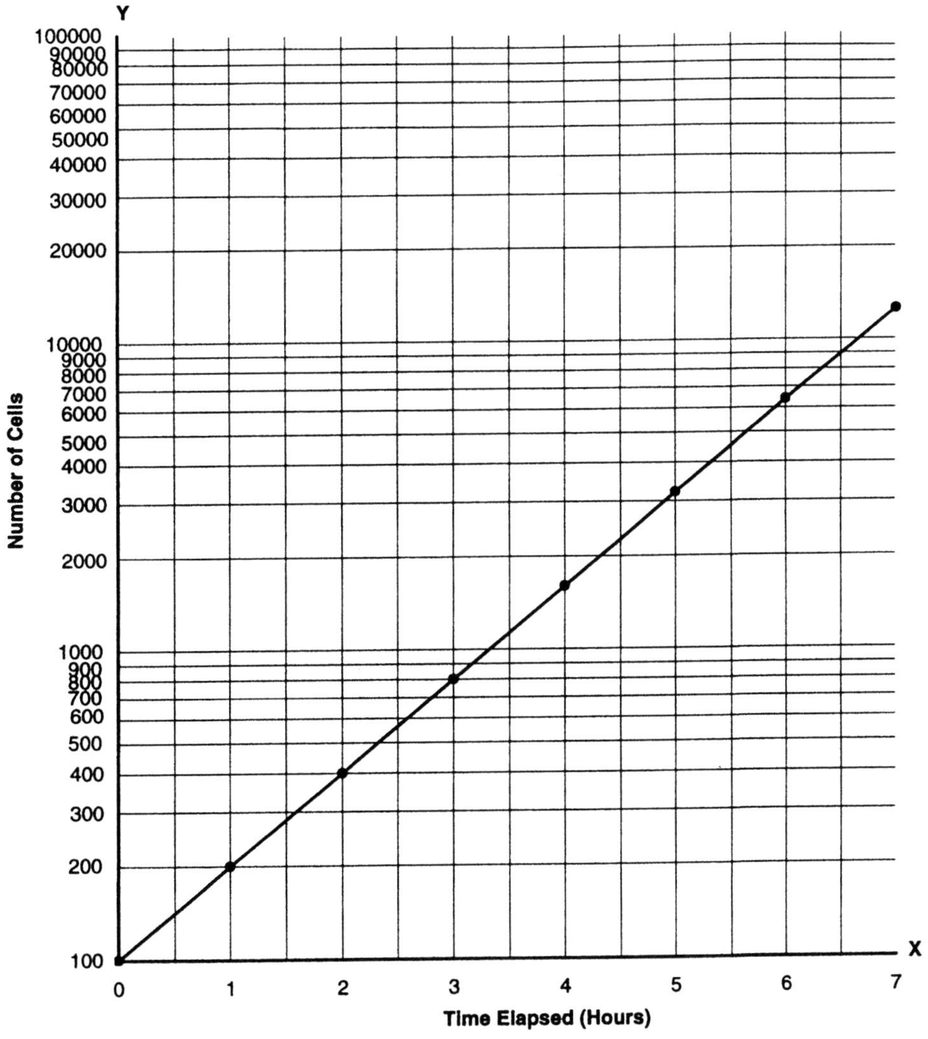


**FIGURE 17.7** Cell growth graphed on semilogarithmic paper.

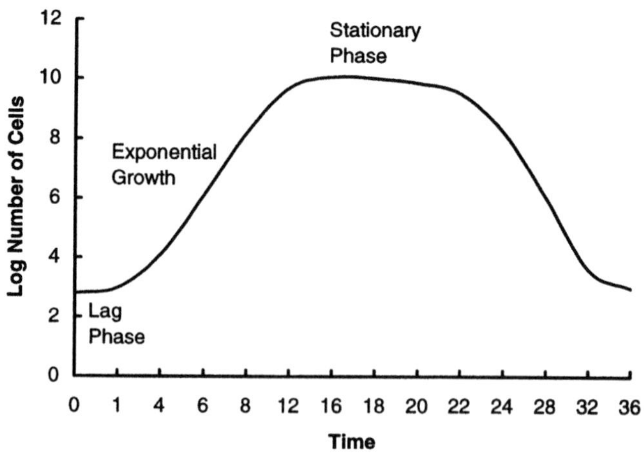


**FIGURE 17.8** The limits to cell growth.

## 17.3 LIMITS TO GROWTH

In principle, all biological populations have the potential to grow exponentially. But if any population continued to grow exponentially for a long enough period of time, it would cover the earth and eventually the universe. In reality, population growth is limited by space, nutrients, waste buildup, and other factors. Cultured cell growth normally looks like the plot in Figure 17.8. When a few cells that are not reproducing rapidly are placed in fresh media, there is initially a lag period as they utilize nutrients and prepare to divide. A period of exponential growth follows the lag period. Eventually, the cells deplete the nutrients in the broth and generate toxic waste products. Reproduction slows and stops and the population declines. Note that in the graphs and calculations we have performed so far in this chapter, we have assumed that the cells are in the phase where their growth is exponential, and we have ignored the lag phase, the stationary phase, and the phase where growth declines.

## 17.4 DETERMINING GENERATION TIME

In the problems introduced so far in this chapter, we assumed that the generation time for a population of cells is known. But this is not always the case. The generation time for any type of cultured cell depends on a number of factors, such as the type and availability of nutrients, temperature, and so on. Therefore, even for commonly cultured cells, the generation time may be unknown. The most intuitive way to determine the generation time for a given population is to prepare a growth curve, and use it to find the time it took the population to double, as illustrated in Figure 17.9.

It is also possible to calculate the doubling time if one knows the number of cells at any two time points – assuming that both time points are in the exponential phase of growth. We can say that the first time point is the beginning timepoint, $N_0$, and the second time point is the ending time point, N. To use these values to determine the generation time requires a bit of algebra. We begin with the familiar Equation 17.1:

$$N = 2^t \left(N_0\right)$$

In this situation, we know the beginning ($N_0$) and ending numbers of cells (N); therefore, the unknown is t. But how do we solve for t, which is an exponent? The algebraic answer is that we begin by taking the log of both sides as follows:

$$N = 2^t \left(N_0\right)$$

$$\log N = t \log 2 + \log N_0$$

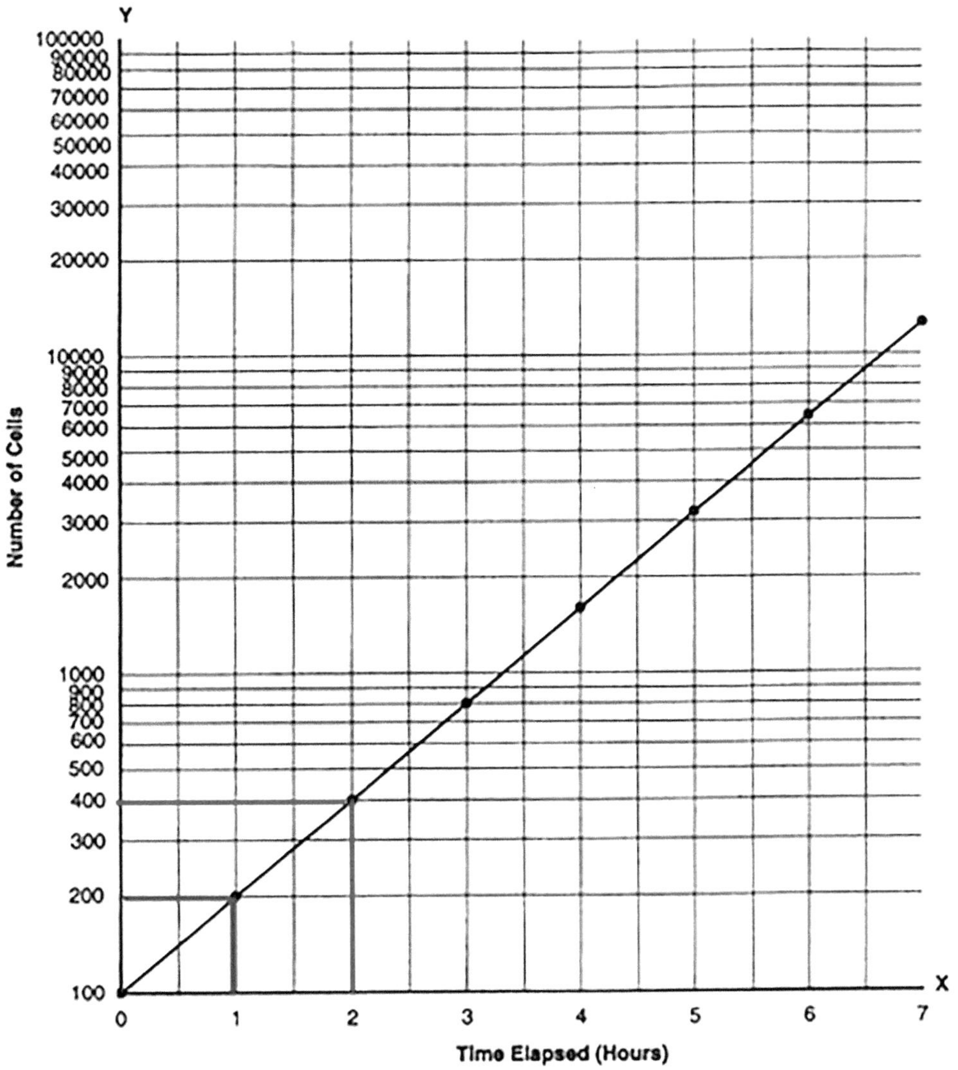


**FIGURE 17.9** Population generation time. During the exponential growth phase, this population doubles every hour, as can be seen in the graph. For example, 200 cells are present at 1 hour and 400 cells are present at 2 hours. Therefore, it took 1 hour for the cell number to double; 1 hour is the generation time.

Next, subtract log $N_0$ from both sides:

$$\log N - \log N_0 = t \log 2$$

Next, divide both sides by log 2:

$$\frac{\log N - \log N_0}{\log\ 2} = t$$

Move t to the left side:

$$t = \frac{\log N - \log N_0}{\log 2}$$

The log of 2 is $\approx$ 0.3010, so:

$$t = \frac{\log N - \log N_0}{0.3010}$$

We will call this Equation 17.2.

We can use this equation, Equation 17.2, to calculate t. Let us illustrate how to use Equation 17.2 with an example. Suppose there are 10,000 cells in a culture at 8:00 AM and there are 80,000 cells in the culture at 11:00 AM. In this example, $N_0=10{,}000$ and $N=80{,}000$. Insert these values into Equation 17.2:

$$t=\frac{\log\ 80{,}000-\log\ 10{,}000}{0.3010}$$

Solving the equation:

$$t=\frac{4.903-\ 4.00}{0.3010}$$

$$t=\frac{0.903}{0.301}\approx \mathbf{3.00}$$

Now, we know that t=3.00. But it is not the doubling or generation time. Rather, recall from Section 17.1 that t is the number of generations that have elapsed, in this case, between 8:00 AM and 11:00 AM. To find the doubling time, we divide the time elapsed by the number of generations.

$$\frac{3\ \text{hour}}{3\ \text{generation}}=\frac{1\ \text{hour}}{1\ \text{generation}}$$

This means the generation time is **1 hour**.

Equation 17.2 summarizes this procedure for calculating the generation time based on the number of cells at two timepoints (assuming that the cells are in the exponential phase of growth).

**EQUATION 17.2: CALCULATING GENERATION TIME**

$$t=\frac{\log N-\log N_0}{0.3010}$$

Step 1. Find the number of cells at any two timepoints. The first number is $N_0$ and the second is N.

Step 2. Take the log of $N_0$ and the log of N.

Step 3. Subtract the log of $N_0$ from the log of N.

Step 4. Divide the result from Step 3 by 0.301. The result is the number of generations that have elapsed.

Step 5. Find the difference between the times at which the population sizes were measured.

Step 6. Divide the elapsed time from Step 5 by the number of generations that have occurred from Step 4. This is the doubling (generation) time.

## Practice Problems

1. ***A new type of cultured cell is being investigated for possible use in manufacturing a product. It is important to know the doubling time. An experiment is performed in which there are initially 5,000 cells. 24 hours later, the cells are counted and there are 71,000 cells. What is the doubling time? (Assume the cells are in the exponential growth phase the entire time.)***
2. ***A new type of nutritional medium is being investigated to see if it promotes the growth of a particular cell type. Cells growing in the original nutritional medium have a doubling time of 7.5 hours. In tests of the new nutritional medium, there were 23,000 cells at 9:00 AM on day 1 and 345,000 cells at 11:00 AM the next day. Compare the generation time with the original and the new medium. (Assume the cells are in the exponential growth phase the entire time.)***
3. ***You purchase CHO cells that will be used for manufacturing a product. Their generation time is 15 hours. The original culture contains 10,000 cells and you need $2 \times 10^6$ cells to begin production. How long will it take to get $2 \times 10^6$ cells? (Ignore any lag phase.)***
4. ***Mammalian cells were cultured over 5 days and the number of cells were counted at various time points. The data are shown in the table below.***
   a. ***Graph these data.***
   b. ***Label the lag phase, exponential growth phase, and stationary phase.***
   c. ***What is the approximate doubling time for these cells during the exponential phase of growth?***

| Time (hours) | Cell Number |
|---|---|
| 0 | $1.41 \times 10^5$ |
| 24 | $1.45 \times 10^5$ |
| 48 | $2.58 \times 10^5$ |
| 72 | $4.08 \times 10^5$ |
| 96 | $6.12 \times 10^5$ |
| 120 | $6.24 \times 10^5$ |
| 144 | $6.28 \times 10^5$ |

### *Answers*

1. $N_0$=5,000 cells and N=71,000 cells. What is the doubling time?
   Using Equation 17.2:

$$t = \frac{\log N - \log N_0}{0.3010}$$

$$t = \frac{\log 71{,}000 - \log 5{,}000}{0.3010}$$

$$t \approx 3.828$$

24 hours / 3.828 ≈ **6.269 hours** = generation time

2. In tests of the new nutritional medium, there were 23,000 cells at 9:00 AM on day 1 and 345,000 cells at 11:00 AM the next day.
   Using Equation 17.2:

$$t = \frac{\log N - \log N_0}{0.3010}$$

$$t = \frac{\log 345{,}000 - \log 23{,}000}{0.3010}$$

$$t \approx 3.91$$

26 hours / 3.91 ≈ **6.654 hours** = generation time

The doubling time in the new nutritional medium is shorter, which might be advantageous if faster cell growth accelerates some desirable process.

3. CHO cells generation time is 15 hours. The original culture contains 10,000 cells and you need $2\times10^6$ cells to begin production. How long will it take to get $2\times10^6$ cells?

$$t=\frac{\log N-\log N_0}{0.3010}$$

$$t=\frac{\log\left(2\times10^6\right)-\log 10{,}000}{0.3010}$$

$$t\approx 7.6446 \text{ doublings}$$

Each doubling requires 15 hours, so it will take (7.6446) (15 hours) ≈ **114.67 hours** to get enough cells.

4. a.b.

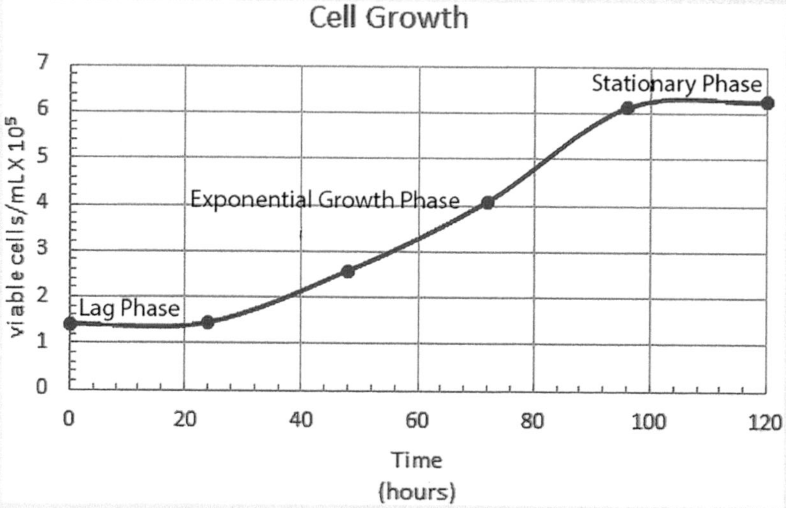


c. Use the viable cell number at any two time points from the exponential portion of the graph. For example, using the time points of 48 and 72 hours:

$$t=\frac{\log N-\log N_0}{0.3010}$$

$$t=\frac{\log 4.1\times10^5-\log 2.6\times10^5}{0.3010}\approx 0.6572$$

24 hours / 0.6572 ≈ **36.52 hours** = generation time

(You may get slightly different answers depending on which points you use.)

It is also possible to read the doubling time directly off the graph. Find two points where the number of cells have doubled, for example, between $2\times10^5$ and $4\times10^5$. Then see how long it took for this to occur. Reading off the graph, there are about $2\times10^5$ cells at 36 hours. There are $4\times10^5$ cells at about 70 hours. 70−36 hours = 34 hours, which is not exactly the same as calculated above but is a reasonable estimate.

## 17.5 THE DECAY OF RADIOISOTOPES

Radioactive substances decay over time so that there is progressively less and less radioactivity present. The **half-life** *of a radioactive substance is the time it takes for the amount of radioactivity to decay to half its original level.* Radioactivity can be measured in various units including disintegrations/minute, curies (Ci), and microcuries (μCi). For example, suppose a solution containing a radioactive substance initially has 400 disintegrations/minute and the half-life of the substance is 1 hour. Then, after 1 hour, there will be 200 disintegrations/minute of radioactivity remaining in the solution. After 2 hours, there will be 100 disintegrations/minute, and so on. The relationship between time elapsed and radioactivity for this example is shown in tabular form in Table 17.4 and is graphed in Figure 17.10.

An exponential equation, Equation 17.3, can be used to calculate the amount of radioactivity remaining after a certain number of half-lives have elapsed:

**EQUATION 17.3 General Equation for Radioactive Decay**

$$N = \left(\frac{1}{2}\right)^t N_0 \text{ or } N = (2)^{-t} N_0$$

where:
N = the amount of radioactivity remaining
t = the number of half-lives elapsed (observe that t in this equation is not time)
$N_0$ = the amount of radioactivity initially
(Recall from Section 1.1 that a negative exponent indicates that the reciprocal of the number should be multiplied times itself.)

**TABLE 17.4 Radioactive Decay (Half-Life = 1 hour)**

| Time Elapsed (hours) | Half-Lives Elapsed | Radioactive Substance Remaining (Disintegrations/Minute) |
|---|---|---|
| 0 | 0 | 400 |
| 1 | 1 | 200 |
| 2 | 2 | 100 |
| 3 | 3 | 50 |
| 4 | 4 | 25 |

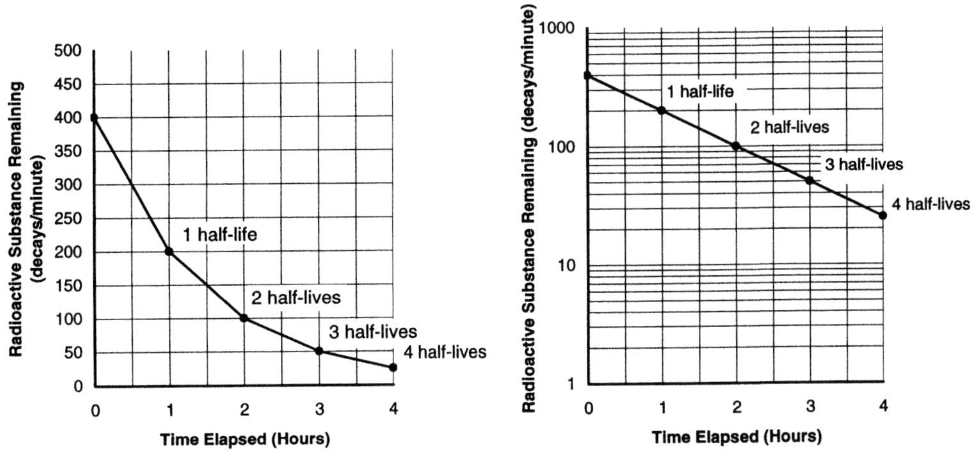


**FIGURE 17.10** The relationship between time elapsed and radioactivity remaining. (a) The relationship on normal graph paper. (b) The relationship plotted on semilogarithmic paper.

For example, let us return to the example of the radioactive solution that has a half-life of one hour and an activity of 400 disintegrations/minute initially. How much radioactivity will remain after 3 hours? We can see from Table 17.4 that there are 50 decays/minute after 3 hours. It is possible to get the same answer by substituting into the Equation 17.3 as follows (3 hours is the same as three half-lives for this substance):

$$N = \left(\frac{1}{2}\right)^3 \left(\frac{400 \text{ disintegrations}}{1 \text{ minutes}}\right) = 50 \text{ disintegrations / minutes}$$

**Example Problem:**

The radioactive isotope, $^{131}$Iodine, has a half-life of 8 days. If you start with 500 μCi of $^{131}$Iodine, how much will remain after 80 days? (A μCi is a unit of radioactivity.)

***Answer:***

**Strategy 1: Using a table**

The answer is 0.4883 μCi or about 0.5 μCi remain.

| Time Elapsed (days) | Half-Lives Elapsed | Radioactive Substance Remaining (μCi) |
|---|---|---|
| 0 | 0 | 500 |
| 8 | 1 | 250 |
| 16 | 2 | 125 |
| 24 | 3 | 62.5 |
| 32 | 4 | 31.25 |
| 40 | 5 | 15.625 |
| 48 | 6 | 7.8135 |
| 56 | 7 | 3.9063 |
| 64 | 8 | 1.9531 |
| 72 | 9 | 0.9766 |
| 80 | 10 | 0.4883 |

**Strategy 2: Using Equation 17.3**

1. Calculate how many half-lives have passed. The half-life of this isotope is 8 days, so the number of half-lives that have passed is: 80/8 = 10.
2. Substitute into Equation 17.3:

$$N = (\tfrac{1}{2})^t (N_0)$$

$$N = (\tfrac{1}{2})^{10} (500 \, \mu\text{Ci})$$

$$\mathbf{N \approx 0.4883 \, \mu Ci}$$

Only about 0.5 μCi remain. Eight days is a relatively short half-life. Isotopes with short half-lives rapidly disappear.

**Example Problem:**

The half-life for the radioisotope $^{32}$P is 14 days. You receive 200 μCi to perform an experiment on March 3. On April 30 you must complete paperwork showing how much $^{32}$P activity remains. How much is present?

*Answer:*

1. Calculate how many half-lives have passed. There are 58 days between March 3 and April 30. The half-live of this isotope is 14 days so the number of half-lives that have passed is: $58/14 \approx 4.143$.
2. Substitute into Equation 17.3:

$$N = (\frac{1}{2})^t (N_0)$$

$$N = (\frac{1}{2})^{4.143} (200\,\mu Ci)$$

$$N \approx 11.32\,\mu Ci$$

The answer to be recorded is **11.32 µCi remain.**

There is similarity between the equations for the decay of radioactivity and the growth of microorganisms. You can see this similarity by comparing Figures 17.3 and 17.10a. Also note the similarity in their equations as shown here:

**A COMPARISON OF THE EQUATIONS FOR BACTERIAL GROWTH AND RADIOACTIVE DECAY**

**The growth of microorganisms**: $N = 2^t (N_0)$

**The decline of radioactivity**: $N = \left(\frac{1}{2}\right)^t N_0$ **or** $N = (2)^{-t} N_0$

where:
$N$ = amount (of bacteria or radioactivity) present after a certain period of time
$t$ = number of generations or number of half-lives
$N_0$ = initial amount (of bacteria or radioactivity)

Observe that in the equation for exponential decay, the exponent is negative while in the equation for exponential growth, the exponent is positive. The equations are the same otherwise.

**Practice Problems**

1. ***There is an insect population in which each adult leaves three offspring and then dies. The generation time is 10 months, that is, the adults reproduce every 10 months. In this type of organism, the adults die after they reproduce. The population begins with 20 adults and reproduces for four generations. The resulting population growth is shown in this table:***

| Generation | Time (months) | Number |
|---|---|---|
| 0 | 0 | 20 |
| 1 | 10 | 60 |
| 2 | 20 | 180 |
| 3 | 30 | 540 |
| 4 | 40 | 1,620 |

a. ***Graph this relationship on a semilog graph.***
b. ***Determine the equation that describes this relationship.***

2. ***The half-life of the radioisotope $^{32}P$ is 14 days. If there are initially 300 μCi of this radioisotope:***
   a. ***How much will be left after 28 days?***
   b. ***How much will be left after 140 days?***
   c. ***How much will be left after 200 days?***
   d. ***How much will be left after 1 year?***

3. ***The half-life of the radioisotope $^{22}Na$ is 2.6 years. If there are initially 600 μCi of this radioisotope, how much will be left after:***
   a. ***1 year***
   b. ***2 years***
   c. ***3 years***

4. ***It is difficult to kill microorganisms. Typically, a solution or material to be sterilized is heated under pressure. The graph below shows the effect of time of exposure to heat and bacterial death (based on information from Perkins, John, J. Principles and Methods of Sterilization in the Health Sciences, 2nd edition, Charles C. Thomas Publishers, 1983).***

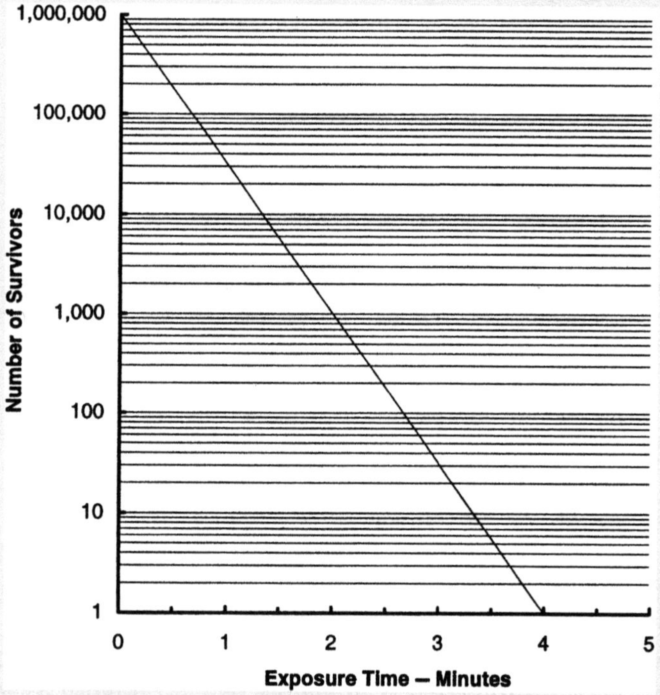


   a. ***About how many bacteria were there at the beginning of the experiment, before exposure to heat?***

b. *About how many bacteria were present after 2 minutes of treatment?*
c. *Why did the investigators show their data on a semilogarithmic plot?*

5. *Label the Y-axis of this semilogarithmic graph.*

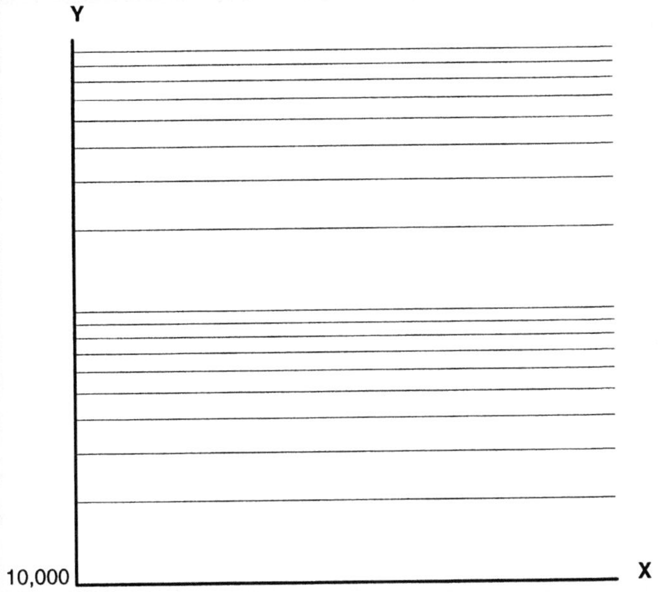


6. *Radioisotopes are used in research settings to make molecules or biological structures detectable. They are similarly used in medicine as tracers. For example, tumors use up to 30 times more sugar than normal tissue. It is possible to inject patients with a radioactive sugar, glucose, and then look for the radioactivity in the patient using a type of scanner called a PET scanner. The radioactive glucose allows the physician to "see" metabolically active areas in the brain which can indicate a brain tumor. The glucose is supplied to the clinic in a radioactive form, abbreviated fdg. The half-life of this compound is 109.7 minutes. Suppose that the supplier makes fdg at 5 AM and supplies it to the hospital with a concentration of 75 mCi/mL. The fdg is administered to an adult male patient at 7:45 AM. The desired dose of radioactivity for an adult male is 10 mCi. How much should be administered to this patient?*
7. *Technetium ($^{99}$mTc) medronic acid is used in nuclear medicine to localize bone metastases (cancer). Its half-life is 6.02 hours. Suppose this material is made at 9:00 AM and administered to a patient at 10:00 AM. The initial preparation contains 65 mCi/mL and a dose of 20 mCi is desired. How much should be administered?*
8. *The graph below shows the radioactive decay of two samples.*
   a. *Is this a linear plot, or a semilogarithmic plot, or a log–log plot?*
   b. *What is the half-life for the sample shown in red (the upper line)?*
   c. *What is the half-life for the sample shown in blue (the lower line)?*
   d. *What is the difference between the two samples?*

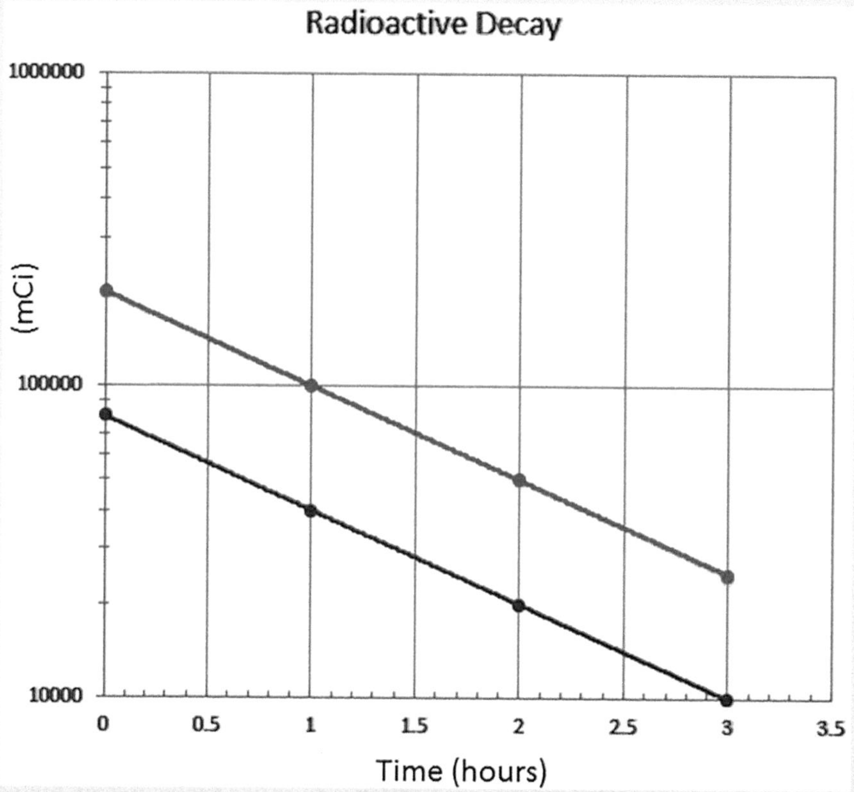


*Answers*

1. a.

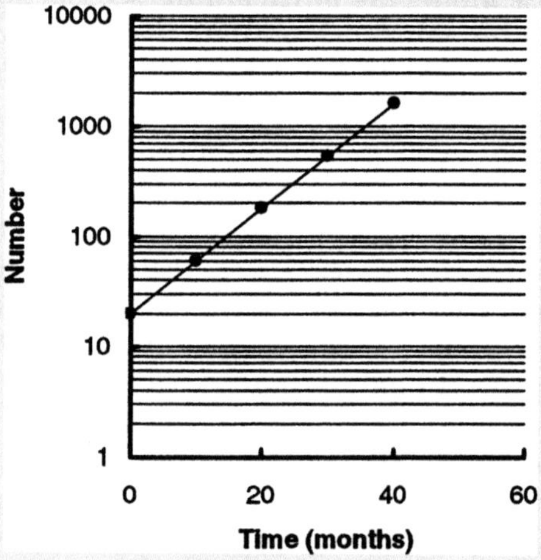


b. $\mathbf{Y = 3^t\ (20)}$ where t=number of generations

2. $N = 1/2^t(N_0)$ $N_0 = 300\ \mu Ci$ ($\mu$Ci is microcuries)

half-life = 14 days

a. t=28/14 days=2 $N_2 = (\frac{1}{2})^2\ (300\ \mu Ci) = \mathbf{75\ \mu Ci}$

b. t=140/14 days=10 $N_{10} = (\frac{1}{2})^{10}\ (300\ \mu Ci) \approx \mathbf{0.293\ \mu Ci}$

c. t=200/14 days≈14.286 $N_{14.286} = (\frac{1}{2})^{14.286}\ (300\ \mu Ci) \approx \mathbf{1.50 \times 10^{-2}\ \mu Ci}$

d. t=365/14 days ≈ 26.071 $N_{26.071} = (\frac{1}{2})^{26.071}\ (300\ \mu Ci) \approx \mathbf{4.26 \times 10^{-6}\ \mu Ci}$

3. a. $N = (\frac{1}{2})^{0.385}(600\,\mu Ci) \approx$ **459 μCi**  b. $N = (\frac{1}{2})^{0.769}(600\,\mu Ci) \approx$ **352 μCi**
   c. $N = (\frac{1}{2})^{1.154}(600\,\mu Ci) \approx$ **270 μCi**

4. a. **$10^6$ bacteria**  b. **$10^3$ bacteria**
   c. Using semilogarithmic paper results in a straight line on the graph that is easier to work with than an exponential graph. It also is used because of the wide range of values needed from 0 to $10^6$.

5.

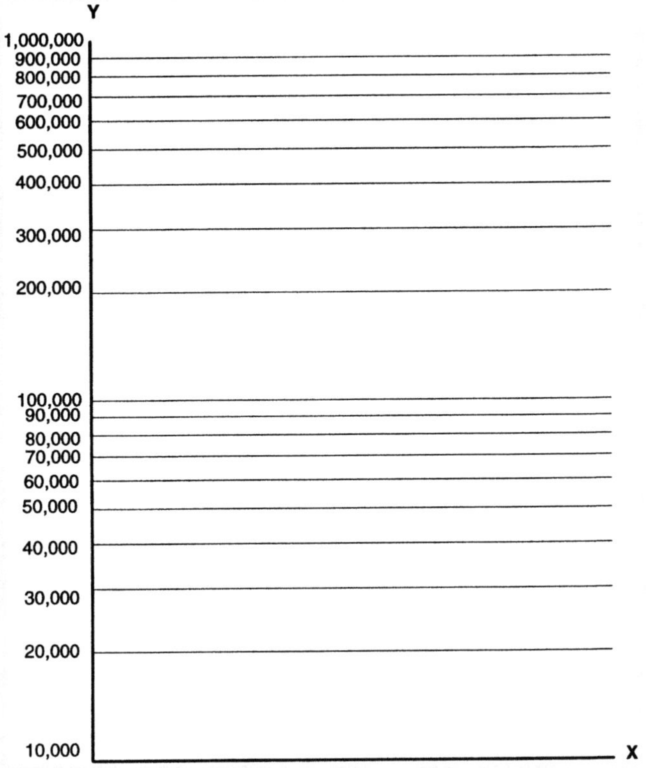


6. The half-life is 109.7 minutes. The manufacturer makes fdg at 5 AM and supplies it with a concentration of 75 mCi/mL. The fdg is administered at 7:45 AM. The desired dose is 10 mCi. How much should be administered to this patient? Two hours and forty five minutes have elapsed since the drug was manufactured = 165 minutes. The half-life is 109.7 minutes so:

$$\frac{165}{109.7} \approx 1.504 \text{ half-lifes}$$

$$N = 1/2^{1.504}\left(75\frac{\text{mCi}}{\text{mL}}\right) \approx 26.4431\text{ mCi/mL}$$

The amount to be administered can be determined by proportions:

$$\frac{26.4431\text{ mCi}}{\text{mL}} = \frac{10\text{ mCi}}{?}$$

**? ≈ 0.3782 mL**

7. Technetium ($^{99m}$Tc) medronic acid half-life is 6.02 hours. It is made at 9:00 AM and administered at 10:00 AM. The preparation contains 65 mCi/mL and a dose of 20 mCi is desired. How much should be administered?

$$\frac{1\text{ hours}}{6.02\text{ hours}} \approx 0.1661 \quad \text{half-lives have elapsed}$$

$$N = 1/2^{0.1661}\left(65\frac{\text{mCi}}{\text{mL}}\right) \approx 57.9312\text{ mCi/mL}$$

$$\frac{57.9312\text{ mCi}}{\text{mL}} = \frac{20\text{ mCi}}{?}$$

$$? \approx \mathbf{0.3452\ mL}$$

8. a. This is a semilogarithmic plot. You can tell because the tick marks on the Y-axis are not evenly spaced but the ones on the X-axis are evenly spaced.
   b., c. Both samples have a half-life of 1 hour. To figure this out, for example, for the red line, observe that at time zero, there are 200,000 mCi present. After 1 hour, there are half that many mCi, that is, 100,000. For the blue line, at 1 hour, there are 40,000 mCi present and at 2 hours 20,000. In both cases, radioactivity declined by half in 1 hour.
   d. The difference between the two samples is in the starting amount. There was more of the red sample to begin with. The slope of the two lines is the same, which means the samples have the same half-life.

## 17.6 CASE STUDY: THE CONCEPT OF "HALF-LIFE" HAS BROADER APPLICABILITY

We have so far talked about the concept of "half-life" only in the context of radioactivity. But the concept is more broadly applicable. For example, the virus SARS-CoV-2 is the agent that causes the illness COVID-19. Transmission of disease occurs primarily through respiratory droplets that are produced by talking, coughing, and sneezing. However, it is thought that people can also be infected by contact with contaminated surfaces and objects. The United States Department of Homeland Security therefore studied the stability of SARS-CoV-2 in simulated saliva, using droplets of varying size deposited on a nonporous surface under a range of temperature and relative humidity conditions. ("Estimated Surface Decay of SARS-CoV-2." *Department of Homeland Security*, 21 December 2020, www.dhs.gov/science-and-technology/sars-calculator.) The scientists used their data to develop a model summarized by Equation 17.4. The equation predicts viral decay, that is, the virus's loss of the ability to infect cells, under certain environmental conditions. They express the result in terms of viral half-life, the amount of time required for infectious virus to decline by half.

**EQUATION 17.4: The Half-Life of Infectious SARS-CoV-2 Virus under Varying Conditions of Temperature and Humidity**

$$\text{Half-life} = 32.43 - 0.63(\text{temperature}) - 0.15(\text{relative humidity})$$

Where:
temperature is expressed in degrees Celsius
Relative humidity is expressed as a percent
The result is in units of hours

Another study showed that infectious SARS-CoV-2 could persist on nonporous surfaces under indoor conditions (23°C, 40% relative humidity), with a maximum half-life approaching 7 hours. However, in this study, they found that bright sunlight rapidly inactivated SARS-CoV-2 dried on stainless steel surfaces with a half-life as short as a little more than 2 minutes. (Ratnesar-Shumate, Shanna, et al. "Simulated Sunlight Rapidly Inactivates SARS-CoV-2 on Surfaces." *The Journal of Infectious Diseases*, vol. 222, no. 2, 2020, pp. 214–22. doi:10.1093/infdis/jiaa274.) The strong deactivating effect of sunlight is one factor that explains why infection rates are much lower when people gather outside rather than inside.

## QUESTIONS

These questions all relate to the virus that causes COVID-19. Other viruses might have different patterns of decay.

**1. a.** Based on Equation 17.4, what is the half-life of infectious virus on a surface when the temperature is 74°F and relative humidity is 40%? How closely does this match the results of the other study that showed, under similar conditions, a viral half-life approaching 7 hours?

**b.** Based on Equation 17.4, what is the half-life of infectious virus on a surface when the temperature is 90°F and relative humidity is 60%?

**c.** Based on the data in this case study, who would appear to be at higher risk for contracting COVID-19, workers in meat-packing plants or bakers?

**2.** Given the result in Question 1, based on Equation 17.4, how long will it take for 90% of virus to be inactivated when the temperature is 74°F and relative humidity is 40%?

**3.** Based on the data in this case study, if there are initially 40,000 viruses present in a bright sunlight situation, how long will it take for 90% of them to be inactivated?

## ANSWERS

1. a. First convert 74°F to °C.

$$\text{Half-life} = 32.43 - 0.63(23.3) - 0.15(40) = \mathbf{11.751\ hours}$$

The equation predicts that the virus has a longer half-life than the 7 hour half-life found in the other study. Perhaps this is because factors in addition to temperature and humidity are important. In fact, the exact nature of the surface on which virus is deposited has been found to strongly impact the half-life of the virus. Yet other unidentified factors might also be important.

b. First convert 90°F to °C.

$$\text{Half-life} = 32.43 - 0.63(32.2) - 0.15(60) = \mathbf{3.144\ hours}$$

Note that this virus is relatively less stable when it is warm and humid than it is when conditions are cold and dry.

c. Based on these data, the virus is more stable, and therefore infectious, in the conditions found in a meat-packing plant. Meat-packing plants are cold and have low relative humidity. There have, in fact, been a number of COVID-19 outbreaks associated with meat and poultry processing facilities. Note, however, that factors in addition to viral stability are likely involved. People who work in these settings are close together over long shifts. Also, workers in these facilities may have additional risk factors, such as high density housing and limited access to protective gear.

2. Given the result in Question 1, how long will it take for 90% of viruses to be inactivated when the temperature is 74°F and relative humidity is 40%?

We can insert numbers for the beginning and ending number of infectious particles. For example, if the beginning number of infectious particles is 10,000, when 90% of them are gone, there will be 1,000 remaining. (When 90% are gone, 10% remain. 10% = (0.1) 10,000 particles = 1,000 particles.)

Equation 17.3 applies to this situation:

$$N = N_0 (0.5)^t$$

$$1{,}000 = 10{,}000 (0.5)^t$$

Take the log of both sides:

$$\log 1{,}000 = \log 10{,}000 + t \log 0.5$$

$$3 = 4 + t \log 0.5$$

$$-1 = t \log 0.5$$

The log of 0.5 is −0.3010, so:

$$t = \frac{-1}{-0.3010} \approx \mathbf{3.3223}$$

Let us consider what this tells us. It means that it requires 3.3223 generations, that is, 3.3223 half-lives, for the number of infectious viruses to be reduced by 90%. We can use the previously determined half-life value for these conditions, that is 11.751 hours. Therefore, assuming the model is correct, it requires: (11.751 hours/1 half-life) (3.3223 half-lives) ≈ 39 hours for infectious virus to be reduced 90% on a surface. In other words, infectious viral particles can linger on surfaces. (If we use the value of a 7 hour half-life, it takes a little over 23 hours for infectious viral particles to be reduced by 90%.)

This result has implications in understanding how people become infected with the virus causing COVID-19. Touching a contaminated surface and then touching one's face is not thought to be the primary method of infection. However, since the virus remains infectious on surfaces for a period time, it is a possible mechanism of infectivity. Note also that the same ideas apply to other viral and bacterial pathogens that might infect a person.

3. If there are initially 40,000 viruses present in a bright sunlight situation, how long will it take for 90% of them to be inactivated?

$$\log 4{,}000 = \log 40{,}000 + t \log 0.5$$

$$3.602 = 4.602 + t \log 0.5$$

$$-1.000 = t \log 0.5$$

The log of 0.5 is −0.3010, so:

$$t = \frac{-1.000}{-0.3010} \approx \mathbf{3.3223}$$

Observe that it again requires about 3.3223 half-lives to reduce the level of virus by 90%. (This is the same value, regardless of the length of the half-life.) But this time the half-life is only about 2 minutes. So, in bright sun, to reduce the level of infectious virus by 90% it takes only (3.3223 half-lives) (2 minutes) ≈ 6.645 minutes, or a little over 6.6 minutes.

# IV

# Introduction to Descriptive Statistics

**Chapters in This Unit**



## INTRODUCTION

The natural world is filled with variability: organisms differ from one another; the weather changes from day to day; and the earth is covered by a mosaic of different habitats. The natural world is also characterized by uncertainty and chance. The outcome of a card game, the weather, the personality of a newborn child are all uncertain. Scientists strive to observe and understand this world that is characterized by variability and uncertainty.

Statistics is a branch of mathematics that has developed over many years to deal with variability and uncertainty. Statistics provides methods to summarize, analyze, and interpret observations of the natural world. Statistical

DOI: 10.1201/9780429282744-21

methods are also used to reach conclusions, based on data, with a certain probability of being right – and a certain probability of being wrong. In this unit, we explore a small area of statistics and its use in summarizing, displaying, and organizing numerical data. We will also see how the tools provided by statistics can be used in a variety of biotechnology workplaces, ranging from basic research laboratories to facilities making large quantities of commercial products.

# Descriptive Statistics: Measures of Central Tendency

18



## 18.1 INTRODUCTION AND TERMINOLOGY

We begin our introduction to statistics with some statistical terminology. In a statistical sense, a **population** *is an entire group of events, objects, results, or individuals all of whom share a unifying characteristic(s).* Examples of populations include all of a person's red blood cells, all the enzyme molecules in a test tube, and all the college students in the United States.

Characteristics of a population often can be observed or measured, such as blood hemoglobin levels, the activity of enzymes, or the heights of students. *Characteristics of a population that can be measured are called* **variables**. They are called "variables" because there is variation among individuals in the characteristic. A population can have numerous variables that can be studied. For example, a given batch of a biopharmaceutical product can be evaluated for its concentration of product, the levels of various impurities, its volume, its weight, and so on. *Observations of a variable are called* **data** (singular "datum").

Observations may or may not be numerical. For example, the concentration of active product in a biopharmaceutical preparation is a type of numerical data. In contrast, electron micrographs of mouse kidney cells are nonnumerical observations. The statistical methods discussed in this unit are used to interpret numerical (quantitative) data.

It is seldom possible to determine the value for a given variable for every member of a population. For example, it is virtually impossible to measure the level of hemoglobin in every red blood cell of a patient. Rather, a **sample** of the patient's blood is drawn, and the hemoglobin level is measured and evaluated.

When a sample is drawn from a population and the value for a particular variable is measured for each individual in the sample, the resulting values constitute a **sample data set**. Since individuals differ from one another, the data set consists of a group of varying values, Figure 18.1.

A set of data without organization is something like letters that are not arranged into words. Like letters of the alphabet, numerical data can be arranged in ways that are meaningful. **Descriptive statistics** *is a branch of statistics that provides methods to organize, summarize, and describe data.*[1]

[1] Another branch of statistics, inferential statistics, provides methods to make predictions about a population based on a sample. That area of statistics is beyond the scope of this book.

DOI: 10.1201/9780429282744-22

Population–All 20-year-old men in the United States

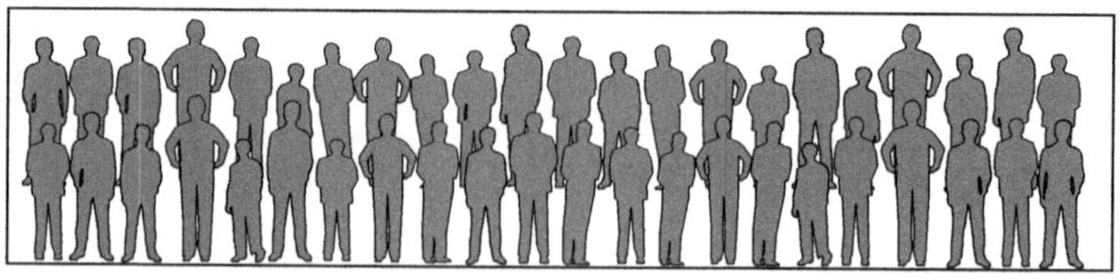

Variables–Many variables could be measured for this population such as: height, hair color, college entrance exam score, and birthplace

Sample–A sample of the population of all 20-year-old men is drawn

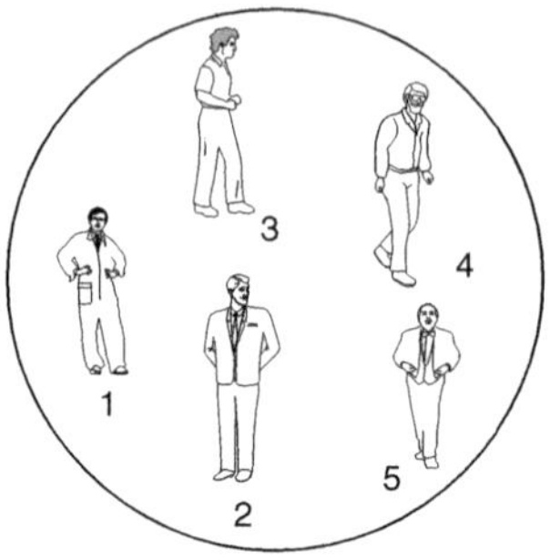


**Data**–Observations are made of the individuals in the sample

| Individual | Height (in cm) | Hair Color | College Exam Score | Birthplace |
|---|---|---|---|---|
| 1 | 172 | brown | 1500 | WI |
| 2 | 173 | blond | none | IL |
| 3 | 169 | black | 1800 | NY |
| 4 | 177 | brown | none | WY |
| 5 | 175 | blond | 1310 | MO |

**FIGURE 18.1** Populations, samples, variables, and data. The population of interest is all 20-year-old men, top. A sample is drawn from this population to represent that population. In this illustration, data for four variables are collected for each individual in the sample.

Consider, for example, the exam scores for a class of students. The variable that is measured is the exam score for each individual. A list of the scores of all the students constitutes the data set. To summarize and describe the performance of the class as a whole, the instructor might calculate the class's average score. The average is an example of a measure that summarizes the data. A measure that describes a sample, such as the average, is sometimes referred to as a "statistic."

The average gives information about the "center" of a data set. There are other measures, such as the median and the mode, that also describe data in terms of its center. *Such measures, which describe the center of a data set, are called* **measures of central tendency**.

Data set A and B both have the same average:

$$A: 4, 5, 5, 5, 6, 6$$

$$B: 1, 2, 4, 7, 8, 9$$

Yet, inspection of these values reveals that the two data sets have a different pattern. The data in A are more clumped about the central value than the data in B. We say that the data in B are more **dispersed**, *that is, spread out.*

Measures of central tendency, such as the average, do not describe the dispersion of a set of observations. Therefore, there are statistical **measures of dispersion** *that describe how much the values in a data set vary from one another.* Common measures of dispersion are range, variance, standard deviation, and coefficient of variation. These measures of dispersion are considered in Chapter 19.

Measures of central tendency and of dispersion are determined by calculation. It is also possible to organize and effectively display data using graphical techniques. Graphical techniques and their interpretation are discussed in Chapter 20.

## 18.2 MEASURES OF CENTRAL TENDENCY

### 18.2.1 THE MEAN OR AVERAGE

Consider a hypothetical data set consisting of these values:

***2, 5, 6, 7, 8, 3, 9, 3, 10, 4, 7, 4, 6, 11, 9***

The simplest way to organize these values is to order them as follows:

***2, 3, 3, 4, 4, 5, 6, 6, 7, 7, 8, 9, 9, 10, 11***

Inspection of the ordered list of numbers reveals that they center somewhere around 6 or 7. The center can be calculated more exactly by determining the average or mean. The mean *is the sum of all the values divided by the number of values.* In this example the mean is calculated as:

$$2+3+3+4+4+5+6+6+7+7+8+9+9+10+11=94$$

***The average or the mean is 94 / 15 ≈ 6.3***

In algebraic notation, the observations are called $\mathbf{X_1, X_2, X_3}$, and so on. In this example there are 15 observations, so the last value is $X_{15}$. The method to calculate the mean can be written compactly as:

$$\textbf{Mean} = \frac{\Sigma X_i}{n}$$

where n = the number of values

$\Sigma$ (the Greek letter "sigma") is short for "add up." $X_i$ means that what is to be added is all the values for the variable, X. Thus:

$$\textbf{Mean} = \frac{\Sigma X_i}{n} = \frac{X_1 + X_2 + X_3 + \cdots + X_n}{n}$$

Statisticians distinguish between the true mean of an entire population and the mean of a sample from that population. The true mean of a population is represented by $\mu$ (the Greek letter "mu"). The mean of a sample is represented by $\bar{x}$ (read as "X bar"), Figure 18.2. In practice, we often do not know the true mean for an entire population. Therefore, the sample mean, or $\bar{x}$ must be used instead of the true population mean.

### 18.2.2 THE MEDIAN OR MIDDLE

The median is another measure of central tendency. When data are sorted in order from lowest to highest, the **median** *is the value such that at least half the values in the data set are at or above it, and at least half are at or below it.* For example, the median for the following values is 6 because half the values in the data set are above six and half are below:

***2, 3, 3, 4, 4, 5, 6, <u>6</u>, 7, 7, 8, 9, 9, 10, 11***

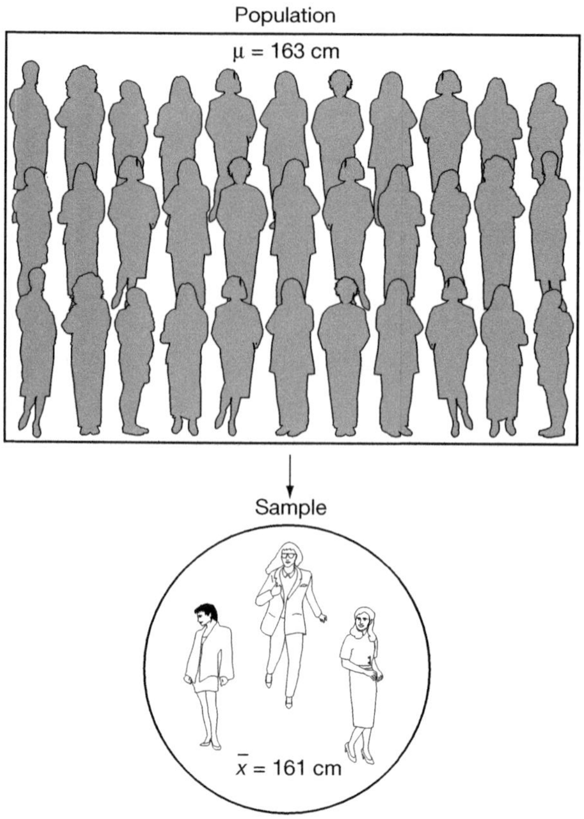


**FIGURE 18.2** The true mean of a population is distinguished from the mean of a sample. The population of interest is all women in the United States (top); the variable of interest is height. The mean height, $\mu$, for all women is 163 cm. A sample of women is drawn, and their heights are measured. The mean height in the sample, $\bar{x}$, is 161 cm.

When there is an even number of values, the median is the average of the 2 central numbers. The median for these values is 7.5 or the average of the numbers 7 and 8:

***3, 5, 7, 8, 9, 11***

Observe that in both of the following data sets the median is five even though their means are quite different:

***2, 3, 4, 5, 6, 7, 8*** $\bar{x} = 5$

***2, 3, 4, 5, 6, 100, 1,000*** $\bar{x} = 160$

### 18.2.3 THE MODE OR MOST COMMON

The **mode** *is the value of the variable that occurs most frequently.* For example, the mode in the following data set is "3" since it appears more often than the other numbers:

***2, 3, 3, 3, 4, 5, 6, 7, 7, 8***

It is possible for a set of data to have more than one mode. *If there are two modes, the data are* **bimodal**. *If there are more than two modes, the data are* **polymodal**. The mode is useful when we are concerned about the "most likely" event when taking data from a population.

Box 18.1 summarizes calculations of these three measures of central tendency – the mean, median, and mode.

**BOX 18.1: Measures of Central Tendency: Calculating the Mean, Median, and Mode**

**To Calculate the Mean:**

Add all the values and divide by the number of values present. $\text{Mean} = \frac{\sum x_i}{n}$

**To Find the Median:**

Order the data values.

If there is an odd number of values, the median is the middle number.

If there is an even number of values, the median is the average of the two middle values.

**To Find the Mode:**

Order the data values.

The mode is the most frequent observation. There may be more than one mode.

**Example:**

Given the data set: **12, 15, 13, 12, 13, 14, 16, 19, 21, 13, 15, 14**

1. Order the data: **12, 12, 13, 13, 13, 14, 14, 15, 15, 16, 19, 21**
2. The mean is $\frac{12+12+13+13+13+14+14+15+15+16+19+21}{12} = 14.75$
3. The median is $\frac{14+14}{2} = 14$
4. The mode is **13**.

**Example Problem:**

Suppose you are investigating the height of college students. You measure the height of every student in your classes and obtain the data shown below.

a. What is the average height of the men in the class?
b. What is the average height of the women in the class?
c. What is the average height of all students in the class?

**Heights of Students in the Class (in cm)**

| Men | | | Women | | |
|---|---|---|---|---|---|
| 175.3 | 176.5 | 177.8 | 162.5 | 166.7 | 155.6 |
| 168.5 | 165.2 | 160.2 | 159.7 | 163.4 | 164.2 |
| 180.9 | 188.9 | 171.6 | 160.1 | 168.6 | 162.6 |
| 175.9 | 174.8 | 179.2 | 162.8 | 158.4 | 174.9 |
| 175.9 | 175.8 | 174.8 | 161.3 | 166.2 | 166.7 |

$n_{men} = 15$ (number of men) $n_{women} = 15$ (number of women)

*Answer:*

d. $\bar{x} = \frac{2621.3\text{ cm}}{15} \approx \mathbf{174.75\text{ cm (men)}}$

e. $\bar{x} = \frac{2453.7}{15} = \mathbf{163.58\text{ cm (women)}}$

f. $\bar{x} = \frac{5075.0\text{ cm}}{30} \approx \mathbf{169.17\text{ cm (men + women)}}$

**Practice Problems**

1. a. ***Ten vials of enzyme were chosen from a batch for quality control testing. What was the sample? What was the population?***
   b. ***The glucose level in a blood sample was measured. What was the sample? What was the population? What was the variable being studied?***
   c. ***The effectiveness of a new drug for treating melanoma was studied in a clinical trial with 100 patients. What was the sample? What was the population? What was the variable being studied?***
2. a. ***Calculate the mean for these test scores.***

   ***83% 71% 97% 99% 75% 83% 92% 98%***

   b. ***The time to completion of an enzyme reaction was determined for six reaction mixtures. Calculate the mean.***

   ***235 seconds 287 seconds 198 seconds 255 seconds 234 seconds 201 seconds***

   c. ***The analyst who performed the enzyme reactions in b tried an alternative assay method and obtained the results below. Calculate the mean for the alternative method.***

   ***245 seconds 235 seconds 256 seconds 228 seconds 237 seconds***

   ***244 seconds 234 seconds 215 seconds***

3. ***(Optional: These calculations are best performed using a calculator that performs statistical functions.) Calculate the mean:***
   a. ***The weights of 33 vials from a lot were sampled. The results in mg are:***

   ***115 133 125 124 87 95 136 146 114 133 139***

   ***177 193 136 177 193 136 123 171 147 153 149***

   ***110 111 121 71 178 173 201 149 94 100 103***

   b. ***The weights of 25 samples were measured. The results are:***

   ***9.27g 9.88g 6.19g 8.38g 9.62g 5.48g 9.71g 9.54g 7.41g 6.76g 9.33g***

   ***8.64g 6.43g 7.66g 9.60g 7.50g 9.89g 7.73g 5.68g 6.74g 8.04g 7.23g***

   ***7.35g 10.82g 8.94g***

4. ***A biotechnology company is developing a new variety of genetically modified fruit tree that is drought resistant. Researchers study the numbers of fruits produced by the trees under a certain condition. What is the mean and median for these data?***

***45 78 25 98 30 32 45 67 45 23***

***44 34 23 78 62 45 35 23 56 25***

5. ***A company plans to grow and market Shiitake mushrooms. The yields of mushrooms obtained in preliminary experiments are shown below and are expressed in kilograms. Calculate the mean and median for these data:***

***38.2 31.7 28.1 29.1 33.4 25.2 18.2 19.7 41.7 26.2 21.0 52.2***

6. ***The average test score for a class of 25 students is 82%. One additional student takes the exam and scores 90%. What is the new average for the class?***

*Answers*

1. a. Sample: **The ten vials**. Population: **All the vials in the batch**.
   b. Sample: **The blood sample tested**. Population: **All the blood in that individual**. Variable: **Glucose level**.
   c. Sample: **100 patients**. Population: **All melanoma patients**. Variable: **Effectiveness of new drug**.
2. a. $\bar{x} = \mathbf{87.25\%}$   b. $\bar{x} = \mathbf{235\ seconds}$   c. $\bar{x} = \mathbf{236.75\ seconds}$
3. a. $n = 33$ $\bar{x} \approx \mathbf{136.76\ mg}$   b. $n = 25$ $\bar{x} \approx \mathbf{8.15\ g}$
4. $n = 20$ $\bar{x} = \mathbf{45.65\ fruit}$   median = **44.5 fruit**
5. $n = 12$ $\bar{x} \approx \mathbf{30.39\ kg}$   median = **28.6 kg**
6. $\Sigma \frac{X}{25} = 82\%$   $\Sigma X = 2{,}050\%$   $2{,}050\% + 90\% = 2{,}140 =$ new total   $\frac{2{,}140}{26} \approx \mathbf{82.3\%}$

# Descriptive Statistics: Measures of Dispersion

19



## 19.1 CALCULATING THE RANGE, VARIANCE, AND STANDARD DEVIATION

Recall that statistical **measures of dispersion** are calculated values that describe how much the values in a data set vary from one another. The **range**, the simplest measure of dispersion, is the difference between the lowest value and the highest value in a set of data:

*2, 3, 3, 3, 4, 4, 5, 6, 7, 7, 8, 9, 9, 10, 11*

***The range is 2 to 11 = 9***

The range is not a particularly informative measure because it is based on only two values from the data set. A single extreme value will have a major effect on the range.

The variance and the standard deviation are more informative measures of dispersion than the range because they summarize information about dispersion based on all the values in the data set. Consider this simple example. Assume the data below are lengths (in mm):

*4, 5, 6, 7, 7, 7, 9, 11*

The mean for these data is 7 mm. An intuitive way to calculate how much the data are dispersed is to take each data point, one at a time, and see how far it is from the mean, Table 19.1. The distance of a data point from the mean is its **deviation**. There is a deviation for each data point; sometimes the deviation is positive, sometimes negative, and sometimes it is zero.

It is useful to summarize all the deviations with a single value. An obvious approach would be to calculate the average of the deviations. However, for any data set, the sum of the deviations from the mean is always zero, as shown in Table 19.1. Therefore, mathematicians devised the approach of squaring each individual deviation value to result in all nonnegative numbers. *The squared deviations can be added together to get the* **total squared deviation** also called the **sum of squares**. In this example, the sum of squares is 34 $mm^2$, Table 19.2.

DOI: 10.1201/9780429282744-23

**TABLE 19.1 Calculation of Deviation from the Mean**

| *Value – Mean* | *Deviation (mm)* |
|---|---|
| First value – mean | =(4 − 7) = −3 |
| Second value – mean | =(5 − 7) = −2 |
| Third value – mean | =(6 − 7) = −1 |
| Fourth value – mean | =(7 − 7) = 0 |
| Fifth value – mean | =(7 − 7) = 0 |
| Sixth value – mean | =(7 − 7) = 0 |
| Seventh value – mean | =(9 − 7) = +2 |
| Eighth value – mean | =(11 − 7) = +4 |
| | *0 = Sum of all the deviations* |

**TABLE 19.2 Calculation of the Sum of Squares**

| *Value-Mean* | *Deviation* | *Deviation Squared (mm²)* |
|---|---|---|
| (4 − 7) | −3 | 9 |
| (5 − 7) | −2 | 4 |
| (6 − 7) | −1 | 1 |
| (7 − 7) | 0 | 0 |
| (7 − 7) | 0 | 0 |
| (7 − 7) | 0 | 0 |
| (9 − 7) | +2 | 4 |
| (11 − 7) | +4 | 16 |
| | | 34 |
| | | *(total squared deviation = the sum of squares)* |

The sum of squares is always a nonnegative number that indicates how much the values in a data set deviate from the mean.

When talking about a population, the **population variance** *is the total squared deviation divided by the number of values:*

$$\text{Variance}(\text{of a population}) = \frac{\text{total squared deviations from the mean}}{\text{n}} = \frac{\Sigma(X_i - \text{mean})^2}{\text{n}}$$

where:

$\Sigma$ = the sum of
$X_i$ = individual value
n = the number of values

In our example, the sum of squares is 34 mm², n is 8, and the population variance is:

$$\text{Variance} = \frac{34\ \text{mm}^2}{8} = 4.25\ \text{mm}^2$$

The standard deviation is calculated by taking the square root of the variance:

$$\text{Standard deviation} = \sqrt{\text{variance}}$$

In our example:

$$\text{Standard deviation} = \sqrt{4.25\ \text{mm}^2} \approx 2.06\ \text{mm}$$

Note that the standard deviation has the same units as the data.

The standard deviation and the variance are values that summarize the dispersion of a set of data around the mean. The larger the variance and the standard deviation, the more dispersed are the data.

**Example Problem:**

A biotechnology company sells cultures of a particular strain of the bacterium *E. coli*. The bacteria are grown up in batches that are freeze dried and packaged into vials. Each vial is expected to contain 200 mg of bacteria. A quality control technician tests a sample of vials from each batch and reports the mean weight and the standard deviation.

Batch Q-21 has a mean weight of 200 mg and a standard deviation of 12 mg. Batch P-34 has a mean weight of 200 mg and a standard deviation of 4 mg. Which lot appears to have been packaged in a more controlled, that is, consistent fashion?

***Answer:***

The standard deviation can be interpreted as an indication of consistency. The standard deviation of the weights in Batch P-34 is less than that of Batch Q-21. Therefore, the values for Batch P-34 are less dispersed than those for Batch Q-21. The packaging of Batch P-34 appears to have been better controlled, and so it is more consistent.

## 19.2 DISTINGUISHING BETWEEN THE VARIANCE AND STANDARD DEVIATION OF A POPULATION AND A SAMPLE

The preceding discussion skipped over a significant detail regarding the calculation of the variance and standard deviation. Statisticians distinguish between the variance and standard deviation of a population and the variance and standard deviation of a sample. *The variance of a population is called* $\sigma^2$ (read as "sigma squared"). *The variance of a sample is called* $\mathbf{S}^2$. *The standard deviation of a population is called* $\sigma$ (sigma). *The standard deviation of a sample is sometimes abbreviated* **S** *and sometimes* **SD**. Terminology relating to populations and samples is summarized in Table 19.3.

The formulas used to calculate the variance and SD of a sample are slightly different than those for a population. In Section 19.1, we showed how to calculate the variance and standard deviation of a population. For a sample, the denominator is n − 1 rather than n. The formulas for variance and SD of a sample are thus:

Variance of a sample $= S^2$:

$$S^2 = \frac{\text{Sum of squared deviations from the mean}}{n-1}$$

$$S^2 = \frac{\Sigma(X_i - \mathbf{x})^2}{n-1}$$

$$\text{Standard deviation}\left(\text{of a sample}\right) = \text{SD} = \sqrt{S^2}$$

$$\text{SD} = \sqrt{\frac{\Sigma(X_i - \mathbf{x})^2}{n-1}}$$

where:

$\Sigma$ = the sum of
$X_i$ = each value
n − 1 = the number of values minus 1

In this text, we are generally looking at data from a sample and so routinely use n − 1 in the denominator of the formula.

**TABLE 19.3 Terminology Relating to Populations and Samples**

| Population | Sample |
|---|---|
| An entire group of events, objects, results, or individuals where each member of the group has some unifying characteristic(s) | A subset of a population that represents the population |
| *Parameters:* | *Statistics:* |
| Measures that describe a population | Measures that describe a sample |
| Mean: $\mu$ | Mean: $\bar{x}$ |
| Variance: $\sigma^2$ | Variance: $S^2$ |
| Standard deviation: $\sigma$ | Standard deviation: **S** or **SD** |

The standard deviation is a widely used statistic and so being able to calculate it for a given set of data is an important skill. Many scientific and graphing calculators are set up to calculate the standard deviation easily. Often the operator can enter the data and then press one key to get the standard deviation for a population and a different key to get the standard deviation for a sample. (Refer to the calculator instructions.) There are also statistical computer programs that are useful for analyzing large sets of data.

**Example Problem:**

The heights for a sample of seven college women are shown below. Calculate the mean ($\bar{x}$), the deviation ($x_i - \bar{x}$) of each value from the mean, the squares of each deviation $(x_i - \bar{x})^2$, the sum of squared deviations ($\Sigma(x_i - \bar{x})^2$), the variance ($S^2$), and the SD.

**Measured Values (cm)**

162.5, 166.7, 155.6, 159.7, 163.4, 164.2, 160.1

*Answer:*

$$\bar{x} \approx \mathbf{161.74\ cm}$$

| $x_i$ Measured Value (cm) | $(x_i - \bar{x})$ Deviation (cm) | $(x_i - \bar{x})^2$ Deviation² (cm²) |
|---|---|---|
| 162.5 | 0.757 | 0.573 |
| 166.7 | 4.96 | 24.6 |
| 155.6 | −6.14 | 37.7 |
| 159.7 | −2.04 | 4.16 |
| 163.4 | 1.66 | 2.76 |
| 164.2 | 2.46 | 6.05 |
| 160.1 | −1.64 | 2.69 |

Sum of squared deviations $\left(\Sigma(x_i - \bar{x})^2\right)$: $\mathbf{78.53\ cm^2}$

$$n - 1 = 6$$

$$S^2 = \frac{78.53\ cm^2}{6} \approx \mathbf{13.09\ cm^2}$$

$$SD = \sqrt{13.09\ cm^2} \approx \mathbf{3.618\ cm}$$

**TABLE 19.4 Weights of Laboratory Mice and Rabbits**

| Weights of Laboratory Mice (g) | Weights of Laboratory Rabbits (g) |
|---|---|
| 32 | 3,178 |
| 34 | 3,500 |
| 24 | 3,428 |
| 33 | 2,908 |
| 36 | 2,757 |
| 30 | 3,100 |
| 36 | 2,876 |
| 36 | 3,369 |
| 30 | 3,682 |
| 34 | 2,808 |
| $\bar{x}$ = **32.5 g** | $\bar{x}$ ≈ **3,161 g** |
| SD ≈ **3.75 g** | SD ≈ **322.83 g** |
| CV ≈ **11.5%** | CV ≈ **10.2%** |

## 19.3 THE COEFFICIENT OF VARIATION (RELATIVE STANDARD DEVIATION)

Table 19.4 shows the weights of laboratory mice and rabbits. Observe that the SD for the rabbits' weights has a higher value than for the mice, but, of course, rabbits weigh more than mice.

The dispersion of a data set can be expressed by the SD as a percentage of the mean. This is called the **coefficient of variation, CV,** or the **relative standard deviation, RSD.** The formula for the CV is:

$$CV = \frac{\text{Standard deviation}\,(100\%)}{\text{Mean}}$$

When the dispersions of the weights of mice and rabbits are expressed in terms of the CV, the value is slightly higher for the mouse data than for the rabbit data. Note that the mean and the SD have units, but the units cancel when the CV is calculated.

Methods of calculating various measures of dispersion for sample data are summarized in Box 19.1.

**BOX 19.1: Measures of Dispersion: The Variance, the Standard Deviation, and the Coefficient or Variation**

To calculate the variance, $S^2$, for a sample, use the equation:

$$S^2 = \frac{\Sigma(X_i - \bar{X})^2}{n - 1}$$

To calculate the standard deviation, SD, for a sample, use the

equation: $SD = \sqrt{\frac{\Sigma\,(X_i - \bar{X})^2}{n - 1}}$

To calculate the coefficient of variation, CV use the

equation: $CV = \frac{\text{Standard deviation (100\%)}}{\text{mean}}$

where:
$\Sigma$ = the sum of
$X_i$ = each value
$\bar{x}$ = the mean
n − 1 = sample size minus 1

**EXAMPLE:**

Given these data from a sample:
1.00 mm, 2.00 mm, 2.00 mm, 3.00 mm, 3.00 mm, 4.00 mm, 4.00 mm, 5.00 mm

$$\bar{x} = 3.00\text{ mm}$$

$$1.\ S^2 = \frac{((1-3)\text{ mm})^2 + ((2-3)\text{ mm})^2 + ((2-3)\text{ mm})^2 + ((3-3)\text{ mm})^2 + ((3-3)\text{ mm})^2 + ((4-3)\text{ mm})^2 + ((4-3)\text{ mm})^2 + ((5-3)\text{ mm})^2}{8-1}$$

$$= \frac{12.00}{7} \approx \mathbf{1.71\ mm^2}$$

2. The SD is the square root of the variance ≈ **1.31 mm**
   *Note that the SD and the variance have units if the data have units.*
3. The CV is:

$$CV = \frac{1.31\text{ mm} \times 100\%}{3.00\text{ mm}} \approx \mathbf{43.67\%}$$

## 19.4 APPLICATION: USING MEASURES OF DISPERSION TO DESCRIBE VARIABILITY

Measures of dispersion are statistical tools that are used to describe the variability, or spread, in a set of data. Consider, for example, hypothetical values obtained by a technician analyzing lead levels in paint samples from houses, Table 19.5. The analyst observes on February 20 that the values from two houses seem to fluctuate more than normal. This observation alerts her to the possibility that there might be a problem in the measurement system. She can analyze the variability in the data using various statistical tools including: the **range**, the **SD**, and the **RSD.**

Table 19.6 shows that the range of values for February 20 is greater than for the other days. The SD and the RSD for the measurement values on February 20 were also higher than on the

**TABLE 19.5 Hypothetical Values Obtained for Lead Levels in Paint Samples**

| Feb. 4 House 1 Window (mg/cm²) | Feb. 4 House 2 Window (mg/cm²) | Feb. 8 House 3 Window (mg/cm²) | Feb. 8 House 4 Window (mg/cm²) | Feb. 8 House 5 Window (mg/cm²) | Feb. 10 House 6 Window (mg/cm²) | Feb. 20 House 7 Window (mg/cm²) | Feb. 20 House 8 Window (mg/cm²) |
|---|---|---|---|---|---|---|---|
| 1.21 | 0.43 | 0.92 | 0.78 | 1.51 | 2.12 | 0.98 | 1.23 |
| 1.18 | 0.40 | 0.93 | 0.67 | 1.43 | 1.99 | 0.78 | 0.21 |
| 1.31 | 0.34 | 0.79 | 0.71 | 1.34 | 2.13 | 0.21 | 0.11 |
| 1.23 | 0.41 | 0.93 | 0.65 | 1.47 | 1.98 | 1.24 | 0.89 |

Some information for this example was taken from Driscoll, J.N., et al. "Field Detection of Lead in Paint and Soil by High-Resolution XRF." *American Laboratory*, March 1995, p. 34H.

**TABLE 19.6 Statistical Analysis of Data in Table 19.5**

| Feb. 4 House 1 Window (mg/cm$^2$) | Feb. 4 House 2 Window (mg/cm$^2$) | Feb. 8 House 3 Window (mg/cm$^2$) | Feb. 8 House 4 Window (mg/cm$^2$) | Feb. 8 House 5 Window (mg/cm$^2$) | Feb. 10 House 6 Window (mg/cm$^2$) | Feb. 20 House 7 Window (mg/cm$^2$) | Feb. 20 House 8 Window (mg/cm$^2$) |
|---|---|---|---|---|---|---|---|
| 1.21 | 0.43 | 0.92 | 0.78 | 1.51 | 2.12 | 0.98 | 1.23 |
| 1.18 | 0.40 | 0.93 | 0.67 | 1.43 | 1.99 | 0.78 | 0.21 |
| 1.31 | 0.34 | 0.79 | 0.71 | 1.34 | 2.13 | 0.21 | 0.11 |
| 1.23 | 0.41 | 0.93 | 0.65 | 1.47 | 1.98 | 1.24 | 0.89 |
| Range = 1.31 − 1.18 = 0.13 | Range = 0.09 | Range = 0.14 | Range = 0.13 | Range = 0.17 | Range = 0.15 | Range = 1.03 | Range = 1.12 |
| Mean ≈ 1.23 | Mean ≈ 0.40 | Mean ≈ 0.89 | Mean ≈ 0.70 | Mean ≈ 1.44 | Mean = 2.06 | Mean ≈ 0.80 | Mean = 0.61 |
| SD ≈ 0.056 | SD ≈ 0.039 | SD ≈ 0.068 | SD ≈ 0.057 | SD ≈ 0.073 | SD ≈ 0.081 | SD ≈ 0.44 | SD ≈ 0.54 |
| RSD ≈ 4.52% | RSD ≈ 9.8% | RSD ≈ 7.7% | RSD ≈ 8.2% | RSD ≈ 5.05% | RSD ≈ 3.93% | RSD ≈ 55% | RSD ≈ 88% |

other days. These results suggest that for some reason the data obtained on February 20 were more variable than on the other dates. There are many possible explanations for this discrepancy. For example, the variability might be due to a characteristic of the houses themselves. Perhaps the windows from which the paint samples were taken had many layers of different paints applied, in which case the variability resulted from nonhomogeneous samples. It is also possible that an instrument was malfunctioning on February 20 and required repair. Perhaps a reagent involved in the measurement procedure had degraded. The technician at this point will want to identify the source of variability and correct any problems that may be present.

**Example Problem:**

A biotechnology company manufactures a particular enzyme that is used to cut DNA strands. The enzyme's activity can be assayed and is reported in terms of "units/mg." Each batch of enzyme is tested before it is sold. The results of repeated tests on four batches of enzyme are shown below.

a. What is the mean activity of the enzyme for each batch?
b. What is the SD for each batch?
c. What is the mean activity for all batches combined?
d. What is the SD for all batches combined?

| Enzyme Activity (units/mg) | | | |
|---|---|---|---|
| **Batch 1** | **Batch 2** | **Batch 3** | **Batch 4** |
| 100,900 | 100,800 | 110,000 | 123,000 |
| 102,000 | 101,000 | 108,000 | 121,000 |
| 104,000 | 100,100 | 107,000 | 119,000 |
| 104,100 | 100,800 | 109,100 | 121,000 |

***Answer:***

Mean of batch 1 = **102,750 units/mg** SD ≈ **1,567 units/mg**
Mean of batch 2 = **100,675 units/mg** SD ≈ **395 units/mg**
Mean of batch 3 = **108,525 units/mg** SD ≈ **1,305 units/mg**
Mean of batch 4 = **121,000 units/mg** SD ≈ **1,633 units/mg**
Mean of all batches ≈ **108,238 units/mg**
SD of all batches ≈ **8,254 units/mg**

Note that there is more variability between the batches than there is within one batch. This is commonly the case. This is reflected in the fact that the SD for all the batches is higher than the SD of any one batch.

**Example Problem:**

A new balance must be purchased for a teaching laboratory. A teacher compares three competing brands by measuring a standard that is 1.0000 g five times on each balance.

a. Which balance is most accurate? Show the percent error for each balance. Percent error was introduced in Chapter 10.3 where it was defined as:

$$\% \text{ Error} = \frac{(\text{True value} - \text{average measured value})}{\text{True value}} (100\%)$$

b. Calculate the SD for the measurements from each balance. Which balance is most consistent?
c. What is the CV for each of the balances?
d. Report the mean value for the standard from each balance ± the SD.
e. Which balance would you buy?

| Brand A (g) | Brand B (g) | Brand C (g) |
|---|---|---|
| 1.0004 | 0.9997 | 1.0003 |
| 1.0005 | 0.9996 | 0.9996 |
| 1.0004 | 1.0003 | 1.0002 |
| 1.0003 | 1.0002 | 0.9995 |
| 1.0005 | 0.9999 | 1.0004 |

*Answer:*

| Balance A | Balance B | Balance C |
|---|---|---|
| Mean ≈ 1.0004 g | Mean ≈ 0.9999 g | Mean = 1.0000 g |
| % error = −0.04% | % error = 0.01% | % error = 0.00% |
| SD ≈ 0.0001 g | SD ≈ 0.0003 g | SD ≈ 0.0004 g |
| CV ≈ 0.01% | CV ≈ 0.03% | CV ≈ 0.04% |
| **Mean ± SD = (1.0004 ± 0.0001) g** | **(0.9999 ± 0.0003) g** | **(1.0000 ± 0.0004) g** |

The percent error is an indication of the accuracy of the balances.

Consistency (absence of variability) is shown by the SD and CV.

Although the mean value of balance C is accurate, its SD is higher than the other two balances, so any single measurement made on balance C is more likely to be inaccurate. Balance A has the best consistency, but all the readings are a bit high. If balance A can be adjusted so that is accurate, it might be a good choice; otherwise, this balance is not acceptable. Balance B might be an acceptable compromise, particularly if it has other qualities that are desirable, such as ruggedness and ease of use.

**Practice Problems**

1. ***Simply by scanning the values in each distribution below, identify the distribution with the largest SD.***
   *A. 1, 16, 17, 19, 20, 20, 22, 25, 30, 39*
   *B. 1, 3, 8, 10, 17, 20, 30, 32, 37, 39*
   *C. 1, 18, 17, 19, 24, 23, 23, 21, 25, 39*
2. ***The incubation time for COVID-19 (the time between being exposed to the illness and developing symptoms) ranges between 2 and 14 days. Based on a sample of 10 people, what is the mean and SD for the incubation time (in days):***
   *7, 9, 4, 12, 8, 8, 6, 10, 11, 4*
3. a. ***Ten measurements of a 10 g standard weight were made. Calculate the SD and CV.***
   *10.001 g 10.000 g 10.001 g 9.999 g 9.998 g*
   *10.000 g 10.002 g 9.999 g 10.000 g 10.001 g*

   b. ***Calculate the SD and CV for these test scores.***
   *75%, 71%, 88%, 99%, 76%, 83%, 89%, 91%*

   c. ***The time to completion of an enzyme reaction was timed in 6 reaction mixtures. Calculate the SD and CV.***
   *235 seconds, 287 seconds, 198 seconds, 255 seconds, 234 seconds, 201 seconds*

   d. ***The analyst who performed the enzyme reactions in c tried an alternative assay method and obtained the results below. Calculate the SD for the alternative method. Compare the two methods***
   *245 seconds, 235 seconds, 256 seconds, 228 seconds, 237 seconds, 244 seconds, 234 seconds, 215 seconds*
4. ***Optional: These calculations are best performed using a calculator that automatically performs statistical functions. Calculate the SD and RSD for the following data sets:***

   a. ***The weights of 33 vials from a lot were sampled. The results in mg are:***
   *115 133 125 124 87 95 136 146 114 133 139 177*
   *193 136 177 193 136 123 171 147 153 149 110 111*
   *121 71 178 173 201 149 94 100 103*

   b. ***The weights of 25 samples were measured. The results are:***
   *9.27 g 9.88 g 6.19 g 8.38 g 9.62 g 5.48 g*
   *9.71 g 9.54 g 7.41 g 6.76 g 9.33 g 8.64 g*
   *6.43 g 7.66 g 9.60 g 7.50 g 9.89 g 7.73 g*
   *5.68 g 6.74 g 8.04 g 7.23 g 7.35 g 10.82 g*
   *8.94 g*

   c. ***The volumes of 19 samples were measured. The results are:***
   *1,022 mL 1,045 mL 1,103 mL 1,200 mL 1,189 mL 1,234 mL*
   *1,043 mL 1,089 mL 1,103 mL 1,020 mL 1,058 mL 1,197 mL*
   *1,201 mL 1,189 mL 1,098 mL 1,155 mL 1,056 mL 1,023 mL*
   *1,109 mL*
5. ***A biotechnology company is developing a new variety of fruit tree and researchers are interested in the number of blossoms produced on each branch of the trees. The following are the total number of blossoms from 20 trees. Find the median, range, and SD for these data:***
   *34 36 29 27 30 35 32 31 39 30 27*
   *44 30 33 43 32 21 35 33 40*
6. ***A company plans to grow and market Shiitake mushrooms. The yields of mushrooms obtained in preliminary experiments are shown below expressed in kilograms. Calculate the median, range, and SD.***
   *38.2, 31.7, 28.1, 29.1, 33.4, 25.2, 18.2, 19.7, 41.7, 26.2, 21.0, 52.2*

***Answers***

1. **B** has the largest SD; it is most dispersed. Observe that the range is the same for all three samples, but A and C clump in the center of the range more than B.
2. The average incubation time based on these data is **7.9 days** and the SD is about **2.7 days**.
3. a. $\overline{X}$ = **10.0001 g** SD ≈ **0.0012 g** CV ≈ **0.012%**
   b. $\overline{X}$ = **84%** SD ≈ **9.49%** CV ≈ **11.29%**
   c. $\overline{X}$ = **235 seconds** SD ≈ **33.56 seconds** CV ≈ **14.28%**
   d. $\overline{X}$ ≈ **237 seconds** SD ≈ **12.26 seconds** CV ≈ **5.18%**
   The means for the two methods are similar. However, the second method is more consistent. Based on this information, the second method seems better.
4. a. n = 33 $\overline{X}$ ≈ **136.76 mg** SD ≈ **32.90 mg** CV ≈ **24.06%**
   b. n = 25 $\overline{X}$ ≈ **8.15 g** SD ≈ **1.47 g** CV ≈ **18.09%**
   c. n = 19 $\overline{X}$ ≈ **1112.32 mL** SD ≈ **71.55 mL** CV ≈ **6.43%**
5. n = 20 $\overline{X}$ ≈ **33.05 blossoms** median = **32.5 blossoms**
   range = 44 − 21 = **23 blossoms** SD ≈ **5.57 blossoms**
6. n = 12 $\overline{X}$ ≈ **30.39 kg** median = **28.6 kg**
   range = 52.2 − 18.2 = **34.0 kg** SD ≈ **9.90 kg**

## 19.5 MORE ABOUT VARIABILITY

We introduced this unit by talking about variability in the natural world. There is always variability in biological systems, and this variability can be problematic in biotechnology settings. It is easy to understand why variability can be a problem if one thinks about manufacturing a biopharmaceutical drug product. Obviously, the dose of the drug must be consistent; variability in that dosage could be life-threatening to patients. Similarly, it is important to reduce variability as much as possible in research laboratories. For example, suppose a researcher is modifying a specific gene and is investigating the effect of the modification on cellular functions. The researcher does not want variability in reagents, instrument performance, procedures, or other factors to unpredictably affect the cells' behavior. Therefore, in virtually all biotechnology settings, it is important to reduce variability as much as possible and to understand the inherent variability in a system. The statistical measures of dispersion that we have described in this chapter are ways of measuring, understanding, and reporting variability.

It is common in a scientific paper or in other technical literature to see a set of data summarized using the mean followed by a measure of dispersion. The smaller the measure of dispersion, the closer the data points are to one another, that is, the less spread out the data points are. This helps the reader evaluate the impact of variability on the data presented. You might encounter a mean reported in any of the following styles:

1. **A mean may be reported as the mean value ± the SD**. For example, in Figure 19.1a, 30.2 pg/mL is the mean and 16.7 pg/mL is the SD at time = 0 (that is, before stem cells were transfused).
2. **You may see a mean reported in a scientific paper as the mean value ± standard error of the mean,** Figure 19.1b. The standard error of the mean (SEM) is not actually a measure of error; rather, it is a measure of dispersion relating to the mean. It is an indication of how much discrepancy there is likely to be in a sample's mean compared to the true mean of the population. The complete meaning of the SEM is outside the scope of this text, but, when encountered in graphs and tables, the simplest way to understand the SEM is to interpret it like the SD: A larger value means there is more variability in the data than a smaller value.

| Measurements of Fibroblast Growth Factor (FGF) and Epidermal Growth Factor (EGF) after Transfusion with Stem Cells (A Study of the Effect of Stem Cells on Nerve Regeneration) | |
|---|---|
| | Mean in units of pg/mL (standard deviation) |
| FGF time 0 | 30.2 (16.7) |
| FGF 7 days after transfusion | 55.4 (12.3) |
| FGF 90 days after transfusion | 30.3 (14.8) |
| EGF time 0 | 428.7 (125) |
| EGF 7 days after transfusion | 601.8 (141.8) |
| EGF 90 days after transfusion | 371.5 (121.9) |

(a)

| | Placebo | Caffeine | Coffee | Decaffeinated Coffee |
|---|---|---|---|---|
| Heart rate (bpm) | 75 ± 6 | 66 ± 4 | 69 ± 5 | 74 ± 5 |
| Systolic BP (mm Hg) | 128 ± 8 | 119 ± 7 | 130 ± 3 | 131 ± 10 |
| Diastolic BP (mm Hg) | 69 ± 2 | 67 ± 2 | 72 ± 3 | 68 ± 3 |

(b)

**FIGURE 19.1** Examples of how the mean is reported in scientific literature. (a) A study of the effects of a stem cell treatment. Values are reported as the mean±the standard deviation. (Excerpted from "Effect of Mesenchymal Stem Cells Transfusion on the Diabetic Peripheral Neuropathy Patients: Study Results." *Clinical Trials.Gov*, clinicaltrials.gov/ct2/show/results/NCT02387749?term=stem+cells&draw=2&view=results.) (b) Baseline data for subjects in a study of the effects of caffeine. (Baseline data compare the groups before coffee is administered.) Data are expressed as the mean ± SEM. (Data are excerpted from: Corti, Roberto, et al. "Coffee Acutely Increases Sympathetic Nerve Activity and Blood Pressure Independently of Caffeine Content." *Circulation*, vol. 106, no. 23, 2002, pp. 2935–40. doi:10.1161/01.cir.0000046228.97025.3a.)

3. **You may see a mean reported in a scientific paper as the mean value and the 95% (or 90% or 99%) confidence interval.** A 95% confidence interval is a range of values that is constructed in such a manner that if 100 random samples were drawn from the population, we would expect 95 of the 100 confidence intervals to include the true mean of the population. It can also be said that "We are 95% confident that $\mu$ is within this range of values." The derivation of a confidence interval is outside the scope of this text, but note that the variability of the data is considered when a confidence interval is calculated: the more variability in the data, the wider the range of the interval.
4. **You may see a mean reported graphically.** The points on the graph in Figure 19.2 represent sample means. The vertical lines are called *error bars.* **Error bars** are not actually about error but rather *provide information about the dispersion of the data.* The error bars may represent±one SD. Error bars may also be used to represent±the SEM or they may show the confidence interval. The interpretation of error bars is customarily explained in the figure caption.

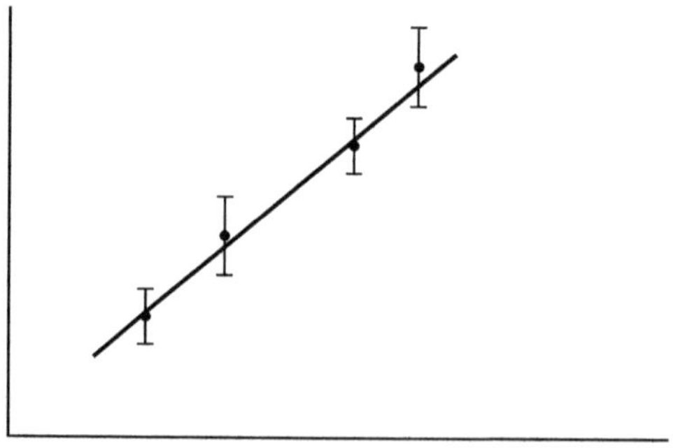

**FIGURE 19.2** Error bars. In this hypothetical experiment, each point on the line in this graph represents the mean of the observations of 20 individuals. The error bar represents ±1 SD.

## Practice Problems

1. *If a flask that is used to measure volume is supposed to be marked at 10.00 mL and is actually marked at 9.98 mL, will this affect its accuracy? Will this affect the SD of a series of measurements made with it?*
2. *A standard sample of human blood serum is prepared that has 38.0 mg/mL of albumin. Technicians from four different laboratories analyze the standard sample four times in one day and obtain the results (in mg/mL) below. Comment on the various laboratories' accuracy and the consistency of their results.*

| Laboratory 1 | Laboratory 2 | Laboratory 3 | Laboratory 4 |
|---|---|---|---|
| 37.1 | 38.3 | 38.6 | 38.7 |
| 37.8 | 38.0 | 37.1 | 39.1 |
| 37.7 | 37.8 | 39.1 | 37.5 |
| 37.4 | 38.2 | 37.0 | 38.2 |

3. *Technicians from Laboratory 2 in Problem 2 (above) repeat the analyses, but this time do analyses over a period of 4 months. Their results are:*
   *37.0 mg/mL, 37.4 mg/mL, 38.1 mg/mL, 37.6 mg/mL*
   *Comment on these results in terms of their SD. Are the results more, less, or equally consistent when the tests are spread over a period of months?*
4. *The table below shows data from a study of blood calcium levels in several individuals:*

| Subject | Mean Calcium Level (mg/L) | # of Observations | Deviation of Results from Mean Values |
|---|---|---|---|
| 1 | 87.5 | 4 | 0.13, 0.19, 0.05, 0.11 |
| 2 | 97.6 | 4 | 0.18, 0.13, 0.10, 0.02 |
| 3 | 104.8 | 4 | 0.09, 0.04, 0.12, 0.06 |

   a. *Calculate the SD for each subject's values.*
   b. *Pool the data and calculate the mean value for blood calcium level based on all subjects.*
5. *A company manufactures buffer solutions for use in calibrating pH meters. A new lot of pH 7.0 buffer was produced. The pH of this new lot was tested on an instrument known to be properly functioning. The results of seven measurements were:*
   *7.12, 7.20, 7.15, 7.17, 7.16, 7.19, 7.15*
   a. *Calculate the mean and SD for these data.*
   b. *Comment on these results if the pH of the buffer is supposed to be 7.00.*
6. *Samples of air in a particular factory were analyzed for lead. Each individual sample was tested three times and samples were taken on three occasions:*

| Sample | Lead (μg/m$^3$) Air |
|---|---|
| 1 | 1.4, 1.3, 1.2 |
| 2 | 2.3, 2.3, 2.1 |
| 3 | 1.6, 1.5, 1.7 |

   a. *Calculate the mean and SD for each sample.*
   b. *Calculate the mean and SD for the pooled set of data.*
   c. *Is the SD higher in a or b? Explain why.*

7. ***A spectrophotometer was used to determine the concentration of protein in a solution. The solution was analyzed six times and the absorbances were:***
***0.956, 0.948, 0.958, 0.991, 0.963, 0.957***
***According to the spectrophotometer manufacturer, the CV of the instrument should not exceed 1%. a. Do these results exceed 1% CV?***
***b. If so, does this indicate that the spectrophotometer is malfunctioning or does not meet its specifications?***

## *Answers*

1. We would expect all the readings made with this flask to be incorrect, but their consistency is unlikely to be affected by the improper marking. Therefore, the accuracy of the flask would be adversely affected but not its consistency or the SD of a series of measurements made with it.
2.

| | Laboratory 1 | Laboratory 2 | Laboratory 3 | Laboratory 4 |
|---|---|---|---|---|
| SD (mg/mL) | 0.316 | 0.222 | 1.06 | 0.690 |
| Mean (mg/mL) | 37.5 | 38.1 | 38.0 | 38.4 |

Laboratories 2 and 3 both have good accuracy but laboratory 2 has the lowest SD and therefore the most consistent results.

3.

| | |
|---|---|
| Mean | 37.5 mg/mL |
| SD | 0.457 mg/mL |

The results from laboratory 2 are more consistent when the assays are completed at one time rather than over 4 months. (Many factors might lead to variability over time. Reagents or samples might slowly degrade, instruments may drift or be replaced, personnel might change, etc.)

4. a. **Subject 1: SD = 0.150 mg/L** **Subject 2: SD ≈ 0.141 mg/L**
**Subject 3: SD ≈ 0.096 mg/L**
b. **Pooled mean ≈ 96.6 mg/L**

5. $\overline{X} \approx 7.16$
**SD ≈ 0.0269**
Given the consistency of these values and the fact that the instrument used to test the buffer was known to be properly working, we can be reasonably confident that the pH of this lot of buffer is about 7.16. This lot of buffer would need to be rejected.

6.

| | Sample 1 | Sample 2 | Sample 3 |
|---|---|---|---|
| $\bar{X}$ | ≈ 1.3 μg/m$^3$ | ≈ 2.2 μg/m$^3$ | 1.6 μg/m$^3$ |
| **SD** | ≈ 0.10 μg/m$^3$ | ≈ 0.12 μg/m$^3$ | 0.10 μg/m$^3$ |

Pooled sample $\bar{X}$ **1.7 μg/m$^3$**
SD **0.42 μg/m$^3$**

As we might expect, the SD is higher for the pooled data since we would expect more variation among samples taken on different occasions than when an individual sample is tested three times. This is because many conditions (such as temperature, humidity, personnel, equipment) can vary from one day to another, leading to variability in results.

7. a. The RSD is ~1.55% which, when rounded, is 2% and is higher than the 1% specification.
   b. This does not necessarily indicate any problem with the spectrophotometer because biological samples are often not homogeneous and are often not stable. Therefore, with biological materials, variability is more likely to be due to the sample than to the instrument.

# Statistics and Graphical Methods of Describing Data

20



## 20.1 USING BAR GRAPHS TO REPRESENT DATA

The previous two statistics chapters introduced calculations (such as the mean and standard deviation) that are used to organize and describe data. This chapter introduces complementary graphical methods to display data. We also introduce frequency distributions in this chapter.

A **bar graph**, also called a **bar chart**, is a familiar and easily understandable graphical method to *portray data using rectangular bars.* This type of graph usually compares two or more different categories. Most often the categories are shown on the X-axis and their values for the variable of interest are shown on the Y-axis, although this is not always the case. Figure 20.1 provides an example of a bar graph.

DOI: 10.1201/9780429282744-24

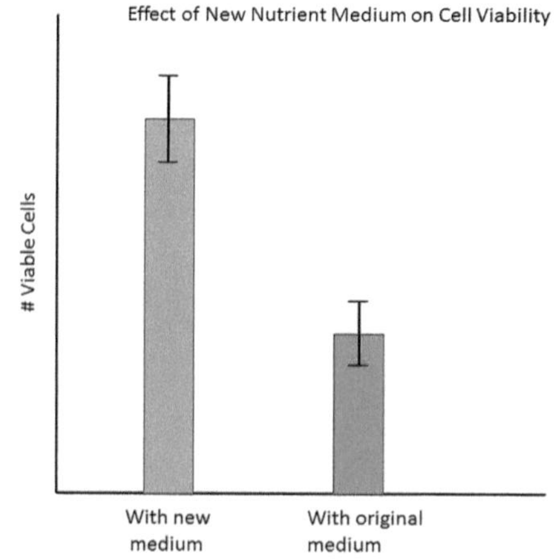


**FIGURE 20.1** Example of a bar graph. Two categories are compared in this graph: viability of cells with a new nutrient medium and viability of cells with an original nutrient medium. This graph suggests that the new medium improves the viability of the cells. The caption for this graph should indicate what the error bars represent. For example, the error bars might indicate the standard deviation of results obtained when the two media were tested in multiple experiments.

## 20.2 THINKING ABOUT VARIABILITY IN EXPERIMENTAL WORK

Let us use bar graphs to illustrate a point about interpreting the results of experimental work. Suppose a beginning researcher was investigating the effect of a drug compound on cell response. The beginning researcher performed an experiment five times with two groups of cells: half of the cells received the experimental compound and the other half did not. In each experiment, the researcher measured the response of the treated cells and of the untreated cells. After the five experiments were completed, the researcher calculated the average response for each of the two groups. The researcher plotted the results on the bar graph shown in Figure 20.2. The heights of the two bars represent the average results for treated and untreated cells based on the results of the five repeated experiments. It might appear from this graph that the drug had some effect because the bar for the treated cells is higher than for the untreated cells.

However, let us further assume this beginning researcher did not use good pipetting technique, and so the volumes of the drug compound measured varied from experiment to experiment. Maybe other factors were also uncontrolled, such as the pH of the reagents, the amounts of salts added to the cell's nutrient medium, and the maintenance of instruments used for analysis. As a result of all these factors, the variability from experiment to experiment was high. In Figure 20.3a, brackets are added to the graph to indicate the dispersion of the

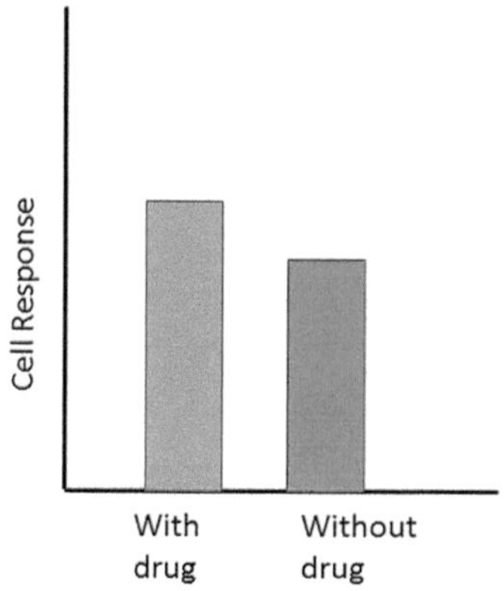


**FIGURE 20.2** Experimental results from a series of five runs comparing cells treated with an experimental drug compound to cells that were untreated. The heights of the two bars represent the average cell response for each of the two groups when a series of five experiments were performed.

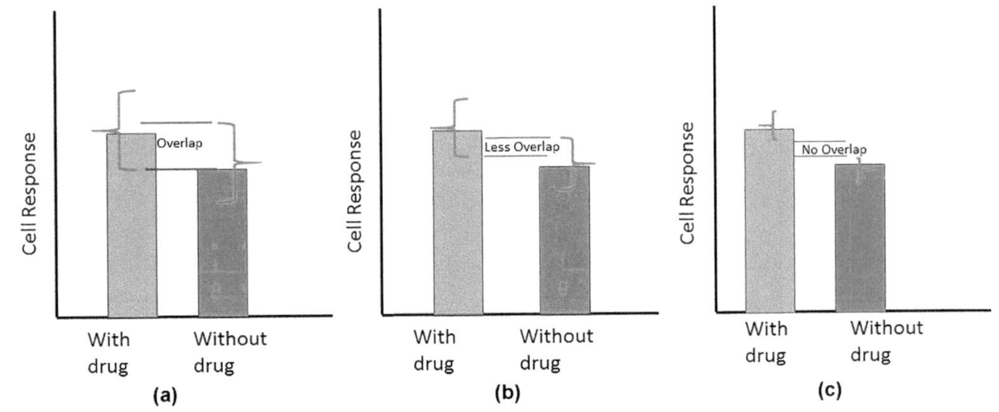


**FIGURE 20.3** Experimental results from a series of five runs comparing cells treated with an experimental drug compound to cells that were untreated. The brackets indicate the range of values that were observed in the five runs. (a) There was considerable variability in the techniques used by the experimenter, resulting in a wide range of experimental results. With so much variability, it is impossible to determine if the drug had any effect. (b) There is less overlap in results of this series of experiments, but it is still difficult to tell if the drug had a meaningful effect. (c) This time there is no overlap in the experimental results, and it would be possible to apply further statistical methods to evaluate whether the drug had a meaningful effect on the cells.

data. The brackets represent the range of the data. (Note that the brackets are *not* error bars, as were described in Section 19.5.) Observe in Figure 20.3a that the range is so wide that, in some runs of the experiment, the results for cells not treated with the experimental drug overlap with the results obtained for treated cells. In the presence of so much experimental variability, it is impossible to determine whether the drug compound of interest had any effect.

Next, suppose that the beginning researcher's technique improves somewhat and the variability due to poor pipetting and other mistakes is reduced, as shown in Figure 20.3b. The range of experimental results, as indicated by the brackets, is reduced, but there is still overlap between the results for treated and untreated cells. In the presence of this much variability in experimental technique, it is still difficult to see if the drug had any effect. The researcher tried again, and the results are shown in Figure 20.3c. This time there is no overlap in the brackets. At this point, when the extraneous sources of variability have been reduced, a difference between the treated and untreated cells can be observed. Other statistical methods (outside the scope of this text) can be applied to see if the difference in the mean values between the treated and untreated cells is likely due to an effect of the experimental drug. Thus, it is evident that researchers must always strive to eliminate, as much as possible, variability that is due to poor measurements, improperly maintained instruments, improperly prepared, reagents, and so on.

As a final note about this example, observe in Figure 20.3c that there is still some variability in the experimental results, as indicated by the brackets. This is expected – biological systems exhibit inherent variability. For example, we would not expect all people to respond in the same way to a drug. Similarly, we would not expect all cultures of cells to respond in exactly the same way.

## 20.3 DESCRIBING DATA: FREQUENCY DISTRIBUTIONS AND GRAPHICAL METHODS

Consider a set of data consisting of the times it took 10 students to run a race (in minutes):

***9.6, 10.3, 9.1, 7.5, 10.9, 7.2, 6.9, 9.5, 8.7, 8.1***

These values are displayed graphically in a **dot diagram** or **dot plot**, Figure 20.4. A dot diagram is a simple graphical technique used to illustrate small data sets. In this technique,

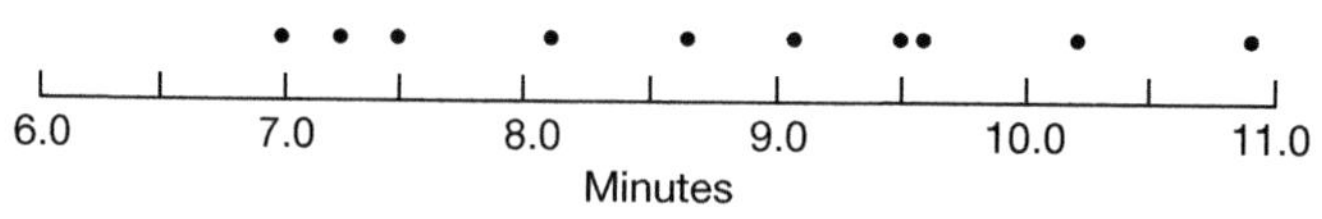


**FIGURE 20.4** A data set displayed as a dot diagram.

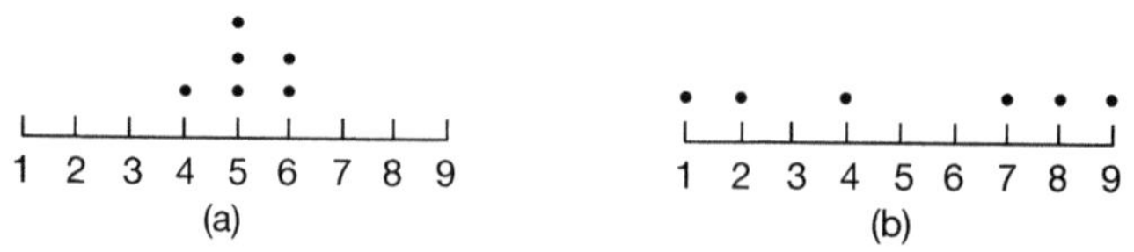


**FIGURE 20.5** Dot diagrams illustrate dispersion. (a) Less dispersed data. The dots are clumped between 4 and 6, a relatively narrow range compared to (b). (b) More dispersed data with a wider range of values than in (a).

each data value is represented as a dot. The dot is situated above the corresponding value on an axis. With a dot diagram it is easy to see the general location and center of the data. The dispersion of data is also evident in such diagrams, Figure 20.5.

A dot diagram is difficult to construct and interpret when a data set is large and there are other graphical methods that are more useful for organizing and displaying large sets of data. For example, suppose a researcher collects data for the weights of a number of field mice, Table 20.1. An informative way to tabulate these data is to list them by frequency, where the frequency *in this case is the number of times a particular value is observed.* Table 20.2 shows the values for the mouse weights and the frequency at which each value occurs.

When the mouse data were collected, they were rounded so that a mouse recorded as 19 g actually might have weighed anywhere between 18.5 g and just under 19.5 g. Weight is a continuous variable, for example, a mouse might weigh 19.0 g or 20.0 g – or anything in between. Therefore, the frequency distribution table could be rewritten with the weights shown as a range or interval, Table 20.3.

Observe in Tables 20.2 and 20.3 that the values for mouse weights have a pattern. Most of the mice have weights in the middle of the range, a few are heavier than average, a few are lighter, Figure 20.6. The term **distribution** *refers to the pattern of variation for a given variable.* It is important to be aware of the patterns or distributions that emerge when data are organized by frequency.

The frequency distribution in Tables 20.2 and 20.3 can be illustrated graphically as a **frequency histogram**, Figure 20.7 (See page 364.). A frequency histogram is a graph where the X-axis is the relevant units of measurement, in this example, weight in grams. The Y-axis is the frequency of occurrence of a particular value in a given interval or class. For example,

**TABLE 20.1 The Weights of 175 Field Mice (Rounded to the Nearest Gram)**

| | | | | | | | | | | | | |
|---|---|---|---|---|---|---|---|---|---|---|---|---|
| 21 | 23 | 22 | 19 | 22 | 20 | 24 | 22 | 19 | 24 | 27 | 20 | 21 |
| 22 | 20 | 22 | 24 | 24 | 21 | 25 | 19 | 21 | 20 | 23 | 25 | 22 |
| 19 | 17 | 20 | 20 | 21 | 25 | 21 | 22 | 27 | 22 | 19 | 22 | 23 |
| 22 | 25 | 22 | 24 | 23 | 20 | 21 | 22 | 23 | 21 | 24 | 19 | 21 |
| 22 | 22 | 25 | 22 | 23 | 20 | 23 | 22 | 22 | 26 | 21 | 24 | 23 |
| 21 | 25 | 20 | 23 | 20 | 21 | 24 | 23 | 18 | 20 | 23 | 21 | 22 |
| 22 | 25 | 21 | 23 | 22 | 24 | 20 | 21 | 23 | 21 | 19 | 21 | 24 |
| 20 | 22 | 23 | 20 | 22 | 19 | 22 | 24 | 20 | 25 | 21 | 22 | 22 |
| 24 | 21 | 22 | 23 | 25 | 21 | 19 | 19 | 21 | 23 | 22 | 22 | 24 |
| 21 | 23 | 22 | 23 | 28 | 20 | 23 | 26 | 21 | 22 | 24 | 20 | 21 |
| 23 | 20 | 22 | 23 | 21 | 19 | 20 | 26 | 22 | 20 | 21 | 22 | 23 |
| 24 | 20 | 21 | 23 | 22 | 24 | 21 | 23 | 22 | 24 | 21 | 22 | 24 |
| 20 | 22 | 21 | 23 | 26 | 21 | 22 | 23 | 24 | 21 | 23 | 20 | 20 |
| 21 | 25 | 22 | 20 | 22 | 21 | | | | | | | |

**TABLE 20.2 Frequency Distribution Table of the Weights of Field Mice**

| Weight (g) | Frequency |
|---|---|
| 17 | 1 |
| 18 | 1 |
| 19 | 11 |
| 20 | 25 |
| 21 | 34 |
| 22 | 40 |
| 23 | 27 |
| 24 | 19 |
| 25 | 10 |
| 26 | 4 |
| 27 | 2 |
| 28 | 1 |

**TABLE 20.3 Frequency Distribution Table of the Weights of Field Mice, with Range**

| Weight (g) | Frequency |
|---|---|
| 16.5–17.4 | 1 |
| 17.5–18.4 | 1 |
| 18.5–19.4 | 11 |
| 19.5–20.4 | 25 |
| 20.5–21.4 | 34 |
| 21.5–22.4 | 40 |
| 22.5–23.4 | 27 |
| 23.5–24.4 | 19 |
| 24.5–25.4 | 10 |
| 25.5–26.4 | 4 |
| 26.5–27.4 | 2 |
| 27.5–28.4 | 1 |

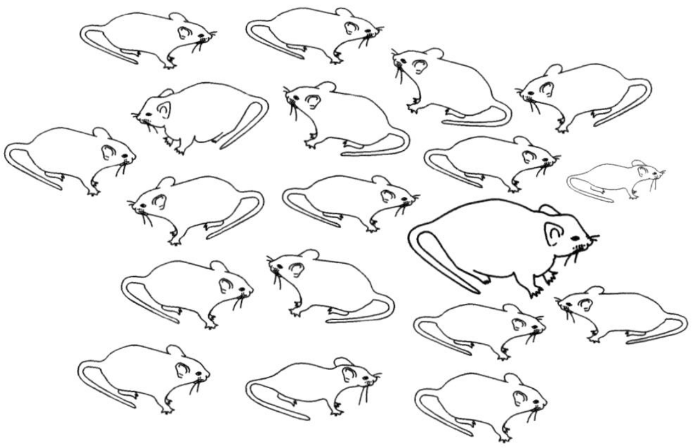

**FIGURE 20.6** Distribution of mouse weights. Most mice are of about average weight, some are a bit heavier, some a bit lighter than others. A few mice are substantially heavier, and a few mice are substantially lighter than average.

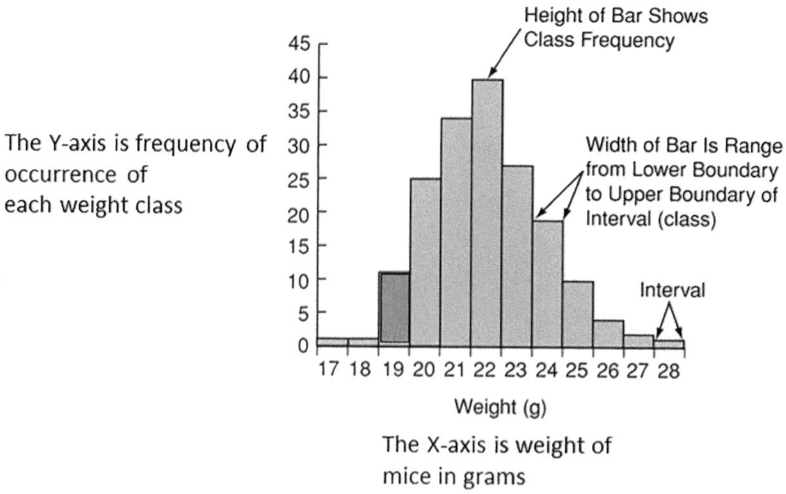


**FIGURE 20.7** Frequency histogram for mouse data.

11 mice are recorded as weighing between 18.5 and 19.4 g. The values for these 11 mice are illustrated as a bar, which is highlighted in orange in the graph above. You can think of the histogram bars as representing individual mice piled up on the number line with each individual sitting above its score.

The mouse data shown above were divided into **classes** or **intervals** of weight, each of which was 1 g in width; for example, 18.5 to just under 19.5 is an interval that is one unit wide. It is not necessary, however, to use intervals that are always one unit wide. If the data span a wide range, you will want to group the values into intervals that are more than one unit in width. It is customary to divide the data into between 5 and 20 intervals, or classes, each of which is the same width. This is illustrated in the following example problem.

A frequency histogram superficially looks much like a bar graph, such as the one in Figure 20.1. However, the two are actually quite different. A frequency histogram shows the

**Example Problem:**

The following are heights in cm of a common prairie aster measured from one field.

a. Prepare a frequency distribution table. To do this, you will need to divide the data into groups. Divide the data into 10–12 classes of equal size and assign each datum value to the proper class.
b. Plot these data as a frequency histogram

| | | | | | | | | | | | |
|---|---|---|---|---|---|---|---|---|---|---|---|
| 151 | 182 | 182 | 162 | 177 | 166 | 197 | 144 | 174 | 160 | 131 | 156 |
| 125 | 170 | 153 | 172 | 146 | 127 | 156 | 140 | 159 | 155 | 158 | 165 |
| 155 | 141 | 180 | 145 | 145 | 150 | 145 | 135 | 105 | 122 | 180 | 152 |
| 161 | 170 | 156 | 150 | 122 | 140 | 133 | 145 | 190 | 165 | 176 | 170 |
| 144 | 160 | 162 | 157 | 155 | 146 | 155 | 143 | 154 | 157 | 141 | 150 |
| 142 | 139 | 138 | 156 | 130 | 126 | 189 | 138 | 103 | 163 | 135 | 158 |
| 151 | 129 | 147 | 153 | 150 | 140 | 146 | 138 | 154 | 138 | 179 | 165 |
| 142 | 140 | 141 | 160 | 125 | 156 | 145 | 159 | 147 | 155 | 189 | 195 |
| 140 | 141 | 160 | 156 | | | | | | | | |

*Answer:*

n = 100 range = 197 to 103 cm, or 94 cm

**FREQUENCY DISTRIBUTION TABLE: (divided into 11 intervals of equal width)**

| Interval | Frequency |
|---|---|
| 100–108 | 2 |
| 109–117 | 0 |
| 118–126 | 5 |
| 127–135 | 7 |
| 136–144 | 19 |
| 145–153 | 19 |
| 154–162 | 26 |
| 163–171 | 8 |
| 172–180 | 7 |
| 181–189 | 4 |
| 190–198 | 3 |

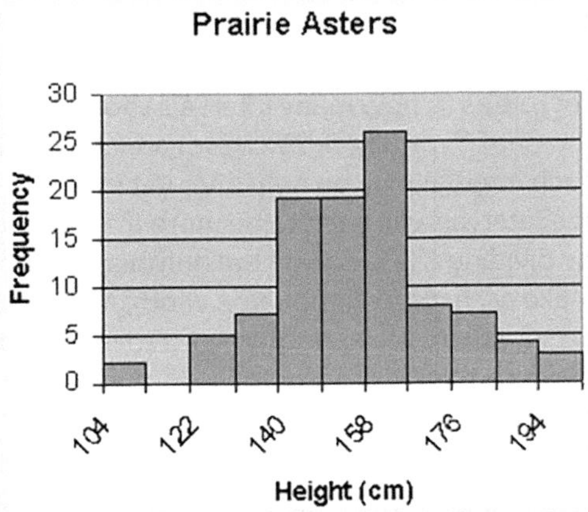


Observe that the intervals in the frequency distribution table are continuous; even if there are no values in an interval, it is still shown on the distribution table and the graph. For example, there are no plants in the interval between 109 and 117, but this class is shown anyway. Also note that each interval is of the same width.

*distribution* of a single variable, for example, height or weight as in Figure 20.7. In contrast, a bar graph is used to *compare two or more categories to one another*, as in Figure 20.1. Remember not to confuse one type of graph with the other.

It is possible to construct a frequency histogram for any data set consisting of the values for a single variable. The procedure for doing so is given in Box 20.1.

**BOX 20.1 Constructing a Frequency Histogram**

Step 1. Divide the range of the data into intervals, or classes. (See notes below.)

Step 2. Count how many observations occurred in each interval.

Step 3. Prepare a frequency table showing each interval and the frequency with which a value fell into that interval.

Step 4. Label the axes of a graph with the intervals on the X-axis and the frequency on the Y-axis.

Step 5. Draw bars where the height of a bar corresponds to the frequency with which a value occurred. Center the bars above the midpoint of the class interval. For example, if an interval is from 0-9 cm, then the bar should be centered at 4.5 cm.

Notes. Some general rules:

a. To divide data into intervals, find the highest and lowest value in the data; this gives you the range. Select the number of classes (intervals) desired. There is no set rule as to how many intervals should be chosen; this will vary depending on the data. Typically, 5–20 classes are used. (If the range of the data is small, then each interval may be only one unit in width. But if the data range is wider, then the intervals will need to be more than one unit.) Find the width of each interval by dividing the range by the number of classes and rounding up.
b. Make each interval the same width, for example, 0–9.9, 10.0–19.9, 20.0–29.9, etc.
c. Be sure there are enough classes to include all the data.
d. Make the classes continuous; do not skip an interval because none of the data fall into it.
e. **Continuous data** *can take any value.* For example, height and time are continuous. A prairie aster might be 100 or 101 cm, or any height in between. **Discrete data**, in contrast, *can only take on certain values.* For example, there might be 20 students in a class or 21, but not any value in between. When data are continuous, the bars on a histogram touch each other, as shown in Figure 20.7, and as shown for the prairie asters. When data are discrete, the bars should be drawn so they do not touch each other.

## 20.4 THE NORMAL FREQUENCY DISTRIBUTION

The same data that are shown in Figure 20.7 are also graphed in a slightly different form, as a **frequency polygon,** in Figure 20.8a. A frequency polygon does not use bars. Rather each class is represented as a single point. The point is placed halfway between the smaller and the larger limit for that class and the points are connected with lines. Figure 20.8a shows the distribution of weights for a sample of only 175 mice. If the weights of a great many laboratory mice were measured, it is likely that the frequency distribution would approximate a bell shape, or normal curve, Figure 20.8b. *The frequency distribution pattern that has a bell shape when graphed is called a* **normal distribution.**

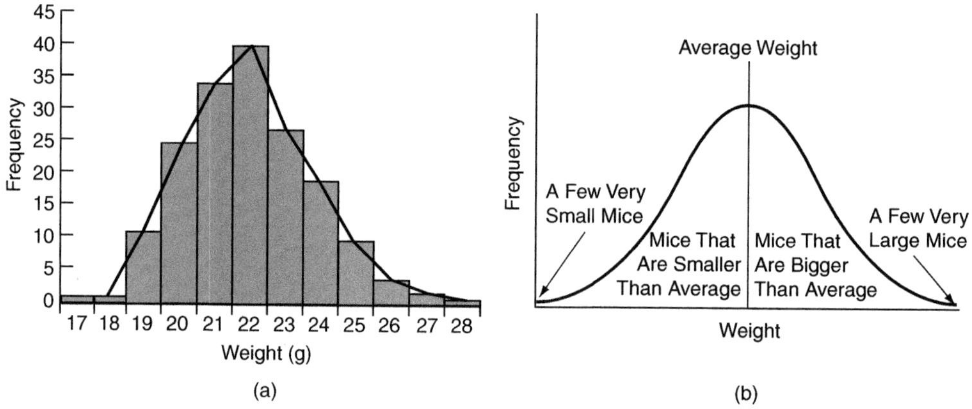


**FIGURE 20.8** The frequency distribution for mouse weights. (a) The weights of 175 mice are graphed both as a frequency histogram and frequency polygon. (b) If a frequency polygon were prepared for a great many mice, the shape of the plot would approach a bell shape. The peak in the center is the average weight. Most of the mice have weights somewhere in the middle of the plot, that is, are around average weight while a few mice are substantially heavier or lighter than average. This distribution pattern is called the normal distribution.

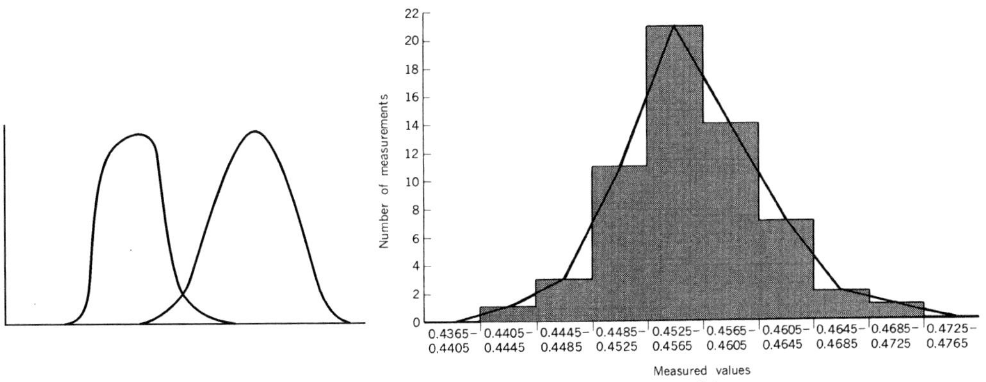


(a) (b)

**FIGURE 20.9** Examples of relationships that approximate a normal curve. (a) An example from chromatography, an analytical technique used to separate and detect various components in a mixture of compounds. Under ideal conditions, each compound appears on the chromatographic printout as an approximately normal curve. (b) The weights of a number of vials from the same batch. The vials vary in weight both because of variability in the manufacturing process and variability that is inherent in repeated measurements. The pattern of variation approximates a normal distribution. If more vials were weighed, we expect the pattern to be even closer to a normal curve.

There are many situations in nature and in the laboratory where the frequency distribution for a set of data approximates a normal curve, Figure 20.9. For example, the height of humans, the weight of animals, and measurements of the same object all tend to be normally distributed.

At this point, it is possible to relate calculated measures of central tendency and measures of dispersion to the graphical techniques in this chapter. The center of the peak of a perfect normal curve is the mean, median, and mode. Values are equally spread out on either side of that central high point, so the graph is symmetrical about the mean. Moreover, the width of the normal curve is related to the standard deviation, Figure 20.10. The more dispersed the data, the higher the value for the standard deviation and the wider the normal curve.

**Example Problem:**

A student weighs himself one morning 25 times on his bathroom scale. The resulting weight values (in pounds) are shown below.

a. Show these data in a frequency table and graphically.
b. Do these data appear to be approximately normally distributed?

| | | | | | | | | |
|---|---|---|---|---|---|---|---|---|
| 159 | 159 | 158 | 161 | 160 | 158 | 159 | 157 | 158 |
| 160 | 159 | 158 | 160 | 159 | 158 | 161 | 160 | 159 |
| 157 | 159 | 162 | 161 | 159 | 158 | 157 | | |

***Answer:***

a. These data can be readily summarized using six classes:

| Recorded Weight (lb) | Frequency |
|---|---|
| 157 | 3 |
| 158 | 6 |
| 159 | 8 |
| 160 | 4 |
| 161 | 3 |
| 162 | 1 |

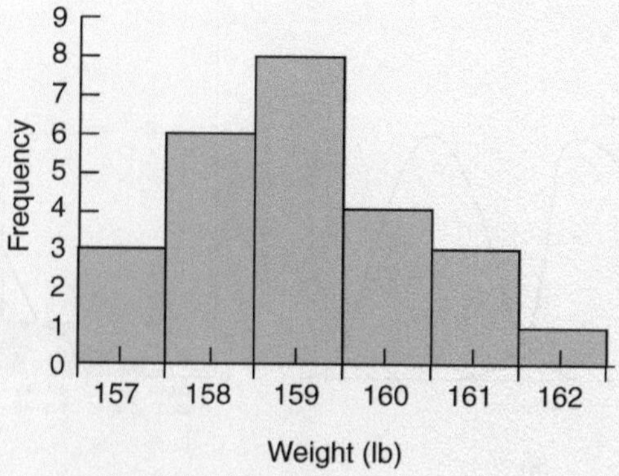

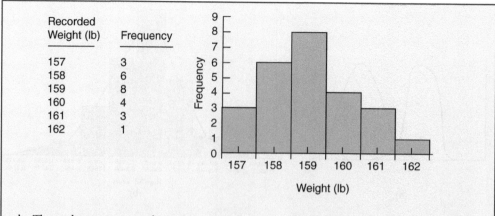

b. These data appear to be approximately normally distributed. In fact, it has been found that if a great many measurements of the same item are made, and if those measurements are made properly, then there is variation in the measurements that tends to be normally distributed.

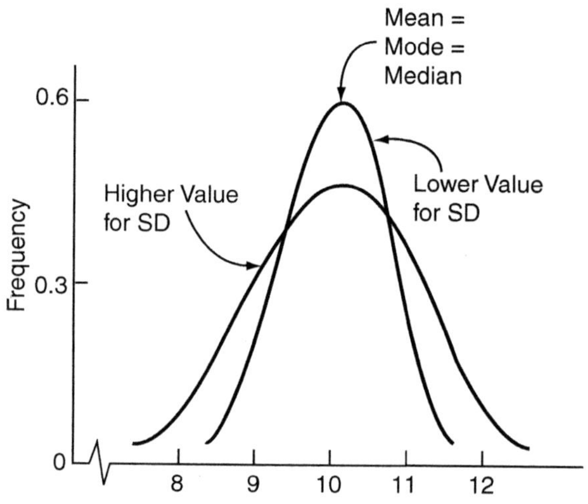


**FIGURE 20.10** The normal curve. When data are perfectly normally distributed, their mean, median, and mode all lie at the X-coordinate of the peak of the distribution plot. The standard deviation determines the width of the curve.

If we know that the pattern of variation for a variable is normally distributed, then we can make certain predictions about individuals. For example, consider a 20-year-old man, Robert Smith, who is from a large population of all 20-year-old men. Height in adults is a variable that is normally distributed. This allows us to predict that Robert is most likely about average height. He is equally likely to be either a bit taller or a bit shorter than average. He is unlikely to be substantially taller or shorter than average, though he might be.

Although data are commonly normally distributed, not all data have a normal distribution. For example, the frequency distribution of a set of data may be **skewed** *in which case the values tend to be clustered either above or below the mean*, Figure 20.11. The frequency distribution in Figure 20.12 is **bimodal** *which means that it has two peaks.* Note that when a distribution is not normal, the mean, the median, and the mode do not coincide.

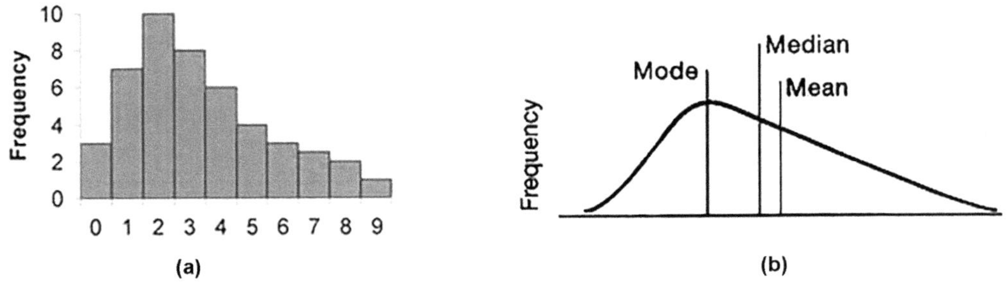


**FIGURE 20.11** Distributions that are skewed.

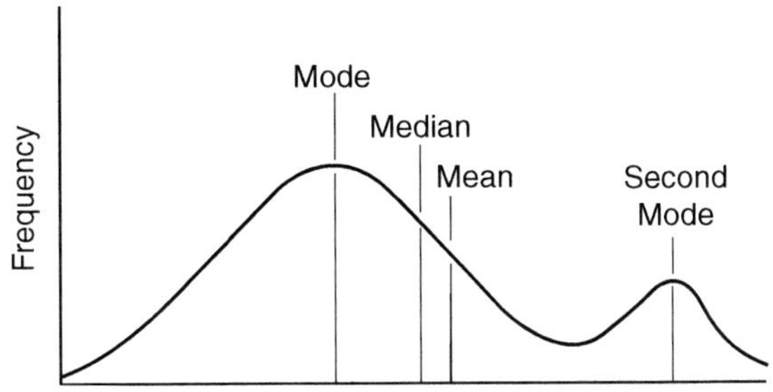


**FIGURE 20.12** A bimodal distribution.

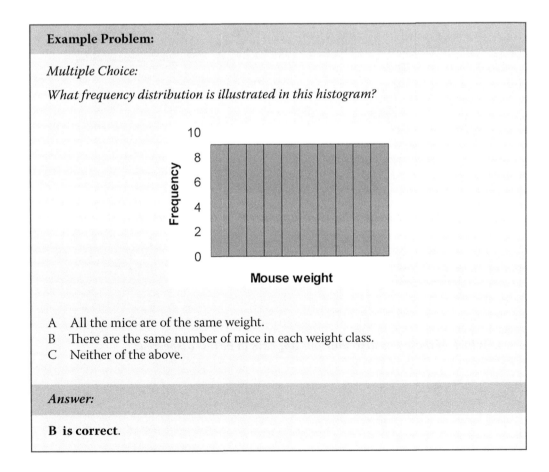

**Example Problem:**

*Multiple Choice:*

*What frequency distribution is illustrated in this histogram?*

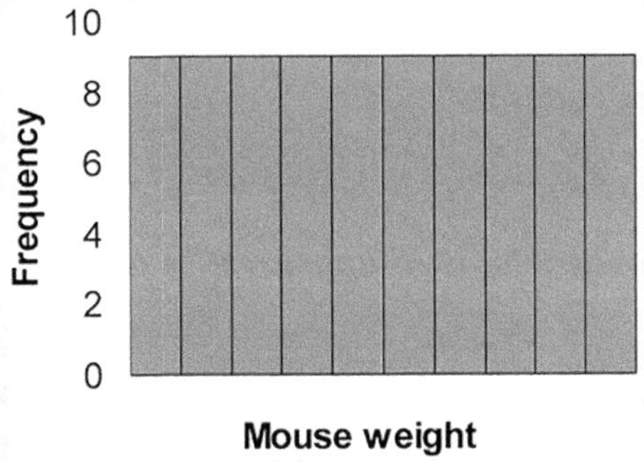


A All the mice are of the same weight.
B There are the same number of mice in each weight class.
C Neither of the above.

***Answer:***

**B is correct.**

## Practice Problems

1. ***For each of the three distributions below, estimate the mean and mode.***

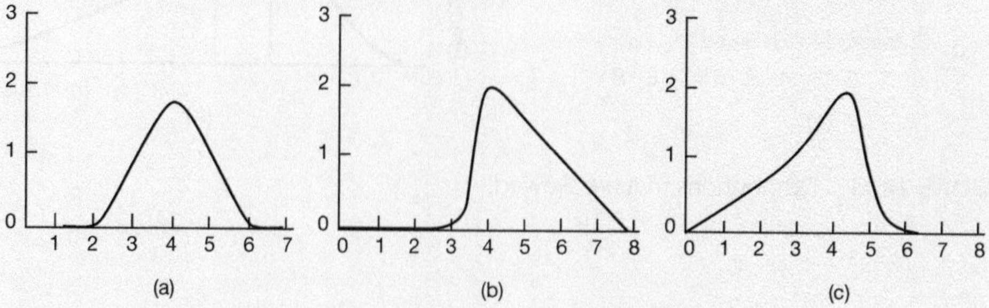


2. ***Which of the frequency histograms below most closely approximates a normal distribution? Which appears to be bimodal? Which appears skewed?***

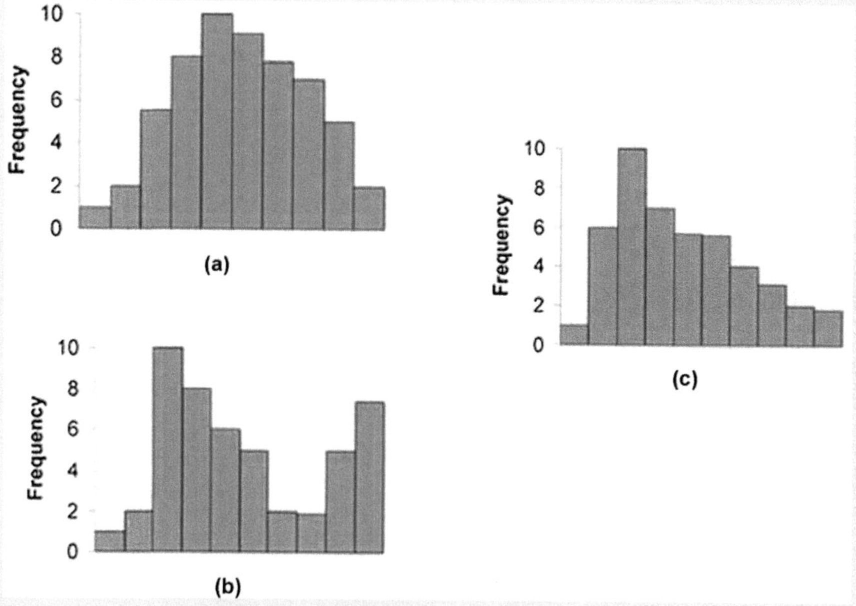


3. ***Which of these two distributions appears to be less dispersed?***

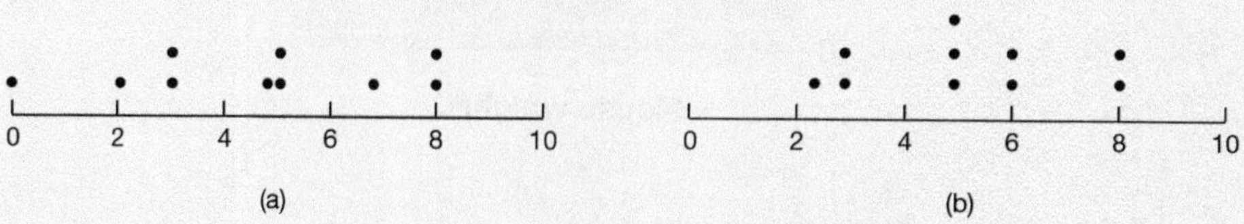


4. ***Which of these two distributions appears to be less dispersed?***

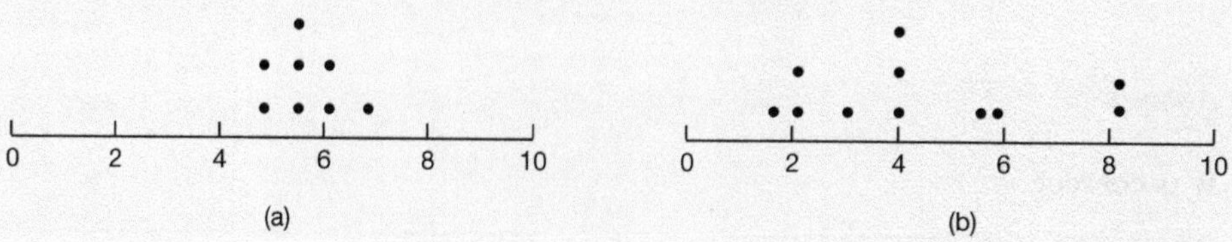

5. ***Which of these two distributions appears to be less dispersed?***

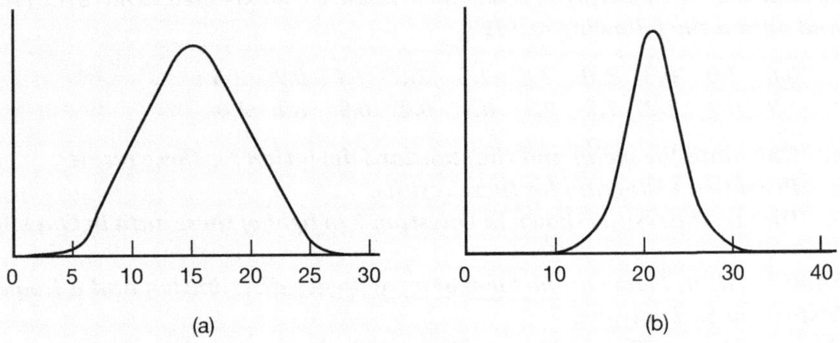


6. ***Which of these two distributions appears to be less dispersed?***

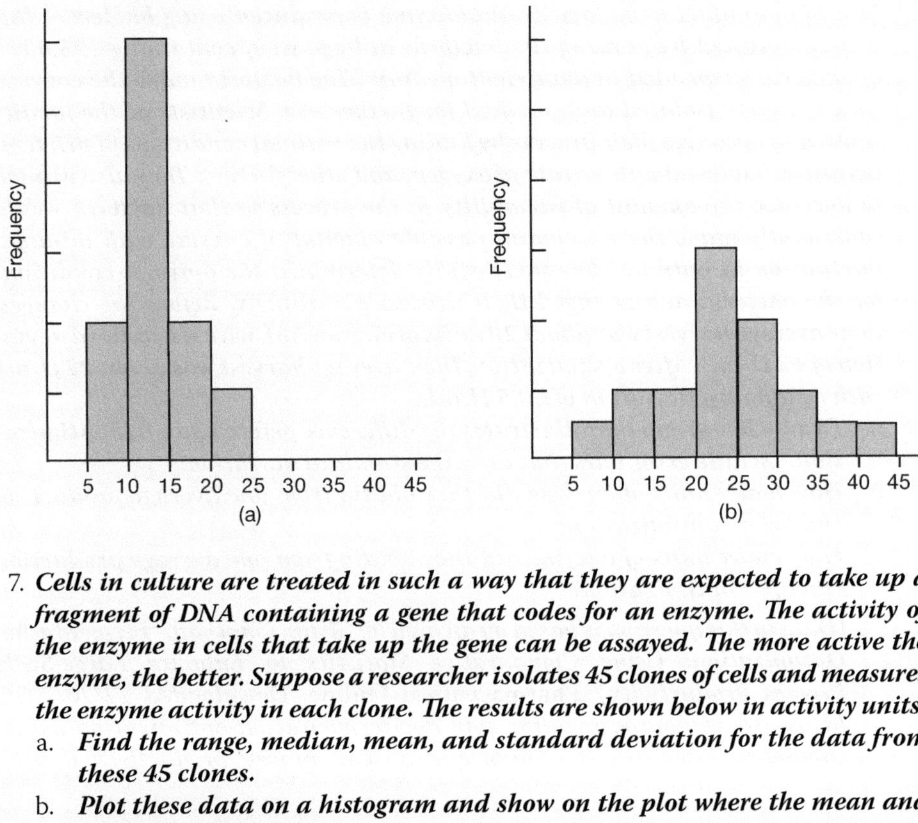


7. ***Cells in culture are treated in such a way that they are expected to take up a fragment of DNA containing a gene that codes for an enzyme. The activity of the enzyme in cells that take up the gene can be assayed. The more active the enzyme, the better. Suppose a researcher isolates 45 clones of cells and measures the enzyme activity in each clone. The results are shown below in activity units.***
   a. ***Find the range, median, mean, and standard deviation for the data from these 45 clones.***
   b. ***Plot these data on a histogram and show on the plot where the mean and median are located.***
   c. ***Do you think these cells have taken up the gene fragment containing the enzyme based on these data? Explain.***

| | | | | | | | | | |
|---|---|---|---|---|---|---|---|---|---|
| *10.4* | *12.2* | *12.0* | *9.1* | *5.8* | *3.2* | *9.8* | *10.1* | *13.0* | *2.1* |
| *9.8* | *10.1* | *1.5* | *7.8* | *5.6* | *2.3* | *9.8* | *10.2* | *9.1* | *12.3* |
| *10.1* | *12.3* | *14.2* | *15.1* | *13.6* | *12.1* | *10.8* | *9.2* | *8.9* | *12.4* |
| *11.0* | *13.1* | *8.9* | *9.4* | *10.2* | *11.3* | *12.8* | *9.0* | *8.6* | *12.3* |
| *12.0* | *2.1* | *0.4* | *10.6* | *13.0* | | | | | |

8. ***Suppose that the assay for enzyme activity (discussed in Question 7) is performed on cultured cells that have not been exposed to the DNA fragment and are not expected to have any enzyme activity at all. In this case, one would***

***expect to see little or no activity when performing the assay. You test this assumption on 20 cultured cell clones that are not expected to have the enzyme and obtain the following results:***

| | | | | | | | | | |
|---|---|---|---|---|---|---|---|---|---|
| *0.0* | *1.0* | *0.3* | *3.0* | *2.8* | *1.2* | *2.3* | *1.1* | *0.9* | *2.5* |
| *1.9* | *0.9* | *2.2* | *1.2* | *0.2* | *0.1* | *0.2* | *0.9* | *1.0* | *2.0* |

a. ***Calculate the mean and the standard deviation for these results.***
b. ***Prepare a histogram for these results.***
c. ***Discuss the results shown in Question 7 in light of these data in Question 8.***

9. ***Show the data below in the form of a frequency distribution and a frequency histogram and polygon.***
   *23 mg 28 mg 22 mg 23 mg 20 mg 19 mg 22 mg 24 mg 26 mg*
   *23 mg 23 mg 24 mg 21 mg 25 mg 24 mg 25 mg 21 mg*

10. ***In a biomanufacturing facility, an enzyme is produced using bacteria. This is accomplished by growing the bacteria in huge vats, containing 125,000 L of bacteria suspended in a nutrient medium. The bacteria make the enzyme, which is later isolated and purified for further use. Scientists at the facility wanted to optimize their process by finding the optimal conditions of pH, temperature, bacterial uptake rate of oxygen, and other factors. They also wanted to decrease the amount of variability in the process so that bacteria would consistently make the maximum possible amount of enzyme with minimal fluctuation in output. They successfully determined the optimal conditions for the bacteria and changed their process accordingly. Before the changes, their average harvest was about 20 units of enzyme/mL with a standard deviation of ±2 U/mL. After optimization, their average harvest was about 22 U/mL with a standard deviation of ±0.5 U/mL.***
    a. ***Draw a bar graph that illustrates the difference before and after optimization. Include error bars that are ± the standard deviation.***
    b. ***How many units of enzyme did they obtain from one average production run before optimization?***
    c. ***How many units of enzyme did they obtain from one average production run after optimization?***
    ***(Data in this question is based on an article: Glynn, Jonathan. "Fermentation Optimization: Using Comparative Statistics to Enhance Large-Scale Process Productivity."*** **Pharmaceutical Online.** ***Downloaded 12/20/2020. https://www.bioprocessonline.com/doc/fermentation-optimization-using-comparative-statistics-to-enhance-large-scale-process-productivity-0001)***

### *Answers*

1. a. Mean ≈ **4**, mode ≈ **4** b. Mean ≈ **5**, mode ≈ **4** c. Mean ≈ **3**, mode ≈ **4**

2. a. Normal b. Bimodal c. Skewed

3. **b** is less dispersed 4. **a** is less dispersed 5. About the same (observe X-axis values)

6. **a** is less dispersed

7. n = 45 $\overline{X}$ ≈ **9.55 activity units.** SD ≈ **3.60 activity units**

Range = 15.1 – 0.4 activity units = **14.7 activity units** Median = **10.1 activity units**

**Frequency Table**

| Interval | Frequency |
|---|---|
| 0–0.9 | 1 |
| 1.0–1.9 | 1 |
| 2.0–2.9 | 3 |
| 3.0–3.9 | 1 |
| 4.0–4.9 | 0 |
| 5.0–5.9 | 2 |
| 6.0–6.9 | 0 |
| 7.0–7.9 | 1 |
| 8.0–8.9 | 3 |
| 9.0–9.9 | 8 |
| 10.0–10.9 | 8 |
| 11.0–11.9 | 2 |
| 12.0–12.9 | 9 |
| 13.0–13.9 | 4 |
| 14.0–14.9 | 1 |
| 15.0–15.9 | 1 |

b.

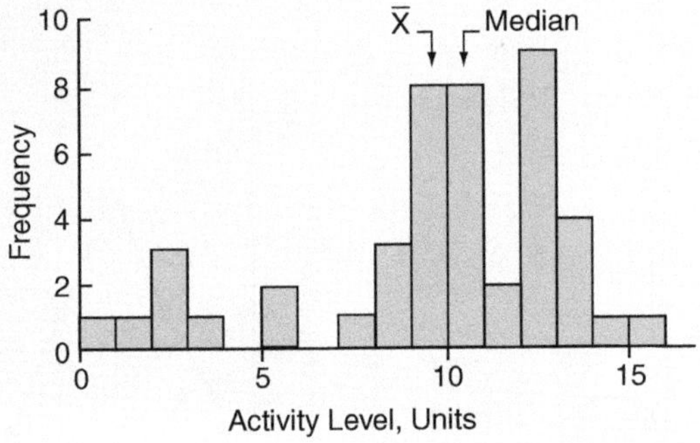


c. Based on just this information, we cannot tell whether the DNA fragment was taken up since we do not know what level of enzyme activity exists in cells that have not been exposed to the fragment.

8. a. $\bar{X} \approx$ **1.29 activity units SD ≈ 0.932 activity units**

| Interval | Frequency |
|---|---|
| 0–0.4 | 5 |
| 0.5–0.9 | 3 |
| 1.0–1.4 | 5 |
| 1.5–1.9 | 1 |
| 2.0–2.4 | 3 |
| 2.5–2.9 | 2 |
| 3.0–3.4 | 1 |

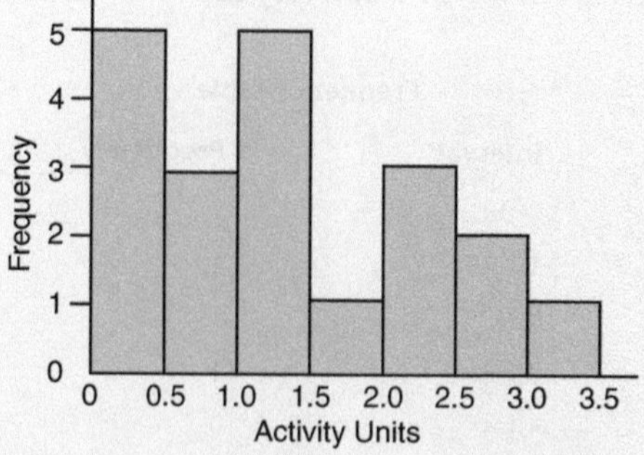


c. There is variation both in the group exposed to the DNA fragment and in the group not exposed. Using this assay, there is a low level of activity exhibited even in clones not exposed to the DNA fragment. However, the mean enzyme activity of the two groups is clearly different. Also, graphically, there is the suggestion that the clones that were exposed to the DNA fell into two categories: (1) those with higher levels of activity and (2) those with lower levels, similar to clones that were not exposed to the DNA. Based on these observations, it appears that some of the exposed cells took up the DNA and some did not. This hypothesis could be investigated by further study.

9.

| Class | Frequency |
|---|---|
| 19–20 | 2 |
| 21–22 | 4 |
| 23–24 | 7 |
| 25–26 | 3 |
| 27–28 | 1 |

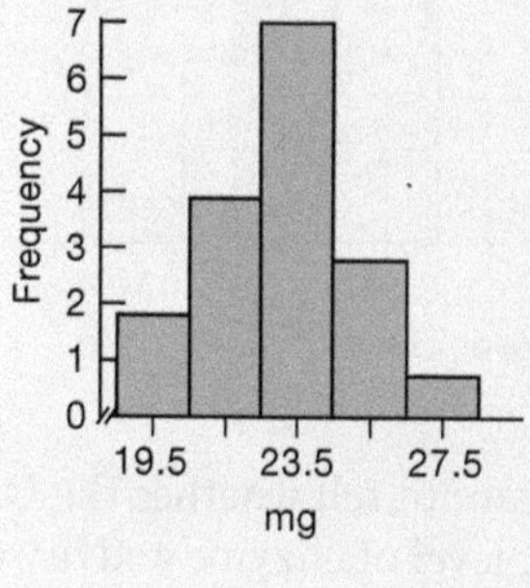


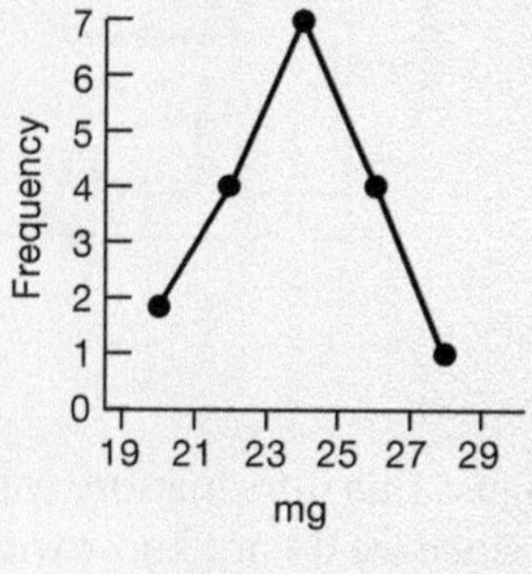


10. a.

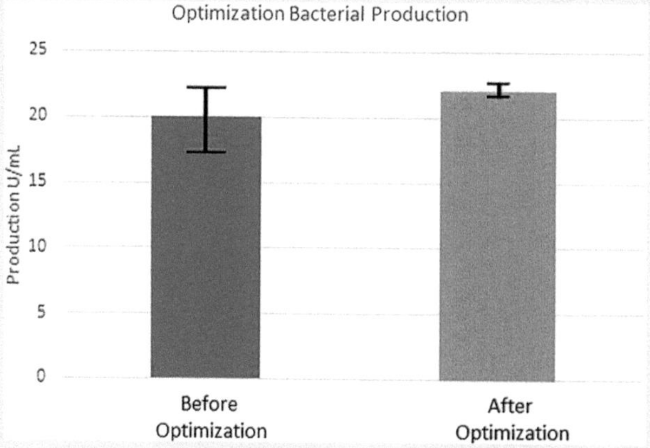

b. Before optimization, they could obtain ≈ **2.50 x 109 U** of enzyme in one production run from a 125,000 L vat.
c. After optimization, they could obtain ≈ **2.75 x 109 U** of enzyme in one production run from a 125,000 L vat. This seems like a minor difference, but if you subtract $2.50 \times 10^9$ U from $2.75 \times 10^9$ U, you will see that after optimization they obtained $2.50 \times 10^8$ U more enzyme than before – which is a significant amount of product.

## 20.5 THE RELATIONSHIP BETWEEN NORMAL DISTRIBUTION AND STANDARD DEVIATION

The normal distribution is extremely important in interpreting and understanding data. Therefore, we will consider some of the features of this distribution in more detail.

The area under any normal curve, by definition, is equal to 100% or 1.0. The center of the peak of a normal curve is the mean. The normal curve is symmetrical; half of the area under the normal curve lies to the right of the mean and half lies to the left of the mean, Figure 20.13.

Figure 20.14 shows four normal probability distributions. The overall pattern of the four curves is the same; each has a peak centered at the mean. Each curve is symmetrical, so that half its area lies to the left of the mean and half to the right; however, the four curves are not identical. Three of the four distributions have different means; therefore, the curves lie at

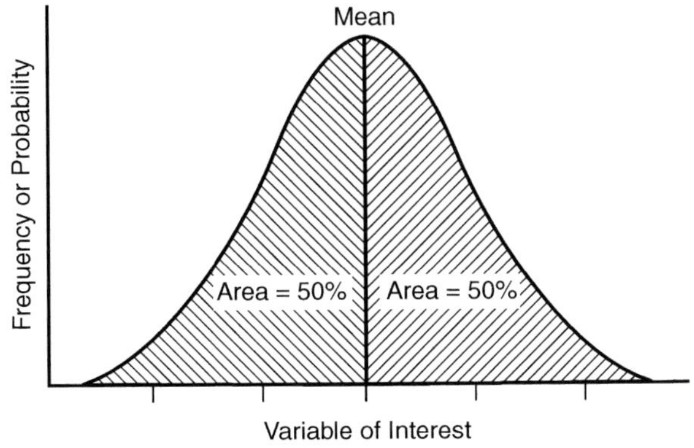


**FIGURE 20.13** The normal curve. The center of the peak is the mean. The variable of interest is plotted on the X-axis, either probability or frequency is on the Y-axis. The normal curve is symmetrical; half its area lies to the left of the mean; half lies to the right.

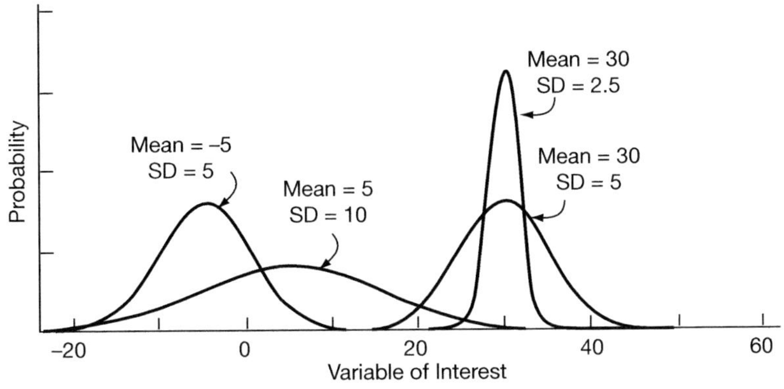


**FIGURE 20.14** The patterns of four normal distributions having different means and different standard deviations. The mean locates the center of the curve along the X-axis. The standard deviation determines how wide or narrow the curve is.

different locations along the X-axis. The curves also differ in width or we could say in their spread. Those with smaller standard deviations are narrower than those with larger standard deviations. Every normal curve is thus described by two characteristics:

1. The mean, which locates the center (or peak) of the curve along the X-axis.
2. The standard deviation, which determines how "fat" or "thin" the curve appears.

The normal curve in Figure 20.15 shows the distribution of heights of men in the United States. Observe that this plot is "marked off" in terms of the standard deviation. The mean height for the population is about 175 cm and the standard deviation is about 7.6 cm. The mean +1 standard deviation equals 175 cm + 7.6 cm = 182.6 cm. The mean −1 standard deviation is 167.4 cm. Observe the location of these two points on the graph. The mean height +2 standard deviations is 190.2 cm and the mean −2 standard deviations is 159.8 cm. Observe these values on the graph and also the location of the mean ± 3 standard deviations.

A graph labeled in terms of standard deviations from the mean can be constructed for any set of data that is approximately normally distributed. There is a certain pattern that is always true of such plots, Figure 20.16. The pattern is such that about 68% of the area under the normal curve lies in the section between the mean +1 standard deviation and the mean − 1 standard deviation. About 95.4% of the total area under the curve lies in the section between the mean + 2 standard deviation and the mean − 2 standard deviation. About 99.7% of the total area under the curve lies in the section between the mean + 3 standard deviation and the mean − 3 standard deviation. The pattern shown in Figure 20.16 is consistent for any normal curve, regardless of how spread out the curve is or the value for the mean.

The relationship between the area under a normal curve and the approximate number of standard deviations from the mean is summarized in tabular form in Table 20.4.

So far, the significance of this discussion of standard deviation and the normal curve may seem obscure; however, it is actually of great practical significance.

1. When a variable is normally distributed, the standard deviation tells us the percent of individuals whose measurements are within a certain range. For example, height in humans is a normally distributed variable; therefore, we know that about 68% of all values measured for height will fall within 1 standard deviation on either side of the mean, as shown in Figure 20.17.
2. When a variable is normally distributed, the mean and the standard deviation can help us determine the probability of obtaining a particular value if a single member of the population is randomly chosen. For example, if a man is picked randomly, there is a 68% probability that his height will be in the range of the mean ± 1 standard deviation.

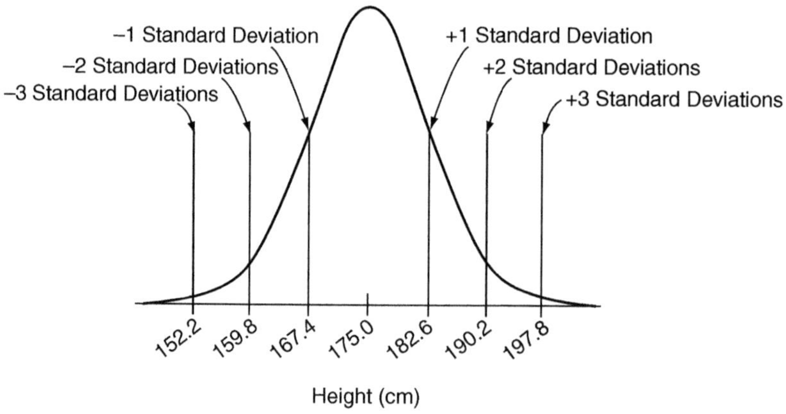


**FIGURE 20.15** The normal curve subdivided in terms of the standard deviation. The frequency distribution for the height of men in the United States in terms of the mean and the standard deviation. (The mean = 175.0 cm; standard deviation = 7.6 cm.)

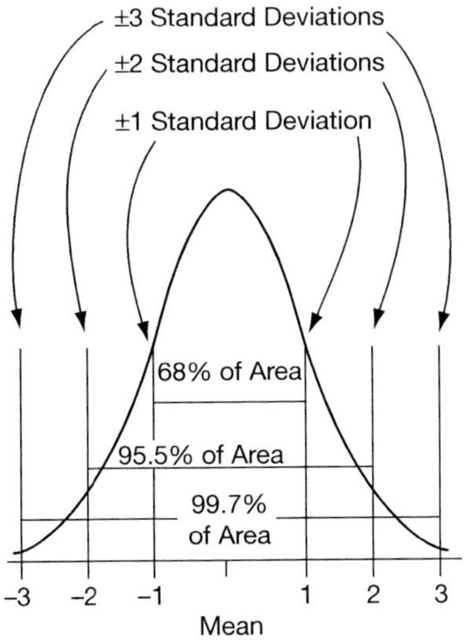


**FIGURE 20.16** The relationship between standard deviation and area under the normal curve. For any normal distribution, about 68% of the area under the curve lies within ±1 standard deviation from the mean; about 95.4% of the area under the curve lies within ±2 standard deviations from the mean; about 99.7% of the area lies within ±3 standard deviations from the mean.

**TABLE 20.4 The Relationship between the Area under a Normal Curve and the Approximate Number of Standard Deviations from the Mean**

| Standard Deviations | Approximate Area Under the Curve (%) |
|---|---|
| ± 1.0 | 68 |
| ± 2.0 | 95 |
| ± 2.6 | 99 |
| ± 3.0 | 99.7 |

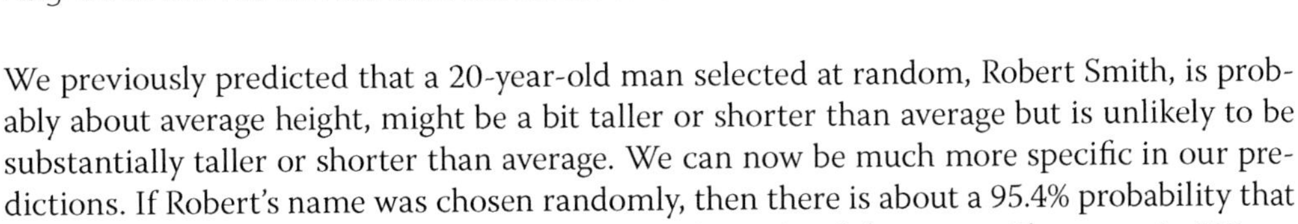


**FIGURE 20.17** Men's height and the normal distribution. About 68% of all men are of a height that falls within 1 standard deviation on either side of the mean. About 95% of men are of a height that falls within 2 standard deviations on either side of the mean.

We previously predicted that a 20-year-old man selected at random, Robert Smith, is probably about average height, might be a bit taller or shorter than average but is unlikely to be substantially taller or shorter than average. We can now be much more specific in our predictions. If Robert's name was chosen randomly, then there is about a 95.4% probability that his height is within 2 standard deviations on either side of the mean. The mean is 175 cm, so there is a 95.4% probability that he is between 159.8 and 190.2 cm tall. If we predict the height of a randomly chosen man to be between 159.8 and 190.2 cm, then, about 4.6% of the time, we expect to be wrong, but about 95.4% of the time we expect to be right. Thus, when data are normally distributed, knowing the mean and standard deviation enables us to make predictions and assign them a certain probability of being correct. We can generalize to say that: **Statistics** provides tools that enable us to make numerical statements and predictions in the presence of chance and variability. Statistics gives answers that are not expressed as "right" or "wrong"; rather, they are expressed in terms of probability.

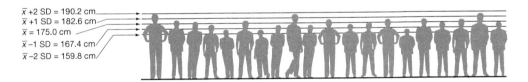

**Example Problem**

For this problem, use the values in Table 20.4.

a. What percent of the area under a perfect normal curve lies between the mean and the mean+1 standard deviation, as shown in the shaded area?

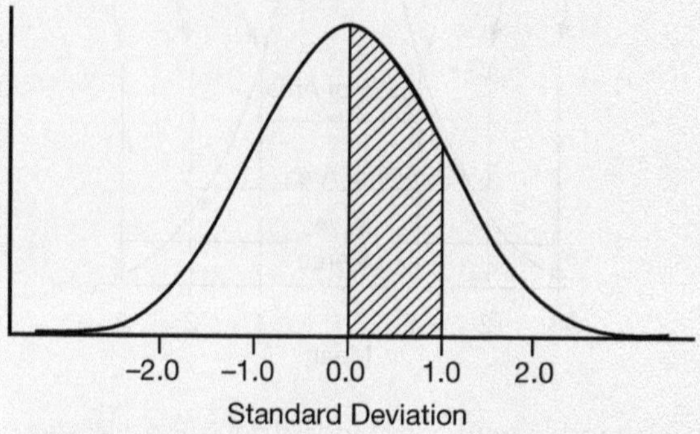


(a)

b. What percent of the area under a perfect normal curve lies in the shaded section in this graph?

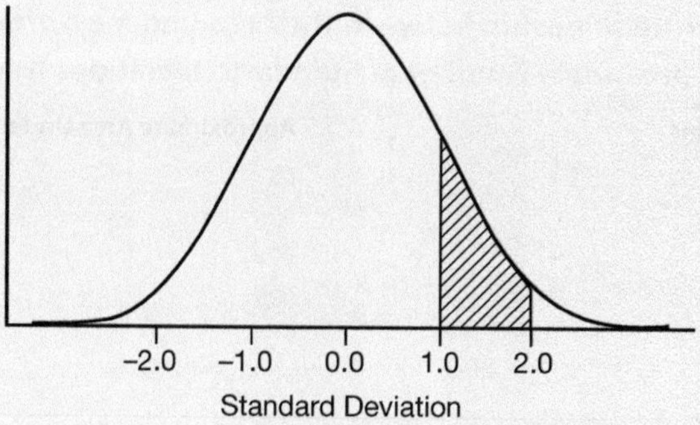


(b)

c. What percent of the area under a perfect normal curve lies in the section shown in this graph?

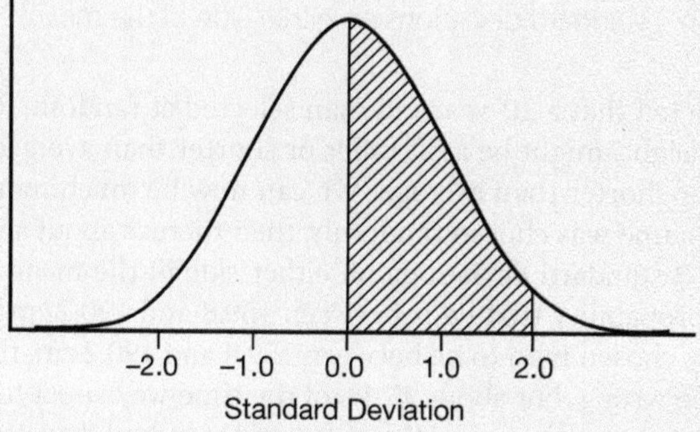


(c)

*Answer:*

Using the values from Table 20.4:

a. About **34%** of the area lies between the mean and+1 standard deviation.
b. About **13.5%** of the area lies between +1 and +2 standard deviations.
c. The area under the curve that lies between the mean and 2 standard deviations is about **47.5%**.

**Example Problem**

The average for US women's height is about 163 cm and the standard deviation is about 6.4 cm. Assuming that women's height is normally distributed:

a. What is the probability that a woman selected at random will have a height between 156.6 and 169.4 cm?
b. What is the probability that a woman selected at random will have a height between 150.2 and 175.8 cm?
c. What percent of women have heights between 143.8 and 182.2 cm?
d. Show the distribution of women's heights graphically.

*Answer:*

a. This is the range of the mean±1 standard deviation (163 cm±6.4 cm). We know that about **68%** of all values can be expected to fall within this range, so there is about a **68%** chance that a woman selected at random will be in this range.
b. This is the range of the mean±2 standard deviations (163 cm±12.8 cm). There is therefore about a **95%** chance that a randomly selected woman will fall in this range.
c. This is the range of the mean±3 standard deviations (163 cm±19.2 cm). About **99.7%** of women will have heights in this range.
d.

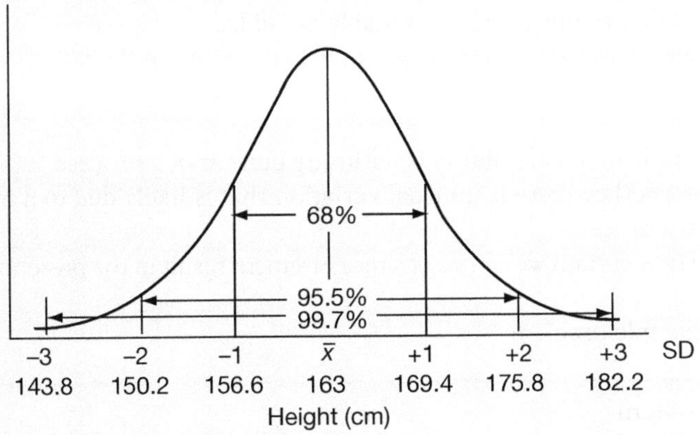

**Example Problem**

The height of adult males is normally distributed with a mean of 175 cm and a standard deviation of 7.6 cm.

a. About what percent of men are taller than 190.2 cm?
b. About what percent of men are shorter than 159.8 cm?

*Answer:*

Roughly 95% of adult men have heights within 2 standard deviations of the mean. This means that a total of about 5% of men are either taller than 190.2 cm or shorter than 159.8 cm. We expect, therefore, that about **2.5%** of men will be taller than 190.2 cm and about **2.5%** of men will be shorter than 159.8 cm.

## 20.6 STATISTICS AND CONTROLLING PRODUCT QUALITY

There are many applications of the ideas discussed so far in this chapter. This section focuses on the application of these principles to the area of ensuring product quality.

It might seem that products made by the same process – or samples of product from the same batch, or measurements of the same sample – ought to be identical. In fact, manufacturers must strive to reduce variability so that products are consistently of high quality. Similarly, as introduced early in this chapter, it is important that researchers identify and reduce factors that cause variability.

Variability is reduced through the development and consistent use of standard procedures, rigorous attention to the quality of solutions and reagents, careful instrument maintenance programs, and so on. In practice, however, even when good practices are implemented, there is always some variability in results. This is partly because there is variability inherent in any process. In addition, measurements vary, even repeated measurements of a single characteristic of a single item. In fact, if there is no variability in a set of measurements relating to a product, then there is likely to be a malfunction or a lack of sensitivity in the system. For example, if the activity of an enzyme product is measured in 10 different vials from a single batch or if the amount of a drug is measured in 25 tablets, then there will inevitably be some variability in the results if a very sensitive detection system is used. The goal is to reduce this variability as much as is reasonably possible.

Statistics provides important tools that can help to maintain the quality of products in the face of this inevitable variability. Statistical tools can be used to:

- determine how much variability is naturally present in a process
- determine whether there is unusual variation that is likely due to a malfunction or problem in a process
- determine how certain we can be of a measurement result in the presence of variability.

Consider this example problem:

**Example Problem**

A technician is responsible for purifying an enzyme product made by fermentation. During the purification process, he checks the amount of protein present. The results of six such measurements made during typical runs were (in grams):

23.5, 31.0, 24.9, 26.7, 25.7, 21.0

One day the technician obtains a value of 15.3 g. Should he be concerned by this value? Another day the technician obtains a value of 32.1 g. Is this value a cause for concern?

*Answer:*

Let us begin by looking at these values in an intuitive way. The six typical values appear to hover around about 25 g±about 5 g. A value of 15.3 g is quite a bit lower than the other values; it is around 10 g below the approximate mean. In contrast, the value 32.1 is not as far from the mean and may therefore be less of a cause for concern.

Let us now apply statistical reasoning to this problem. The six measurements that were made during normal runs are assumed to represent values obtained when the purification process was working properly. The mean for these six values is 25.5 g and their standard deviation is 3.36 g. Based on the normal distribution, we expect about 95% of the values to fall by chance within 2 SD of the mean. The range that includes two standard deviations is 18.8–32.2 g. Thus, based on the normal distribution, the value of 15.3 g is clearly unexpected on the basis of chance alone and is therefore cause for concern. The value of 32.1 g does not immediately suggest there is a problem (although, if it signals the beginning of an upward trend, there might in fact be a problem in the process).

Note that in this example the technician is applying statistical thinking to his everyday work. He is taking advantage of knowledge about normal distributions and about variability to identify potential problems.

## 20.7 CONTROL CHARTS

There is a common graphical quality control method that extends the reasoning demonstrated in the preceding example problem. This is the use of **control charts**. A control chart is a graph that is used to understand and monitor how a process changes over time. We introduce control charts with an example. A biotechnology company uses a fermentation process in which bacteria produce an enzyme that is sold for use in food processing. The pH of the bacterial broth must be controlled over time; otherwise, the pH tends to drop and production of the enzyme diminishes. A preliminary fermentation run that successfully produced enzyme was performed. The pH was monitored throughout the run and the resulting values are shown in Table 20.5.

**TABLE 20.5 The pH during Fermentation in Preliminary Studies**

| Time | pH |
|---|---|
| 0800 | 7.22 |
| 0830 | 7.13 |
| 0900 | 6.84 |
| 0930 | 6.93 |
| 1000 | 7.12 |
| 1030 | 7.33 |
| 1100 | 7.04 |
| 1130 | 6.79 |
| 1200 | 6.94 |
| 1230 | 7.03 |
| 1300 | 7.22 |

Let us assume that this fermentation process is tested more times and that the pattern of variability illustrated in Table 20.5 is characteristic of successful runs. The mean hovers around pH 7.05 and the SD is 0.17 pH units. When the company begins to produce this enzyme for sale, the pattern of pH variability should be similar to that observed in the preliminary, successful tests. In a production setting, ***a variable that has the same distribution over time is said to be* in statistical control *or is simply* in control**. Production processes should be consistent; therefore, having "in control" processes is critical.

A control chart is a graphical representation of the variability in a process over time. A control chart for the data in Table 20.5 is shown in Figure 20.18. When a control chart is constructed, a line is drawn across the chart at the mean (in this case, at pH 7.05). A second line is drawn at $\bar{x}+2$ SD (in this example, at 7.39). A third line is drawn on the graph at $\bar{x}-2$ SD (in this example at 6.71). Two more lines are drawn at $\bar{x}\pm3$ SD (pH 7.56 and 6.54, respectively).

The lines drawn across the control chart have names. The line at $\bar{x}-2$ SD is called the **lower warning limit, LWL.** The line at $\bar{x}+2$ SD is called the **upper warning limit, UWL.** The **lower control limit, LCL,** is $\bar{x}-3$ SD and the **upper control limit, UCL,** is $\bar{x}+3$ SD.

The use of control charts is based on the important assumption that the inherent variability in production processes is approximately normally distributed. Given that this is the case, then about 95% of all observations are expected to fall within ±2 SD of the mean; therefore, the warning limits define the range in which about 95% of all values are predicted to lie. One pH observation falling outside the warning limits is not a cause for concern because about 5% of the time, values may fall outside these limits simply because of chance variability. Two or more points outside the warning limits, however, may indicate a problem in the process. The control limits define the range in which 99.7% of all points should lie. The probability that an observation, by chance, would fall outside the control lines is only 3 in 1000. It is important, therefore, to find the problem if a value outside these action lines is obtained.

When a process is in control, its control chart has features illustrated in Figure 20.18. All the points are between the upper and lower warning limits. About half the points are above the mean and half below. It is also important that there is no trend where the points seem to be increasing in pH over time or decreasing in pH over time.

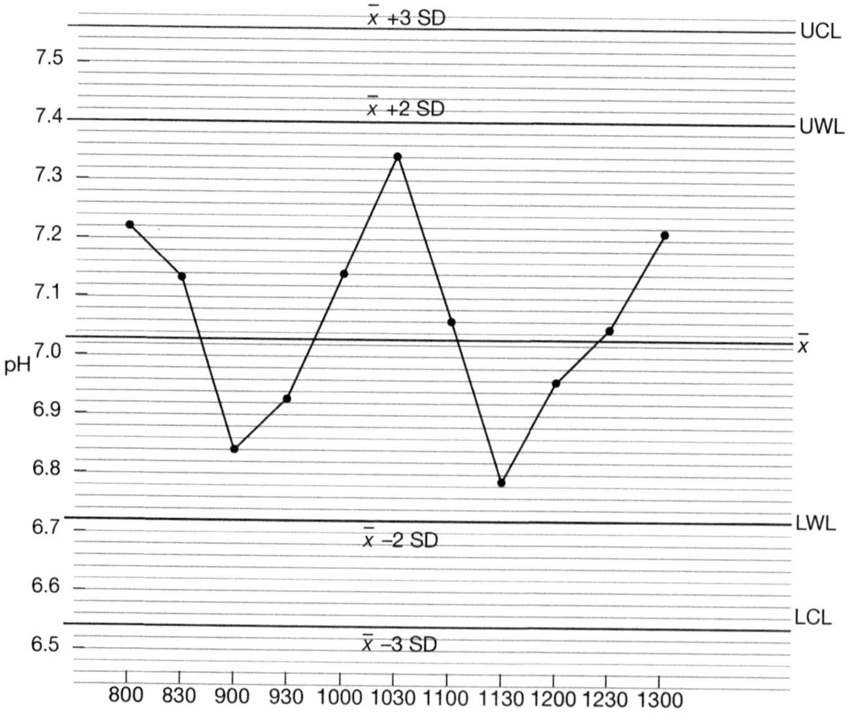


**FIGURE 20.18** A control chart for pH values from a fermentation run.

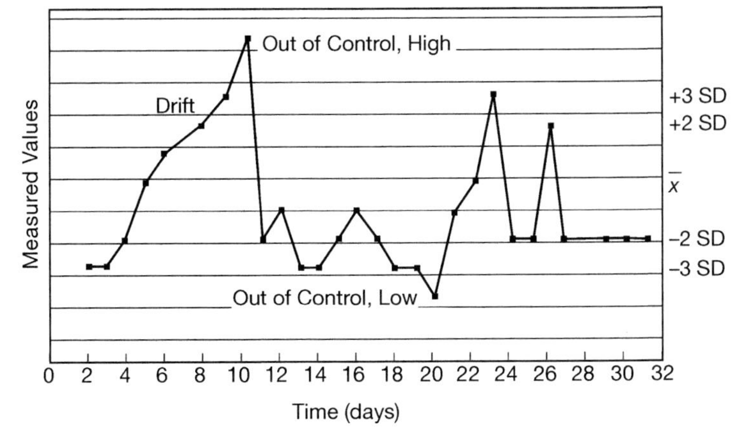


**FIGURE 20.19** A control chart illustrating possible problems.

A control chart helps operators distinguish between variation that is inherent in a process and variation that is due to a problem and should be investigated.

*A point that has a value much higher or much lower than the rest of the data is called an* **outlier.** For example, an aberrant pH value in the fermentation process might indicate that the bacteria are not growing properly and that enzyme production is likely to be adversely affected. In the real world, outliers may or may not signal that a process is out of control. Outliers are sometimes simply errors in how a test was performed. Errors might include, for example, improperly removing and preparing the sample, using a malfunctioning instrument, or inattentiveness on the part of the analyst. An aberrant pH reading might also be due to a malfunction in the pH meter – a testing error. In production settings, the initial investigation of an outlier looks at whether it is simply due to testing error.

Figure 20.19 is a control chart that illustrates several problems. On days 7–10, the process is showing an upward trend. At day 10, there is a high point that is outside the control limits. At day 20 there is a point that exceeds the LCL. When these types of problems are observed, the cause(s) of the deviations would be investigated.

**Example Problem**

The company that produces an enzyme by fermentation performs a production run. The following pH data are obtained. Prepare a control chart for these data. Is the process in control during this run? (Note that the expected pattern of variability in this process was determined in preliminary studies; therefore, use the same mean, standard deviation, UWL, LWL, UCL, and LCL as in Figure 20.18.)

| Time | pH |
|---|---|
| 0800 | 7.34 |
| 0830 | 7.22 |
| 0900 | 7.27 |
| 0930 | 6.88 |
| 1000 | 7.02 |
| 1030 | 7.01 |
| 1100 | 6.78 |
| 1130 | 6.88 |
| 1200 | 6.76 |
| 1230 | 6.57 |
| 1300 | 6.54 |

*Answer:*

The points for this run are plotted on a control chart. Observe that the data shows a downward trend. Moreover, the final point is close to the control limit. These data strongly suggest that the process is not in control.

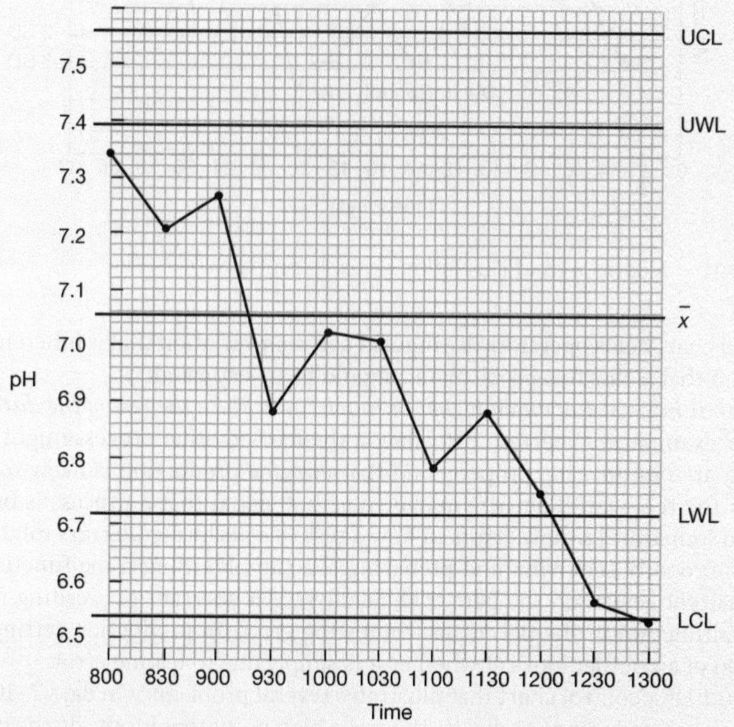


Control charts are a statistical tool based on an understanding of variability and the normal distribution. Control charts allow operators to quickly distinguish between inherent, expected variability in measurement values and variation that is caused by a problem in a process. As long as the values remain within the limits of expected variability, the process is considered to be in control and variation is assumed to be due to chance alone. If a value falls outside the range predicted by chance, or if the values begin to be consistently high or low, then there may be a problem in the production process that needs to be examined. There are many types and forms of control charts other than the one illustrated here. The basic purpose of a control chart is the same, however, regardless of the details of its construction.

**Practice Problems**

***Where applicable, use the values in Table 20.4 (see page 377).***

1. ***As a trouser manufacturer, you are interested in the average height of adult males in your town. You take a random sample of five male customers and find the mean to be 5 ft 10 in. and the standard deviation to be 3 in. How certain are you of the following statements and why?***
   a. ***The average height of the population is between 0 and 50 ft.***
   b. ***The average height of the population is between 4 and 7.5 ft.***
   c. ***The next new adult male customer will be between 5 ft 7 in and 6 ft 1 in.***
   d. ***The average height of the entire male population is 5 ft 10 in.***

2. ***The average for US women's height is about 163 cm and the standard deviation is about 6.4 cm. Assuming that women's height is normally distributed:***
   a. ***What is the probability that a woman selected at random will be shorter than 150.2 cm?***
   b. ***What is the probability that a woman selected at random will be taller than 169.4 cm?***

3. ***A pharmaceutical company finds that the average amount of drug in each vial is 110 µg with a standard deviation of 6.1 µg.***
   a. ***About what percent of all vials can be expected to have between 94.1 and 125.9 µg of drug?***
   b. ***What is the likelihood that a vial selected at random will have more than 122.2 µg of drug?***
   c. ***What percent of all the vials are expected to have a value between 103.9 and 116.1 µg?***
   d. ***Suppose 1,000 vials are checked. About how many of them would be predicted to have more than 125.9 µg?***

4. ***A technician customarily performs a certain assay. The results of eight typical assays are:***

   ***32.0 mg, 28.9 mg, 23.4 mg, 30.7 mg, 23.6 mg, 21.5 mg, 29.8 mg, 27.4 mg***
   a. ***If the technician obtains a value of 18.1 mg, should he be concerned? Base your answer on estimation without performing actual calculations.***
   b. ***Perform statistical calculations to determine whether the value 18.1 mg is out of the range of two standard deviations.***

5. ***A technician customarily counts the number of leaves on cloned plants. The results of nine such counts in successful experiments are:***

   ***75, 54, 55, 61, 71, 67, 51, 77, 71***
   a. ***If the technician obtains a count of 79, is this a cause for concern? Base your answer on estimation without performing actual calculations.***
   b. ***Perform statistical calculations to determine whether 79 leaves is out of the range of 2 SD.***

6. ***Examine this control chart. Discuss the points on March 22, April 15, May 31, and June 23.***

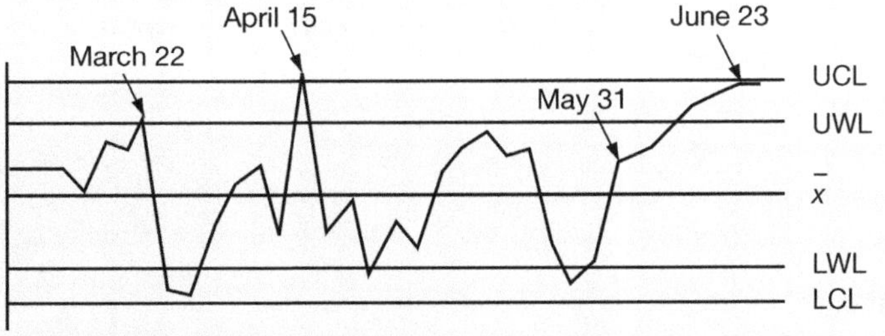


7. ***Suppose a biotechnology company is using bacteria to produce an antibiotic. During production of the drug, the pH of the bacterial broth must be adjusted so that it remains optimal; otherwise, production of the antibiotic diminishes. Preliminary studies were performed to determine the optimal pH. The results of a successful preliminary study are shown in the following table.***

| Time | pH |
|---|---|
| 0800 | 6.12 |
| 0830 | 5.13 |
| 0900 | 5.84 |
| 0930 | 6.53 |
| 1000 | 6.12 |
| 1030 | 6.23 |
| 1100 | 6.04 |
| 1130 | 5.79 |
| 1200 | 5.94 |
| 1230 | 6.03 |
| 1300 | 6.12 |

a. ***Calculate the mean pH and the SD.***
b. ***Construct a control chart with a central line, UWL, LWL, UCL, and LCL.***

***The enzyme goes into production and periodic samples of the broth are assayed for pH. The results are shown in the following table.***

| Time | pH |
|---|---|
| 0800 | 6.54 |
| 0830 | 6.12 |
| 0900 | 5.87 |
| 0930 | 5.18 |
| 1000 | 4.95 |
| 1030 | 4.89 |
| 1100 | 5.03 |
| 1130 | 5.43 |
| 1200 | 5.34 |
| 1230 | 5.37 |
| 1300 | 5.38 |

c. ***By simply observing these points, what can you say about the process?***
d. ***Plot these data on the control chart.***
e. ***Comment on the process; did it ever reach the warning level or action required levels?***

## *Answers*

1. a. **100%.**
   b. Very certain. Common sense is sufficient to know this.
   c. Based on the standard deviation of the sample, we would expect 68% of customers to be in this range; however, a sample of 5 is too small to draw firm conclusions.
   d. Not very certain due to the small sample size.

2. a. **2.5%** b. **16%**

3. a. **99%** b. **2.5%** c. **68%** d. **0.5%**

4. a. The average appears to be in the mid-twenties and hovers at around ±5. 18.1 mg is lower than any typical value. Yes, the technician should be concerned.
   b. Mean ≈ 27.16 mg, SD ≈ 3.87 mg. The mean − 2 SD is 19.4; therefore, 18.1 mg is outside the range of 2 SD and probably should be investigated.

5. a. The values appear to hover around 65 leaves, give or take about 10. It is difficult to tell whether 79 is a cause for concern although this value is higher than all the other values.
   b. Mean ≈ 64.7 leaves. The mean + 2 SD = 84.1; therefore, 79 does not appear to be unreasonable.

6. On several occasions, such as on March 22, the points lie outside the warning range; however, because later points are within the expected range, this is probably due to normal variation. The point on April 15 is out of the control range and therefore the process should be checked for problems. The points between May 31 and June 23 display an upward trend and June 23 is very close to the UWL. This pattern would likely cause the process to be checked.

7. a. Mean = **5.99 pH units**, SD ≈ **0.35 pH units.**
   b.

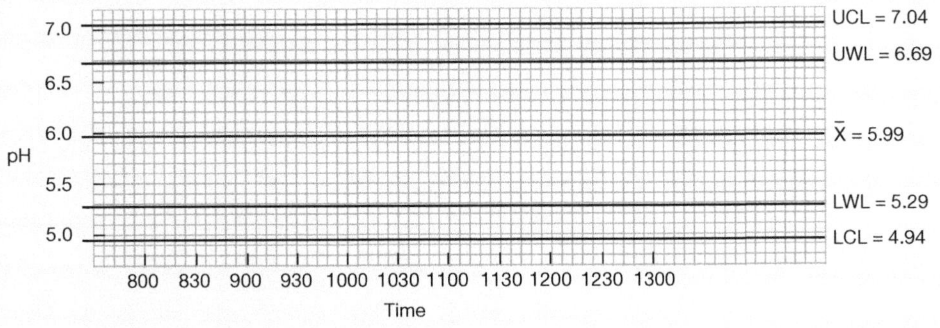


   c. The pH values tend to decline with time.
   d.

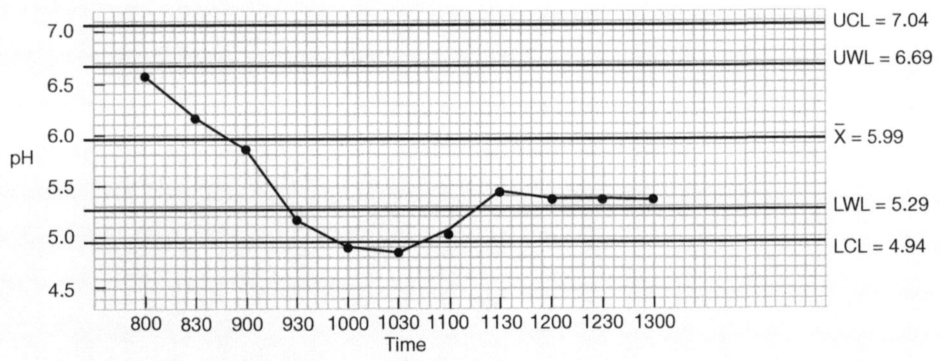


   e. This process tended downward from the beginning, eventually reaching the LCL. Action should have been taken at 1000 (and maybe it was) causing the pH to rise.

# V

# Biotechnology Applications

**Chapters in This Unit**



DOI: 10.1201/9780429282744-25

## INTRODUCTION

Something attracted you to biotechnology; otherwise, you would not be working through these math calculations. Perhaps you became interested in biotechnology because the science that underlies biotechnology is fascinating. Perhaps you became interested in biotechnology because you enjoy working in the laboratory performing molecular biology procedures, running experiments, or growing cells. So far in this text, we have not talked very much about molecular biology techniques, cell culture, or other topics that might be the ones that first attracted you to biotechnology. In this unit, we will turn our attention to these methodologies; that is, we will explore calculations involving cell culture, manipulation of genetic material, and isolation of proteins.

You will find that the math tools used in the calculations in this unit are the same math tools we have already discussed in this text. These tools include the following:

- Ratios and proportions are particularly important. Remember that concentration is a ratio. Cell density, as will be explored in Chapter 21, is also a ratio. When you see ratios, remember that proportional expressions are often a tool that you can use to solve problems.
- The $C_1V_1 = C_2V_2$ equation will also make a frequent appearance. This is because many biological solutions are prepared as concentrated stocks that must be diluted before use. The $C_1V_1 = C_2V_2$ equation is the main tool for this calculation task.
- Molecular biologists often work with extremely small amounts and concentrations of biological molecules. Therefore, you will encounter calculations involving metric prefixes that might be initially unfamiliar, such as micro-, nano-, and pico-.
- Calculations involving the preparation of biological solutions (as discussed in Chapters 12 and 13) are critically important in almost all molecular biology and cell culture procedures.

Thus, the calculation tools explored in earlier chapters will enable you to perform most of the routine calculations encountered in sophisticated molecular biology laboratories and biotechnology production settings.

Chapter 21 begins the unit by exploring common calculations associated with cell culture (growing cells in vessels outside of any organism). Chapters 23 and 24 introduce routine calculations associated with various molecular biology techniques, particularly those involving DNA or RNA. We devote two chapters (Chapters 24 and 25) to the important technique, the polymerase chain reaction (PCR). PCR is based on the exponential amplification of DNA and therefore takes us into calculations involving exponents and logarithms. However, we have already introduced these concepts in previous chapters, particularly Chapter 17, so the PCR calculations should feel familiar. Chapter 26 finishes the text by talking about proteins. People sometimes forget about proteins, but it is said that "DNA is the flash, but proteins are the cash." Proteins are the major products that biotechnology brings to the world, such as biopharmaceutical drugs to treat cancer, drugs to treat diabetes and other diseases, enzymes to perform useful tasks (like cleaning our laundry), and many other valuable materials. Proteins are not only important commercially, but they are also the molecules that do the work of our cells. It is because of proteins that we can move, think, and act. Understanding protein structure and function is the goal of many basic research laboratories. Thus, we end this text with protein-related calculations.

# Common Calculations Relating to Animal Cell Culture Techniques

21



## 21.1 INTRODUCTION

This chapter is about common calculations associated with animal cell culture. In **animal cell culture**, living cells derived from the tissue of multicellular animals are maintained in cell culture medium inside petri-style dishes, the wells of multi-well plates, flasks, or other vessels, Figures 21.1–21.3. Maintaining cells outside of an organism requires stringent conditions of bacterial sterility, appropriate nutrition, constant temperature, and the like. There

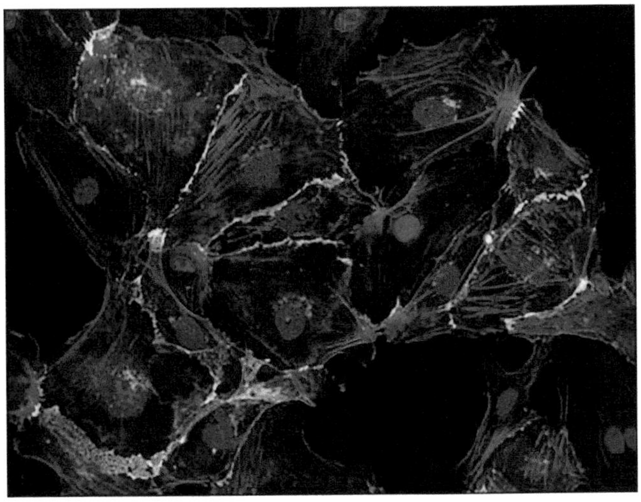

**FIGURE 21.1** Cultured cells viewed with a fluorescent light microscope. Cultured cells were stained to show their nuclei (blue), actin filaments that are involved in shape and motility (red), and a protein involved in developmental processes (green). (Illustration reproduced courtesy of Cell Signaling Technology, Inc. http://www.cellsignal.com)

DOI: 10.1201/9780429282744-26

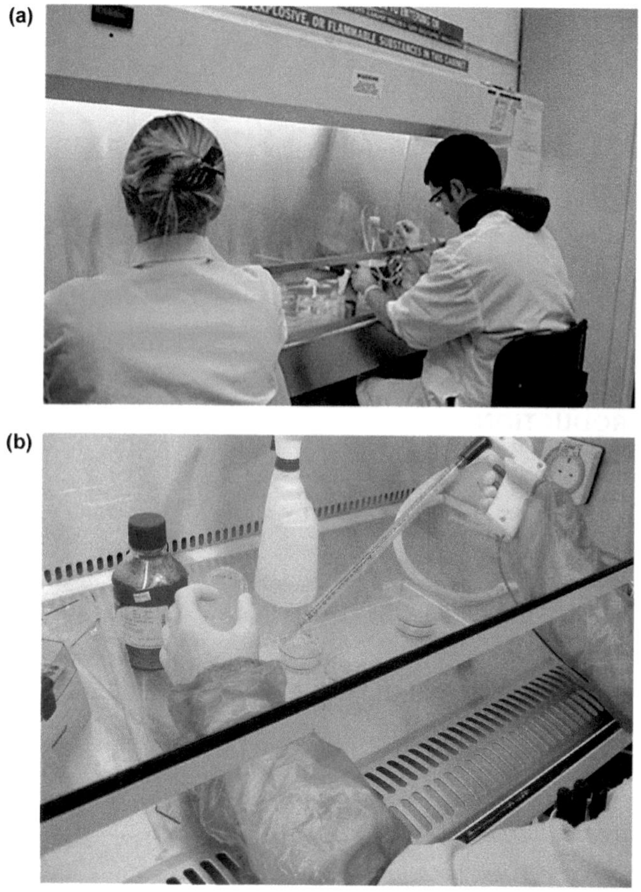


**FIGURE 21.2** Performing cell culture. Cultured cells are readily contaminated by stray microorganisms from the air, dust, surfaces, people, and so on. Therefore, cultured cells are manipulated within special hoods, as shown in (a), that provide an aseptic environment. The biologist in (b) is adding culture medium to cultured cells that have just been manipulated.

are a vast number of applications of cell culture, ranging from basic research into the intricacies of cellular function to the production of large quantities of commercially valuable drugs and enzymes.

Cultured cells grow by cell division: one cell divides to form two, the two divide to become four, and so on. As they divide and grow, the cells consume the nutrients in the culture medium, which is supplied and replenished by the cell culturist.

When cells are used as "factories" to make drugs and enzymes, they are usually grown in large vats, suspended in a nutrient medium (variously called growth medium, culture medium, or simply, medium). These vats may be relatively small, and hold a few liters of suspended cells, or several stories tall, holding thousands of liters of suspended cells. When animal cell lines are maintained in the laboratory for experimental purposes, the methods are somewhat different and generally are much smaller in scale. Cell culturists working in laboratories think in terms of milliliters, not liters. Although the calculations in this chapter are relevant in a production setting, this chapter is primarily concerned with laboratory-scale cell culture.

In a laboratory, cultured animal cells commonly are grown as a single cell layer in which each cell is moored by proteinaceous strands to the surface of their plastic or glass vessel. Culture medium is added to the vessel to nourish the cells. These moored cells are said to be adherent. Adherent cells spread across the surface of their vessel as they divide. *When the surface of the vessel is entirely covered by a layer of cells, the cells are said to be* **confluent.** At this point the cells stop growing, and it is necessary to **subculture** or **split** them. This process is also called **passaging** the cells. Subculturing involves:

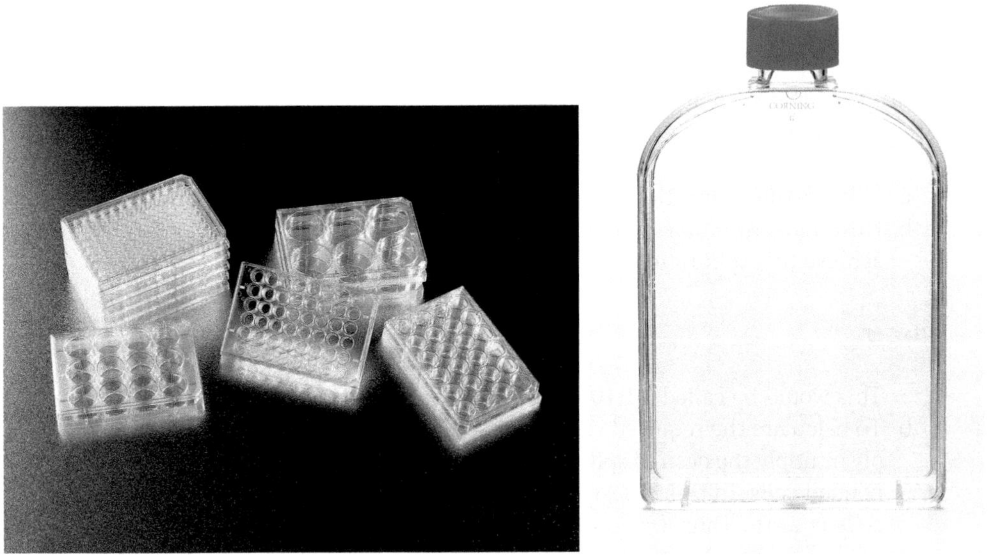

(a) (b)

**FIGURE 21.3** Vessels for culturing cells in a laboratory. (a) These culture plates contain wells; each well can contain a certain volume of growth medium with suspended cells. There are 6-well plates, 12-well plates, and so on. (b) This type of culture vessel is called a T-flask. T-flasks come in various sizes. For example, a T-75 flask has an interior surface area of 75 $cm^2$ to which cells can adhere and grow. (Copyright 2019 Corning Incorporated.)

- breaking the bonds that attach the cells to the culture vessel, usually by adding enzymes (often trypsin) that break the protein attachments.
- removing the cells from the dish, also called "harvesting."
- suspending the cells in fresh cell culture medium.
- dividing the cells into new vessels so they are present at a lower cell density.

The new vessels are said to be **seeded** with, or **inoculated** with, cells. The new vessels are put back into an incubator where the cells reattach to the vessel surfaces, begin dividing, and again reach confluency. When the cells again become confluent, they must be subcultured another time, and the cycle continues. If all goes well, it is possible to start out with relatively few cells and, after a series of passages, eventually have a great many cells.

## 21.2 SIMPLE CELL SPLITS

Consider a common situation where adherent cells reach confluency every few days, and the contents of one vessel are split into three to ten new vessels. The number of new culture vessels required depends on the type of cells, their growth characteristics, the number of cells ultimately desired, and other factors.

At this point, it is important to talk about terminology. If, for example, all the cells from one vessel are *equally divided into three new vessels*, they are, in essence, diluted. Using the dilution terminology introduced in Chapter 14, **this is a 1/3 split ratio**. Each new vessel will now contain one third (1/3) of the cells. However, in conventional cell culture usage, this would be termed a 1:3 split ratio. Similarly, a split ratio of 1:4, in conventional cell culture usage, could be achieved by taking the cells from one vessel and splitting them into four new vessels. A split ratio of 1:8, in conventional usage, could be achieved by taking the cells from one vessel and dividing them equally into eight new vessels. As you will see in the practice problems below, the math involved in working with split ratios is simplified by using the 1/3 terminology, that is, a division sign rather than a colon. However, it is important to understand what people mean when they use various terminology (or notation) conventions.

**Example Problem:**

A culture dish of cells is harvested. The cells are centrifuged into the bottom of a centrifuge tube and then are resuspended in 2 mL of fresh growth medium. A 1/10 split ratio is desired.

a. What is the conventional cell culture terminology for this split ratio?
b. How many milliliters of the suspended cells are placed onto each new plate to achieve this split ratio?

***Answer:***

a. This would be called a **1:10 split ratio** in conventional terminology.
b. To calculate the required volume of cell suspension for each new vessel, simply multiply the desired split (expressed as a fraction) times the volume of suspended cells. In this case, the split ratio is 1/10 and the volume of suspended cells is 2 mL. Thus, (1/10) (2 mL) = 0.2 mL. So, **0.2 mL** of suspended cells are seeded onto each new plate.

In this situation, it would be possible to begin with the cells from one plate and end with 10 plates of cells. (Sometimes cells are discarded, if there are too many to use.)

Fresh growth medium is then also added to each plate to whatever final volume is needed. For example, a 100 mm cell culture dish is typically filled with 10 mL of growth medium. So, 9.8 mL of fresh growth medium would be added to each of the plates, along with its 0.2 mL of suspended cells, for a total volume of 10 mL per plate. (In practice, for convenience, 10 mL, rather than 9.8 mL, of fresh medium might be added to each plate.) This problem is sketched in Figure 21.4.

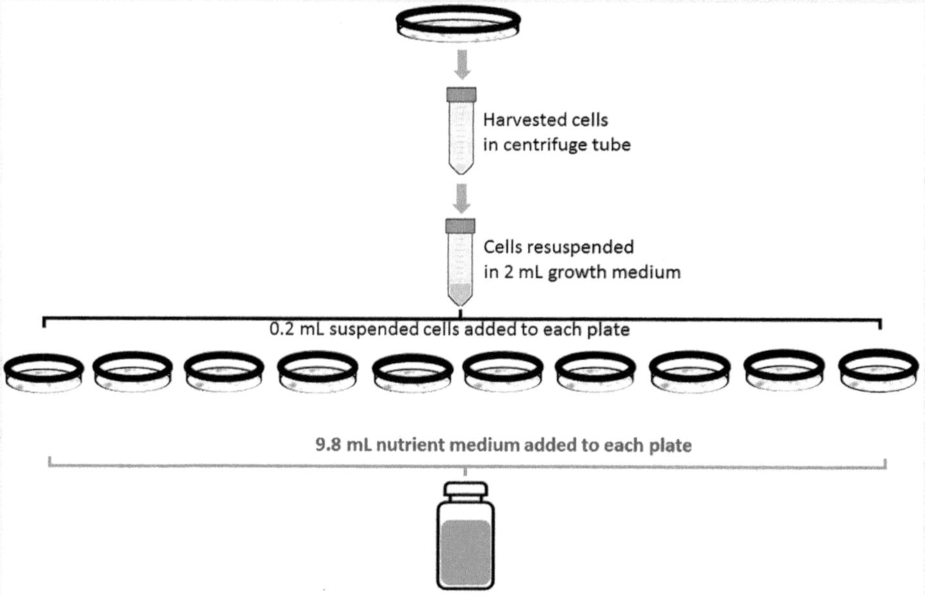


**FIGURE 21.4** A 1/10 cell split where cells are resuspended in 2 mL of nutrient medium and divided into ten cell culture dishes. In this situation, the culture dishes require 10 mL total volume, although this does not enter into the calculation of how to do the split.

**Example Problem:**

A plate of cells is harvested and subsequently suspended in a volume of 10 mL of culture medium. To get a 1/10 split ratio (in conventional terminology a 1:10 split), a culturist would transfer (1/10) (10 mL) = 1 mL to each of ten new plates or flasks. The density of cells on the new plates is now 1/10th of what it was before. The culturist would then add a volume of additional growth medium to the new vessels that is recommended for that size vessel.

a. Given harvested cells suspended in 10 mL culture medium, how could the culturist obtain a 1/5 (1:5 in conventional terminology) split ratio? How many new vessels can be seeded at this density?
b. Given harvested cells suspended in 10 mL culture medium, how could the culturist obtain a 1/2 split ratio? How many new vessels can be seeded at this density?

*Answer:*

a. Given that the cells are suspended in 10 mL of fresh medium, to achieve a 1/5 split ratio:
   (1/5) (10 mL) = **2 mL**. So, put 2 mL of cell suspension into the new vessels.
   Add the recommended amount of growth medium based on the size of the vessels. Five new vessels can be seeded at this density, each of which now has one fifth the density of cells that were present on the original plate.
b. Given that the cells are suspended in 10 mL of fresh medium, to achieve a 1/2 split:
   (1/2) (10 mL) = **5 mL**. So, put 5 mL of cell suspension into the new vessels.
   Add the recommended amount of growth medium based on the size of the vessels. Two new vessels can be seeded at this density, each of which now has one half the density of cells that were present on the original plate.

**Practice Problems**

1. ***A flask of cells is harvested, and the cells are resuspended in 10 mL of fresh growth medium. A 1/10 split is desired.***
   a. ***How many mL of resuspended cells are placed in each new flask?***
   b. ***If each flask is to have 30 mL of growth medium, how much additional fresh growth medium is required for each plate?***

2. ***A dish of cells is harvested, centrifuged, and resuspended in 5 mL of fresh growth medium. A 1/10 split is desired.***
   a. ***How many mL of resuspended cells are placed on each new dish?***
   b. ***If each dish is to have 10 mL of growth medium, how much additional fresh growth medium is required for each dish?***

3. ***A flask of cells is harvested, and the cells are resuspended in 10 mL of fresh growth medium. A 1/3 split is desired.***
   a. ***How many mL of resuspended cells are placed in each new flask?***
   b. ***How many flasks can be seeded?***
   c. ***If each flask requires 15 mL of medium, how much additional growth medium should be added to each flask?***

4. ***You are growing MDCK cells in a 6-well plate (refer to Figure 21.3a). (MDCK cells are derived from canine kidney and are commonly used experimentally.) MDCK cells have a doubling time of nearly 24 hours. All the cells are in one well of the plate. You observe the cells with a microscope and estimate that they cover about 80% of the surface of the well, that is, they are at 80% confluency. It is time to split the cells and you decide to split them into four new wells of the plate. 2 mL is the recommended volume in each well of a 6-well plate.***
   a. ***How much cell culture medium will you need in total for your split into four wells?***
   b. ***What will be the approximate confluency (that is, the percent of the plate that is covered by cells) in each well after they are split?***
   c. ***What do you estimate the confluency will be at the same time on the next day after splitting?***

5. ***You are following a protocol that tells you to harvest the cells from a flask and resuspend them into 100 mL of cell culture medium.***
   a. ***The protocol says to do a 1:2 split. How many mL of cells go into each new flask?***
   b. ***The protocol says to do a 1:5 split. How many mL of cells go into each new flask?***
   c. ***The protocol says to do a 1:10 split. How many mL of cells go into each new flask?***

6. ***You are following a protocol that says to harvest your cells and resuspend them in 5 mL of fresh culture medium.***
   a. ***The protocol says to do a 1:4 split. How many mL should you remove and place in each new vessel?***
   b. ***The protocol says to do a 1:5 split. How many mL should you remove and place in each new vessel?***

*Answers*

1. a. (1/10) (10 mL) = 1 mL. So, **1 mL** of resuspended cells is added to each new flask.
   b. **29 mL** of growth medium. (In practice this might be rounded to 30 mL.)

2. a. (1/10) (5 mL) = **0.5 mL** of resuspended cells are added to each new dish.
   b. **9.5 mL** of growth medium. (In practice this might be rounded to 10 mL.)

3. a. (1/3) (10 mL) ≈ **3.33 mL** of resuspended cells will be placed in each new flask.
   b. **3 flasks**
   c. **11.67 mL**, but this would probably be rounded to 12 mL.

4. a. (4 wells) (2 mL/well) = **8 mL**.
   b. **20%**
   c. About **40%**

5. This protocol is using conventional cell culture terminology.
   a. Using this conventional terminology, a 1:2 split means removing **50 mL** of cells and placing them in each new flask. (In this chapter, we call this a 1/2 split, so it means taking (100 mL) (1/2) = **50 mL**.)
   b. A 1:5 split means taking **20 mL** into each new flask.
   (In this chapter, we call this a 1/5 split, so it means taking (100 mL) (1/5) = 20 mL.)
   c. A 1:10 split means taking **10 mL** into each new flask.
   (In this chapter, we call this a 1/10 split, so it means taking (100 mL) (1/10) = 10 mL.)

6. a. (5 mL) (1/4) = **1.25 mL**   b. (5 mL) (1/5) = **1 mL**

## 21.3 THE CONCEPT OF CELL DENSITY

In cell culture we often talk about **cell density**, *expressed as the number of cells/mL*. For adherent cells, **cell density** can also be defined as the *number of cells/surface area.* (We will explore cell density expressed as cells/surface area in Section 21.5.) Calculations involving cell density will be familiar to you because we have discussed many analogous situations. For example, previous chapters have explored problems relating to the number of grams of solute required per milliliter of solution, and dosage problems relating to the milligrams of drug administered per kilogram body weight. The underlying math in all these varied situations is the same, and ratios and proportions provide a useful tool for calculations. Try the following practice problems to get comfortable applying familiar calculation tools to cell density problems.

*Practice Problems*

1. ***Cells are present in a cell culture dish at a density of $2.5\times10^5$ cells/mL of cell culture medium. The dish contains 10 mL of culture medium total. How many cells are in the dish altogether?***

2. ***Cells are present in a cell culture flask at a density of $3.4\times10^4$ cells/mL of cell culture medium. The flask contains 45 mL of medium total. How many cells are present in the flask?***

3. ***You need to remove $1.4\times10^6$ cells from a suspension containing $2.6\times10^5$ cells/mL. How many mL of the suspension should you remove?***

4. ***A cell culture flask contains 45 mL of cells at a density of $2.4\times10^5$ cells/mL.***
   - a. ***How many cells are present altogether in the flask?***
   - b. ***How many cells are present in 0.1 mL of medium from this flask?***

5. ***You need $5\times10^7$ cells for an experiment. You have 25 cell culture plates, each with 10 mL of volume. Each plate has cells at a density of approximately $6\times10^5$ cells/mL. How many plates do you need to harvest to get at least $5\times10^7$ cells?***

6. ***You have a 2 mL suspension of cells at a density of $5.5\times10^6$ cells/mL. You add 3 mL of fresh growth medium to the suspension. What is the density of cells now?***

7. ***You have a 5 mL suspension of cells at a density of $3.1\times10^6$ cells/mL. You add 5 mL of fresh growth medium to the suspension. What is the density of cells now?***

*Answers*

1. If there are $2.5\times10^5$ cells in 1 mL, then how many are in 10 mL? This can be solved using proportions:

$$\frac{2.5\times10^5 \text{ cells}}{1 \text{ mL}} = \frac{?}{10 \text{ mL}} \qquad ? = \mathbf{2.5\times10^6} \text{ cells}$$

2. If there are $3.4\times10^4$ cells in 1 mL, how many are there in 45 mL? This can also be solved using proportions, like the problem above. But here is a unit canceling strategy:

$$\left(\frac{3.4\times10^4 \text{ cells}}{1 \cancel{\text{mL}}}\right)\left(\frac{45 \cancel{\text{mL}}}{1}\right) \approx \mathbf{1.5\times10^6} \text{ cells}$$

3. If you have $2.6\times10^5$ cells in 1 mL, then how many mL are required to get $1.4\times10^6$ cells? By proportions:

$$\frac{2.6\times10^5\text{cells}}{1\,\text{mL}}=\frac{1.4\times10^6\text{cells}}{?} \qquad ?\approx\mathbf{5.4\,mL}$$

4. A cell culture flask contains 45 mL of cells at a density of $2.4\times10^5$ cells/mL.
   a. How many cells are present altogether in the flask? Let's use unit canceling:

$$\left(\frac{2.4\times10^5\text{ cells}}{\cancel{\text{mL}}}\right)\left(\frac{45\,\cancel{\text{mL}}}{1}\right)\approx\mathbf{1.1\times10^7\ cells}$$

   b. How many cells are present in 0.1 mL of medium from this flask? Let's use unit canceling:

$$\left(\frac{2.4\times10^5\text{ cells}}{\cancel{\text{mL}}}\right)\left(\frac{0.1\,\cancel{\text{mL}}}{1}\right)=\mathbf{2.4\times10^4\ cells}$$

5. The total number of cells on each plate is about:

$$\left(\frac{6\times10^5\text{ cells}}{\cancel{\text{mL}}}\right)\left(\frac{10\,\cancel{\text{mL}}}{1\text{ plate}}\right)=\frac{6\times10^6\text{ cells}}{1\text{ plate}}$$

You need $5\times10^7$ cells total. If each plate has $6\times10^6$ cells, then how many plates are required to get $5\times10^7$ cells?

$$\frac{6\times10^6\text{ cells}}{1\text{ plate}}=\frac{5\times10^7\text{ cells}}{?} \qquad ?\approx\mathbf{8.333}$$

This means you need to harvest **9 plates** to get enough cells.

6. You have $\left(\frac{5.5\times10^6\text{ cells}}{1\,\text{mL}}\right)\left(\frac{2\,\text{mL}}{1}\right)=1.1\times10^7$ cells total.

If you add 3 mL of medium, you have $\frac{1.1\times10^7\text{ cells}}{5\,\text{mL}}=\mathbf{2.2\times10^6\ cells/mL}$

You might want to observe that the $C_1V_1=C_2V_2$ equation can be used to perform this calculation.

$C_1$, the original concentration is $\frac{5.5\times10^6\text{ cells}}{1\,\text{mL}}$

$V_1$, the original volume, is 2 mL
$C_2$, the final concentration is ?
$V_2$, the final volume is 5 mL
Plugging into the $C_1V_1=C_2V_2$ equation:

$$\underset{C_1}{\left(\frac{5.5\times10^6\text{ cells}}{1\,\cancel{\text{mL}}}\right)}\underset{V_1}{(2\,\cancel{\text{mL}})}=\underset{C_2\ V_2}{?\ (5\text{ mL})}$$

$$\mathbf{?=2.2\times10^6\ cells/mL}$$

7. You have $\left(\frac{3.1\times10^{6}\text{ cells}}{1\ \cancel{\text{mL}}}\right)\left(\frac{5\ \cancel{\text{mL}}}{1}\right)=1.55\times10^{7}$ cells total.

If you add 5 mL of medium, you have $\frac{1.55\times10^{7}\text{ cells}}{10\text{ mL}}\approx\mathbf{1.6\times10^{6}\ cells/mL}$

(The $C_1V_1=C_2V_2$ equation also applies here.)

## 21.4 USING A HEMOCYTOMETER

Section 21.3 talked about cell density. Determining the density of cells in a culture at regular intervals is a good way to monitor their growth and health, and allows a specific density of cells to be seeded into each new culture vessel when cells are passaged (subcultured). In order to know cell density, it is necessary to have some means of counting the cells. How are cells counted? An individual cell is too small to see with the naked eye, and tens of thousands of cells are likely to be present in each milliliter of growth medium. There are cell counting instruments that automate cell counting. But many laboratories do not have these expensive instruments, and cells are counted by the cell culturist using a hemocytometer and a microscope. A **Neubauer hemocytometer**, Figure 21.5, *is a special modified microscope slide that is used to determine the concentration of cells in a suspension of cells.*

The hemocytometer contains two identical wells, or chambers, into which a small volume of the cell suspension is pipetted, Figure 21.5a. Each chamber is manufactured to hold an exactly specified volume of liquid. Observe in Figure 21.5b that when you view the hemocytometer under a microscope, you see that the bottom surface of each well is marked off into a grid pattern. The grid consists of nine larger squares that are further subdivided into smaller squares. The four corner large squares are subdivided into 16 smaller squares.

Each of the nine larger squares has dimensions of 1 mm×1 mm×0.1 mm. Therefore, the volume of fluid over each of these large squares is 0.1 $mm^3$. (Volume is length times width times height.) The units of $mm^3$ are not helpful to us, so they are converted to units of mL: 0.1 $mm^3=10^{-4}$mL.

The process of counting cells with a hemocytometer is:

**Step 1. Remove some of the cell suspension and dilute it with trypan blue.**

Some of the cell culture suspension is removed and is diluted with the dye, trypan blue, and possibly also with sterile medium. Trypan blue is used so that living cells can be distinguished from dead ones. Living cells exclude the dye, but it readily passes through the membrane of dead cells. Thus, living cells are clear while dead cells are blue.

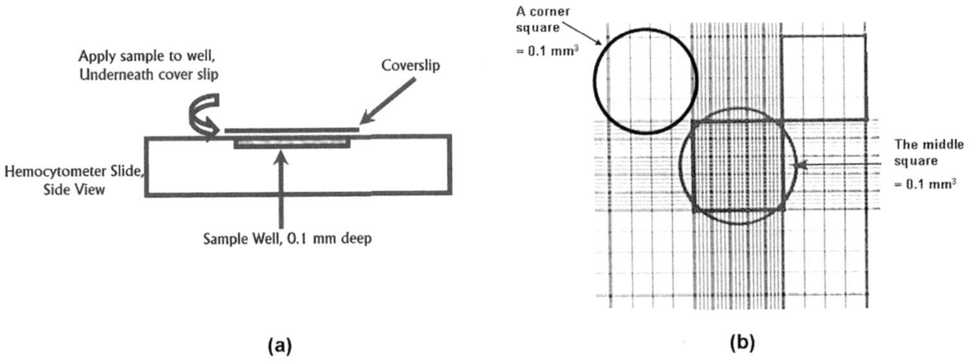


**FIGURE 21.5** The hemocytometer, used for counting cells. (a) Side view of the slide. (b) Top view of one of the two grids as it appears under a microscope.

**Step 2. Apply the mixture to the hemocytometer.**

A cover slip is placed on top of the hemocytometer slide. The cell suspension is mixed well and then is carefully applied under the cover slip into both wells of the hemocytometer in such a way that each chamber is exactly filled.

**Step 3. Count the cells.**

Using a microscope, all the cells located over the four large corner squares and the center square in one of the chambers are counted. A separate tally is kept of the viable (living) and non-viable (dead) cells. Sometimes the cells in both chambers are counted, either to make sure that the counts are comparable, or to count more cells if necessary. (Some analysts try to count enough squares to get at least 100 cells, others aim for at least 200 cells.)

**Step 4. Calculate percent viability.**

The percent of viable cells is calculated.

**Step 6. Calculate the concentration of viable cells.**

The concentration of viable cells per milliliter is calculated using Equation 21.1.

**EQUATION 21.1 Calculation of the Number of cells/mL from Hemocytometer Counts**

$$\frac{\text{Number of viable cells}}{1\text{ mL}} = \left(\frac{\#\text{ viable cells}}{\#\ \cancel{\text{squares}}}\right)\frac{1\ \cancel{\text{square}}}{10^{-4}\text{ mL}}(\text{reciprocal of dilution})$$

Observe that $\frac{1}{10^{-4}} = 10^4$

therefore, this equation can be rewritten as:

$$\frac{\text{Number of viable cells}}{1\text{ mL}} = \left(\frac{\#\text{ viable cells}}{\#\ \cancel{\text{squares}}}\right)\left(\frac{10^4\ \cancel{\text{square}}}{1\text{ mL}}\right)(\text{reciprocal of dilution})$$

Consider the parts of this equation:

- The number of viable cells per mL is what we want to know.
- We need to know the average number of cells per square. Suppose you count the number of cells in five squares. Then, the # of viable cells in five large squares/five gives the average number of cells per large square. If you count only the four corner squares and not the center square, then you divide the total number of viable cells by four instead of five to get the average number of cells per large square.
- We multiply by $1/10^{-4}$ mL (which equals $10^4/1$ mL) because each square has a volume of $10^{-4}$ mL.
- The dilution must be considered when calculating the number of cells per milliliter. In this situation, we use the reciprocal of the dilution (expressed as a fraction, see Chapter 14.7), since we are calculating back from the concentration of cells in a diluted sample to the concentration of cells in the original solution.

**Example:**

200 μL of a cell suspension is removed from a plate of cells.
300 μL of sterile diluent is added to the suspension.
500 μL of trypan blue is added.
The total volume is thus 1,000 μL.

The total number of viable cells in the four corner plus center squares is 245.
The total number of non-viable cells in these squares is 55.

**Calculations:**

1. The total number of cells counted = 245 + 55 = 300.
2. The percent viable cells = 245/300 ≈ **81.7%**
3. The average number of viable cells per square = 245/5 = 49.
4. The dilution is 200 µL/ (200 µL + 300 µL + 500 µL) = 200 µL /1,000 µL = 1/5.
5. The reciprocal of the dilution is 5/1 or 5.
6. Applying Equation 21.1, the concentration of viable cells in the original dish is:

$$\frac{\text{Number of viable cells}}{\text{mL}} = \left(\frac{\text{\# viable cells counted}}{5\ \cancel{\text{squares}}}\right)\left(\frac{10^4\ \cancel{\text{square}}}{1\ \text{mL}}\right)(\text{reciprocal of dilution})$$

$$= \left(\frac{245\ \text{cells}}{5\ \cancel{\text{squares}}}\right)\left(\frac{10^4\ \cancel{\text{square}}}{1\ \text{mL}}\right)(5) = \mathbf{2,450,000\ cells/mL}$$

$$= \mathbf{2.45 \times 10^6\ cells/mL}$$

**Example Problem:**

You are performing experiments relating to cancer-causing agents using cells in culture. A cell culture dish contains a suspension of treated mouse cells. You remove 0.5 mL of the cell suspension to a tube and add 0.5 mL of trypan blue. You apply the diluted cells to a hemocytometer and count the viable and non-viable cells in the four corner and in the center large squares. There are 171 clear cells and 5 blue cells.

a. What is the average number of viable cells per square?
b. What is the percent viability?
c. What is the reciprocal of the dilution?
d. What is the concentration of viable cells in the original cell culture dish?

***Answer:***

a. The average number of viable cells per square = 171/5 = **34.2**
b. The percent viability = 171/176 ≈ **97%**.
c. The dilution, expressed as a fraction, is 0.5 mL/1.0 mL or 1/2. The reciprocal is 2/1 or **2**.
d. Applying Equation 21.1, the concentration of viable cells in the original solution =

$$\frac{\text{Number of viable cells}}{\text{mL}} = \left(\frac{\text{\# viable cells}}{5\ \cancel{\text{squares}}}\right)\left(\frac{10^4\ \cancel{\text{square}}}{1\ \text{mL}}\right)(\text{reciprocal of dilution})$$

$$= \left(\frac{171\ \text{cells}}{5}\right)\left(\frac{10^4}{1\ \text{mL}}\right)(2) = \mathbf{6.84 \times 10^5\ cells/mL}$$

*Practice Problems*

1. ***You have a suspension of treated cells. You remove 0.5 mL of the cell suspension to a tube and add 0.5 mL of trypan blue. You apply the diluted cells to a hemocytometer and count the viable and non-viable cells in the four corners and in the center large squares. There are 456 clear cells and 25 blue cells.***
   a. ***What is the average number of viable cells per square?***
   b. ***What is the percent viability?***
   c. ***What is the reciprocal of the dilution?***
   d. ***What is the density of viable cells in the original cell culture dish?***

2. ***You have a cell culture flask containing 75 mL of a suspension of treated cells. You remove 0.2 mL of the cell suspension to a tube and add 0.5 mL of trypan blue and 0.3 mL of sterile medium. You apply the diluted cells to a hemocytometer and count the viable and non-viable cells in the four corner squares. There are 226 clear cells and 25 blue cells. You do not count the center square because you have already counted enough cells.***
   a. ***What is the average number of viable cells per square?***
   b. ***What is the percent viability?***
   c. ***What is the reciprocal of the dilution?***
   d. ***What is the density of viable cells in the original cell culture dish?***
   e. ***How many viable cells are there altogether in the original 75 mL?***

3. ***You have a cell culture dish containing 20 mL of a suspension of treated cells. You remove 0.1 mL of the cell suspension to a tube and add 0.4 mL of trypan blue. You apply the diluted cells to a hemocytometer and count the viable and non-viable cells in the four corner and in the center large squares. There are 126 clear cells and 15 blue cells.***
   a. ***What is the average number of viable cells per square?***
   b. ***What is the percent viability?***
   c. ***What is the reciprocal of the dilution?***
   d. ***What is the density of viable cells in the original cell culture dish?***
   e. ***How many viable cells are there altogether in the original 20 mL?***

*Answers*

1. a. The average number of viable cells per square = 456/5 = **91.2 cells/square**
   b. The percent viability = 456/481 ≈ **94.8%.** c. The reciprocal of the dilution is **2.**
   d. By Equation 21.1, the density of viable cells in the original solution = (91.2) (2) $(10^4)$ ≈ **$1.82 \times 10^6$ viable cells/mL.**

2. a. The average number of viable cells per square = 226/4 = **56.5 cells/square**
   b. The percent viability = 226/251 ≈ **90.0%.** c. The reciprocal of the dilution is **5.**
   d. By Equation 21.1, the density of viable cells in the original solution = (56.5) (5) $(10^4)$ = **$2.825 \times 10^6$ cells/mL.**
   e. ($2.825 \times 10^6$ cells/mL) (75 mL) ≈ **$2.12 \times 10^8$ viable cells total**

3. a. The average number of viable cells per square = 126/5 = **25.2 cells/square**
   b. The percent viability = 126/141 ≈ **89.4%.** c. The reciprocal of the dilution is **5.**
   d. By Equation 21.1, the density of viable cells in the original solution = (25.2) (5) $(10^4)$ ≈ **$1.26 \times 10^6$ cells/mL.**
   e. ($1.26 \times 10^6$ cells/mL) (20 mL) = **$2.52 \times 10^7$ viable cells total**

## 21.5 SPLITTING CELLS AND SEEDING PLATES AT SPECIFIC CELL DENSITIES

In Section 21.2, we talked about splitting cells without counting them. In these situations, the cells are, for example, split 1/3 (1:3 in conventional terminology) or 1/2 (1:2 in conventional terminology). However, it is often more reliable to count the cells first, and then determine the proper split ratio to obtain a desired density of cells.

**Example Problem:**

You have 5 mL of resuspended cells at a density of $2\times10^5$ cells/mL.

a. How many 100 mm plates can you seed (inoculate) if you want $2\times10^5$ cells/plate?
b. How many mL of the cell suspension should be seeded on each plate?

***Answer:***

a. Your total number of cells is:

$$(5\text{ mL})(2\times10^5\text{ cells/mL}) = 1\times10^6\text{ cells}$$

You want $2\times10^5$ cells/plate, how many plates can you seed? You can use proportions to solve this:

$$\frac{2\times10^5\text{ cells}}{1\text{ plate}} = \frac{1\times10^6\text{ cells}}{?} \qquad \mathbf{? = 5\ plates}$$

So, you have enough cells for 5 plates.

b. This is a simple calculation where you have $2\times10^5$ cells/mL and you want $2\times10^5$ cells to seed each plate. Therefore, you can add **1 mL** of cells to each plate.

***Practice Problems***

1. ***A flask of cells is harvested, centrifuged, and resuspended in 10 mL of fresh growth medium. The cells are counted and there are 4.5 × $10^4$ viable cells/mL.***
   a. ***How many flasks can you seed at a density of 5 × $10^4$ cells/flask?***
   b. ***How many mL of the resuspended cells will you seed into each flask?***

2. ***A plate of cells is harvested, centrifuged, and resuspended in 5 mL of fresh growth medium. There are 6 × $10^3$ viable cells/mL. You want to seed new plates at a density of 2 × $10^3$ cells/plate.***
   a. ***How many cell culture plates can you seed at a density of 2 × $10^3$ cells/plate?***
   b. ***How many mL of the resuspended cells will you seed onto each plate?***

3. *You have $6 \times 10^4$ cells/mL in a volume of 2 mL.*
   a. *How many cell culture plates can you seed at a density of $3 \times 10^3$ cells/mL if each plate will have a final volume of 4 mL?*
   b. *How many mL of the resuspended cells will you seed onto each plate?*

4. *You are going to perform an assay that requires 20,000 cells in each well of a 6-well plate. Each well holds 4 mL of volume. You have $8 \times 10^5$ cells that are suspended in 1 mL of fresh growth medium. You decide to make 28 mL of a cell suspension that will have 20,000 cells/4 mL. You will be able to pipette 4 mL into each well of the plate and there should be four mL left over. How much cell suspension and how much fresh medium should you combine to get 28 mL of cells with a concentration of 20,000 cells/4 mL?*

5. *Adherent cells are often grown in flasks that can be purchased in various sizes (for example, as shown in Figure 21.3b). Each size flask provides a certain interior surface area for cell growth. For adherent cells in these flasks, cell density is often expressed as # cells/cm², rather than cells/mL.*

   *For Corning Brand cell culture flasks, the recommended volume of cell culture medium is between 0.2 and 0.3 mL/cm² growth area. The average yield of cells from a 100% confluent culture is $1 \times 10^5$ cells/cm². Fill in Table 21.1a for the recommended volume of medium and the average cell yield. (The first row is completed for you as an example.)*

6. *You are beginning an experiment by thawing a vial of frozen MDCK cells. The cells have been frozen in 1 mL aliquots and each aliquot contains roughly $1 \times 10^6$ cells. It is recommended that you seed the cells into cell culture flasks at a density between $2 \times 10^3$ and $1 \times 10^4$ viable cells/cm². (Observe that the recommended seeding density is expressed in units of cells/cm².)*
   a. *Refer to Table 21.1a in Practice Problem 5. If you take all the cells and place them in one T-25 flask, the seeding density is $1 \times 10^6$ cells/25 cm² = $4 \times 10^4$ cells/cm². Is this density in the recommended range?*
   b. *Refer to Table 21.1a. What is the seeding density if you thaw the cells and plate them all into a T-75 flask? Is this density in the recommended range?*
   c. *Refer to Table 21.1a. What is the seeding density if you thaw the cells and plate them all into a T-150 flask? Is this density in the recommended range?*

7. *You have a T-25 flask with CHO cells. (CHO cells are derived from Chinese hamster ovary and are widely used to manufacture pharmaceuticals.) The cells appear to be about 80% confluent and have a doubling time of about 22 hours. You count the cells with a hemocytometer and find there are about*

**TABLE 21.1a Typical Cell Yields and Recommended Volumes of Medium for Corning Flasks**

| Flask Name | Flask Internal Surface Area | Average Cell Yield | Recommended Volume |
|---|---|---|---|
| T-25 | 25 cm² | $2.5 \times 10^6$ | 5–7.5 mL |
| T-75 | 75 cm² | | |
| T-150 | 150 cm² | | |
| T-175 | 175 cm² | | |

***$2.2 \times 10^6$ viable cells available in the flask. You want to transfer the cells to an appropriate flask(s) and expand them to $7.0 \times 10^6$ cells, enough cells for an experiment. The suggested seeding density is between $2.5 \times 10^3$ and $1.8 \times 10^4$ cells/cm$^2$.***

a. ***What would the seeding density be if you divided the available cells into two T-75 flasks (answer will be in cells/cm$^2$). Is this in the acceptable range?***
b. ***What would be the estimated percent confluency in each flask if you seed the available cells into two T-75 flasks? (To perform this calculation, refer to Table 21.1b to find the approximate yield of a T-75 flask at 100% confluency.)***
c. ***After 44 hours, what would you estimate the confluency to be in each flask?***
d. ***How many cells would you estimate that you will have in each flask after 44 hours? How many cells will you have in total?***
e. ***After 44 hours will you have enough cells for your experiment?***

8. ***You are ready to freeze down some of your CHO cells for long-term storage in liquid nitrogen. You have a T-150 flask with cells at 70% confluency. You will freeze the cells in 1 mL aliquots at a concentration of $1 \times 10^6$ cells/mL.***
   a. ***Based on your estimate of confluency, about how many cells are available to freeze down?***
   b. ***After removing the cells from the flask and collecting them in the bottom of a centrifuge tube, how much freezing medium will you need to resuspend the cells to the appropriate concentration?***
   c. ***About how many tubes of cells can you freeze?***

9. ***Suppose you have a suspension with 620,000 cells/mL. You want to inoculate a T-75 flask with 2,500 cells/cm$^2$. How much volume should you pipette into the T-75 flask?***

10. ***Let us think about cell splits that are based on T-flask surface area. For example, suppose you are growing cells in T-25 flask. If you remove all the cells and place them in a T-75 flask, which has three times more area than a T-25 flask, then you have split them 1/3 (1:3 using conventional terminology). You could also split them 1/3 by dividing the contents of the single flask into three T-25 flasks.***
    a. ***If you take the cell contents of a T-75 flask and put the cells into a T-150 flask, what is the split? Express your answer using with a / and with a colon (:).***
    b. ***If you take the cell contents of a T-75 flask and place them into two T-75 flasks, what is the split? Express your answer using with a / and with a colon (:).***
    c. ***If you take the cell contents of a T-25 flask and place them into a T-175 flask, what is the split? Express your answer using with a / and with a colon (:).***

11. ***Suppose you want to do a 1/6 cell split. You have your cells in a culture dish with a 57 cm$^2$ surface area. You are going to use a new culture dish with a surface area of 145 cm$^2$. (Assume that the new dish has three times the surface area of the original dish, although 57 cm$^2$ times 3 is not exactly 145 cm$^2$.)***
    a. ***If you simply move the cells into the new dish, what is the split ratio? Observe that you have not achieved your desired 1/6 split ratio.***
    b. ***Suppose that you have resuspended your cells in 10 mL of fresh culture medium. How many mL of this cell suspension should you add to the 145 cm$^2$ dish to get a total split ratio of 1/6?***

***Answers***

1. a. How many flasks can you seed at a density of $5\times10^4$ cells/flask?
   Total number of cells is:

$$\left(\frac{4.5\times10^4 \text{ cells}}{1\ \cancel{\text{mL}}}\right)\left(10\ \cancel{\text{mL}}\right)=4.5\times10^5 \text{ cells}$$

$$\frac{5\times10^4 \text{ cells}}{1 \text{ flask}}=\frac{4.5\times10^5 \text{ cells}}{?} \quad \mathbf{?=9\ flasks}$$

   b. How many mL of the resuspended cells will you seed into each flask to get $5\times10^4$ cells?

$$\frac{4.5\times10^4 \text{ cells}}{1 \text{ mL}}=\frac{5\times10^4 \text{ cells}}{?} \quad \mathbf{?\approx 1.1\ mL}$$

2. a. Total number of cells is:

$$\left(\frac{6\times10^3 \text{ cells}}{1\ \cancel{\text{mL}}}\right)\left(5\ \cancel{\text{mL}}\right)=3\times10^4 \text{ cells}$$

$$\frac{2\times10^3 \text{ cells}}{1 \text{ plate}}=\frac{3\times10^4 \text{ cells}}{?} \quad \mathbf{?=15\ plates}$$

   b. How many mL of the resuspended cells will you seed into each flask?

$$\frac{6\times10^3 \text{ cells}}{1 \text{ mL}}=\frac{2\times10^3 \text{ cells}}{?} \quad \mathbf{?\approx 0.33\ mL}$$

3. a. If each plate has a volume of 4 mL, each plate needs:

$$\left(3\times10^3 \text{ cells}/\cancel{\text{mL}}\right)\left(4\ \cancel{\text{mL}}\right)=1.2\times10^4 \text{ cells}$$

   Have a total of $\left(6\times10^4 \text{ cells}/\cancel{\text{mL}}\right)\left(2\ \cancel{\text{mL}}\right)=1.2\times10^5$ cells

$$\frac{1.2\times10^4 \text{ cells}}{1 \text{ plate}}=\frac{1.2\times10^5 \text{ cells}}{?} \quad \mathbf{?=10\ plates}$$

   b. $\dfrac{6\times10^4 \text{ cells}}{1 \text{ mL}}=\dfrac{1.2\times10^4 \text{cells}}{?}$ **? = 0.2 mL for each plate**

4. Your preparation needs to have 20,000 cells/4 mL. Then, when you add 4 mL into each well, it will have the desired # of cells, that is, 20,000.
   20,000 cells/4 mL = 5,000 cells/mL. This is the cell density needed.
   You need 28 mL of suspension at this density, which means you need a total of (5,000 cells/mL) (28 mL) = 140,000 cells
   Use a proportion equation to calculate how to obtain 140,000 cells from your 1 mL suspension:

$$\frac{8\times10^5 \text{ cells}}{1 \text{ mL}}=\frac{140{,}000 \text{ cells}}{?} \quad \mathbf{?=0.175\ mL} \text{ of the resuspended cells}$$

So, take **0.175 mL** of the resuspended cells and add **27.825 mL (in practice, 28 mL)** of fresh culture medium.

You might want to observe that the $C_1V_1 = C_2V_2$ equation can be used to perform this calculation.

$C_1$, the original concentration is $\frac{8 \times 10^5 \text{ cells}}{1 \text{ mL}}$

$V_1$, the original volume, is ?

$C_2$, the final concentration is 20,000/4 mL

$V_2$, the final volume is 28 mL

Plugging into the $C_1V_1 = C_2V_2$ equation:

$$C_1 \quad V_1 = \quad C_2 \; V_2$$

$$\left(\frac{8 \times 10^5 \text{ cells}}{1 \text{ mL}}\right) ? = \frac{20{,}000}{4 \text{ mL}} (28 \text{ mL})$$

**? = 0.175 mL of cell suspension**

5.

**TABLE 21.1B Typical Cell Yields and Recommended Volumes of Medium for Corning Flasks**

| Flask Name | Flask Internal Surface Area | Average Cell Yield | Recommended Volume |
|---|---|---|---|
| T-25 | 25 $cm^2$ | $2.5 \times 10^6$ cells | 5–7.5 mL |
| T-75 | 75 $cm^2$ | $7.5 \times 10^6$ cells | 15–22.5 mL |
| T-150 | 150 $cm^2$ | $1.5 \times 10^7$ cells | 30–45 mL |
| T-175 | 175 $cm^2$ | $1.75 \times 10^7$ cells | 35–52.5 mL |

6. a. $1 \times 10^6$ cells/25 $cm^2$ = **$4 \times 10^4$ cells/$cm^2$** No, this exceeds the recommended density.

   b. $1 \times 10^6$ cells/75 $cm^2 \approx$ **$1.3 \times 10^4$ cells/$cm^2$** No, this exceeds the recommended cell density.

   c. $1 \times 10^6$ cells/150 $cm^2 \approx$ **$6.67 \times 10^3$ cells/$cm^2$** Yes, this is in the recommended range for cell density.

7. a. You will have $1.1 \times 10^6$ cells in each of the two T-75 flasks.
   $1.1 \times 10^6$/75 $cm^2 \approx$ **$1.47 \times 10^4$ cells/$cm^2$** Yes, this is acceptable.

   b. At 100% confluency you expect $7.5 \times 10^6$ cells.

$$(1.1 \times 10^6 \text{ cells})/(7.5 \times 10^6 \text{ cells}) \approx 0.1467$$

   Expressed as a percent, this is **14.67% or about 15%.**

   c. 44 hours/22 hours = 2 doublings. 15% × 2 × 2 ≈ **60%**

   d. $(1.1 \times 10^6$ cells) (2) (2) = $4.4 \times 10^6$ cells per T-75 flask

$$(4.4 \times 10^6 \text{ cells per T-75 flask}) \text{ (2 flasks)} = \mathbf{8.8 \times 10^6 \text{ cells total}}$$

   e. The goal is to have $7.0 \times 10^6$ cells, so there are more than enough to move forward.

8. a. From Table 21.1b, at 100% confluency, a T-150 flask has about $15 \times 10^6$ cells. But you have cells at 70% confluency: $(15 \times 10^6)$ (0.7) = **$10.5 \times 10^6$ cells** = number of cells in the flask

b. Goal is to resuspend the cells in sufficient freezing medium to have $1\times10^6$ cells/mL.

$$\frac{10.5\times10^6 \text{ cells}}{?}=\frac{10^6 \text{ cells}}{1 \text{ mL}} \quad ?=\mathbf{10.5\,mL\ of\ freezing\ medium\ required}$$

c. You will have 10.5 mL of freezing medium with cells. Each tube will have 1 mL so can freeze 10.5 tubes. It is likely that you would just **freeze 10 tubes with a little left over, since partially filled tubes are not typically used.**

9. You have 620,000 cells/mL. You want to inoculate a T-75 flask with 2,500 cells/cm$^2$.
   Multiply the density desired times the surface area:
   (2,500 cells/cm$^2$) (75 cm$^2$/1 flask) = 187,500 cells/flask, which is the number of cells that will go into the T-75 flask.
   Calculate the volume of cell suspension with which to inoculate a T-75 flask:

$$\frac{620{,}000 \text{ cells}}{1 \text{ mL}}=\frac{187{,}500 \text{ cells}}{?} \quad ?\approx\mathbf{0.3024\,mL}$$

might round this to 0.3 mL, which can be measured easily

10. a. If you take the cell contents of a T-75 flask and put the cells into a T-150 flask, the split is a **½ or 1:2** using conventional terminology.
    b. If you take the cell contents of a T-75 flask and place them into two T-75 flasks, the split is a **½ or 1:2** using conventional terminology.
    c. If you take the cell contents of a T-25 flask and place them into a T-175 flask, the split is a **1/7 or 1:7** using conventional terminology.

11. You want to do a 1/6 cell split. You have your cells in a culture dish with a 57 cm$^2$ surface area.
    You are going to use a new culture dish with a surface area of 145 cm$^2$ that you are assuming has three times the surface area as the original dish.
    a. If you simply move the cells into the new dish, you will have a **1/3 split**. This does not sufficiently dilute the cell density. To get a 1/6 split, you need a further split of 1/2.
    b. You need a further **1/2 split**. You have your cells in 10 mL of suspension. Therefore, if you use half of this volume, that is, 5 mL, and place it in the new dish, you will have the desired split.

## 21.6 FINDING THE MATH: FOLLOWING A WRITTEN CELL CULTURE PROCEDURE

Cell culturists often follow written procedures (also called protocols) that describe how to perform particular tasks, such as how to split cells, how to prepare culture plates, how to prepare cells to be frozen for storage, and so on. Often the procedures are written in a general way so that they are useful regardless of the type and size of culture vessel you are using, or the cell density you might have, or the cell density that you might want, or other factors that can vary. Therefore, before beginning to follow a procedure, it is important to review the steps and look for any calculations that you might need to perform to tailor the procedure for your own situation. The following problems provide excerpts from cell culture procedures. To carry out these procedures, certain calculations are required. If you have never actually performed cell culture, it is not essential that you understand exactly how you would perform each step; just find the math and perform the calculations. Much of the math required is just ratios and proportions, so you already have the skills you need.

**Protocol I: Preparing for Transfection.**

**Transfection** means *to introduce a gene of interest into cells.* The purpose of transfection is usually to cause the transfected cells to make the protein for which that gene codes. You are going to perform a transfection procedure and have purchased cells for that purpose from a company that provides you with the following information:

> CHO cells grown in suspension are one of the most important cell lines for producing proteins in a biomanufacturing environment. Successful cell growth of these cells is dependent on proper growth medium composition and appropriate cell maintenance. With proper culture technique, the cells can reach densities of 1 or $2\times10^7$ cells/mL. The doubling time is typically 24 hours for adherent CHO cells but can decrease to nearly half that for suspension CHO cells. This poses a challenge with regard to cell maintenance because suspended cells will quickly consume nutrients and will starve if not regularly split to lower cell densities and provided with fresh growth medium.
>
> We recommend splitting suspension CHO cultures to a cell density of $2\times10^6$ cells/mL almost every day if the cells will be used for transfection experiments. To avoid coming into laboratory on the weekends, you can split to a lower density of $0.3\times10^6$ cells/mL on Friday; this will prevent overgrowth during the days the cells are not passaged. For best results, only cells that have been recently split to $2\times10^6$ cells/mL should be transfected.
>
> Maintain cell densities between $0.3\times10^6$ cells/mL and $8\times10^6$ cells/mL and do not exceed $10\times10^6$ cells/mL.
>
> For optimal transient transfection and protein expression in suspension CHO cells, it is crucial that cells are split the day before transfection, preferably daily for two or more days before transfection. We recommend splitting the cells to a density of $2\times10^6$ cells/mL the day before transfection. On the day of transfection, split the cells to $4\times10^6$ cells/mL.

**Questions for Protocol I: Preparing for Transfection**

> a. You plan to transfect the cells next Wednesday. Today is Friday. You count the cells, and you have $5.7\times10^6$ cells/mL in a culture vessel that holds 50 mL of suspended cells. What volume of cell suspension should you seed into a fresh culture vessel of the same size? What volume of fresh culture medium should you add to the fresh vessel?
>
> b. On Monday you count the cells, and you have $4.6\times10^6$ cells/mL. What volume of cell suspension should you seed into a fresh culture vessel of the same size? What volume of fresh culture medium should you add?
>
> c. On Tuesday you count the cells, and you have $6.8\times10^6$ cells/mL. What volume of cell suspension should you seed into one or more fresh culture vessels of the same size? What volume of fresh culture medium should you add?
>
> d. On Wednesday, the day of transfection, you count the cells, and you have $7.6\times10^6$ cells/mL. What volume of cell suspension should you seed into a fresh culture vessel of the same size? What volume of fresh culture medium should you add?
>
> (Information for this question is derived from "Tips from the Bench: Cell Culture Tip." *Mirus Bio LLC.* www.mirusbio.com/tech-resources/tips/maintain-suspension-cho-cells)

**Protocol II: Harvesting Cells**

You are following the procedure below to harvest the cells from a T-75 flask.

**HARVESTING CELL PROTOCOL**

Step 1. Aspirate (remove) the culture medium from the flask.
Step 2. Rinse the flask with phosphate buffered saline (PBS) by adding 1 mL of PBS per each 5 $cm^2$.
Step 3. Tilt the flask to coat the surface with PBS.
Step 4. Aspirate the PBS.
Step 5. Repeat the rinse.
Step 6. Add 2 mL of 1X trypsin-EDTA per each 25 $cm^2$ to the flask.

### Questions for Protocol II: Harvesting Cells

a. Highlight each step where you will need to perform a calculation.
b. Perform the required calculation(s). Assume that you have a stock solution of 10× trypsin-EDTA.

### Protocol III: Plate Coating Matrix

You are working with stem cells. These cells require plate coating matrix. Plate coating matrix is applied to the bottom surface of cell culture plates to help the stem cells adhere properly to the plates. In this procedure, you will open a vial of plate coating matrix and dilute it to the proper concentration. You dilute it by adding the proper volume of cell culture nutrient medium. Therefore, you need to measure out two things: the plate coating matrix from the vial and the proper amount of nutrient medium.

- You want enough plate coating matrix to coat two 6-cm cell culture plates.
- Plate coating matrix comes from the manufacturer dissolved in aqueous solution.
- The manufacturer tells you that each 6-cm cell culture plate requires 2 mL of plate coating matrix diluted in culture medium at a concentration of 150 µg/mL.
- This procedure is sketched in Figure 21.6a and the label from your vial of plate coating matrix is shown in Figure 21.6b.

### Questions for Protocol III: Plate Coating Matrix

a. How much plate coating matrix will you need to remove from the vial?
b. How much cell culture medium is required to dilute the plate coating matrix?

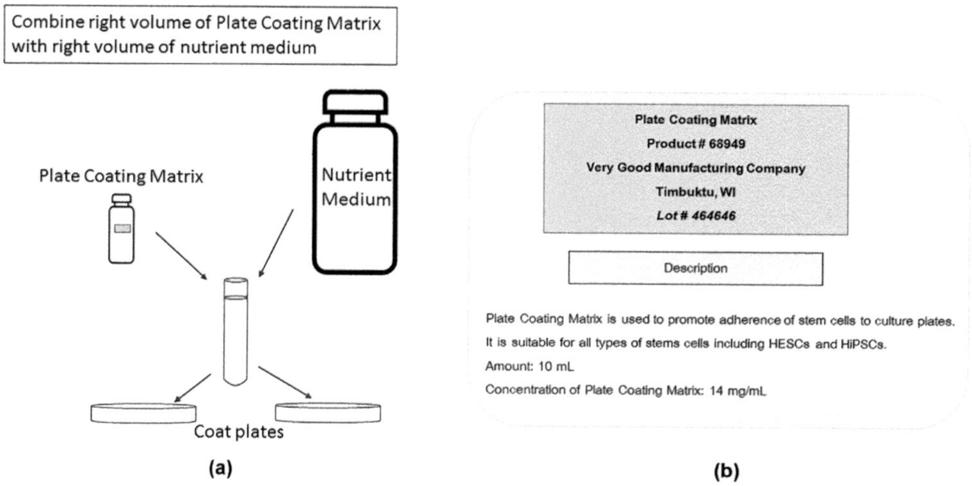


**FIGURE 21.6** Plate coating matrix. (a) The overall procedure. (b) The label from the plate coating matrix vial.

**Answers**

**Protocol I: Preparing For Transfection**

a. Friday: You have $5.7\times10^6$ cells/mL. On Fridays, it is recommended to split the cells to a density of $0.3\times10^6$ cell/mL. You are putting the cells into a fresh 50 mL culture vessel. To calculate how many cells you need in total for a 50 mL culture:

$$(0.3\times10^6 \text{cell}/\cancel{\text{mL}})(50\ \cancel{\text{mL}}) = 1.5\times10^7 \text{ cells}$$

You have suspended cells at a density of $5.7\times10^6$ cells/mL. To calculate how many mL of this cell suspension you need, you can use a proportion equation:

$$\frac{5.7\times10^6 \text{cells}}{1 \text{ mL}} = \frac{1.5\times10^7 \text{cells}}{?}$$

$$? \approx 2.6\,\text{mL}$$

**Therefore, you need 2.6 mL of suspended cells and 47.4 mL of culture medium.**

b. On Monday, you have $4.6\times10^6$ cells/mL. The directions recommend maintaining the cells normally to $2\times10^6$ cells/mL (except on Fridays). To calculate how many cells you need in total for your 50 mL culture:

$$(2\times10^6 \text{cell}/\cancel{\text{mL}})(50\ \cancel{\text{mL}}) = 1.0\times10^8 \text{ cells}$$

You have suspended cells at a density of $4.6\times10^6$ cells/mL. To calculate how many mL of this cell suspension you need, you can again use a proportion equation:

$$\frac{4.6\times10^6 \text{cells}}{1 \text{ mL}} = \frac{1.0\times10^8}{?}$$

$$? \approx 21.7\,\text{mL}$$

**Therefore, you need 21.7 mL of suspended cells and 28.3 mL of culture medium.**

c. On Tuesday, you count the cells, and you have $6.8\times10^6$ cells/mL. You want $2.0\times10^6$ cells/mL in the new vessel. To calculate how many cells you need in total for your 50 mL culture:

$$(2\times10^6 \text{cell}/\cancel{\text{mL}})(50\ \cancel{\text{mL}}) = 1.0\times10^8 \text{ cells}$$

You have suspended cells at a density of $6.8\times10^6$ cells/mL. To calculate how many mL of this cell suspension you need, you can again use a proportion equation:

$$\frac{6.8\times10^6 \text{cells}}{1 \text{ mL}} = \frac{1.0\times10^8 \text{cells}}{?}$$

$$? \approx 14.7\,\text{mL}$$

**Therefore, you need 14.7 mL of suspended cells and 35.3 mL of culture medium.**

d. On Wednesday, the day of transfection, you count the cells, and you have $7.6\times10^6$ cells/mL. According to the directions, on the day of transfection, you want $4\times10^6$ cells/mL. To calculate how many cells you need in total for your 50 mL culture:

$$(4.0\times10^6 \text{cell}/\cancel{\text{mL}})(50\ \cancel{\text{mL}}) = 2.0\times10^8 \text{ cells}$$

You have suspended cells at a density of $7.6\times10^6$ cells/mL. To calculate how many mL of this cell suspension you need, you can again use a proportion equation:

$$\frac{7.6\times10^6\,\text{cells}}{1\ \text{mL}}=\frac{2.0\times10^8\,\text{cells}}{?}$$

$$?\approx 26.3\ \text{mL}$$

**Therefore, you need 26.3 mL of suspended cells and 23.7 mL of culture medium**

**Protocol II: Harvesting Cells**

a. Highlight each step where you will need to perform a calculation.

> **HARVESTING CELL PROTOCOL**
>
> Step 1. Aspirate (remove) the culture medium from the flask.
> Step 2. Rinse the flask with PBS by adding 1 mL of PBS per each 5 cm$^2$.
> Step 3. Tilt the flask to coat the surface with PBS.
> Step 4. Aspirate the PBS.
> Step 5. Repeat the rinse.
> Step 6. Add 2 mL of 1X trypsin-EDTA per each 25 cm$^2$ to the flask.

b. You are using a T-75 flask. In Step 2, you need:

$$\left(\frac{75\ \text{cm}^2}{5\ \text{cm}^2}\right)\left(\frac{1\ \text{mL PBS}}{5\ \text{cm}^2}\right)=15\ \text{mL PBS for the wash}$$

You will need another 15 mL to repeat the wash in Step 5, so be sure to have enough.

In Step 6, you need to dilute the trypsin-EDTA. Before you can do so, you must calculate the volume required:

$$\left(\frac{75\ \text{cm}^2}{1}\right)\left(\frac{2\ \text{mL trypsin}-\text{EDTA}}{25\ \text{cm}^2}\right)=6\ \text{mL trypsin}-\text{EDTA}$$

You have 10X trypsin-EDTA. Use the $C_1V_1=C_2V_2$ equation to calculate how much 10X stock is needed:

(10X) (?) = (1X) (6 mL)

**? = 0.6 mL** of the stock

Dilute the trypsin-EDTA with 5.4 mL of diluent (typically sterile PBS)

**Protocol III: Using Plate Coating Matrix**

You are working with stem cells and require plate coating matrix. The plate coating matrix helps the cells adhere properly to the plate surface.

You want to coat two 6-cm cell culture plates and each requires 2 mL of plate coating matrix. This means that you need 4 mL of dissolved plate coating matrix.

You need plate coating matrix at a concentration of 150 µg/mL = 0.150 mg/mL

**You need 4 mL for the two plates:**

(0.150 mg/mL) (4 mL) = 0.6 mg (This is the amount of plate coating matrix you need.)

From the label, you know there are 14 mg/mL in the undiluted vial of plate coating matrix, so you need:

$$\frac{14\ \text{mg}}{1\ \text{mL}}=\frac{0.6\ \text{mg}}{?}$$

? ≈ 0.0429 mL = **42.9 µL**

a. So, take 43 µL from the plate coating matrix vial. (It is not possible to accurately pipette exactly 42.9 µL.)
b. Take 4 mL of nutrient medium and dilute the plate coating matrix in it.

# Amount and Concentration of Nucleic Acids

22



## 22.1 INTRODUCTION AND BRIEF REVIEW OF NUCLEIC ACID STRUCTURE

**DNA** (**deoxyribonucleic acid**) *is a biological molecule that carries the inherited information that determines the structure, function, and behavior of a cell.* Biotechnologists frequently manipulate DNA for many purposes and in many ways. This chapter introduces some of the math calculations that arise when working with DNA. (Most of this discussion is also relevant to manipulations of RNA, ribonucleic acid, an important biological molecule that is related to DNA.) To understand the calculations in this chapter, you need to know a little bit about the structure of DNA and RNA; here is a brief review (consult any biology book to learn more).

*DNA and RNA, which are* **nucleic acids**, are long molecules composed of subunits held together by chemical bonds, Figure 22.1. *The subunits of DNA and RNA are called* **nucleotides**. A nucleotide consists of a nitrogen-containing base, a sugar molecule (ribose in RNA and deoxyribose in DNA), and a phosphate group, all chemically bonded together to form a subunit, Figure 22.1a. There are five types of bases: guanine, G; adenine, A; cytosine, C; thymine, T; and uracil, U. Guanine, adenine, cytosine, and thymine are found in DNA; RNA has uracil instead of thymine. *A single nucleotide subunit is referred to as a* **base**, abbreviated **b**, because each type of nucleotide is distinguished by its particular nitrogen-containing base.

DOI: 10.1201/9780429282744-27

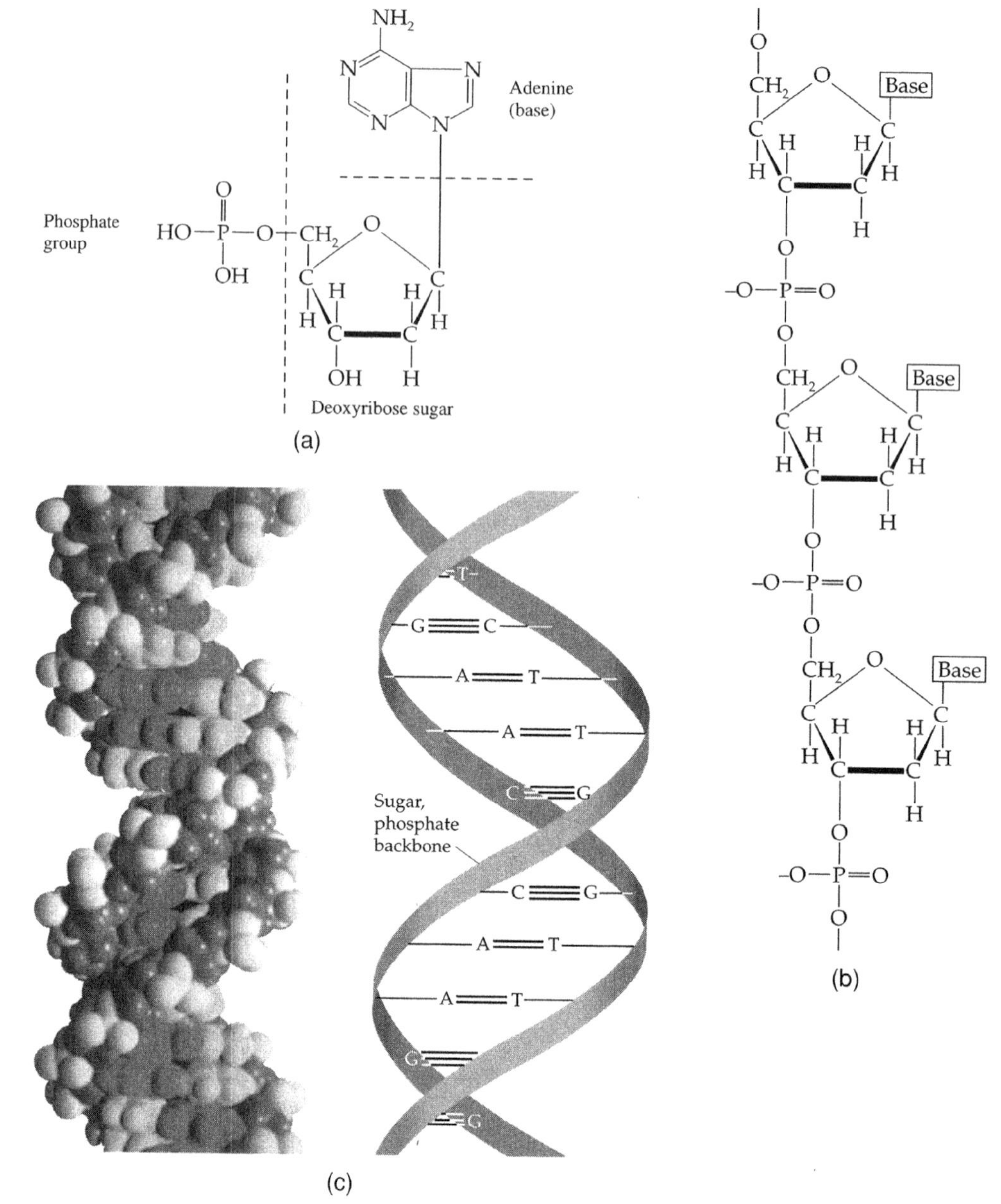


**FIGURE 22.1** The structure of DNA. (a) The subunit of DNA is the nucleotide, which consists of a sugar, a phosphate group, and a nitrogenous base, in this case, adenine. (b) The subunits of DNA are connected by covalent phosphodiester bonds between the phosphate group on one nucleotide and the sugar on the next. The bases extend out to the side. When nucleotides come together to form a phosphodiester bond, a water molecule is lost. (c) Chromosomal DNA is a double helix consisting of two strands of DNA held together by hydrogen bonds between complementary bases.

When nucleotide subunits come together to form a strand of DNA or RNA, phosphodiester bonds form that link one subunit to the next, Figure 22.1b. A water molecule is lost each time a phosphodiester bond forms because the sugar of one nucleotide loses an OH group and the phosphate group of the adjacent nucleotide loses an H.

DNA typically is double-stranded, that is, two strands of DNA lie side by side, held together by hydrogen bonds between nitrogen-containing bases, and twisted into the famous "double-helix" form, Figure 22.1c. In double-stranded DNA, a guanine is always paired with a cytosine on the other strand, and adenine always lies across from thymine. Guanine and cytosine are said to be **complementary** to one another, and adenine and thymine are **complementary** to one another. *A pair of opposing nucleotides are called a* **base pair,** abbreviated **bp**. The human genome consists of about $3.2 \times 10^9$ base pairs organized into 23 chromosomes. *A short strand of nucleotides,* say, 15–40 bases or base pairs, is called an **oligonucleotide.** An oligonucleotide with 15 base pairs might be termed a "15mer."

RNA molecules in nature are shorter than those of DNA and do not form double-stranded helices, although they do sometimes fold with complementary bases across from one another.

The continuity of life on earth depends on the fact that DNA can be replicated (reproduced) in cells. During replication, the two strands of DNA separate from one another and each acts as a template from which a complementary strand is synthesized. The result is two daughter double-stranded DNA molecules. This copying of DNA is an enzymatic reaction catalyzed by DNA polymerase enzymes. The enzymes require **primers,** *short strands of DNA or RNA, that attach to the template DNA and provide a starting point for the polymerase enzymes.* (We will also consider DNA replication in Chapters 24 and 25.)

Moving from the cell's interior to the molecular biology laboratory, there are various forms of DNA that biotechnologists manipulate. These varieties of DNA are mentioned in the math problems in this text:

- **Genomic DNA** *is chromosomal DNA.* Sometimes molecular biologists extract all (or most of) the DNA from a mass of cells. Sometimes shorter segments of genomic DNA are used.
- **Template DNA** *is usually a piece of genomic DNA that is of interest and that will be copied in a reaction.*
- **Vector DNA** *is a DNA molecule that has the ability to replicate and into which molecular biologists insert a fragment of DNA of interest.* The vector then carries the DNA of interest into a host cell (such as a bacterial cell) where the DNA is produced or expressed (made into protein).
- **Plasmids** *are small, circular DNA molecules that were originally isolated from bacteria and are commonly used as vectors.*
- **Viral DNA** *is isolated from viruses and is sometimes used as a vector.*
- **Primers** *are short pieces of DNA that bind to template DNA during replication and provide a start-point for DNA replication enzymes.* Primers are found naturally in cells and are also synthesized in the laboratory for use in molecular biology procedures.

Many of the math skills required when manipulating DNA and RNA are the same as were previously explored in this book. These skills include: comfort with metric prefixes (Chapter 3), ability to convert between units (Chapter 7), understanding moles and molarity (Chapter 12), ability to dilute a substance to the proper concentration (Chapter 14), ability to make a reagent with multiple components (Chapter 13), understanding how spectrophotometry is used to quantify the amount or concentration of an analyte in a solution (Chapter 16), and understanding exponential relationships (Chapter 17).

## 22.2 REACTION MIXTURES

When working with nucleic acids, you will often need to set up a **reaction mixture**. You are probably familiar with the term "reaction" from a chemistry class, but biologists use the term "reaction mixture" in a particular way. When biologists use this term, there is an enzyme (enzymes are proteins) involved in catalyzing (promoting) a reaction. Substrates (which are molecules) are converted into molecular products in the presence of enzymes:

$$\text{Substrate(s)} \xrightarrow{\text{Enzyme}} \text{Product(s)}$$

Many molecular biology procedures depend on reactions catalyzed by enzymes. Molecular biologists set up these reactions in a test tube by combining the enzyme with its substrate(s)

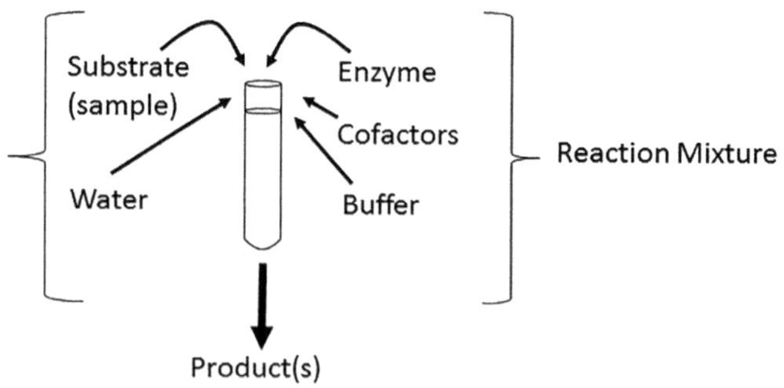


**FIGURE 22.2** Enzymatic molecular biology procedures require setting up a reaction mixture.

plus any necessary buffers, salts, and cofactors (chemicals) that the enzyme requires to function properly. The mixture is combined in water, Figure 22.2. *The aqueous mixture of molecules in the test tube is called the* **reaction mixture.** The *p*olymerase *c*hain *r*eaction (PCR) is an important example of a procedure that requires a reaction mixture. **PCR** *is used to create millions of copies of an original DNA sequence.* As the name suggests, PCR involves a chain of reactions that are catalyzed by an enzyme. PCR is so important that Chapters 24 and 25 are devoted to it.

PCR is not the only enzyme-catalyzed reaction that is used by molecular biologists. You might be familiar with DNA restriction digests. These are enzyme-catalyzed reactions that break a DNA molecule into smaller pieces, using enzymes called restriction endonucleases. We mention restriction digests here because DNA restriction analysis is one of the first skills taught in most biotechnology courses.

Another common example of an enzyme-catalyzed reaction is when RNA is transcribed (converted into) into DNA, termed cDNA (complementary DNA). For example, the virus that causes the illness, COVID-19, has an RNA genome. When people are tested to see if they have contracted this virus, it is common to first transcribe a portion of the virus's RNA genome into DNA. An assay is then used that detects viral cDNA.

In all these enzymatic procedures, molecular biologists must prepare the components for a particular reaction mixture and then combine them in a test tube in the proper proportions. In some cases, the reaction mixture includes a component that is labeled to allow analysts to detect the results of the reaction. Fluorescence is a common type of label; we will see how fluorescence is used in PCR in Chapter 25. Radioisotopes are also sometimes used as a label. Molecules that have incorporated a radioactive substance can be detected in the laboratory using specialized techniques.

This chapter introduces calculations relating to preparing reaction mixtures with DNA. There are various ways to express the concentration and amount of nucleic acids in reaction mixtures, and therefore it is often necessary to perform conversions between these different expressions. We will spend some time in this chapter on these conversions. We will also introduce common spectrophotometric methods of determining the concentrations of nucleic acids in a solution. But first, it is necessary to spend some time talking about the terms "amount" and "concentration" as they apply to nucleic acids.

## 22.3 AMOUNT AND CONCENTRATION

Chapters 11 and 12 talked about "amount" and "concentration" of solutes in solutions. Understanding the distinction between amount and concentration is also vital when dealing with nucleic acids and reaction mixtures. Recall that an amount is how much of a substance of interest is present, for example, a teaspoon, gram, or mole. A concentration is the amount of a substance of interest per total volume (or occasionally per total mass). Concentration might be expressed, for example, as µg/mL, molarity, or percent. Table 22.1a and b shows in overview how amounts and concentrations of DNA/RNA are commonly expressed, and then

**TABLE 22.1a Expressions of *Amount* of Nucleic Acids**

| Type of Expression | Expression | Abbreviation | Conversion Factors |
|---|---|---|---|
| AMOUNT, units relating to "bases" | Bases | b | 1 b (sodium salt) ≈ 330 D (when incorporated into a DNA/RNA strand) |
| | Base pairs | bp | 1 bp (sodium salt) ≈ 660 D (when incorporated into a DNA/RNA strand) |
| | Kilobases | Kb | 1 Kb double-stranded DNA = 1,000 bp ≈ $6.6 \times 10^5$ D<br>1 Kb single-stranded DNA = 1000 b ≈ $3.3 \times 10^5$ D |
| | Megabases | Mb | $1\,\text{Mb} = 1{,}000{,}000\,(\text{million or } 10^6)\,\text{bp}$ |
| | Gigabases | Gb | $1\,\text{Gb} = 1{,}000{,}000{,}000\,(\text{billion or } 10^9)\,\text{bp}$ |
| AMOUNT, units relating to g | Grams | g | $1\,\text{g} = 10^3\,\text{mg} = 10^6\,\mu\text{g} = 10^9\,\text{ng} = 10^{12}\,\text{pg}$ |
| | Milligrams | mg | $1\,\text{mg} = 1/1{,}000\,\text{g} = 10^{-3}\,\text{g}$ |
| | Micrograms | µg | $1\,\mu\text{g} = 1/1{,}000{,}000\,\text{g} = 10^{-6}\,\text{g}$ |
| | Nanograms | ng | $1\,\text{ng} = 1/1{,}000{,}000{,}000\,\text{g} = 10^{-9}\,\text{g}$ |
| | Picograms | pg | $1\,\text{pg} = 1/1{,}000{,}000{,}000{,}000\,\text{g} = 10^{-12}\,\text{g}$ |
| AMOUNT, units relating to moles | Moles | mol | $1\,\text{mol} = 6.0221 \times 10^{23}$ atoms or molecules $= 10^3\,\text{mmol} = 10^6\,\mu\text{mol} = 10^9\,\text{nmol} = 10^{12}\,\text{pmol}$ |
| | Millimoles | mmol | $1\,\text{mmol} = 1/1{,}000\,\text{mol} = 10^{-3}\,\text{mol}$ |
| | Micromoles | µmol | $1\,\mu\text{mol} = 1/1{,}000{,}000\,\text{mol} = 10^{-6}\,\text{mol}$ |
| | Nanomoles | nmol | $1\,\text{nmol} = 1/1{,}000{,}000{,}000\,\text{mol} = 10^{-9}\,\text{mol}$ |
| | Picomoles | pmol | $1\,\text{pmol} = 1/1{,}000{,}000{,}000{,}000\,\text{mol} = 10^{-12}\,\text{mol}$<br>1 pmol of a 1 Kb DNA fragment ≈ 0.66 µg |
| AMOUNT, units relating to daltons | Daltons | D or Da | $1\,\text{D} = 1.6605 \times 10^{-24}\,\text{g}$ |
| | Kilodaltons | KD | 1 KD = 1,000 D |

**TABLE 22.1b Expressions of *Concentration* for Nucleic Acids**

| Type of Expression | Expression | Abbreviation | Conversion Factors |
|---|---|---|---|
| CONCENTRATION, units expressed as a fraction | | µg/mL | |
| | | mg/mL | |
| | | ng/mL | |
| | | pg/mL | |
| CONCENTRATION, units relating to molarity | molar | M | 1 mol/L |
| | millimolar | mM | $1\,\text{mM} = 10^{-3}\,\text{M}$ |
| | micromolar | µM | $1\,\mu\text{M} = 10^{-6}\,\text{M}$ |
| | nanomolar | nM | $1\,\text{nM} = 10^{-9}\,\text{M}$ |
| | picomolar | pM | $1\,\text{pM} = 10^{-12}\,\text{M}$ |

subsequent sections of this chapter explore these expressions in more detail. Table 22.1a and b also provides conversion factors that you will need in later problems.

## 22.4 UNITS OF "BASES"

Nucleic acids are frequently described in terms of how many bases (b) or pairs of bases (bp) are present in a strand or molecule. We have not previously encountered this expression of amount because it is unique to nucleic acids. A stretch of DNA might consist, for example, of 500 nucleotide subunits, b, if the DNA is single-stranded; or 500 complementary nucleotide pairs, bp, if the DNA is double-stranded. *1,000 bases or base pairs is called a* **kilobase**, abbreviated **Kb.** This terminology can be ambiguous because 1 Kb refers to 1000 nucleotide *pairs* if the DNA is double-stranded and 1,000 nucleotides if it is single-stranded. It is usually safest to assume that DNA is double-stranded, if it is not specified. Therefore, 1 Kb usually (but not always) means 2,000 nucleotides total. A **megabase, Mb** is 1,000,000 (million) bp or b. A **gigabase, Gb,** is 1,000,000,000 (billion) bp or b.

**Example Problem:**

How many nucleotides are present in 3.5 Kb of DNA? (Assume double-stranded DNA.)

*Answer:*

There are 3,500 nucleotide *pairs* or 7,000 nucleotides.

**Practice Problems**

1. ***A particular gene is 1.2 Kb in length. How many nucleotides does it have? (Assume double-stranded DNA.)***
2. ***Epstein-Barr is a common virus that occasionally causes the disease infectious mononucleosis ("mono"). The entire genome of the Epstein-Barr virus consists of about 0.0172 ×10⁶ bp of DNA.* E. coli *is a kind of bacterium that inhabits everyone's gut. (A few strains of* E. coli *cause disease but the majority of* E. coli *are harmless and may even be necessary for good health.) The genome of* E. coli *bacteria consists of about 4.6 × 10⁶ base pairs. The genome of humans consists of about 3.2 billion base pairs. Express the genome sizes of Epstein-Barr virus,* E. coli *bacteria, and humans with units of:***
   a. ***Kb*** b. ***Mb***

*Answers*

1. A gene that is 1.2 Kb in length has: (1,200) (2) = **2,400 nucleotides**
2. a. Epstein-Barr: **172 Kb** *E. coli*: **4,600 Kb** human: **$3.2 \times 10^6$ Kb**
   b. Epstein-Barr: **0.172 Mb** *E. coli*: **4.6 Mb** human: **$3.2 \times 10^3$ Mb**

## 22.5 GRAMS, MILLIGRAMS, MICROGRAMS, NANOGRAMS, AND PICOGRAMS

Molecular biologists manipulate very small amounts of nucleic acids, so it is common to speak of grams (g), milligrams (mg), micrograms (μg), nanograms (ng), and picograms (pg), see Table 22.1a. It is therefore essential to be familiar with these metric prefixes. Before leaving this section, memorize the definitions of milli-, micro-, nano-, and pico- and be able to convert between them.

**Example Problem:**

A reaction mixture contains 1 µg of DNA. How much does it contain in units of:

a. g b. mg c. ng d. pg

***Answer:***

As with all unit conversion problems, different strategies are possible. Four strategies are illustrated here:

a. $1\ \mu g = \mathbf{10^{-6}\ g}$ (Memorize this conversion. See Table 22.1a.)
b. You might use the unit canceling method based on the conversion factors in Table 22.1a:

$$1\ \cancel{\mu g}\left(\frac{1\ \text{mg}}{10^{-3}\ \cancel{g}}\right)\left(\frac{1\ \cancel{g}}{10^{6}\ \cancel{\mu g}}\right) = 0.001\ \text{mg} = \mathbf{10^{-3}\ mg}$$

c. You might do this in your head, knowing that a µg ($10^{-6}$ g) is 1,000 times larger than an ng:

$$1\ \mu g = 1{,}000\ \text{ng} = \mathbf{10^{3}\ ng}$$

d. You might use proportions. With the conversion factors in Table 22.1a, this will require two steps. First, convert 1 µg to units of g. Then, convert that value to picograms:
From Table 22.1a:

$$1\ \mu g = 1 \times 10^{-6}\ g$$

$$\frac{1\ g}{10^{12}\ pg} = \frac{1 \times 10^{-6}\ g}{?} \quad \mathbf{? = 1 \times 10^{6}\ pg}$$

**Practice Problems**

1. ***Convert 2.3 mg to units of:***
   a. ***g*** b. ***µg*** c. ***ng*** d. ***pg***
2. ***A procedure calls for 10 pg of DNA template. How much does it contain in units of:***
   a. ***g*** b. ***mg*** c. ***µg*** d. ***ng***
3. ***1 ng =*** ____________ ***µg =*** ____________ ***pg =*** ____________ ***g***
4. ***1.5 pg =*** ____________ ***ng =*** ____________ ***µg =*** ____________ ***g***

***Answers***

1. a. $\mathbf{2.3 \times 10^{-3}\ g}$ b. $\mathbf{2.3 \times 10^{3}\ \mu g}$ c. $\mathbf{2.3 \times 10^{6}\ ng}$ d. $\mathbf{2.3 \times 10^{9}\ pg}$
2. a. $\mathbf{1 \times 10^{-11}\ g}$ b. $\mathbf{1 \times 10^{-8}\ mg}$ c. $\mathbf{1 \times 10^{-5}\ \mu g}$ d. $\mathbf{1 \times 10^{-2}\ ng}$
3. $1\ \text{ng} = \mathbf{10^{-3}}\ \mu g = \mathbf{10^{3}\ pg} = \mathbf{10^{-9}}\ g$
4. $1.5\ \text{pg} = \mathbf{1.5 \times 10^{-3}\ ng} = \mathbf{1.5 \times 10^{-6}}\ \mu g = \mathbf{1.5 \times 10^{-12}}\ g$

## 22.6 MOLES, MILLIMOLES, MICROMOLES, NANOMOLES, AND PICOMOLES

Recall that a **mole** *of any atom or molecule contains about 6.022 × $10^{23}$ particles of that atom or molecule.* (Mole is the SI unit for the amount of substance.) Nucleic acids are typically added to reaction mixtures in very low concentrations, so it is common to speak of:

- millimoles, mmol
- micromoles, µmol
- nanomoles, nmol
- picomoles, pmol

We will return later in this chapter to moles and molarity calculations; at this point, practice converting between the various units.

**Example Problem:**

A mixture contains 10 µmol of DNA. How much does it contain in units of:

a. mol b. mmol c. nmol d. pmol

*Answer:*

a. $10\ \mu\text{mol} = \mathbf{10 \times 10^{-6}\ mol = 1 \times 10^{-5}\ mol}$ (Table 22.1a)
b. Unit canceling method:

$$10\ \cancel{\mu\text{mol}}\left(\frac{1\ \text{mmol}}{10^{-3}\ \cancel{\text{mol}}}\right)\left(\frac{1\ \cancel{\text{mol}}}{10^{6}\ \cancel{\mu\text{mol}}}\right) = \mathbf{0.01\ mmol = 10^{-2}\ mmol}$$

c. A micromole is 1,000 times larger than a nanomole:

$$10\ \mu\text{mol} = 10 \times 10^{3}\ \text{nmol} = \mathbf{1 \times 10^{4}\ nmol}$$

d. Proportions: From Table 22.1a: $10\ \mu\text{mol} = 1 \times 10^{-5}\ \text{mol}$

$$\frac{1\ \text{mol}}{10^{12}\ \text{pmol}} = \frac{1 \times 10^{-5}\ \text{mol}}{?} \qquad \mathbf{? = 1 \times 10^{7}\ pmol}$$

**Practice Problems**

1. ***Convert 35 mmol to units of:***
   a. ***mol*** b. ***µmol*** c. ***nmol*** d. ***pmol***
2. ***A reaction mixture contains 100 pmol of template DNA. How much does it contain in units of:***
   a. ***mol*** b. ***mmol*** c. ***µmol*** d. ***nmol***
3. ***1 nmol =__________ µmol =__________ pmol =__________ mol***
4. ***1.5 pmol =__________ nmol =__________ µmol =__________ mol***

*Answers*

1. a. $\mathbf{3.5 \times 10^{-2}}$ **mol** b. $\mathbf{3.5 \times 10^{4}}$ **μmol** c. $\mathbf{3.5 \times 10^{7}}$ **nmol**
   d. $\mathbf{3.5 \times 10^{10}}$ **pmol**
2. a. $\mathbf{1 \times 10^{-10}}$ **mol** b. $\mathbf{1 \times 10^{-7}}$ **mmol** c. $\mathbf{1 \times 10^{-4}}$ **μmol**
   d. $\mathbf{1 \times 10^{-1}}$ **nmol**
3. **1 nmol =** $\underline{\mathbf{10^{-3}}}$ **μmol =** $\underline{\mathbf{10^{3}}}$ **pmol =** $\underline{\mathbf{10^{-9}}}$ **mol**
4. **1.5 pmol =** $\underline{\mathbf{1.5 \times 10^{-3}}}$ **nmol =** $\underline{\mathbf{1.5 \times 10^{-6}}}$ **μmol =** $\underline{\mathbf{1.5 \times 10^{-12}}}$ **mol**

## 22.7 CONCENTRATION EXPRESSED AS A FRACTION

It is common to see the concentration of nucleic acids expressed in terms of μg/mL, μg/μL, ng/mL, and so on. The example problems illustrate typical calculations associated with these types of expressions. The examples and practice problems also show how dilutions are frequently required when working with the very low amounts/concentrations that are typical of nucleic acid procedures.

**Example Problem:**

DNA is present in a stock solution at a concentration of 1 μg/mL.

You need 50 ng of DNA for a reaction. How much of the stock solution do you need?

*Answer:*

First, observe that weight is expressed both in units of ng (50 ng) and μg (1 μg/mL). Convert the weight units to the same unit, either both to ng or both to μg. In this example, let us convert μg to ng:

$1\ \mu g = 10^3$ ng. So the stock contains DNA at a concentration of 1 μg/mL = $10^3$ ng/mL.

Then, it is possible to use a proportion equation; if the stock solution contains $10^3$ ng in each mL, how many mL are needed to get 50 ng?

$$\frac{10^3\ \text{ng}}{1\ \text{mL}} = \frac{50\ \text{ng}}{?} \qquad \mathbf{? = 0.05\ mL = 50\ \mu L}$$

As an alternative strategy, note that 1 μg/mL = 1 ng/μL. (Both the numerator and denominator are divided by 1,000.)

Now, using a proportion, determine the volume required to get 50 ng:

$$\frac{1\ \text{ng}}{1\ \mu\text{L}} = \frac{50\ \text{ng}}{?} \qquad \mathbf{? = 50\ \mu L}$$

**Example Problem:**

DNA is present in a stock solution at a concentration of 1 µg/mL.

You need 50 pg of DNA for a reaction. How much of the stock do you need?

***Answer:***

Convert the weights to the same unit: 1 µg/mL = $10^6$ pg/mL

$$\frac{10^6 \text{ pg}}{1 \text{ mL}} = \frac{50 \text{ pg}}{?} \quad \mathbf{? = 0.00005\ mL = 0.05\ \mu L}$$

It is not possible to accurately pipette this volume, so the stock needs to be diluted. There is no standard way to decide how much to dilute the stock nor how much volume to make, since your strategy will depend on how much stock you have, how many times you will be removing 50 pg, and other factors.

If you dilute the stock so that it is 100 times less concentrated, then you will need to remove 5 µL of it instead of 0.05 µL. 5 µL can be dispensed with a micropipette, so this is a reasonable dilution. Decide how much volume of the dilution to make, for example, 200 µL. Recall from Section 14.5 that we can use proportions to calculate how to make this dilution:

$$\frac{1}{100} = \frac{?}{200\ \mu\text{L}} \quad ? = 2\ \mu\text{L}$$

This means that you remove 2 µL of the 1 µg/mL stock and bring it to 200 µL by adding 198 µL of buffer or water.

What is the concentration of DNA in the diluted solution? (Use Equation 14.2, introduced in Section 14.6)

$$(\text{Original concentration})\ (\text{dilution}) = \text{concentration in the diluted sample}$$

$$\left(\frac{1\times10^6 \text{ pg DNA}}{1 \text{ mL}}\right)\left(\frac{1}{100}\right) = \frac{1\times10^4 \text{pg DNA}}{1 \text{ mL}}$$

How much of the diluted solution is needed? It is possible to use a proportion equation to calculate this:

$$\frac{1\times10^4 \text{ pg}}{1 \text{ mL}} = \frac{50 \text{ pg}}{?} \quad \mathbf{? = 0.005\ mL = 5\ \mu L}$$

**Example Problem:**

DNA is present in a stock solution at a concentration of 1 µg/mL.

Your recipe calls for you to remove 200 µL from the DNA stock solution and put it into a reaction mixture. How many µg will you add to the reaction mixture?

***Answer:***

Let us solve this with the unit canceling strategy:

$$(\text{Volume removed})(\text{concentration of stock solution})(\text{conversion factor})$$

$$= \mu\text{g removed from stock}$$

$$\left(\frac{200\ \cancel{\mu L}}{1}\right)\left(\frac{1\ \mu g\ DNA}{1\ \cancel{mL}}\right)\left(\frac{1\ \cancel{mL}}{1{,}000\ \cancel{\mu L}}\right) = \mathbf{0.2\ \mu g\ DNA}$$

If you prefer proportions, here is a proportions strategy: Make the units of volume consistent by converting mL to µL and then use a proportion equation:

$$\frac{1\ \mu g\ DNA}{1{,}000\ \mu L} = \frac{?}{200\ \mu L} \qquad \mathbf{? = 0.2\ \mu g\ DNA}$$

**Example Problem:**

Enzyme concentrations are often expressed as units of enzyme activity/volume, for example, 2 U/mL. (Be careful not to confuse the abbreviation of unit, U, with micro, µ.) A catalog states that the concentration of an enzyme is 5 U/µL. You need 1.25 U/reaction tube. You plan to perform 25 reactions. How many microliters of enzyme do you need altogether?

***Answer:***

By proportions:

$$\frac{5\ U\ enzyme}{1\ \mu L} = \frac{1.25\ U}{?} \qquad ? = 0.25\ \mu L$$

You need (0.25 µL/reaction tube) (25 tubes) = **6.25 µL total.**

**Practice Problems**

1. ***You have a solution of 100 μg/mL of DNA.***
   a. ***You need 2 mg of DNA for a reaction, how much of the solution should you take?***
   b. ***You need 35 μg of DNA for a reaction, how much of the solution should you take?***
   c. ***You need 0.3 mg of DNA for a reaction, how much of the solution should you take?***
   d. ***You need 50 μg of DNA for a reaction, how much of the solution should you take?***
2. ***A reaction mixture calls for 5 U of HindIII enzyme. The enzyme comes from the manufacturer at a concentration of 10 U/μL. How much do you need?***
3. ***A procedure calls for 100 ng of DNA/μL of reaction mixture. Your stock solution is 1 μg DNA/μL. How much of the stock do you need if your reaction mixture will be 20 μL?***
4. ***This is a recipe modified from the Promega Corporation "Protocols and Applications Guide, Second Edition." Promega Corporation is a company that makes products for research in molecular biology. (Do not worry about the nature of the constituents of this buffer, nor its purpose, since we will focus only on calculations.)***

| **Assay Buffer** | |
|---|---|
| **Genomic DNA (1 μg/μL)** | **10 μL** |
| **Sau3A 1 10X buffer** | **45 μL** |
| **1 mg/mL acetylated BSA** | **50 μL** |
| **Water** | **340 μL** |
| **Total volume** | **445 μL** |

***If you have a solution of genomic DNA at a concentration of 4 mg/mL, how could you dilute it to a concentration of 1 μg/μL (because that is the concentration specified in the recipe)?***

5. ***In this chart from Promega Corporation, it shows that 1.2 μg of pGEM® (a plasmid vector) are present at a concentration of 50 ng/μL. How many μL of pGEM are in the kit?***

| ***pGEM®-T Easy Vector System*** | |
|---|---|
| ***1.2 μg pGEM®-T easy vector*** | ***50 ng/μL*** |
| ***Control insert DNA*** | ***12 μL*** |
| ***2X Rapid ligation buffer*** | ***200 μL*** |
| ***T4 DNA ligase*** | ***100 U*** |

*Answers*

1. a. $\frac{100\ \mu g}{1\ mL} = \frac{2{,}000\ \mu g}{?}$ $\quad ? = \mathbf{20\ mL}$

   b. $\frac{100\ \mu g}{1\ mL} = \frac{35\ \mu g}{?}$ $\quad ? = 0.35\ mL = \mathbf{350\ \mu L}$

   c. $\frac{100\ \mu g}{1\ mL} = \frac{300\ \mu g}{?}$ $\quad ? = \mathbf{3\ mL}$

   d. $\frac{100\ \mu g}{1\ mL} = \frac{50\ \mu g}{?}$ $\quad ? = 0.5\ mL = \mathbf{500\ \mu L}$

2. A reaction mixture calls for 5 U of HindIII enzyme, which comes from the manufacturer at a concentration of 10 U/µL.

$$\frac{10 \text{ units enzyme}}{1\,\mu\text{L}} = \frac{5 \text{ units enzyme}}{?} \quad ? = \mathbf{0.5\,\mu L}$$

It is generally considered to be poor practice to dispense 0.5 µL (although modern micropipettes carefully used may be accurate at this low volume). One might therefore dilute the stock, for example, 2 µL of stock with 18 µL of buffer or water. **5 µL of the diluted enzyme solution** will then be needed for the reaction mixture.

3. A procedure calls for 100 ng of DNA/µL of reaction mixture. Stock solution is 1 µg/µL. How much of the stock is needed if your reaction mixture will be 20 µL?
   First, calculate how much DNA is needed, based on the volume of the reaction mixture. A unit canceling strategy is:

$$\left(\frac{100 \text{ ng DNA}}{\cancel{1\,\mu\text{L reaction mixture}}}\right)\left(20\ \cancel{\mu\text{L reaction mixture}}\right) = 2{,}000 \text{ ng DNA}$$

The stock is present at 1 µg/µL = 1,000 ng/µL so, using proportion strategy:

$$\frac{1{,}000 \text{ ng}}{\mu\text{L}} = \frac{2000 \text{ ng}}{?} \quad ? = \mathbf{2\,\mu L}$$

4. First, note that 4 mg/mL = 4 µg/µL
   Decide how much volume to make of the 1 µg/mL solution, for example, 100 µL.

$$C_1 \qquad V_1 = C_2 \qquad V_2 \qquad \text{(See Chapter 13.1 for an explanation of this equation.)}$$

$$(4\,\mu\text{g}/\mu\text{L}) \quad ? = (1\,\mu\text{g}/\mu\text{L}) \quad (1\,00 \text{ mL})$$

$$\mathbf{? = 25\,\mu L}$$

   So, take **25 µL** of the original DNA stock solution and add **75 µL** of water or buffer.

5. The concentration of pGEM is 50 ng/µL = $50 \times 10^{-3}$ µg/µL = 0.05 µg/µL
   If there are 0.05 µg in 1 µL, then 1.2 µg would require how many µL?

$$\frac{0.05\,\mu\text{g}}{1\,\mu\text{L}} = \frac{1.2\,\mu\text{g}}{?} \quad \mathbf{? = 24\,\mu L}$$

## 22.8 MOLAR CONCENTRATIONS

Molecular biologists deal with very low concentrations of DNA and RNA, so concentration is often expressed in units of millimolar, mM; micromolar, µM; nanomolar, nM; and picomolar, pM. By definition:

- 1 M = 1 mol/L
- 1 mM = 1 mmol/L
- 1 µM = 1 µmol/L
- 1 nM = 1 nmol/L
- 1 pM = 1 pmol/L

**Example Problem:**

You have a stock solution that is 100 nM. (a) Convert this to µM. (b) Convert this to pM. (c) Convert this to nmol/L. (d) Convert this to nmol/µL.

***Answer:***

a. A nmol is 1,000 times smaller than a µmol.
   So: $100\text{ nM} = 100 \times 10^{-3}\ \mu\text{M} = \mathbf{1 \times 10^{-1}\ \mu M}$
b. A nmol is 1,000 times larger than a pmol.
   So: $100\text{ nM} = 100 \times 10^{3}\text{ pM} = \mathbf{1 \times 10^{5}\ pM}$
c. By definition: 100 nM = **100 nmol/L**
d. We need units of µL in the denominator, so convert the units of L to µL:

$$100\text{ nmol}/\text{L} = 100\text{ nmol}/10^{6}\ \mu\text{L} = 100 \times 10^{-6}\text{ nmol}/\mu\text{L} = \mathbf{1 \times 10^{-4}\ nmol/\mu L}$$

**Example Problem:**

a. Convert 1 µmol/mL to units of mM
b. Convert 1 pmol/µL to units of µM. (This conversion sometimes arises in calculations relating to PCR primers.)

***Answer:***

a. 1 µmol/mL to mM
   **Strategy 1:**
   Multiply the numerator and denominator by 1,000 to get L in the denominator:

$$= 1 \times 10^{3}\ \mu\text{mol}/10^{3}\text{ mL} = 1\text{ mmol}/\text{L}$$

   By definition, 1 mmol/L = **1 mM**
   **Strategy 2: Unit Canceling**

$$\frac{1\ \cancel{\mu\text{mol}}}{1\ \cancel{\text{mL}}}\left(\frac{10^{3}\ \cancel{\text{mL}}}{1\text{ L}}\right)\left(\frac{1\text{ mmol}}{10^{3}\ \cancel{\mu\text{mol}}}\right) = \frac{1\text{ mmol}}{1\text{ L}} = \mathbf{1\ mM}$$

b. 1 pmol/µL to µM
   **Strategy 1:**
   Multiply the numerator and denominator by $10^6$ to get L in the denominator:

$$= 1 \times 10^{6}\text{ pmol}/\text{L} = 1\ \mu\text{mol}/\text{L} = \mathbf{1\ \mu M}$$

   **Strategy 2: Unit Canceling**

$$\frac{1\ \cancel{\text{pmol}}}{1\ \cancel{\mu\text{L}}}\left(\frac{10^{6}\ \cancel{\mu\text{L}}}{1\text{ L}}\right)\left(\frac{1\ \mu\text{mol}}{10^{6}\ \cancel{\text{pmol}}}\right) = \frac{1\ \mu\text{mol}}{1\text{ L}} = \mathbf{1\ \mu M}$$

**Example Problem:**

A 50 μL PCR reaction mixture contains primers at a concentration of 0.2 μM. How much primer is in the reaction mixture? (a) Express your answer in units of μmol. (b) Express your answer in units of pmol. Observe that the answers are amounts, not concentrations.

***Answer:***

a. By definition, a 0.2 μmolar solution has 0.2 μmol of primer per liter.

So, how many μmol are in the 50 μL reaction volume?

We could set this up as a proportion, but first we need to express the volumes with the same units, such as, L, or μL, or mL. Let us use mL:

$$1\text{ L} = 1{,}000\text{ mL} \qquad 50\ \mu\text{L} = 50\times10^{-3}\text{ mL}$$

Now, setting up the proportion:

$$\frac{0.2\ \mu\text{mol}}{1{,}000\text{ mL}} = \frac{?}{50\times10^{-3}\text{ mL}} \qquad \mathbf{? = 1\times10^{-5}\ \boldsymbol{\mu}mol}$$

Alternatively, by unit canceling:

$$\left(\frac{50\ \cancel{\mu\text{L}}}{1}\right)\left(\frac{0.2\ \mu\text{mol}}{1\ \cancel{\text{L}}}\right)\left(\frac{1\ \cancel{\text{L}}}{10^{6}\ \cancel{\mu\text{L}}}\right) = \mathbf{1\times10^{-5}\ \boldsymbol{\mu}mol}$$

b. 1 μmol = $10^6$ pmol so, how many picomoles is $10^{-5}$ μmol?

$$\frac{1\ \mu\text{mol}}{10^{6}\text{ pmol}} = \frac{1\times10^{-5}\ \mu\text{mol}}{?} \qquad ? = 1\times10^{1}\text{ pmol} = \mathbf{10\ pmol}$$

**Practice Problems**

1. ***Convert 200 pM to:***
   a. ***molar concentration*** b. ***μM concentration*** c. ***nM concentration***
2. ***Convert 0.002 M to:***
   a. ***pM concentration*** b. ***μM concentration*** c. ***nM concentration***
3. a. ***Convert 100 μmol/L to a μM concentration.***
   b. ***Convert 50 pmol/μL to a pM concentration.***
   c. ***Convert 35 pmol/μL to a nM concentration.***
4. ***A reaction mixture contains 50 μL of DNA at a concentration of 500 nM. How many nanomoles are present?***
5. ***A stock solution of DNA is 500 nM and you need 20 picomoles for a reaction. How much of the stock do you need?***

*Answers*

1. a. $200\ \text{pM} = 200 \times 10^{-12}\ \text{M} = \mathbf{2 \times 10^{-10}\ M}$
   b. $200\ \text{pM} = 200 \times 10^{-6}\ \mu\text{M} = \mathbf{2 \times 10^{-4}\ \mu M}$
   c. $200\ \text{pM} = 200 \times 10^{-3}\ \text{nM} = \mathbf{2 \times 10^{-1}\ nM}$
2. a. $0.002\ \text{M} = 0.002 \times 10^{12}\ \text{pM} = \mathbf{2 \times 10^{9}\ pM}$
   b. $0.002\ \text{M} = 0.002 \times 10^{6}\ \mu\text{M} = \mathbf{2 \times 10^{3}\ \mu M}$
   c. $0.002\ \text{M} = 0.002 \times 10^{9}\ \text{nM} = \mathbf{2 \times 10^{6}\ nM}$
3. a. Convert 100 µmol/L to a µM concentration. 1 µM = 1 µmol/L.
   100 µmol/L = **100 µM.**
   b. Convert 50 pmol/µL to a pM concentration. By definition, 1 pM = 1 pmol/L.
   We need units of L in the denominator. If we multiply the denominator by $10^6$ to get units of L, we must also multiply the numerator by $10^6$:

$$\left(50\ \text{pmol} \times 10^6\right) / \left(1\ \mu\text{L} \times 10^6\right) = 5 \times 10^7\ \text{pmol} / 1\ \text{L}$$

   So this is $\mathbf{5 \times 10^7\ pM}$.
   c. Convert 35 pmol/µL to a nM concentration. By definition, 1 nM = 1 nmol/L.
   We need units of L in the denominator. If we multiply the denominator by $10^6$ to get units of L, we must also multiply the numerator by $10^6$:

$$\frac{35\ \text{pmol} \times 10^6}{1\ \mu\text{L} \times 10^6} = \frac{3.5 \times 10^7\ \text{pmol}}{1\ \text{L}}$$

$$3.5 \times 10^7\ \text{pmol} / \text{L} = 3.5 \times 10^4\ \text{nmol} / \text{L} = \mathbf{3.5 \times 10^4\ nM}$$

   Alternatively, by unit canceling:

$$\left(\frac{35\ \cancel{\text{pmol}}}{1\ \cancel{\mu\text{L}}}\right)\left(\frac{10^6\ \cancel{\mu\text{L}}}{1\ \text{L}}\right)\left(\frac{1\ \text{nmol}}{10^3\ \cancel{\text{pmol}}}\right) = \frac{3.5 \times 10^4\ \text{nmol}}{1\ \text{L}} = \mathbf{3.5 \times 10^4\ nM}$$

4. A reaction contains 50 µL of DNA at a concentration of 500 nM. How many nanomoles are present?
   500 nM means there are 500 nmol in 1 L. So how many nmol are in 50 µL?

$$\frac{500\ \text{nmol}}{10^6\ \mu\text{L}} = \frac{?}{50\ \mu\text{L}} \qquad \mathbf{? = 0.025\ nmol}$$

   Alternatively, by unit canceling:

$$\left(\frac{50\ \cancel{\mu\text{L}}}{1}\right)\left(\frac{500\ \text{nmol}}{1\ \cancel{\text{L}}}\right)\left(\frac{1\ \cancel{\text{L}}}{10^6\ \cancel{\mu\text{L}}}\right) = \mathbf{2.5 \times 10^{-2}\ nmol}$$

5. A stock solution is 500 nM and you need 20 pmol for a reaction. How much of the stock do you need?
   By definition, 500 nM means there are 500 nmol in 1 L.
   This means there are $500 \times 10^3$ pmol/L.
   If there are $500 \times 10^3$ pmol/$10^6$ µL, then how many µL will have 20 pmol?

$$\frac{500 \times 10^3\ \text{pmol}}{10^6\ \mu\text{L}} = \frac{20\ \text{pmol}}{?} \qquad \mathbf{? = 40\ \mu L\ of\ stock}$$

## 22.9 UNITS OF DALTONS

The mass[1] of one atom of an element is equal to the combined mass of its protons and neutrons (the electrons' mass are so slight that they are usually ignored). A periodic table provides the atomic mass for every element. The atomic masses in the periodic table are reported in units of "atomic mass units" or "Daltons," abbreviated D or Da. For example, the atomic mass of carbon is 12.01; this means *one* atom of carbon has a mass of 12.01 Daltons.

It is possible to convert daltons to the more familiar unit of grams by using a conversion factor. A dalton is approximately equal to the mass of a hydrogen atom. (It is defined as 1/12th the mass of a $^{12}$carbon nucleus, which is about the same as the mass of a hydrogen atom.) Of course, the mass in grams of one hydrogen atom is a really small number: $1.6605 \times 10^{-24}$ g. So, the conversion factor to convert daltons to grams is:

$$1\,\text{D} = 1.66054 \times 10^{-24}\ \text{g}$$

How many daltons are there per gram?

$$\frac{1\,\text{D}}{1.66054 \times 10^{-24}\ \text{g}} = \frac{?}{1\,\text{g}} \qquad \mathbf{? \approx 6.02214 \times 10^{23}}$$

$$6.02214 \times 10^{23}\,\text{D} = 1\,\text{g}$$

Observe that there are $6.02214 \times 10^{23}$ D in 1 g. The number $6.02214 \times 10^{23}$ should look familiar – it is **Avogadro's number**, *the number of molecules or atoms in a mole of any substance.*

$$1\ \text{mole} \approx 6.02214 \times 10^{23}\ \text{atoms or molecules}$$

**Example Problem:**

How much does a mole of hydrogen weigh in units of grams?

***Answer:***

By definition, 1 D is approximately equal to the mass of 1 hydrogen atom.

There are $6.02214 \times 10^{23}$ atoms in a mole of hydrogen.

Each atom weighs 1 D, so a mole of hydrogen weighs $6.02214 \times 10^{23}$ D.

The conversion factor for converting daltons to grams is:

1 dalton ≈ $1.66054 \times 10^{-24}$ g

$$\frac{1\,\text{D}}{1.66054 \times 10^{-24}\ \text{g}} = \frac{6.02214 \times 10^{23}\ \text{D}}{?} \qquad \mathbf{? \approx 1\,g}$$

[1] Note that weight and mass are not synonyms and it is correct to speak of gram molecular *mass* in the context of molarity. However, it is common practice to speak of "atomic weight," "molecular weight," and "formula weight," as we do in this book.

**Example Problem:**

How much does a mole of NaCl weigh in units of grams? The molecular weight of 1 molecule of NaCl is 58.44 D.

***Answer:***

There are $6.02214 \times 10^{23}$ molecules in a mole of NaCl.

Each one weighs 58.44 D, so a mole of NaCl weighs:

$$(58.44\,\text{D})(6.02214 \times 10^{23}\text{ molecules}) \approx 3.519339 \times 10^{25}\,\text{D}$$

The conversion factor for converting daltons to grams is:

$$1\,\text{D} \approx 1.66054 \times 10^{-24}\,\text{g}$$

$$\frac{1\,\text{D}}{1.66054 \times 10^{-24}\,\text{g}} = \frac{3.519339 \times 10^{25}\,\text{D}}{?} \quad \mathbf{? \approx 58.44\,g}$$

So, one mole of NaCl weighs 58.44 g. Observe that a single *molecule* of NaCl weighs 58.44 D and a *mole* of NaCl weighs 58.44 g.

You can see that the mass of a *single atom or molecule* is its atomic mass or its formula mass in units of *daltons*. A *mole* of any atom or compound has the same numerical value but in units of *grams*. For this reason, the terms dalton and MW or FW are often used interchangeably.

## 22.10 THE MOLECULAR WEIGHTS OF OLIGONUCLEOTIDES

In Chapter 12, we talked about making solutions at a certain molar concentration. Recall that to convert between units of weight (such as grams or micrograms) and molarity, it is necessary to know the molecular or formula weight of the substance of interest. In Chapter 12, we found that it is usually possible to find the formula or molecular weight of a chemical compound simply by looking at its container. The molecular weight of a specific chemical compound is always the same. DNA and RNA are different however, first because their sequence varies depending on the source and second because the length of a DNA molecule can vary greatly. A DNA molecule may consist of anywhere from a few nucleotides to billions of base pairs. An oligonucleotide with 20 bases has a much lower MW than intact genomic DNA from a human cell. For these reasons, there is no single MW for all DNA or RNA molecules.

Let us consider how to find the MW of DNA (or RNA), first for oligonucleotides of known sequence and second for other types of DNA. Oligonucleotides are short segments of DNA that are often synthesized in a laboratory. Primers for PCR are a type of oligonucleotide; they are single-stranded. It is relatively simple to find the molecular weight of primers and other synthesized oligonucleotides by adding the weights of all the nucleotides present. Table 22.2 shows the MW of individual nucleotides that have been incorporated into a nucleic acid. When nucleotides form phosphodiester bonds, a water is lost so the MW of the incorporated bases is about 18 D less than that of solitary nucleotides. When oligonucleotides are synthesized, the last nucleotide in the chain is generally lacking a $PO_4$ group, rather it has a single H in that position. Also, synthesized oligonucleotides usually have an OH group at the other end of the chain. A correction factor is usually included to account for the chemistry that occurs during synthesis. This correction factor is commonly 61.96, which is subtracted from the total weight of the nucleotides. Thus, the formula to determine the MW of a DNA oligonucleotide is Equation 22.1:

**EQUATION 22.1 To Determine the MW of a DNA Oligonucleotide**

$$MW = (N_c \times 289.18) + (N_a \times 313.22) + (N_t \times 304.21) + (N_g \times 329.22) - 61.96$$

where:

$N_c$ is the number of cytosines
$N_a$ is the number of adenines
$N_t$ is the number of thymines
$N_g$ is the number of guanines
−61.96 is the correction factor

**TABLE 22.2 Molecular Weights of Nucleotides Incorporated into Nucleic Acids**

| | | | |
|---|---|---|---|
| A in DNA | 313.22 D | A in RNA | 329.22 D |
| C in DNA | 289.18 D | C in RNA | 305.18 D |
| T in DNA | 304.21 D | U in RNA | 306.20 D |
| G in DNA | 329.22 D | G in RNA | 345.22 D |
| A+T | 313.22+304.21 = 617.43 | | |
| G+C | 289.18+329.22 = 618.40 | | |

Data from: Roskams, Jane, and Linda Rodgers. *Lab Ref: A Handbook of Recipes, Reagents, and Other Reference Tools for Use at the Bench*. 1st ed., Cold Spring Harbor Laboratory Press, 2002.

**Practice Problems**

1. ***What is the MW for a single-stranded DNA oligonucleotide with the sequence: GCTCCTACAAATGCCATCA?***
2. ***What is the MW for a single-stranded DNA oligonucleotide with the sequence: GATAGTGGGATTGTGCGTCA?***

*Answers*

1. $MW = (7 \times 289.18) + (6 \times 313.22) + (4 \times 304.21) + (2 \times 329.22) - 61.96 \approx$ **5717**
2. ≈**6228**

## 22.11 THE MOLECULAR WEIGHT OF DNA BASED ON FRAGMENT LENGTHS

There are situations where the exact sequence of a DNA or RNA molecule is unknown but its length, or approximate length, in bases or base pairs is known. There are helpful conversion factors to convert between nucleic acid length and MW. These conversion factors are estimates since the exact MW of a DNA or RNA molecule depends on its exact sequence. A single nucleotide, on average, has a molecular weight of approximately 330 D (or 330 g/mole) and so a base pair on average has a weight of approximately 660 D (or 660 g/mole). These conversion factors enable you to do a variety of helpful conversions. (Note that these are the values from: Sambrook, et al. *Molecular Cloning: A Laboratory Manual.* 2nd ed., Cold Spring Harbor Laboratory Press, 1989. Other references use somewhat different average molecular weights, for example, 649 D for double-stranded and 325 D for single-stranded DNA.)

Suppose you have a double-stranded DNA molecule that is 100 bp long. Its MW is approximately 100 bp × 660 D/bp = 66,000 D. That means that one mole of this oligonucleotide would weigh 66,000 g. So, for this molecule:

- 1 M is 66,000 g/L
- 1 mM is 66 g/L
- 1 μM is 0.066 g/L
- 1 nM is $6.6 \times 10^{-5}$ g/L
- 1 pM is $6.6 \times 10^{-8}$ g/L

Looking at these values, you can see why molecular biologists work with micro-, nano-, and picomolar concentrations of DNA and RNA.

**Example Problem:**

The β-globin gene consists of about 2,000 bp. (β-globin is a subunit of hemoglobin, the protein that allows red blood cells to carry oxygen.) How much does *one* copy of this gene weigh?

a. In units of D?
b. In units of g?

***Answer:***

a. An average bp weighs 660 D. So, the gene weighs

$$\left(\frac{660\text{ D}}{1\ \cancel{\text{bp}}}\right)(2{,}000\ \cancel{\text{bp}}) = \mathbf{1.32 \times 10^6\ D}$$

b. Using the conversion factor between D and grams:

$$\frac{1\text{ D}}{1.66054 \times 10^{-24}\text{ g}} = \frac{1.32 \times 10^6\text{ D}}{?} \quad ? \approx \mathbf{2.19 \times 10^{-18}\ g}$$

**Example Problem:**

Vectors are DNA molecules that carry a DNA segment of interest into a foreign cell. Suppose you buy a vial of the plasmid vector pBR322, which is 4,361 bp in length. The manufacturer tells you that the vial contains 10 μg of vector. You are following a procedure that calls for 1 pmol of vector, so you want to convert 10 μg to pmol. How many picomoles do you have?

***Answer:***

You can calculate the molecular weight of this vector based on the fact that on the average each bp has a MW of 660 g/mol. There are 4,361 bp, so the MW of this vector is:

$$\left(\frac{660\text{ g/mole}}{1\ \cancel{\text{bp}}}\right)(4{,}361\ \cancel{\text{bp}}) = 2.87826 \times 10^6\text{ g/mole}$$

You have 10 μg, how many moles is this?

Begin by making the units of weight consistent: $10\ \mu g = 10 \times 10^{-6}$ g

Now, you can use a proportion equation:

If 1 mole weighs $2.87826 \times 10^6$ g, then how many moles is $10 \times 10^{-6}$ g?

$$\frac{2.87826 \times 10^6\ g}{1\ mol} = \frac{10 \times 10^{-6}\ g}{?} \quad \mathbf{? \approx 3.47 \times 10^{-12}\ mol = 3.47\ pmol}$$

So, your tube contains about **3.47 pmol**.

Alternatively, by unit canceling:

$$\left(\frac{10\ \cancel{\mu g}}{1\ vial}\right)\left(\frac{1\ g}{10^6\ \cancel{\mu g}}\right)\left(\frac{1\ \cancel{mol}}{2.87826 \times 10^6\ g}\right)\left(\frac{10^{12}\ pmol}{1\ \cancel{mol}}\right) \approx \frac{\mathbf{3.47\ pmol}}{\mathbf{vial}}$$

**Example Problem:**

Sequencing DNA means to determine the nucleotide order of a molecule of DNA. Promega Corporation's *Protocols and Applications Guide*, 2nd ed., provides the following instructions for setting up one of the enzymatic reactions involved in sequencing. (Do not worry about the nature of the constituents of this reaction since we will focus only on calculations.)

In a microcentrifuge tube, combine the following:

| | |
|---|---|
| Primer (Primer Table) | 10 pmol |
| γ-labeled ATP | 10 pmol |
| Polynucleotide kinase 10X buffer | 1 μL |
| T4 polynucleotide kinase enzyme (5–10 U/μL) | 5 U |
| Sterile water | To final volume 10 μL |

The primer table, found in the same publication, relates to the primer. It conveniently shows how much primer to add to the reaction mixture in units of ng to get 10 pmol. Note that the table is based on average molecular weights, since the exact sequence of the primer is not considered. Note also that primers are single-stranded. We show the primer table below as Table 22.3.

In this Example Problem, we consider how Table 22.3 is derived. Here is part of it:

**Amount of Sequencing Primer (ng) Needed to Equal 10 pmol**

| Primer Length | ng Primer Equal to 10 pmol |
|---|---|
| 15 b | 50 ng |
| 16 b | 53 ng |
| 17 b | 56 ng |
| 18 b | _____ |
| ... | |

a. How was it determined that a 15 b primer requires 50 ng to equal 10 pmol?
b. Fill in the blank for the 18 base long primer (without looking at Table 22.3).

***Answer:***

a. Let us begin by considering why 50 ng = 10 pmol for a 15 base long primer. First, find the MW of a 15 base primer:

$15 \text{ base} \times \frac{330 \text{ D}}{\text{base}} = 4950 \text{ D}$ This means that a *mole* of the primer weighs 4,950 g.

To get the units of moles and picomoles to match: $1 \text{ mol} = 10^{12} \text{ pmol}$

Using a proportion, we know that 1 mole is 4950 g, so how much is 10 pmol?

$$\frac{4{,}950 \text{ g}}{1 \times 10^{12} \text{ pmol}} = \frac{?}{10 \text{ pmol}} \quad ? = 4.95 \times 10^{-8} \text{ g} \approx 50 \times 10^{-9} \text{ g} = \mathbf{50\ ng}$$

b. Using the same logic for the 18 b primer:

$\text{MW} = (18 \text{ bases})\left(\frac{330 \text{ D}}{\text{base}}\right) = 5{,}940 \text{ D}$ This means that a *mole* of the primer weighs 5,940 g.

$$\frac{5{,}940 \text{ g}}{1 \times 10^{12} \text{ pmol}} = \frac{?}{10 \text{ pmol}} \quad ? = 5.94 \times 10^{-8} \text{ g} \approx 59 \times 10^{-9} \text{ g} = \mathbf{59\ ng}$$

Alternatively, here is part b using the unit canceling strategy:

$$\left(\frac{10 \cancel{\text{pmol}}}{1}\right)\left(\frac{1 \cancel{\text{mol}}}{10^{12} \cancel{\text{pmol}}}\right)\left(\frac{5{,}940 \cancel{\text{g}}}{1 \cancel{\text{mol}}}\right)\left(\frac{10^{9} \text{ ng}}{1 \cancel{\text{g}}}\right) = 59.4 \text{ ng} \approx \mathbf{59\ ng}$$

**TABLE 22.3 Amount of Primer (in nanograms) Needed to Equal 10 pmol**

| Primer Length | Nanograms of Primer Equal to 10 pmol |
|---|---|
| 15 b | 50 ng |
| 16 b | 53 ng |
| 17 b | 56 ng |
| 18 b | 59 ng |
| 19 b | 63 ng |
| 20 b | 66 ng |
| 24 b | 80 ng |

Data from: *Promega Protocols and Applications Guide*, 2nd ed., Promega Corporation.

**Practice Problems**

1. ***A particular gene is 1.3 Kb in length. There are two copies of the gene in every cell. A human has about $10^{13}$ cells. How much of this particular gene is present in a human in units of μg?***
2. ***There are about $3.2 \times 10^{3}$ Mb in the human genome. How much does the DNA in one human cell weigh in units of μg? Remember that each cell contains 2 copies of every gene, so every cell contains about $6.4 \times 10^{3}$ Mb of DNA.***

3. ***Forensic scientists are working to find methods to analyze DNA present in extremely low quantities, for example, in the saliva residue on a licked stamp. If scientists can successfully analyze the DNA in only 10 cells, how much DNA is this in units of µg?***
4. ***Lambda (λ) is a virus that is commonly used in molecular biology. Lambda DNA can be purchased in a vial containing 250 µg of DNA. The length of a single lambda DNA molecule is 48,502 bp. How many λ molecules are present in the vial?***
5. ***You buy a vector that is 5,386 bp in size. The manufacturer tells you there are 50 µg of vector in your tube. Your procedure calls for 2 pmol of vector, so you want to see how many picomoles your tube contains. Convert 50 µg to picomoles.***
6. ***How many ng are required to get 10 pmol of a primer (single-stranded) that is 20 b in length?***
7. ***You have 1 nmol of a plasmid that is 1,000 D. How many µg do you have?***
8. ***You have a 1 µg of a preparation of genomic DNA that is 160,000 D. How many molecules do you have?***

*Answers*

1. A gene is 1.3 Kb in length. There are two copies of the gene in every cell. A human has about $10^{13}$ cells. How much of this particular gene is present in a human in units of µg?

   A 1.3 Kb gene has a MW of: (1300 bp) (660 D/bp) = 858,000 D
   There are two copies per cell, so:

$$(858{,}000\ \text{D/copy})\ (2\ \text{copies/cell}) = 1.716 \times 10^{6}\ \text{D/cell}$$

   There are about $10^{13}$ cells in a human, so there are:

$$\left(\frac{1.716\times10^{6}\ \text{D}}{1\ \text{cell}}\right)\left(10^{13}\text{cell}\right)=1.716\ \times\ 10^{19}\ \text{D}$$

$$1\ \text{D}\approx1.66054\times10^{-24}\ \text{g}$$

$$\left(1.716\times10^{19}\ \text{D}\right)\left(\frac{1.66054\times10^{-24}\ \text{g}}{1\ \text{D}}\right)\approx2.849487\times10^{-5}\ \text{g}\approx\mathbf{28.5\ \mu g}$$

   This can also be conveniently solved using the unit canceling method in one long expression:

$$\left(\frac{1{,}300\ \cancel{\text{bp}}}{1\ \cancel{\text{copy}}}\right)\left(\frac{660\ \cancel{\text{D}}}{\cancel{\text{bp}}}\right)\left(\frac{2\ \cancel{\text{copy}}}{\cancel{\text{cell}}}\right)\left(10^{13}\ \cancel{\text{cell}}\right)\left(\frac{1.66054\times10^{-24}\ \text{g}}{1\ \cancel{\text{D}}}\right)$$

$$\approx2.849\times10^{-5}\ \text{g}\approx\mathbf{28.5\ \mu g}$$

2. There are about $3.2 \times 10^{3}$ Mb in the human genome. How much does the DNA in one human cell weigh in units of µg? Each cell contains 2 copies of every gene.

$$6.4\times10^{3}\ \text{Mb}=6.4\times10^{9}\ \text{bp/cell}$$

   By proportions:

$$\frac{660\ \text{D}}{1\text{bp}}=\frac{?}{6.4\times10^{9}\ \text{bp}}\qquad ?=4.224\times10^{12}\ \text{D}$$

$$\frac{1\,\text{D}}{1.66054\times10^{-24}\,\text{g}}=\frac{4.224\times10^{12}\,\text{D}}{?}\quad ?\approx7.0141\times10^{-12}\,\text{g}\approx\mathbf{7.0\times10^{-6}\ \mu g}$$

3. If scientists can successfully analyze the DNA in 10 cells, how much is this in units of μg?

   This is simply the answer to Question 2 times 10 cells:

$$\frac{7.0141\times10^{-6}\,\mu\text{g}}{\cancel{\text{cell}}}(10\,\cancel{\text{cell}})\approx\mathbf{7.0\times10^{-5}\ \mu g}$$

4. A vial of λ DNA (48,502 bp) contains 250 μg. How many λ molecules are present in the vial?

   First, determine the weight of a single molecule of λ DNA:
   A single molecule weighs:

$$\left(\frac{660\,\text{D}}{1\,\text{bp}}\right)(48{,}502\,\text{bp})\approx3.201\times10^{7}\,\text{D}$$

Convert this to units of grams and then μg:

$$\frac{1\,\text{D}}{1.66054\times10^{-24}\,\text{g}}=\frac{3.201\times10^{7}\,\text{D}}{?}\quad ?\approx5.3154\times10^{-17}\,\text{g}=5.3154\times10^{-11}\,\mu\text{g}$$

1 molecule weighs $5.3154\times10^{-11}$ μg, so how many molecules are in 250 μg?

$$\frac{5.3154\times10^{-11}\,\mu\text{g}}{1\,\text{molecules}}=\frac{250\,\mu\text{g}}{?}\quad ?\approx\mathbf{4.70\times10^{12}\ molecules}$$

5. A vector is 5,386 bp in size; there are 50 μg/tube. Convert 50 μg to picomoles.

   First, determine the weight of a single molecule of vector DNA:
   A single molecule weighs:

$$\frac{660\,\text{D}}{1\,\text{bp}}(5386\,\text{bp})\approx3.55476\times10^{6}\,\text{D}$$

This means that 1 mole of this vector weighs $3.55476\times10^{6}$ g

$$1\,\text{pmol weighs }3.55476\times10^{-6}\,\text{g}=3.55476\,\mu\text{g}$$

If 1 pmol is 3.55476 μg, then how many pmol is 50 μg?

$$\frac{1\,\text{pmol}}{3.55476\,\mu\text{g}}=\frac{?}{50\,\mu\text{g}}\quad ?\approx\mathbf{14\ pmol}$$

6. How many ng are required to get 10 pmol of a primer (single-stranded) that is 20 bases in length?

$$\text{A single molecule weighs}\left(\frac{330\,\text{D}}{1\,\cancel{\text{b}}}\right)(20\,\cancel{\text{b}})\approx6{,}600\,\text{D}$$

This means that 1 mole of this vector weighs 6600 g

$$1\,\text{pmol weighs }6600\times10^{-12}\,\text{g}=6.6\,\text{ng}$$

Then, 10 pmol weighs **66 ng**

You could also read this off of Table 22.3.

7. You have 1 nmol of a plasmid that is 1,000 D. How many μg do you have?
   1 mole = 1,000 g of this plasmid

$$1\,\text{nmol} = 1 \times 10^{-6}\,\text{g} = \mathbf{1\,\mu g}$$

8. You have 1 μg of a preparation of genomic DNA that is 160,000 D. How many molecules do you have?

$$1\,\text{mol} = 160{,}000\,\text{g} = 160{,}000 \times 10^{6}\,\mu\text{g}$$

$$\frac{1\,\text{mol}}{160{,}000 \times 10^{6}\,\mu\text{g}} = \frac{?}{1\,\mu\text{g}}$$

$$? = 6.25 \times 10^{-12}\,\text{mol}$$

$$\frac{1\,\text{mol}}{6.022 \times 10^{23}\,\text{molecules}} = \frac{6.25 \times 10^{-12}\,\text{mol}}{?}$$

$$? \approx \mathbf{3.76 \times 10^{12}\ molecules}$$

## 22.12 SPECTROPHOTOMETRIC ANALYSIS OF DNA, RNA AND PROTEINS

Consider the situation in which an analyst isolates DNA from cells or another natural source. The isolated DNA may be broken into different size fragments and the sequence of the DNA is unknown. How can the analyst determine the amount or concentration of DNA in the preparation? Spectrophotometry provides a quick and commonly used method to estimate the concentration of DNA, RNA, and sometimes proteins in the sample. (Spectrophotometry is introduced in Chapter 16.) Nucleic acids and proteins absorb ultraviolet light at a wavelength of 260 nm. Table 22.4 provides spectrophotometric conversions for nucleic acids. This table assumes the use of a 1 cm cuvette.

The relationships in Table 22.4 are based on average absorptivity constants for DNA, RNA, and proteins. These relationships are estimates because different DNA and RNA fragments actually have different absorptivity constants. Proteins vary even more in their absorptivity constants, depending on their composition. (Protein absorptivity constants will

**TABLE 22.4 Nucleic Acid Spectrophotometric Conversions**

If a sample containing pure double-stranded DNA has an absorbance of 1 at 260 nm, then it contains approximately **50 μg/mL of double-stranded DNA**[a]

If a sample containing pure single-stranded DNA has an absorbance of 1 at 260 nm, then it contains approximately **36 μg/mL of DNA**[a]

If a sample containing pure RNA has an absorbance of 1 at 260 nm, then it contains approximately **40 μg/mL of RNA**[a]

If a sample containing pure synthesized oligonucleotide has an absorbance of 1 at 260 nm, then it contains approximately **33 μg/mL of single-stranded oligonucleotides**[a]

Values for proteins vary. A very rough estimate is that if a sample containing pure protein has an absorbance of 1 under specified conditions, then it contains approximately 1 mg/mL of protein. For example, it is reported that 1 mg/mL of bovine serum albumin had an absorbance value of 0.7. 1 mg/mL of antibodies was found to have an absorbance between 1.35 and 1.2. (Harlow, Ed, and David Lane. ***Antibodies: A Laboratory Manual***. 1st ed., Cold Spring Harbor Laboratory Press, 1988.)

[a] Values from: Roskams, Jane, and Linda Rodgers. ***Lab Ref: A Handbook of Recipes, Reagents, and Other Reference Tools for Use at the Bench***. 1st ed., Cold Spring Harbor Laboratory Press, 2002.

be considered in more detail in Chapter 26.) Using these estimated relationships is a "short-cut" method that provides quick (though not entirely accurate) estimates of protein, DNA, or RNA concentration. Note also that the method is useful for DNA/RNA concentrations from roughly 5 to 100 µg/mL. More concentrated DNA solutions can be diluted, but less concentrated ones must be quantitated using other methods.

You may see the abbreviation OD, the optical density at a specified wavelength, or $A_{260}$, meaning the absorbance at 260 nm, or the term absorbance unit, AU. These expressions are all different ways to express the absorbance of a substance in a spectrophotometer.

**Example Problem:**

A scientist isolated DNA from bacterial cells and was interested in estimating the amount of DNA present in the preparation. The preparation had a volume of 2 mL. The scientist removed 50 µL from the preparation and added 450 µL of buffer and then read the absorbance of the dilution at a wavelength of 260 nm. The absorbance was 0.65. Assuming the sample was pure, about how much double-stranded DNA was present in the original 2,000 µL preparation?

***Answer:***

Recall from Chapter 16 that absorbance is proportional to concentration. Therefore, a proportion equation can be set up based on the relationship that a sample containing 50 µg/mL of pure double-stranded DNA has an absorbance of 1:

$$\frac{1}{50\ \mu g/mL} = \frac{0.65}{?} \quad ? = 32.5\ \mu g/mL$$

Considering that the preparation was diluted, the concentration was:

(10) (32.5 µg/mL) = 325 µg/mL

To estimate the amount of DNA in the original preparation, note that there were 2 mL of isolated product and the concentration of DNA in that preparation was about 325 µg/mL. Therefore, the 2 mL of the original preparation had about:

(2 mL) (325 µg/mL) = **650 µg double-stranded DNA.**

**Example Problem:**

Using the relationships in Table 22.4 (which are based on certain specified conditions, such as a 1 cm cuvette), what is the absorptivity constant for double-stranded DNA? Use Beer's law, as was explained in Chapter 16.

***Answer:***

If a sample containing pure double-stranded DNA has an absorbance of 1 under specified conditions, then it contains approximately 50 µg/mL of double-stranded DNA.

Beer's law

$A = \alpha b C$

$1 = \alpha\ (1\ cm)\ (50\ \mu g/1\ mL)$

Rearranging this equation:

$$\alpha = \frac{1\ mL}{50\ \mu g\ cm} = \mathbf{0.02\ mL/(\mu g\ cm)}$$

Note that the units of this constant are essential. If we had begun with units other than "µg/mL," we would have a different constant with different units.

**TABLE 22.5 Molar Extinction Coefficients[a] for the Four dNTPs[b] found in DNA**

| dNTP | Wavelength (nm) | Molar Absorptivity Constant |
|---|---|---|
| dATP | 259 | 15,400 L/mol·cm |
| dCTP | 271 | 9,100 L/mol·cm |
| dGTP | 253 | 13,700 L/mol·cm |
| dTTP | 260 | 7,400 L/mol·cm |

[a] Molar extinction coefficients are absorptivity constants with units of L/mol·cm.

[b] dNTP stands for any of the four nucleotide subunits that make up DNA. There are four dNTPs, each with a different base: adenine (dATP), cytosine (dCTP), guanine (dGTP), and thymine (dTTP).

Data from: Roskams, Jane, and Linda Rodgers. *Lab Ref: A Handbook of Recipes, Reagents, and Other Reference Tools for Use at the Bench*. 1st ed., Cold Spring Harbor Laboratory Press, 2002.

There might be a situation where you want to use spectrophotometry to determine the molar concentration of a solution of dNTPs. Table 22.5 shows the molar extinction coefficients for the four dNTPs found in DNA.

**Example Problem:**

The molar absorptivity constant for dATP at 259 nm is 15,400 L/mole·cm. You have a solution that is supposed to be 100 mM dATP. You serially dilute the solution by taking 10 μL of the stock and adding 990 μL buffer. You then take 10 μL of this dilution and add 990 μL of buffer. The absorbance of the final dilution is 0.130 in a 1 cm cuvette. Based on the absorbance value, was the original solution actually 100 mM?

***Answer:***

Substituting into the equation for Beer's law:

$$A = \alpha \quad b \quad C$$

$$0.130 = \frac{(15,400\ \text{L})(1\ \cancel{\text{cm}})C}{1\ \text{mol} \cdot \cancel{\text{cm}}}$$

The cm cancel:

$$0.130 = \frac{(15,400\ \text{L})C}{1\ \text{mol}}$$

Solving for the concentration:

$$C = \frac{0.130}{\frac{(15,400\ \text{L})}{1\ \text{mol}}}$$

$$C = (0.130)\left(\frac{1\ \text{mol}}{15,400\ \text{L}}\right)$$

$$\approx 8.44 \times 10^{-6}\ \frac{\text{mol}}{\text{L}}$$

Next, multiply by the reciprocal of the final dilution. The total dilution was:

$$(10/1,000)\ (10/1,000)\ =\ 1/10,000$$

So, the reciprocal of the dilution is 10,000/1 or just 10,000

$$\left(\frac{8.44 \times 10^{-6}\text{mol}}{1\text{ L}}\right)(10{,}000) = \left(8.44 \times 10^{-2}\text{ mol}\right)/\text{L} = \mathbf{84.4\ mmol/L}$$

So, based on absorbance, the stock is 84.4 mM instead 100 mM. Note, however, that spectrophotometry provides approximate values when quantifying DNA.

**Practice Problems**

1. a. ***A sample of double-stranded DNA had an absorbance of 3 (at a wavelength of 260 nm). Since spectrophotometers are not reliable when the absorbance is so high, the analyst diluted the sample by mixing 1.0 mL of the DNA solution with 9.0 mL of buffer. This time the absorbance reading was 1.25. What was the approximate concentration of the DNA in the original sample?***
   b. ***A sample of purified RNA had an absorbance of 2.4. Therefore, the analyst diluted it by mixing 1.0 mL of the RNA solution with 4.0 mL of buffer. The absorbance was 0.63. Approximately what concentration of RNA was in the original sample?***
2. a. ***A sample of reasonably pure double-stranded DNA has an absorbance of 0.85. What is the approximate concentration of DNA in the solution?***
   b. ***A sample of reasonably pure RNA has an absorbance of 3.8. The analyst dilutes the sample by adding 1 part sample to 9 parts buffer. The absorbance is then 0.69. What is the concentration of RNA in the original solution?***
3. ***Based on the relationships given in this section and assuming a 1 cm cuvette, what is the absorptivity constant for RNA?***

*Answers*

1. a. C = 50 µg/mL (1.25) = 62.5 µg/mL
   10 (62.5 µg/mL) = **625 µg/mL** = concentration of DNA in the original sample
   b. C = (0.63) (40 µg/mL ) = 25.2 µg/mL
   5 (25.2 µg/mL) = **126 µg/mL** = concentration of RNA in the original sample
2. a. Concentration = 50 µg/mL (0.85) = **42.5 µg/mL**
   b. 40 µg/mL (0.69) = 27.6 µg/mL 10 (27.6 µg/mL) = **276 µg/mL**
3. From Beer's law: A = α b C 1 = α (1 cm) (40 µg/mL)

$$\alpha = \frac{1\text{ mL}}{40\ \mu\text{g cm}} = \mathbf{0.025\ mL/(\mu g\ cm)}$$

## 22.13 FINDING THE MATH: SETTING UP REACTION MIXTURES

Molecular biologists often follow written procedures (also called protocols) that describe how to set up a reaction mixture. As we saw with cell culture protocols, before beginning to follow a procedure, it is important to review the steps and look for any calculations that you might need to perform to tailor the procedure for your own situation. The following problems provide excerpts from procedures involving a reaction mixture. To prepare the reaction mixture, certain calculations are required. If you have never actually performed these molecular biology procedures, it is not essential that you understand exactly how you would perform each step; just find the math and perform the calculations. Much of the math required is just ratios and proportions, plus knowledge of how to prepare biological buffers and other solutions with the proper concentrations of solute. Thus, you already have the math skills you need.

### Reaction Mixture I: A PCR Reaction Mixture

Below are the directions for preparing a certain reaction mixture (derived from: Bloom, Mark, et al. *Laboratory DNA Science*. 1st ed., Benjamin Cummings, 1995.) (Do not worry at this point about the purpose of the various components of the mixture.)

**"RECIPE" FOR TPA-25 PCR MIXTURE**

| | |
|---|---|
| • PCR buffer (10 mM Tris-HCl, 50 mM KCl, and 1.5 mM $MgCl_2$, pH 8.3) | 5.6 μL |
| • Deoxynucleotide mix (purchased from supplier at correct concentration) | 9 μL |
| • Primers (12.5 pmol/μL) | 1.1 μL |
| • Taq polymerase (at a concentration of 25 U/mL)* | ____ |
| • Purified water (as required to get total volume of 45 μL) | ____ |

*The label for the Taq DNA polymerase is shown in Figure 22.3.

**Questions:**

a. Highlight each place in the "Recipe" for TPA-25 PCR mix where you will need to perform a calculation to prepare the reaction mixture properly.
b. Perform the required calculations to make the PCR buffer. Note that with normal laboratory equipment, it would be impossible to make only 5.6 μL of this buffer. In practice, this buffer would be made in advance as a stock solution. Perform the calculations to make 100 mL of a 10X stock solution of PCR buffer. Use a web browser to find any formula weights that you might need.

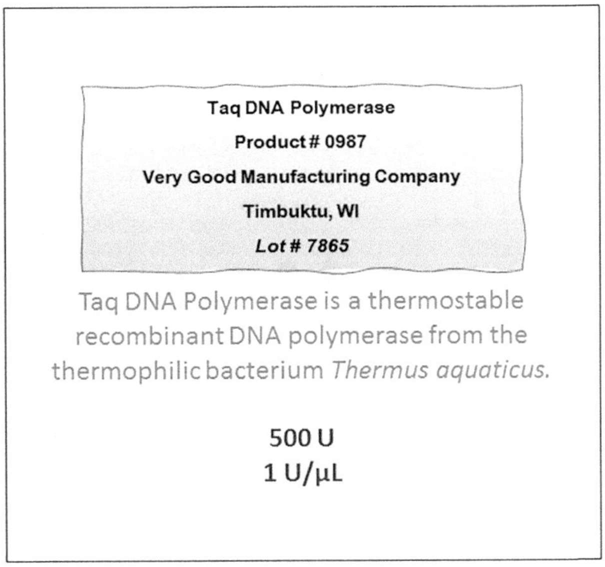
Taq DNA Polymerase
Product # 0987
Very Good Manufacturing Company
Timbuktu, WI
Lot # 7865
Taq DNA Polymerase is a thermostable recombinant DNA polymerase from the thermophilic bacterium Thermus aquaticus.
500 U
1 U/μL

**FIGURE 22.3** The label from the vial of Taq DNA polymerase.

c. How much of the TPA-25 primers are in the reaction mixture in units of pmol?
d. How much of the TPA-25 primers are in the reaction mixture in units of pmol/μL?
e. How much Taq DNA polymerase is required?
f. What else needs to be calculated?

### Reaction Mixture II: RNAi

A reaction mixture associated with an RNAi procedure is shown below. **RNAi** *is a process in which RNA molecules inhibit the expression or translation of a specific gene by neutralizing mRNA molecules.* It is not necessary at this time to understand RNAi or to know the purpose of the components of the reaction mixture – we are interested in the math calculations required to set up the reaction mix.

**"RECIPE" FOR RNAi REACTION MIXTURE**

**Prepare the Following Stocks:**
Dithioerythritol (10 mM)
Magnesium Acetate (0.1 M)
Tris-acetate (1 M pH 7.8)
*Prepare Tris-acetate by adjusting the pH of Tris base with glacial acetic acid*

**Set up a 45 μL Reaction Containing:**
0.3 mM each ATP, CTP, and GTP (you have a stock mixture that contains 1 mM of each)
2 mM Dithioerythritol
10 mM Magnesium acetate
50 mM Tris-acetate
0.02 mM tritiated UTP*
1 μg TMV RNA**

*Figure 22.4 shows the label from the vial of tritium-labeled UTP. This is a radioactive material. Ci is a unit of radioactivity.

**Assume that you prepared the TMV RNA in your laboratory. You used a spectrophotometric method to determine its concentration. You removed 10 μL of the preparation and added 90 μL of buffer. You measured the absorbance of the diluted TMV RNA preparation and found an absorbance of 1.22.

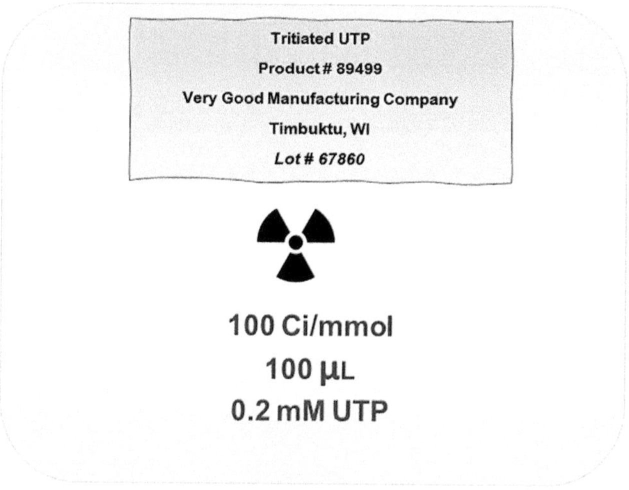


**FIGURE 22.4** The label from the vial of tritium-labeled UTP.

**Questions:**

a. How would you make each of the three stock solutions? Find any required formula weights by using a web browser. Perform the calculations to make **100 mL** of each stock solution.
b. How would you set up the reaction mixture?
c. How many µCi of radioactivity will be in your final reaction mix?

## Answers

## Reaction Mixture I

a.

**"RECIPE" FOR TPA-25 PCR MIX**

| | |
|---|---|
| • PCR buffer (10 mM Tris-HCl, 50 mM KCl, and 1.5 mM MgCl2, pH 8.3) | 5.6 µL |
| • Deoxynucleotide mix (purchased from supplier at correct concentration) | 9 µL |
| • Primers (12.5 pmol/µL) | 1.1 µL |
| • Taq polymerase (at a concentration of 25 U/mL) | _____ |
| • Purified water (as required to get total volume of 45 µL) | _____ |

b. **PCR Buffer**: If necessary, review Chapters 12 and 13 for information about making a solution, such as PCR buffer.

PCR buffer has three components that are combined together in purified water. The first is 10 mM Tris-HCl at pH 8.3. To determine how much Tris base powder is required, use Equation 12.1 (assuming you want to make 100 mL):

Solute required = (grams/mole) (molarity) (volume)

$$\left(\frac{121.0\text{ g}}{1\ \cancel{\text{mol}}}\right)\left(\frac{0.100\ \cancel{\text{mol}}}{1\ \cancel{\text{L}}}\right)(0.100\ \cancel{\text{L}}) = \mathbf{1.211\ g = grams\ of\ solute\ required}.$$

Equation 12.1 is used three times, once for each solute. Thus, 100 mL of a 10X stock solution could be made as follows:

Step 1. For 100 mL of 100 mM Tris solution (FW 121.1), weigh out 1.211 g of Tris base. Dissolve in about 60 mL of water and adjust the pH to 8.3 with HCl. Do not BTV yet.
Step 2. 100 mL of 500 mM KCl (FW 74.55) requires 3.7275 g, weigh out add to the Tris solution.
Step 3. 100 mL of 15 mM MgCl2 (FW 95.211) requires 0.1428 g, weigh out and add to the Tris solution.
Step 4. Dissolve all the components and BTV 100 mL. Check pH.

c. and d. The TPA-25 primers exist as a stock at a concentration of 12.5 pmol/µL. 1.1 µL of the stock is removed and added to the reaction mix: (12.5 pmol/µL) (1.1 µL) = **13.75 pmol**

The total volume of the mixture is 45 µL. 13.75 pmol/45 µL ≈ **0.3056 pmol/µL**

e. **The Taq Polymerase**:

Need 25 U/mL but the entire volume is 45 µL. Using proportions to calculate the number of units required:

$$\frac{25\text{ U}}{1\text{ mL}} = \frac{?}{0.045\text{ mL}}$$

$$\mathbf{? = 1.125\ U}$$

From the label, we know there is 1 U/µL, so we need 1.125 µL. In practice, this would be rounded, perhaps to 1.5 µL or possibly to 2 µL. It is not unusual to add a little extra enzyme to a reaction mix.

f. **Water**:

The total volume needs to be 45 μL. Thus,

| | |
|---|---|
| PCR buffer | 5.6 μL |
| Deoxynucleotide mix | 9 μL |
| Primers | 1.1 μL |
| Taq polymerase | 1.1 μL |
| | 16.8 μL |

So, we need **28.2** μL of water. (If extra enzyme is added, then the water would be reduced.)

### Reaction Mixture II

a. Making the stock solutions:

(Chapter 13 introduces the use of stock solutions.)

| **Prepare the Following Stocks: (For 100 mL of each stock)** | |
|---|---|
| Use Equation 12.1 three times to determine how much solute is required to make each of the three stock solutions | |
| 10 mM dithioerythritol (FW 154.253) | **Mix 0.1543 g in water, BTV 100 mL** |
| 0.1 M magnesium acetate (FW 142.394) | **Mix 1.4239 g in water, BTV 100 mL** |
| 1 M Tris-acetate (pH 7.8) (FW 121.1) | **Weigh out 12.11 g of Tris base. Dissolve in about 60 mL of water and adjust the pH to 7.8 with glacial acetic acid. BTV 100 mL** |

b. To set up the reaction mixture:

| **To Set Up a 45 μL Reaction Containing These Components** | |
|---|---|
| 0.3 mM each ATP, CTP, and GTP (Note that all three are purchased together as a mixture.) | $C_1V_1 = C_2V_2$<br>(1 mM) (?) = (0.3 mM) (45 μL)<br>**? = 13.5 μL**<br>**This is the amount of the stock mixture required** |
| 2 mM dithioerythritol | $C_1V_1 = C_2V_2$<br>(10 mM) (?) = (2 mM) (45 μL)<br>**? = 9 μL** |
| 10 mM magnesium acetate | $C_1V_1 = C_2V_2$<br>(0.1 M) (?) = (0.01 M) (45 μL)<br>**? = 4.5 μL** |
| 50 mM Tris-acetate | $C_1V_1 = C_2V_2$<br>(1 M) (?) = (0.05 M) (45 μL)<br>**? = 2.25 μL** |
| 0.02 mM tritiated UTP | $C_1V_1 = C_2V_2$<br>(0.2 mM) (?) = (0.02 mM) (45 μL)<br>**? = 4.5 μL** |
| 1 μg TMV RNA | From Table 22.4, 1 absorbance unit is roughly 40 μg/mL of RNA. So:<br>$\frac{1\text{ AU}}{40\ \mu\text{g/mL}} = \frac{1.22}{?}$<br>? = 48.8 μg/mL<br>But the sample was diluted 10X, so the concentration of TMV RNA is about 488 μg/mL<br>You need 1 μg:<br>$\frac{488\ \mu\text{g}}{1\text{ mL}} = \frac{1\ \mu\text{g}}{?}$<br>**? ≈ 0.002 mL = 2 μL** |

c. In the final reaction mixture, have 45 μL of tritiated (radioactive) UTP at a concentration of 0.02 mM.

How many millimoles are in the 45 μL? By definition, 0.02 mM = 0.02 mmol/L.

$$\frac{0.02\ \text{mmol}}{10^6\ \mu\text{L}} = \frac{?}{45\ \mu\text{L}}$$

$$? = 9 \times 10^{-7}\ \text{mmol}$$

The label says there are 100 Ci per mmol

$$\frac{100\ \text{Ci}}{1\ \text{mmol}} = \frac{?}{9 \times 10^{-7}\ \text{mmol}}$$

$$? = 9 \times 10^{-5}\ \text{Ci} = \mathbf{90\ \mu Ci}$$

Alternatively, by unit canceling:

$$\left(\frac{45\ \cancel{\mu\text{L}}}{1}\right)\left(\frac{0.02\ \cancel{\text{mmol}}}{1\ \cancel{\text{L}}}\right)\left(\frac{100\ \text{Ci}}{1\ \cancel{\text{mmol}}}\right)\left(\frac{1\ \cancel{\text{L}}}{10^6\ \cancel{\mu\text{L}}}\right) = 9 \times 10^{-5}\ \text{Ci} = \mathbf{90\ \mu Ci}$$

# Calculations Relating to Common Molecular Biology Techniques

23



## 23.1 RESTRICTION DIGESTS

This chapter considers the calculations associated with several common molecular biology techniques. The first is the digestion of DNA with restriction enzymes, the second is electrophoresis, and the third is transformation.

A **restriction digest** is an enzymatic reaction in which DNA is cut with specialized enzymes, called **restriction endonucleases**, *that recognize a specific DNA sequence and cleave the DNA at that site.* For example, the restriction enzyme BamHI recognizes and cuts a specific sequence in double-stranded DNA as illustrated in Figure 23.1. Whenever BamHI finds this sequence in a strand of DNA, it cuts the DNA leaving two fragments. BamHI always recognizes the same sequence of DNA and always cuts in the same way.

A segment of DNA can be cut with one or more restriction enzyme(s) in the same restriction digest mixture. The number and size(s) of fragments formed depends on the sequence

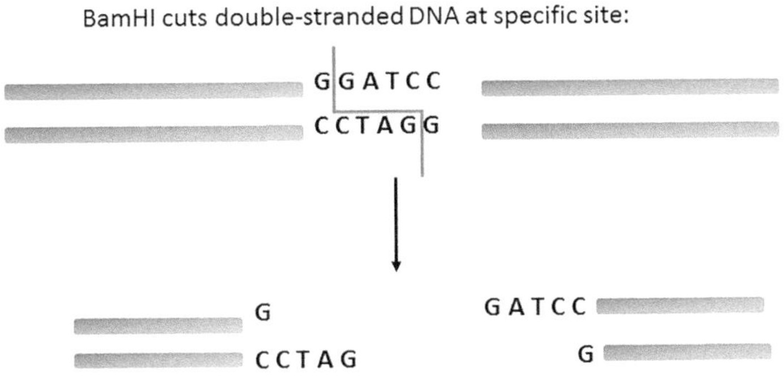


**FIGURE 23.1** BamHI cuts double-stranded DNA wherever there is a specific sequence of bases. BamHI recognizes the sequence: GGATCC.

DOI: 10.1201/9780429282744-28

of the DNA, the recognition sequence(s) of the restriction enzyme(s), and the length of the DNA present initially.

**Example Problem:**

A DNA molecule has three restriction sites: two are recognized by the enzyme BamH1 and the other is recognized by HindIII. The DNA molecule is shown in Figure 23.2 diagrammatically as a line with numbers. These numbers represent base pairs. The total length of the molecule is 5 Kb. The diagram shows that BamHI cuts the molecule at 550 bp and at 2,500 bp while HindIII cuts at 4,800 bp.

a. How many fragments are produced when this molecule is cut with the two enzymes?
b. What is the length of the fragments formed?

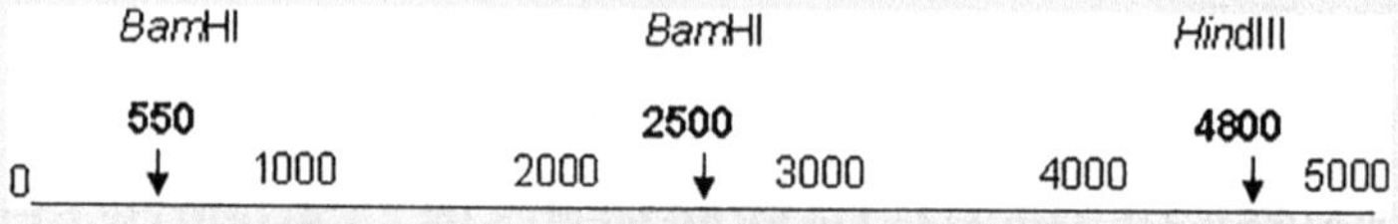


**FIGURE 23.2** Restriction digest Example Problem sketch.

*Answer:*

a. BamHI cuts twice and HindIII cuts once resulting in **four fragments.**
b. The first fragment is from 0 to 550 bp, that is, **550 bp long.**
   The second fragment is from 550 to 2,500 bp, that is, **1,950 bp.**
   The third fragment is from 2,500 to 4,800, that is, **2,300 bp.**
   The fourth fragment is from 4,800 to 5,000, that is, **200 bp.**

**Practice Problem**

***A circular DNA molecule is shown in Figure 23.3. It is 4,800 bp total in length. It has two sites recognized by the restriction enzyme EcoRI and one site recognized by the restriction enzyme HaeIII.***

a. ***How many fragments are produced when this molecule is cut with the two enzymes?***
b. ***What is the length of the fragments formed?***

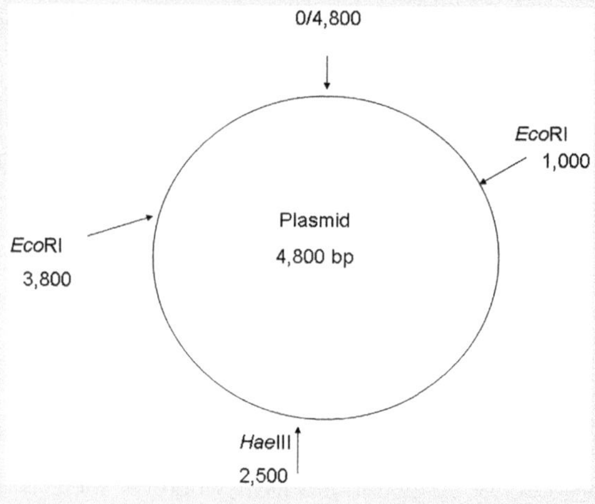


**FIGURE 23.3** Sketch for restriction digest Practice Problem.

*Answers*

a. There will be three fragments after digestion:
b. Fragment 1: (1,000 – 0) bp + (4,800 – 3,800) bp = **2,000 bp**
Fragment 2: (2,500 – 1,000) bp = **1,500 bp**
Fragment 3: (3,800 – 2,500) bp = **1,300 bp**

## 23.2 SETTING UP RESTRICTION DIGESTS

Many procedures in molecular biology take advantage of reactions catalyzed by enzymes (see Section 22.2 for an introduction to reaction mixtures). Digesting (cutting) DNA with restriction enzymes is an example of an enzymatic reaction. Enzymatic reactions require that various components be mixed together in a tube at the proper concentrations. The components of reaction mixtures vary, depending on the procedure, but generally include:

- a nucleic acid sample
- the enzyme(s) that performs the required task
- buffer, salts, and cofactors
- water

The components of reaction mixtures are usually purchased or prepared as stock solutions at a particular concentration that are stored until needed. When a reaction is performed, the proper volume of each component's stock solution is added to the mixture to achieve the proper final concentration of that component. Thus, some calculations are involved in preparing reaction mixtures.

The main components of a restriction digest are shown in Table 23.1. To perform a restriction digestion reaction, the analyst combines the components in small tubes (microfuge tubes), Figure 23.4. Inside each tube there are billions of DNA molecules of whatever sample type one is digesting (for example, human genomic DNA, a plasmid vector, or lambda virus). Given enough time and the proper conditions, the restriction enzyme(s) that have been added to each tube will cut all of those DNA molecules in exactly the same places resulting in billions of DNA fragments of specific lengths. This ability to use restriction enzymes to cut DNA molecules selectively and efficiently in specific ways provides one of the most powerful tools in molecular biology.

Box 23.1 outlines the steps in performing a restriction digest, which is then discussed in more detail below.

**TABLE 23.1 The Major Components of a Restriction Digest Reaction**

| Component | Purpose | Final Amount or Concentration in Reaction Mixture |
|---|---|---|
| *Restriction buffer* | Controls the pH, usually contains $Mg^{++}$ which is an enzyme cofactor, and controls salt concentration | 1X |
| *DNA* | Whatever DNA is to be digested | 0.2–1 µg is common |
| *Restriction enzyme(s)* | Enzyme(s) that cut DNA at specific nucleotide sequences | 1 unit/µg is common |
| *Water* | Brings reaction mixture to the right volume to ensure that buffer and enzyme are at the appropriate concentration; 20 µL volume is common | |

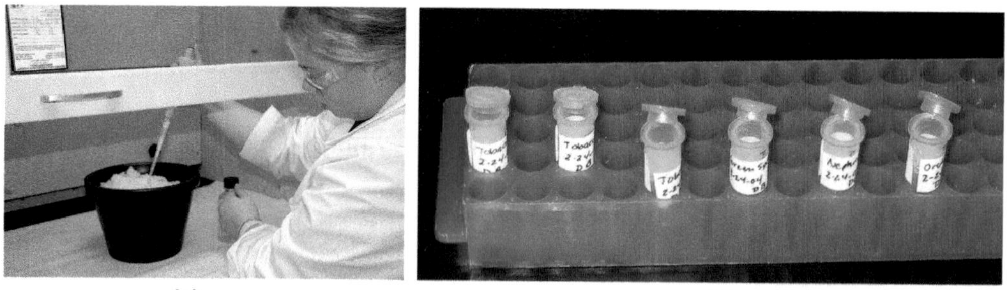

(a) (b)

**FIGURE 23.4** Preparing a restriction digest. (a) The analyst removes stock solutions that are kept on ice and places them into microfuge tubes. (b) In this illustration, six reaction mixtures are being prepared.

**BOX 23.1 Performing a Restriction Digest**

Step 1. Select and purchase enzyme(s). Purchase or prepare buffer that is recommended for the enzyme(s).

Step 2. Decide how much DNA to digest.

Step 3. Determine how much restriction enzyme to use.

Step 4. Determine the total volume of the restriction digest mixture.

Step 5. Determine the volume of restriction buffer required.

Step 6. Determine the volume of water required.

Step 7. Combine the components of the restriction digest mixture.

Step 8. Incubate at the recommended temperature for recommended time.

**Step 1. Select and Purchase Enzyme(s) and Buffer.**

The first steps in restriction analysis are to select and purchase enzyme(s) that cut the DNA in ways that work for the application. Once the enzymes have been chosen, then a buffer that is recommended for the enzyme(s) can be purchased or prepared. These components are stored until needed for a restriction digestion.

**Step 2. Decide How Much DNA to Digest.**

Typical restriction enzyme reactions contain 0.2–1 μg of DNA in a volume of 20 μL or less.

**Example Problem:**

Suppose you decide to cut 1 μg of pBR322 (pBR322 is a plasmid). Your stock concentration of pBR322 is 0.5 μg/μL. How much stock solution should you add to the reaction mixture?

***Answer:***

(1 μg pBR322) (1 μL/0.5 μg pBR322) = **2 μL of pBR322 stock solution required**

**Step 3. Determine How Much Restriction Enzyme to Use.**
Restriction enzyme units are usually defined as the amount of enzyme required to completely digest 1 μg of DNA in one hour in the recommended buffer and at the recommended temperature – although the definition of a unit may vary somewhat with different manufacturers. Observe that the amount of enzyme required depends on the amount of DNA to be digested and the duration of the digest. If you decide to digest 1 μg of DNA in 1 hour, you could use one unit of enzyme. But if you must digest 1 μg of DNA in 30 minutes, then use two units. Restriction digests generally use at least 1 unit of enzyme per μg of DNA, regardless of the duration of the reaction. Commercial preparations of enzyme usually have a concentration in the range of 4–20 U/μL. (Be careful not to confuse the abbreviation for "unit," U, with the abbreviation for "micro," μ.)

**Example Problem:**

You want to digest your 1 μg of pBR322 plamid DNA with NaeI restriction enzyme. The concentration of enzyme is 4 U/μL. How much enzyme is needed? (Assume you are working at the recommended temperature.)

***Answer:***

Assuming that you want 1 unit of enzyme for each μg of DNA, you want 1 unit. The enzyme is at a concentration of 4 U/μL:

$$1\,\text{U}\left(\frac{1\,\mu\text{L}}{4\,\text{U}}\right) = \mathbf{0.25\,\mu L}$$

This means that you want to add 0.25 μL of the enzyme stock. However, this volume is too low to pipette accurately. You might dilute your enzyme stock solution. It is also common to add 1 μL of the undiluted enzyme stock, even though this is more enzyme than is necessary. An excess of enzyme helps ensure that the restriction reaction goes to completion, and it is readily added with a standard micropipette. (Do not overdo it by adding way too much enzyme. A ten-fold excess of enzyme is plenty, and the enzymes are often expensive.)

**Step 4. Determine the Total Volume of the Restriction Digest Mixture.**
The volume of the digest is determined partly by the volume of enzyme required. Restriction enzymes are often stored in a buffer containing glycerol. The glycerol helps maintain enzyme activity during storage but can inhibit enzyme activity during the digestion. Therefore, the volume of restriction enzyme used should never be greater than 10% of the volume of the restriction digest and keeping it below 5% is good practice.

**Example Problem:**

For the Example Problem above, in which 1 µL of restriction enzyme will be used in a restriction digest, what should be the reaction volume if the enzyme is: (a) 10% of the total volume and (b) 5% of the total volume?

***Answer:***

a. To calculate the answer:
   1 µL is 10% of what volume?
   1 µL = (0.10) (?)
   10 µL = ?
   which means that 1 µL is 10% of **10 µL**, so the restriction digest would take place in a volume of **10 µL** total.

b. To calculate the answer:
   1 µL is 5% of what volume?
   1 µL = (0.05) (?)
   20 µL = ?
   which means that 1 µL is 5% of **20 µL**, so the restriction digest would take place in a volume of **20 µL** total, which is a typical restriction digest volume.

**Step 5. Determine the Volume of Restriction Buffer Required.**
Restriction enzyme buffers are usually provided by the manufacturer or are prepared as a 10X stock. This means that the stock solution of buffer is at ten times the working concentration. Therefore, you must dilute the buffer in your digest to the final 1X working concentration.

**Example Problem:**

You are going to perform a restriction digest with a total volume of 20 µL. Your restriction buffer stock is 10X. How much buffer should you use to get a 1X concentration in the final mixture?

***Answer:***

This is a situation where you are going from a more concentrated to a less concentrated solution, so the $C_1V_2 = C_2V_2$ equation applies:

$$C_1 \quad V_1 = C_2 \quad V_2$$

$$(10X) \quad (?) = (1X) \quad (20\,\mu L) \qquad \mathbf{? = 2\,\mu L}$$

Use **2 µL of the 10 X buffer.**

**Step 6. Determine the Volume of Water Required.**
Once you have determined how much of each of the other components should be used, it is easy to calculate the appropriate amount of water to add to get the desired final volume of restriction mixture.

**Example Problem:**

You are going to perform a restriction digest with these components; how much water is required?

? μL of water
2 μL of plasmid DNA
2 μL of 10X restriction buffer
+1 μL of restriction enzyme
20 μL total volume

*Answer:*

Solving for ? above, add **15 μL** of water to the digest.

**Step 7. Prepare the Restriction Digest Mixture and Incubate.**
Combine the ingredients of the mixture with the restriction enzyme as the last component. Restriction enzymes are sensitive to buffer conditions and temperature. By adding the enzyme last, you ensure that the enzyme only encounters the correct buffer conditions. Additionally, restriction enzymes should be kept in the freezer until just before addition, and digests should be kept on ice until you are ready to incubate them at the appropriate temperature. Incubate the restriction digest mixture at the appropriate temperature for the time required.

**Practice Problems**

1. ***Fill in this table with the amounts of each component to add to a restriction digest.***

**Restriction Digest Mixture, Practice Problem 1**

| Component | Stock Concentration | Final Amount or Concentration | Amount of Stock to Add |
|---|---|---|---|
| *plasmid pBR322* | 1 μg/μL | 1 μg | |
| *buffer* | 5X | 1X | |
| *EcoRI enzyme* | 10 U/μL | | 1 μL |
| *water* | | As much as necessary to get final volume of 20 μL total | |

2. ***You want to cut 10 μg of the plasmid pBR322 with the restriction enzyme, EcoRI. You have plasmid at a stock concentration of 2 μg/μL, restriction buffer at a concentration of 10X, and EcoR1 at a concentration of 4 U/μL. Assume you want a 1 hour digestion. Do not use less than 1 μL of enzyme, and do not allow the enzyme to be more than 5% of the restriction digest volume. What are the components of the reaction mixture? Show your answer in a table like that in problem 1 above.***

3. ***You need to cut 200 ng of the plasmid pBR322 with the restriction enzyme, XhoI. The plasmid stock concentration is 0.1 μg/μL. Restriction buffer is present at a concentration of 4X and the enzyme is at a concentration of 5 U/μL. Assume you want a 1 hour digestion. Do not use less than 1 μL of enzyme, and do not allow the enzyme to be more than 5% of the restriction digest volume. What are the components of the reaction mixture? Show your answer in a table like that in problem 1 above.***

4. ***Lambda (λ) is a virus that is commonly used in molecular biology and it is often used as a marker when DNA electrophoresis is run (see Section 23.4). Suppose that 5 μg of lambda DNA is digested using restriction enzymes. The length of a single lambda DNA molecule is 48,502 bp. How many λ molecules are present in the restriction digest? (Hint: refer to Section 22.11).***

## *Answers*

1.

**Restriction Digest Mixture, Practice Problem 1**

| Component | Stock Concentration | Final Amount or Concentration | Amount of Stock to Add |
|---|---|---|---|
| plasmid pBR322 | 1 μg/μL | 1 μg | 1 μL |
| buffer | 5X | 1X | 4 μL |
| EcoRI enzyme | 10 U/μL | 10 U | 1 μL |
| water | | to final, total volume of 20 μL | 14 μL |

2.

**Restriction Digest Mixture, Practice Problem 2**

| Component | Stock Concentration | Final Amount or Concentration | Amount of Stock to Add |
|---|---|---|---|
| plasmid pBR322 | 2 μg/μL | 10 μg | 5 μL |
| buffer | 10X | 1X | 5 μL |
| EcoRI enzyme | 4 U/μL | 10 U | 2.5 μL |
| water | | to final, total volume of 50 μL | 37.5 μL |

3.

**Restriction Digest Mixture, Practice Problem 3**

| Component | Stock Concentration | Final Amount or Concentration | Amount of Stock to Add |
|---|---|---|---|
| plasmid pBR322 | 0.1 μg/μL | 200 ng | 2 μL |
| buffer | 4X | 1X | 5 μL |
| XhoI enzyme | 5 U/μL | 5 U | 1 μL |
| water | | to final, total volume of 20 μL | 12 μL |

4. **Strategy 1:**

First, determine the weight of a single molecule of λ DNA:

A single molecule weighs $\left(\frac{660\text{ D}}{1\text{ bp}}\right)(48{,}502\text{ bp}) \approx 3.201 \times 10^7\text{ D}$

Convert this to units of grams and then μg:

$$\frac{1\text{ D}}{1.6605 \times 10^{-24}\text{ g}} = \frac{3.201 \times 10^7\text{D}}{?}$$

$? \approx 5.3155 \times 10^{-17}\text{g} = 5.3155 \times 10^{-11}\mu\text{g}$

If 1 molecule weighs 5.3155 ×10$^{-11}$ then how many molecules are in 5 μg?

$$\frac{5.3155 \times 10^{-11}\mu g}{1 \text{ molecule}} = \frac{5\ \mu g}{?} \qquad \textbf{?} \approx \textbf{9.41} \times \textbf{10}^{\textbf{10}} \textbf{ molecules}$$

**Strategy 2:**

Calculate the MW of one mole of lambda DNA:

$660 \times 48502 = 3.201132 \times 10^7$

So, one mole weighs $3.201132 \times 10^7$ g. Then how many moles is 5 μg?

$$\frac{3.201132 \times 10^7 \text{ g}}{1 \text{ mol}} = \frac{5 \times 10^{-6} \text{ g}}{?} \qquad ? \approx 1.5619 \times 10^{-13} \text{mol}$$

One mol has $6.02214 \times 10^{23}$ molecules, so how many molecules are in $1.5619 \times 10^{-13}$ mol?

$$\frac{1 \text{ mol}}{6.02214 \times 10^{23} \text{ g}} = \frac{1.5619 \times 10^{-13} \text{ mol}}{?} \qquad \textbf{?} \approx \textbf{9.41} \times \textbf{10}^{\textbf{10}} \textbf{ molecules}$$

## 23.3 ELECTROPHORESIS

**Agarose gel electrophoresis** is a common molecular biology technique in which DNA fragments are separated from one another on the basis of their size and are also stained with dyes that allow them to be visualized and photographed. There are many situations in which agarose gel electrophoresis is performed; one of the most common is to separate and visualize the DNA fragments that are formed in a restriction digest. Figure 23.5 shows a diagrammatic representation of electrophoresis.

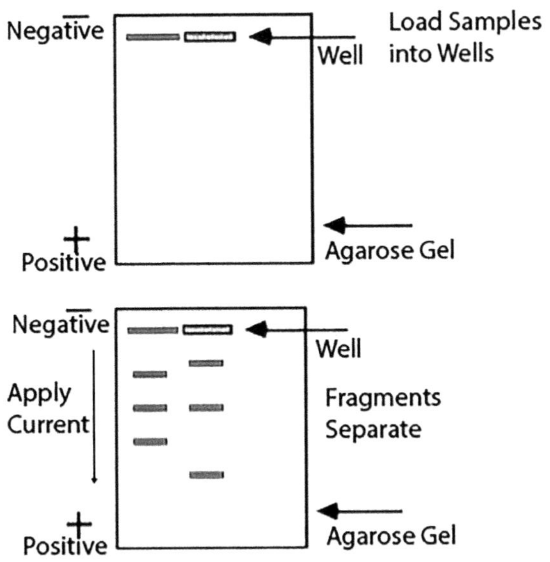


**FIGURE 23.5** A diagrammatic representation of electrophoresis. The samples are loaded into wells in a gel-like matrix, to which an electrical current is applied. DNA moves away from the negative pole, toward the positive pole at a rate that is inversely proportional to the log of the size of the DNA fragment. The result is that DNA fragments separate from one another, with the largest fragments at the top of the gel and the smaller ones lower down.

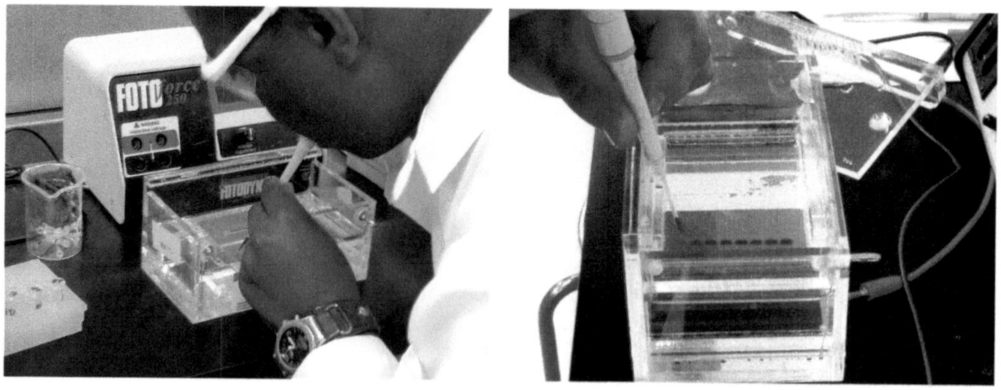


(a) (b)

**FIGURE 23.6** Electrophoresis. (a) An analyst is loading the samples into an agarose gel that is resting in a plastic gel box. After the samples are loaded, the box will be connected to the power supply and a current will be applied to the gel. (b) A closer view of the gel and the sample wells. (A blue dye has been added to the samples to make them easier to see.)

Agarose gel electrophoresis uses a gelatin-like matrix made of agarose. The gel is placed in a plastic box and is covered with a salt/buffer solution. The gel contains "wells," or indentations, into which samples can be placed, one sample in each well Figure 23.6. (A typical agarose gel might have wells for eight samples.) After the samples are loaded into the wells, the box is covered, and electrodes are attached to the box so that an electrical current can be applied to the gel. DNA in aqueous solution is negatively charged. Therefore, when current is applied to the gel, the DNA molecules move through the gel matrix away from the negative electrode toward the positive electrode. Smaller DNA fragments maneuver more quickly through the gel matrix than larger ones, so the fragments separate from one another based on their sizes. The small fragments move farther away from the wells than the larger fragments. The rate at which a DNA fragment moves through an agarose gel is inversely proportional to the $\log_{10}$ of its size in base pairs. After the fragments have had time to migrate through the gel, the current is turned off, the gel is removed from the box, and a stain is used that makes the DNA fragments visible.

## 23.4 ANALYSIS OF THE SIZE OF FRAGMENTS IN AN AGAROSE GEL

Examine the agarose gel picture in Figure 23.7a. Eight samples were loaded onto this gel, electrical current was applied, the DNA fragments migrated, and the gel was then stained with ethidium bromide. Ethidium bromide attaches to DNA and glows when exposed to UV light. Thus, the white bands that you see on the gel are DNA fragments that are stained with ethidium bromide. The small numbers running across the top of the gel, 1–8, mark the location of the wells into which the samples were loaded. Sample 1 was loaded into well 1; sample 2 was loaded into well 2; and so on. Sample 1 migrated down the gel in "lane" 1; sample 2 migrated down the gel in lane 2; and so on. Lane 1, where sample 1 was run, has one DNA band. Lanes 2, 3, and 8 also have one band that ran the same distance as the band in lane 1. This tells us that there is a DNA fragment in samples 1, 2, 3, and 8 that is the same size or about the same size (has the same number of bp). Lanes 4, 6, and 7 contain no DNA bands because these were negative control lanes. Lane 5 contains a commercially produced molecular weight marker mixture. This mixture contains eight DNA fragments whose sizes are known. Figure 23.7b is provided by the manufacturer of the molecular weight markers and specifies the sizes of each of the fragments. When the marker mixture is subjected to electrophoresis, the eight fragments separate from one another and provide a tool to determine the sizes of the bands in the sample lanes. Box 23.2 outlines the general steps in analyzing the results of an electrophoresis gel followed by an example that demonstrates how to use the molecular weight markers to determine the size of the bands in lanes 1, 2, 3, and 8 in Figure 23.7.

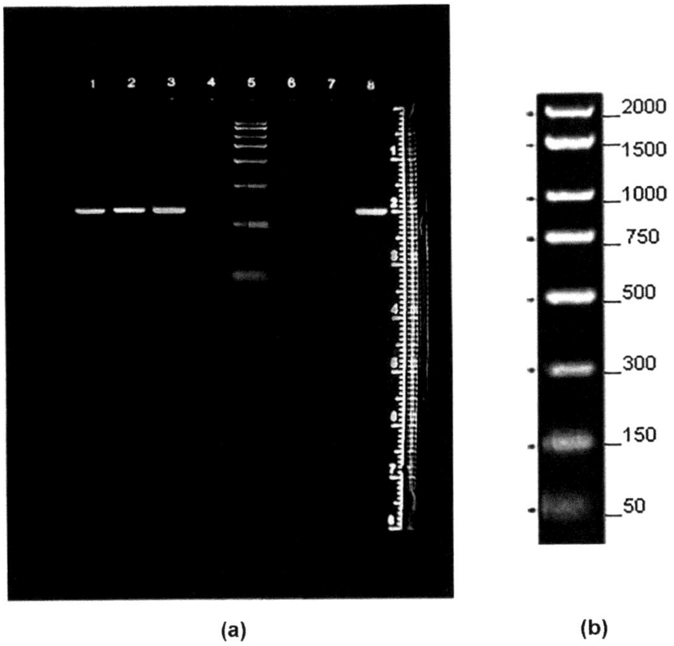


**FIGURE 23.7** Agarose gel electrophoresis. (a) An agarose gel, gel 1, after electrophoresis and staining. (b) The molecular weight standards in lane 5, from the manufacturer, Novagen. The sizes of the eight marker fragments, from bottom (smallest) to top (largest), in base pairs are: 50, 150, 300, 500, 750, 1,000, 1,500, and 2,000.

**BOX 23.2 Analyzing the Results of DNA Electrophoresis**

Step 1. Determine the distance of migration of each band.

Step 2. Plot a standard curve based on the molecular weight markers. The X-axis is linear and is the distance migrated by the fragments in millimeters. The Y-axis is logarithmic and is the DNA fragment length in base pairs.

Step 3. Use the standard curve to determine the sizes of the sample fragments.

**Step 1. Determine the Distance of Migration for Every Band.**
The first step in determining the size of the sample bands is to measure how far each band (DNA fragment) in the molecular weight marker lane migrated in the gel. Also measure the distance migrated by bands in the sample lanes. For consistency, measure the distance in millimeters from the bottom edge of the well to the bottom edge of each band. You can see that a ruler is conveniently displayed on the right side of the gel in Figure 23.7a to facilitate this measurement. Table 23.2 shows the size and distance migrated for each band of the molecular weight marker in Figure 23.7a. Remember that the largest size DNA fragments are at the *top* of the gel (migrate least far); smaller DNA fragments migrate further through the gel.

**Step 2. Plot a Standard Curve Based on the Molecular Weight Markers.**
Figure 23.8 shows the molecular weight marker data from Table 23.2 plotted on regular graph paper. Observe that the relationship is not linear. If you refer back to Figure 17.10, you will see that the relationship between distance migrated and fragment size looks similar to the

**TABLE 23.2 Molecular Marker Migration, Gel 1**

| Size (bp) | Distance Migrated (mm) |
|---|---|
| 2,000 | 3 |
| 1,500 | 3.5 |
| 1,000 | 5.5 |
| 750 | 7 |
| 500 | 10.5 |
| 300 | 15 |
| 150 | 22.5 |
| 50 | 32.5 |

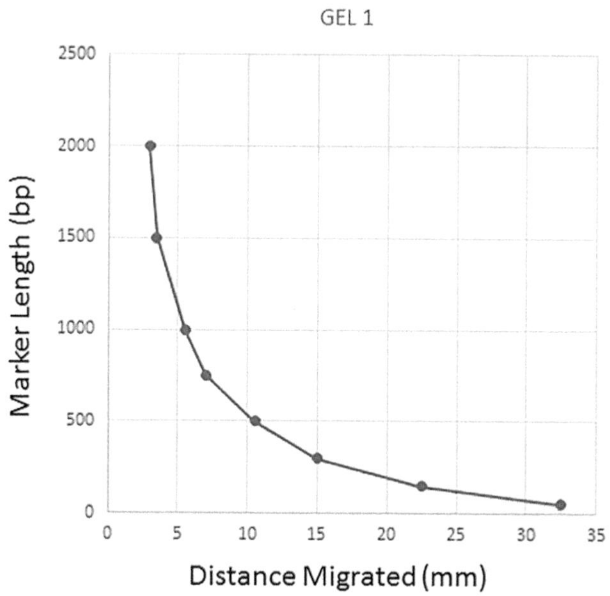


**FIGURE 23.8** Molecular weight standard data from Table 23.2 plotted on regular graph paper.

relationship between radioactive substance remaining and time elapsed – both are exponential relationships. Recall also from Chapter 17 that plotting such relationships on semilogarithmic paper provides a linear plot. Figure 23.9 shows the molecular weight marker data plotted again, but this time as a semilogarithmic plot. The X-axis (linear) is the distance migrated by the fragments in millimeters and the Y-axis (logarithmic) is the DNA fragment length in base pairs. (It is common practice to plot these graphs with distance migrated on the X-axis.) Observe that three-cycle semilogarithmic paper is necessary to plot these data. (Refer back to Chapter 17 for more information about semilogarithmic graphs.) In principle, the relationship between distance migrated and fragment length should be linear when plotted on a semilogarithmic graph. Note that this is a reasonable description for the smaller fragments, but there is a slight deviation from a linear relationship for the larger ones. This is commonly observed.

**Step 3. Use the Standard Curve to Determine the Sizes of the Sample Fragments.**
Determine the base-pair length for the bands in the sample lanes by finding their distance migrated on the X-axis of the standard curve graph. With a ruler, extend a vertical line from this point to its intersection with the best-fit data line on the standard curve. Then take the ruler and extend a horizontal line from this point to the Y-axis to determine the length of the DNA in that band. This is a simple example because lanes 1, 2, 3, and 8 only have one band, and it migrated 20 mm in each of these lanes. Figure 23.10 illustrates how to read off its size from the standard curve. You can see that a distance of migration of 20 mm corresponds to a size of about 200 bp.

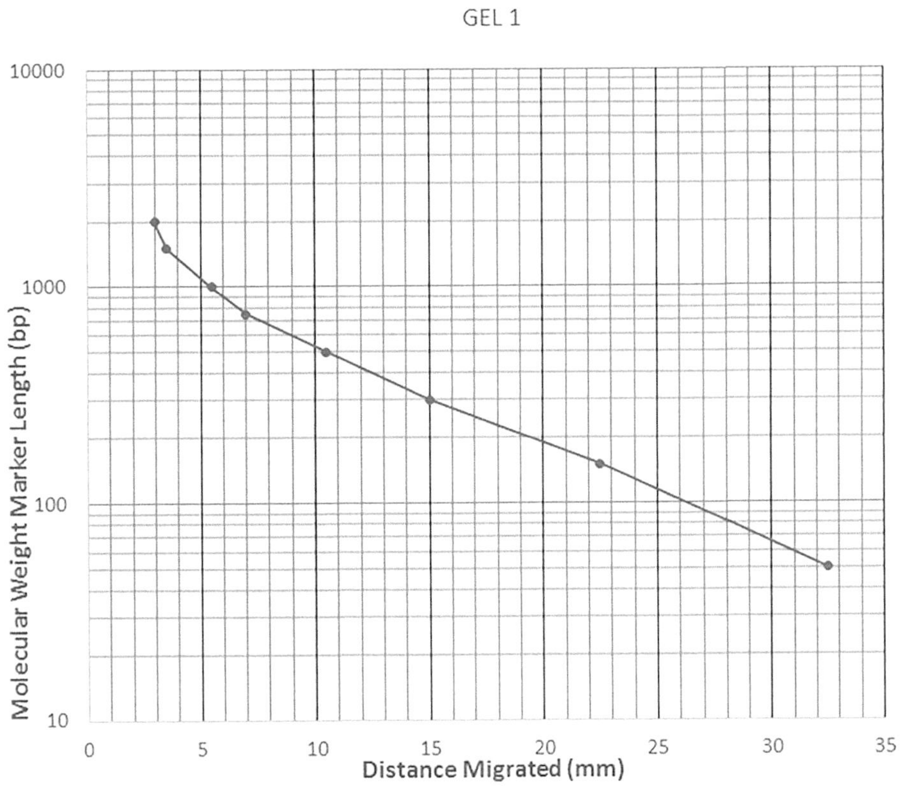


**FIGURE 23.9** Molecular weight standard data from Table 23.2 plotted as a semilogarithmic plot.

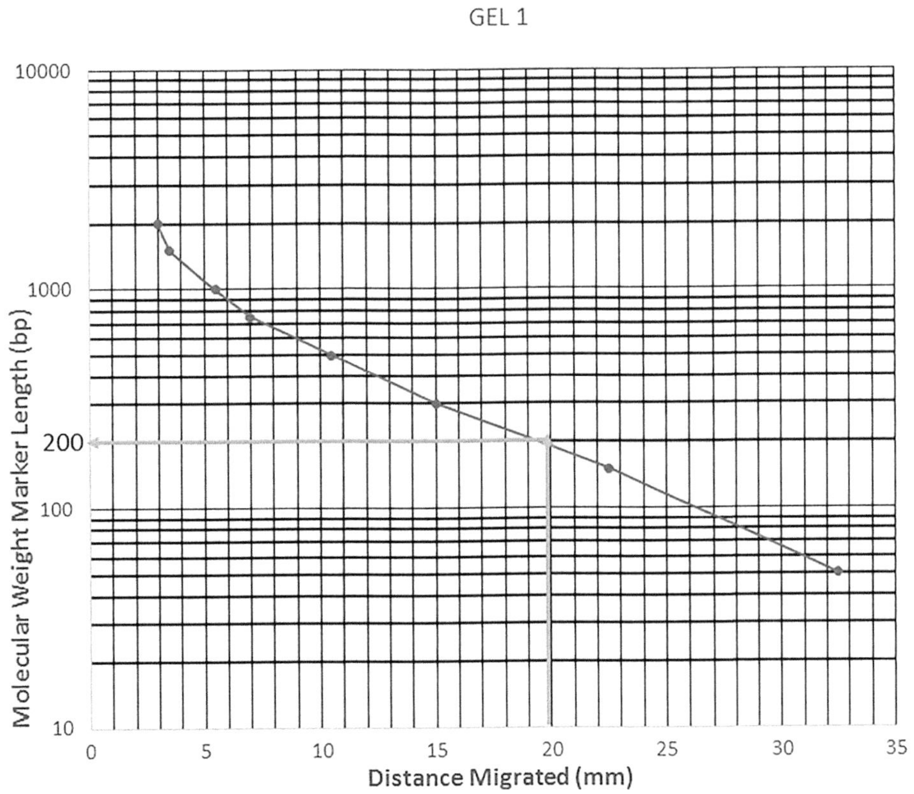


**FIGURE 23.10** Using a standard curve based on molecular weight standards to determine the molecular weight (in bp) of sample DNA fragments. In the example illustrated here, a fragment migrated 20 mm, corresponding to a length of about 200 bp.

## Practice Problem

***Determine the size (in bp) of the band in lane 8 of the gel shown in Figure 23.11. There are molecular weight markers in lane 5 that are the same as the molecular weight markers in Figure 23.7b.***

### *Answer*

Fill in a table for the molecular weight markers (your values might be slightly different):

**Practice Problem**
**Analysis of Electrophoresis Data**

| Size (bp) | Distance Migrated (mm) |
|---|---|
| 2,000 | 4 |
| 1500 | 5 |
| 1000 | 7.5 |
| 750 | 10 |
| 500 | 14 |
| 300 | 21 |
| 150 | 30.5 |
| 50 | 43.5 |

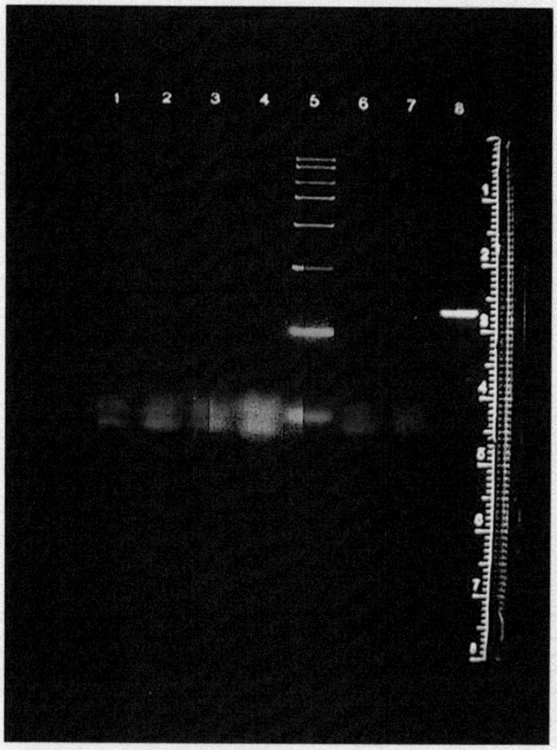


**FIGURE 23.11** Gel results for Practice Problem determining length of DNA fragment in a sample.

Graph the data on a semilogarithmic plot, Figure 23.12. The band in lane 8 is at about 27.5 mm. Reading off the graph, this band is about **190 bp**.

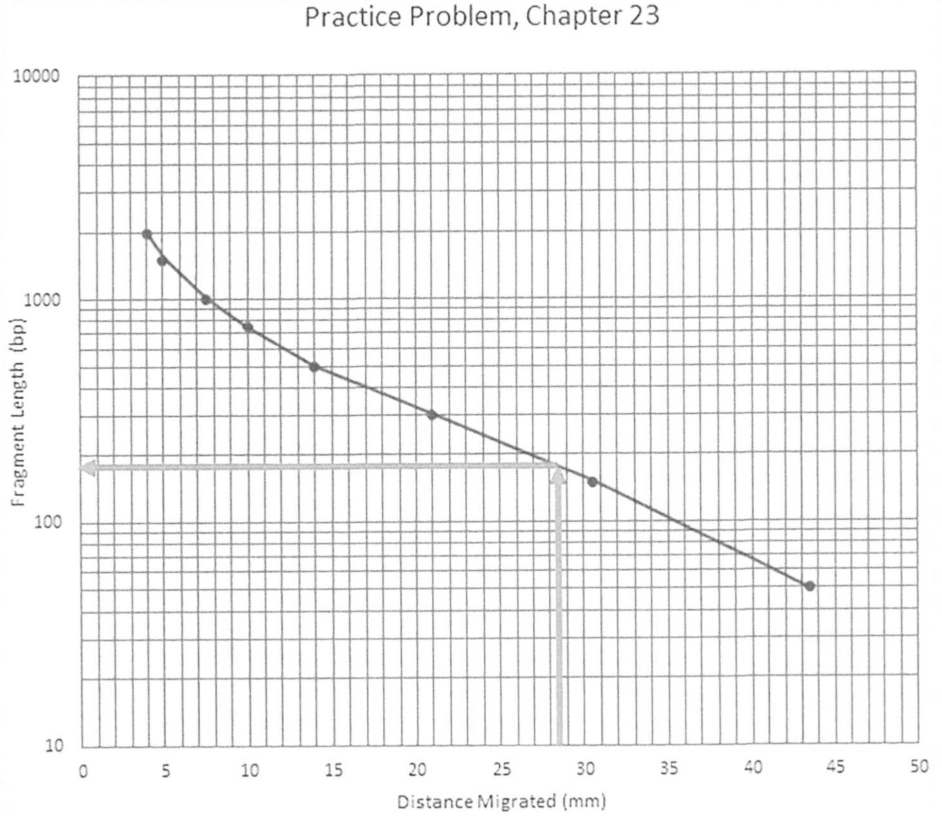

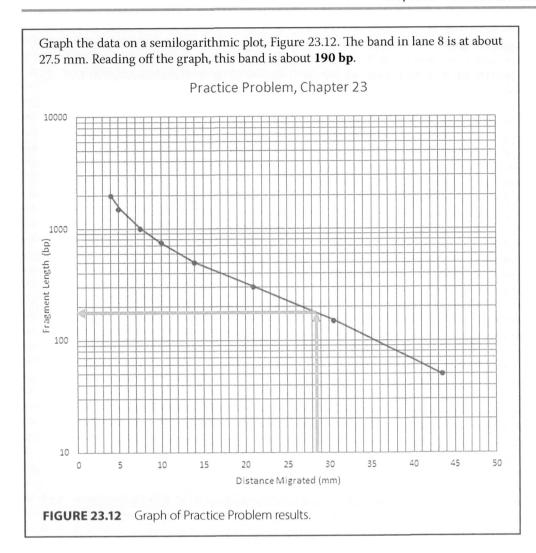

**FIGURE 23.12** Graph of Practice Problem results.

## 23.5 DETERMINING HOW MUCH DNA TO LOAD ONTO AN AGAROSE GEL

Before samples are placed in the wells, loading dye is added to them. Loading dye serves several functions, including adding color to the samples to make them easier to see when loading into the gel. Also, the progress of the electrophoresis run can be monitored by watching the dye move down the gel.

The volume that is loaded onto each well of an agarose gel depends on the size of the wells, which varies depending on the electrophoresis set-up one is using. 10 µL is a common well volume. It is necessary to consider how much DNA should be contained in that volume. If too much DNA is loaded into a well, the bands will be "streaky," but if too little DNA is added, the bands will not be visible. The maximum amount of DNA that can be applied depends on the number of fragments in the sample and the sizes of the fragments. The general range is 0.2–10 µg DNA/well when ethidium bromide staining is used (there are other stains as well). Simple samples, such as plasmid digests, require about 0.2–0.5 µg/well. Complex samples containing a number of DNA fragments of different sizes, for example, digests of mammalian DNA, require 5–10 µg/well. Water is added to the mixture, if necessary, to bring the mixture to the desired volume.

**Example Problem:**

You are preparing a sample for electrophoresis. The concentration of DNA in your sample is 0.8 µg/µL and you want to load 1 µg onto the gel. You have 10X loading dye. The manufacturer of your electrophoresis apparatus states that the volume of each sample should be 10 µL. How will you prepare this sample for electrophoresis?

*Answer:*

The loading dye is 10X and you want it to be 1X in the mixture, so this is a $C_1V_1 = C_2V_2$ problem:

$$C_1 \quad V_1 = C_2 \quad V_2$$

$$(10X)\ (?) = (1X)\ (10\,\mu L) \qquad ? = 1\,\mu L$$

Calculate how much of your DNA sample is required to get 1 µg:

$$\frac{0.8\,\mu g}{\mu L} = \frac{1\,\mu g}{?} \qquad ? = 1.25\,\mu L$$

Combine the following and load it onto your gel:

| | |
|---|---|
| DNA sample | **1.25 µL** |
| Loading dye | **1 µL** |
| Water | **7.75 µL** |
| | **10 µL** |

Note that you might round these volumes to volumes that are easier to pipette accurately. For example, you might use 2 µL of DNA sample and 7 µL water.

**Practice Problems**

1. ***You are preparing a DNA sample for electrophoresis. The concentration of DNA in your sample is 0.5 µg/µL and you want to load 1 µg of DNA. You will be loading 10 µL total volume into each well. Your loading dye is 5X. How should you prepare your sample?***
2. ***You are preparing a DNA sample for electrophoresis. The concentration of DNA in your sample is 70 ng/µL and you want to load 0.25 µg of DNA. You will be loading 10 µL total volume into each well. Your loading dye is 6X. How should you prepare your sample?***

*Answers*

1. First determine how much DNA sample is required:

$$\frac{0.5\,\mu g}{1\,\mu L} = \frac{1\,\mu g}{?} \qquad ? = 2\,\mu L$$

For the loading dye:

$$C_1 \quad V_1 = C_2 \quad V_2$$

$$(5X)\ (?) = (1X)\ (10\,\mu L) \qquad ? = 2\,\mu L$$

So, combine the following and load it onto your gel:

| | |
|---|---|
| DNA sample | **2 μL** |
| Loading dye | **2 μL** |
| Water | **6 μL** |
| | **10 μL** |

2. First determine how much DNA sample is required:

$$\frac{0.07\,\mu g}{1\,\mu L} = \frac{0.25\,\mu g}{?} \quad ? \approx 3.6\,\mu L$$

For the loading dye:

$$\begin{array}{cccc} C_1 & V_1 = C_2 & V_2 & \\ (6X) & (?) = (1X) & (10\,\mu L) & ? \approx 1.7\,\mu L \end{array}$$

So, combine the following and load it onto your gel:

| | |
|---|---|
| DNA sample | **3.6 μL** |
| Loading dye | **1.7 μL** |
| Water | **4.7 μL** |
| | **10 μL** |

## 23.6 VARIATION ON A THEME: DECIDING HOW MUCH PROTEIN TO LOAD ON A POLYACRYLAMIDE GEL

Agarose gel electrophoresis is a type of electrophoresis commonly used to separate DNA fragments from one another. **Polyacrylamide gel electrophoresis (PAGE)** *is another type of electrophoresis that is commonly used to separate proteins of different sizes from one another* (and sometimes is also used for DNA separations). The same principles apply to loading proteins into the wells in a PAGE gel, that is, the proper amount of protein and loading dye/sample buffer must be calculated. These problems relate to proteins.

**Example Problem:**

Sample buffer (with loading dye) is added to each protein sample before PAGE. The sample buffer is stored as a 5X stock. If each sample well is loaded with 50 μL total volume, how much of the loading buffer should be used for each sample?

***Answer:***

This is a simple $C_1V_1 = C_2V_2$ problem:

$$\begin{array}{ccc} C_1 & V_1 = C_2 & V_2 \\ (5X) & (?) = (1X) & (50\,\mu L) \end{array}$$

$$\mathbf{? \approx 10\,\mu L}$$

**Example Problem:**

You have been purifying a protein of interest that was isolated from bacteria and you now have samples from each stage of the purification process. You want to run the samples using PAGE because this is a good way to evaluate the purity of the protein at each stage of the purification.

To prepare each sample for PAGE, you want to combine:

a. Sample buffer: sample buffer is kept as a 5X stock
b. Either 50 µg of protein or 20 µg of protein depending on the purity of the preparation (more is added when the protein is contaminated with impurities)
c. Water to a volume of 50 µL

You have five samples of protein from the purification procedure, each sample contains protein at a different concentration, as shown in the table below. Fill in the table to show:

a. how much sample buffer is required
b. how much protein sample is required
c. how much water is required

**Example Problem**

| Sample | Protein concentration | Amount Protein to Load into Well | Sample Buffer Required | Volume of Protein Required | Water to a Volume of 50 µL |
|---|---|---|---|---|---|
| Unpurified protein | 10 mg/mL | 50 µg | 10 µL | 5 µL | 35 µL |
| First stage of purification | 20 mg/mL | 20 µg | | | |
| Second stage of purification | 1.5 mg/mL | 20 µg | | | |
| Third stage of purification | 0.5 mg/mL | 20 µg | | | |
| Control protein | 1 mg/mL | 20 µg | | | |

***Answer:***

a. 10 µL of sample buffer is required, as calculated in the Example Problem above.
b. For example, for unpurified protein:

The protein is present at a concentration of 10 mg/mL = 10 µg/µL.
You want 50 µg. If there are 10 µg in 1 µL, how many µL are required to get 50 µg?
By proportions:

$$\frac{10\ \mu g}{1\ \mu L} = \frac{50\ \mu g}{?} \qquad \mathbf{? = 5\ \mu L}$$

For example, for unpurified protein, 10 µL of sample buffer is required, 5 µL of protein sample, and so **35 µL** of water is needed to bring the volume to 50 µL.

**Example Problem, Answer**

| Sample | Protein Concentration | Amount Protein to Load into Well | Sample Buffer Required | Volume of Protein Required | Water to a Volume of 50 μL |
|---|---|---|---|---|---|
| Unpurified protein | 10 mg/mL | 50 μg | 10 μL | 5 μL | 35 μL |
| First stage of purification | 20 mg/mL | 20 μg | 10 μL | 1 μL | 39 μL |
| Second stage of purification | 1.5 mg/mL | 20 μg | 10 μL | 13.3 μL | 26.7 μL |
| Third stage of purification | 0.5 mg/mL | 20 μg | 10 μL | 40 μL | 0 |
| Control protein | 1 mg/mL | 20 μg | 10 μL | 20 μL | 20 μL |

## Practice Problem

***Fill in this table assuming that you want:***

a. ***10 μL of 5X sample buffer for each well***
b. ***20 μg of protein***
c. ***Water to a volume of 50 μL***

**Practice Problem**

| Sample | Protein Concentration | Amount Protein to Load into Well | Sample Buffer Required | Volume of Protein Required | Water to a Volume of 50 μL |
|---|---|---|---|---|---|
| Unpurified protein | 2 mg/mL | 20 μg | 10 μL | | |
| First stage of purification | 4 mg/mL | 20 μg | 10 μL | | |
| Second stage of purification | 2.5 mg/mL | 20 μg | 10 μL | | |
| Third stage of purification | 0.75 mg/mL | 20 μg | 10 μL | | |
| Control protein | 1 mg/mL | 20 μg | 10 μL | | |

### *Answer*

**Practice Problem**

| Sample | Protein Concentration | Amount Protein to Load into Well | Sample Buffer Required | Volume of Protein Required | Water to a Volume of 50 μL |
|---|---|---|---|---|---|
| Unpurified protein | 2 mg/mL | 20 μg | 10 μL | 10 μL | 30 μL |
| First stage of purification | 4 mg/mL | 20 μg | 10 μL | 5 μL | 35 μL |
| Second stage of purification | 2.5 mg/mL | 20 μg | 10 μL | 8 μL | 32 μL |
| Third stage of purification | 0.75 mg/mL | 20 μg | 10 μL | 26.7 μL | 13.3 μL |
| Control protein | 1 mg/mL | 20 μg | 10 μL | 20 μL | 20 μL |

## 23.7 QUANTITATION OF DNA USING GEL ELECTROPHORESIS

Section 22.12 discussed the use of spectrophotometry to estimate the quantity of DNA or RNA in a sample. It is also common to use gel electrophoresis to estimate the quantity of DNA in a sample. This is done by comparing the intensity of a DNA band on an ethidium bromide-stained agarose gel to the intensity of a band containing a known amount of DNA. The intensity of staining of a band is proportional to how much DNA is in the band. For example, if band A is twice as intensely stained with ethidium bromide as band B, then band A has twice the amount of DNA as band B. If, for example, band B is known to contain 75 ng of DNA, then band A must contain approximately 150 ng of DNA. In this method, we compare the intensity only. It does not matter how far the band has migrated on the gel.

Box 23.3 outlines the steps in quantifying DNA using electrophoresis, which is then discussed in more detail below. Figure 23.13 sketches the overall procedure.

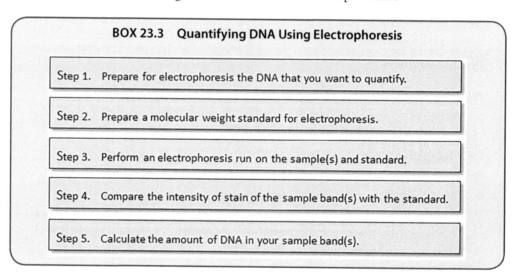

**BOX 23.3 Quantifying DNA Using Electrophoresis**

Step 1. Prepare for electrophoresis the DNA that you want to quantify.

Step 2. Prepare a molecular weight standard for electrophoresis.

Step 3. Perform an electrophoresis run on the sample(s) and standard.

Step 4. Compare the intensity of stain of the sample band(s) with the standard.

Step 5. Calculate the amount of DNA in your sample band(s).

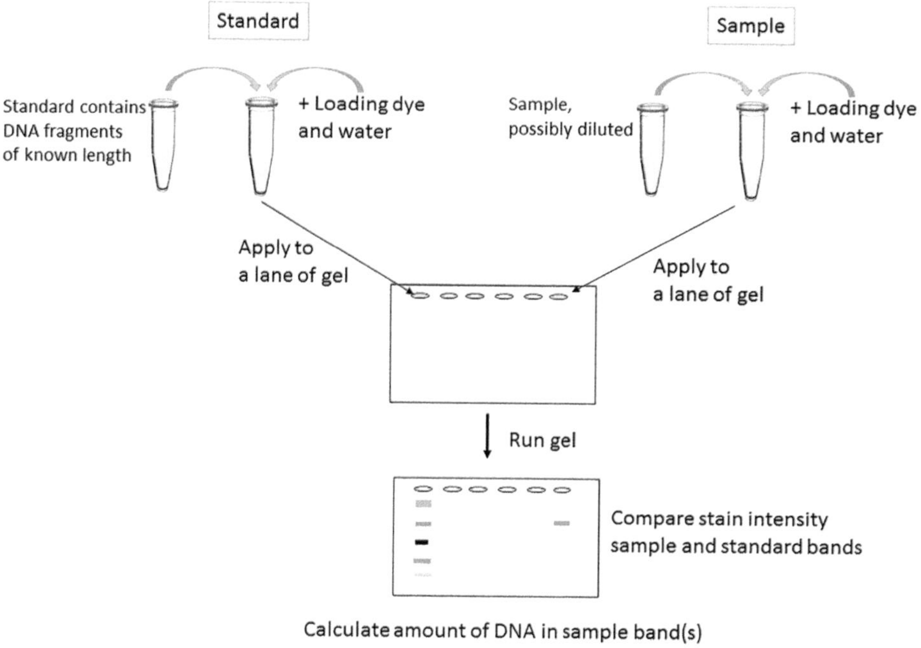


**FIGURE 23.13** The general procedure for quantifying DNA by electrophoresis. This method requires a standard whose original length is known and that has been cut into fragments of varying, known lengths.

Here is an example to illustrate this method of quantifying DNA by electrophoresis.

**Step 1. Prepare for Electrophoresis the DNA that You Plan to Quantify.**
You want to estimate how much DNA is present in a DNA sample. The sample is prepared for electrophoresis by combining some of it, say, 1 μL, with loading dye and water:

1 μL DNA
8 μL water
<u>1 μL loading dye</u>
10 μL total

**Step 2. Prepare a Molecular Weight Standard for Electrophoresis.**
There are various molecular weight standards that can be used for this purpose. Lambda (λ) DNA digested with HindIII restriction enzyme is a commonly used standard because it is readily available and inexpensive. The λ standard is prepared as follows for electrophoresis:

1 μL λ DNA (500 ng/μL stock concentration)
8 μL water
<u>1 μL loading dye</u>
10 μL total

Figure 23.14 is from the manufacturer of the λ standard. It shows the sizes of the fragments in the λ standards mixture.

**Step 3. Perform an Electrophoresis Run on the Sample and the Standard.**
The DNA sample and the standard are run on a gel and stained with ethidium bromide.

**Step 4. Compare the Intensity of the Sample Band(s) with the Standard.**

**Step 5. Calculate the Amount of DNA in Your Sample Fragment Band.**
Suppose, for example, that after electrophoresis your DNA sample has only one band and that band matches the 9416 bp band in the lambda standard lane in intensity of staining. Then:

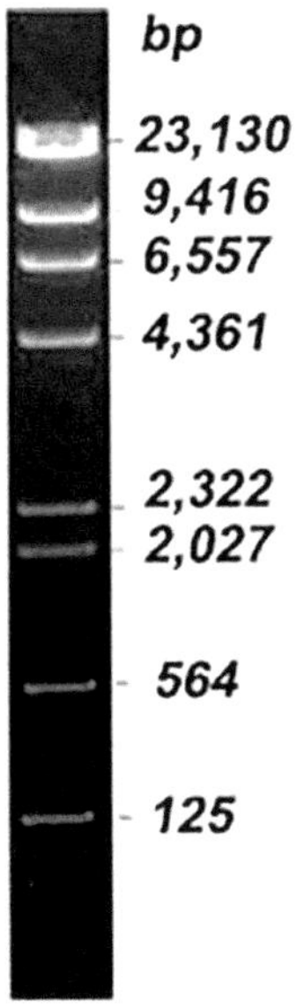


**FIGURE 23.14** A lambda standard that can be used for quantifying DNA.

1. The 9,416 bp band of the lambda digest represents only a fraction of the total lambda DNA loaded onto the gel, that is:

$$\frac{\mathbf{9,416\ bp}}{\mathbf{48,502\ bp}} \approx \mathbf{0.1941}$$

(Remember that the total length of the λ DNA is 48,502 bp.)
2. How much λ DNA was loaded? 1 µL of a 500 ng/µL stock = 500 ng
Of the 500 ng of λ DNA loaded onto the gel, 0.1941 of it is the 9416 bp fragment.
So the 9416 bp lane contains: 500 ng (0.1941) ≈ **97 ng**
3. This means your sample band also has about 97 ng. Since you loaded 1 µL onto the gel, it has a concentration of about **97 ng/µL.**

**Example Problem:**

You have 100 µL of a buffered solution containing a DNA fragment amplified by PCR. You want to determine the amount and concentration of amplified DNA in this solution using agarose gel electrophoresis. Here is what you do:

Step 1. a. Dilute a portion of the sample 1/10, for example, 1 µL of DNA sample + 9 µL water.

b. The diluted sample is prepared by combining 4 µL of it with loading dye and water:

4 µL DNA sample
5 µL water
1 µL loading dye
10 µL total

Step 2. The standard is prepared. You use a restriction digested standard that contains eight fragments of known sizes. You take:

1 µL standard DNA (250 ng/µL stock concentration)
8 µL water
1 µL loading dye
10 µL total

Step 3. You run electrophoresis on the sample and the standard and then stain the resulting gel with ethidium bromide. You obtain the result shown in Figure 23.15 below.

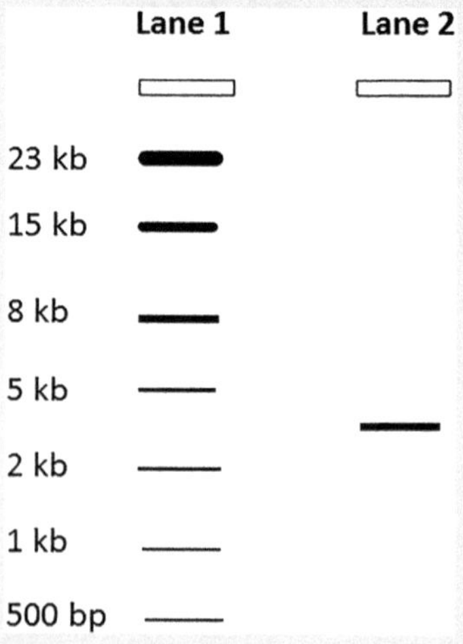


**FIGURE 23.15** The result of the Practice Problem gel.

Step 4. You compare the intensity of the sample band with the standard and decide that the sample band matches the 8 Kb standard fragment in intensity.

a. Sketch this procedure. You can use Figure 23.13 as a model or create a sketch that makes sense to you.
b. What is the concentration of DNA in your sample?
c. What is the amount of DNA in your sample?

***Answer:***

a. A sketch is shown in Figure 23.16.
b. First, you must determine the total amount of DNA loaded in the standard lane. If you add all the fragment sizes together, you obtain 54,500 bp.

The 8 Kb standard fragment is 8,000/54,500 of the total DNA in the standard lane. So, it contains: (250 ng) (8,000 bp/54,500 bp) ≈ 36.7 ng in band.
This means your sample band also contained about 36.7 ng of DNA.
That 36.7 ng was in a volume of 4 µL, so the concentration of DNA in your sample was:
Concentration = 36.7 ng/4 µL of DNA = 9.175 ng/µL
The sample had been diluted 1/10, so the concentration in the undiluted sample was:
(9.175 ng/µL) (10) ≈ **91.8 ng/µL**

c. The total amount of DNA that you had in the original 100 µL was:
Amount DNA isolated: (100 µL) (91.8 ng/µL) = **9180 ng DNA**

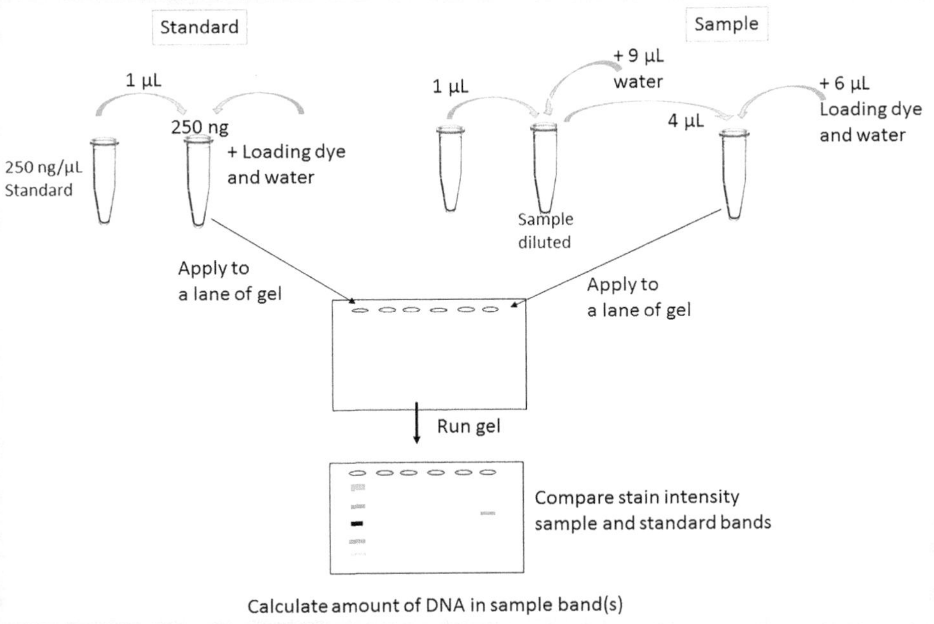


**FIGURE 23.16** Practice Problem sketch.

**Practice Problem**

***You want to estimate how much DNA is present in a DNA sample. You are not sure how much of the sample to load on the gel, so you prepare it three times with different amounts of sample each time as follows:***

| *Preparation A* | *Preparation B* | *Preparation C* |
|---|---|---|
| ***1 μL DNA*** | ***2 μL DNA*** | ***3 μL DNA*** |
| ***8 μL water*** | ***7 μL water*** | ***6 μL water*** |
| ***1 μL loading dye*** | ***1 μL loading dye*** | ***1 μL loading dye*** |
| ***10 μL total*** | ***10 μL total*** | ***10 μL total*** |

***You also prepare λ DNA digested with HindIII restriction enzyme as follows:***

***1 μL λ DNA (500 ng/μL stock concentration)***
***8 μL water***
***1 μL loading dye***
***10 μL total***

***You run all four preparations on an agarose gel: the three DNA preparations and the λ standard digest. After electrophoresis and staining, you do not see a band at all in the lane with sample preparation A, you see a faint band for sample preparation B, and the band for sample preparation C band matches the 4,361 band of the lambda standard. About how much DNA is present in your DNA sample? Express your answer as an amount and as a concentration (lambda is 48,502 bp).***

*Answer*

The band you see for preparation C matches the 4361 band of the λ digest. This band represents a portion of the total lambda DNA loaded onto the gel, that is:

$$\frac{4,361\text{ bp}}{48,502\text{ bp}} \approx 0.0899$$

How much λ DNA was loaded? 1 μL of a 500 ng/μL stock = 500 ng
Of the 500 ng of λ DNA loaded onto the gel, 0.0899 of it is the 4361 bp fragment.
So, the 4361 bp lane contains: (500 ng) (0.0899) ≈ 45 ng
This means your sample band also has about **45 ng** (amount). Since you loaded 3 μL onto the gel, it has a concentration of about **15 ng/μL**.

## 23.8 TRANSFORMATION EFFICIENCY

This section discusses a somewhat different problem in molecular biology, the calculation of transformation efficiency. This relates to a situation where a DNA gene, or sequence of interest, has been inserted into a vector, typically a plasmid, that can be taken up by bacterial cells, for example, by *E. coli* bacteria. The bacteria are prepared in such a way that they are able to take up the plasmid (are "competent"). The bacteria then are incubated with the plasmid vector under specialized conditions that promote the uptake of the vector. When a cell takes up plasmid vector, it is said to be "transformed." **Transformation efficiency** *is the number of transformed bacteria per μg of plasmid DNA.* The process of calculating transformation efficiency is summarized in Box 23.4 followed by an example. The example is sketched in Figure 23.17.

**BOX 23.4 Calculating Transformation Efficiency**

Step 1. Mix the plasmid DNA with the bacteria to be transformed.

Step 2. Apply the bacterial cells onto a Petri plate.

Step 3. Incubate the bacteria overnight to allow growth.

Step 4. Count the resulting bacterial colonies on the Petri plate.

Step 5. Calculate the transformation efficiency.

**Example**:

**Step 1. Mix the Plasmid DNA with the Bacteria to Be Transformed.**
Assume that your gene of interest has been inserted into the plasmid pBR322 and your plasmid DNA stock solution has a concentration of 20 ng plasmid DNA/μL. You remove 10 μL from the plasmid stock solution and add it to another tube that contains 190 μL of *E. coli* cells. You apply a brief heat shock to the cells, which facilitates plasmid uptake. Then you add

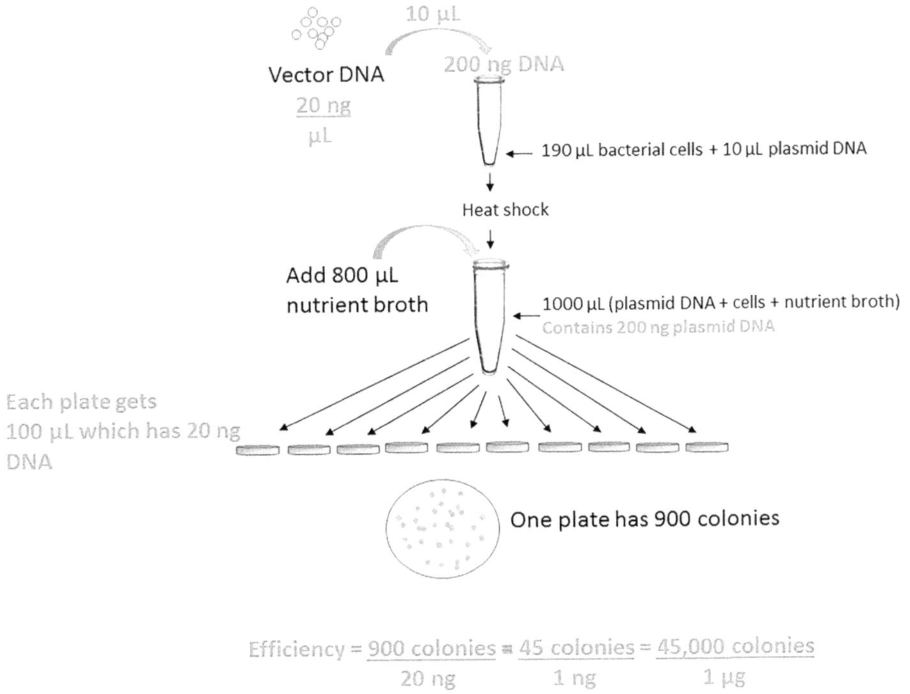


**FIGURE 23.17** An example of transformation efficiency calculation.

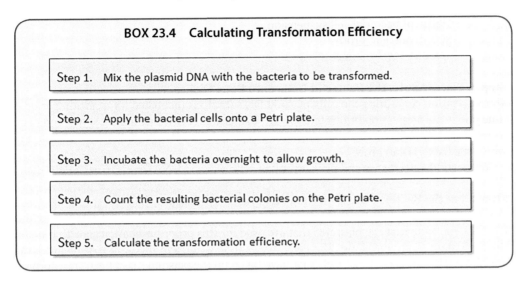

800 μL of nutrient broth (nutrient medium) to the mixture to promote recovery of the bacterial cells. You now have a tube containing:

10 μL of plasmid DNA stock
190 μL of bacterial cell suspension
800 μL nutrient broth
1,000 μL total volume

**Step 2. Plate (Apply) the Bacterial Cells onto Petri Dishes.**
The suspension containing the cells/plasmid DNA/broth is incubated for a certain period of time under the proper conditions to allow the bacteria to recover from heat shock and begin to replicate the plasmid. Then the bacteria are plated onto Petri dishes with nutrient agar where the bacteria can grow.

You take 10 Petri dishes and plate 100 μL of cells/plasmid DNA/broth to each Petri dish.

**Step 3. Let the Bacteria Grow on the Petri Plates Overnight.**
You incubate your ten Petri dishes overnight under conditions that support the growth of the bacteria. Note that the plasmids that are used for this procedure have a gene that makes them resistant to an antibiotic. The Petri dishes have a nutrient medium that includes this antibiotic. Therefore, bacterial cells that have taken up the plasmid (have been transformed) can grow on the Petri dishes. Many of the bacteria may not have been transformed and they will die because the antibiotic on the Petri dishes will kill them.

**Step 4. Count Colonies**
Individual bacteria are too small to see with the naked eye. But when bacteria have been incubated overnight and have undergone many cell divisions, there are so many cells on the Petri dish that they are visible. A colony is a discrete rounded mass of bacteria, large enough to see, where each colony is assumed to have arisen from a single bacterial cell that divided many times.

Suppose the next day you look at one of the Petri plates and you count 900 bacterial colonies.

**Step 5. Calculate the Transformation Efficiency.**
Let us consider only the plate on which you counted 900 colonies. Transformation efficiency is the number of transformed bacteria per μg of plasmid DNA. Thus, we need to know two things to calculate the transformation efficiency: the number of transformed bacteria and the μg of plasmid DNA that were used to transform those bacteria. The first part is easy. There are 900 colonies; each is assumed to have arisen from a single transformed bacterial cell. It is a bit more complex to calculate how many μg of plasmid DNA were used to transform those bacterial cells.

1. Calculate how much plasmid DNA was added to the 190 μL of *E. coli* cells:
   (10 μL) (20 ng/μL) = 200 ng plasmid was added to the *E. coli* cells.
2. Calculate the total volume of the plasmid/cell suspension:

$$\text{Volume} = \text{volume of DNA stock solution} + \text{volume of } E.\,coli \text{ cells}$$
$$+ \text{volume of nutrient broth}$$
$$= 10\ \mu\text{L} + 190\ \mu\text{L} + 800\ \mu\text{L} = 1{,}000\ \mu\text{L}$$

3. Calculate what portion of the total volume was plated onto the Petri dish with 900 colonies:

$$\text{Plated fraction} = (100\ \mu\text{L})/(1{,}000\ \mu\text{L}) = 0.1$$

4. You started with 200 ng of plasmid DNA, but only 0.1 of that total plasmid was added to the bacteria on the Petri dish with 900 colonies:

$$\text{plasmid DNA} = (0.1)\,(200\text{ ng}) = 20\text{ ng}$$

5. Calculate the transformation efficiency:

$$\text{Efficiency} = 900\text{ colonies}/20\text{ ng plasmid DNA} = 45\text{ colonies}/1\text{ ng} = \mathbf{45{,}000\ colonies/\mu g}$$

**Practice Problem**

***E. coli is to be transformed with the plasmid vector pBR322. A gene of interest has been incorporated into the plasmids. The vector is present at a concentration of 0.01 µg plasmid DNA/µL. 15 µL of this plasmid vector is removed and added to another tube that contains 185 µL of* E.coli *cells. After a brief heat shock, you add 800 µL of nutrient broth to the mixture. You now have one tube with:***

***15 µL of plasmid DNA stock***
***185 µL of bacterial cell suspension***
***800 µL nutrient broth***
***1,000 µL total volume***

***You then allow the cells to incubate under the correct conditions to promote plasmid uptake by the bacterial cells. Then, you:***

***Plate 50 µL of the suspension onto a Petri dish with nutrient agar and antibiotic, and you allow the dish to incubate overnight.***
***You also plate 100 µL of the suspension onto another Petri dish and incubate it overnight.***
***On the first Petri dish you count 430 colonies, on the second 910 colonies.***

a. ***Sketch this problem. You can use the basic scheme shown in Figure 23.10 or make a sketch that makes sense to you.***
b. ***Calculate the average transformation efficiency based on these two plates.***

*Answer*

a. Sketches may vary.
b. The steps to perform this calculation are:

1. Calculate how much plasmid DNA was added to the 185 µL of *E. coli* cells:
(15 µL) (0.01 µg/µL) = **0.15 µg plasmid** was added to the *E. coli* cells.

2. Calculate the total volume of the plasmid/cell suspension:
Volume = volume of DNA stock solution + volume of *E. coli* cells + volume of nutrient broth
= 15 µL + 185 µL + 800 µL = **1,000 µL**

3. Calculate what portion of the total volume was plated onto each Petri dish:
First Petri dish:
Plated fraction = 50 µL/1,000 µL = **0.05**

Second Petri dish:
Plated fraction = 100 μL/1,000 μL = **0.1**

4. You started with 0.15 μg of plasmid DNA, but on the first dish 0.05 of that total plasmid was added to the bacteria:
   Plasmid DNA = (0.05) (0.15 μg) = **0.0075 μg**
   On the second Petri dish:
   Plasmid DNA = (0.1) (0.15 μg) = **0.015 μg**

5. Calculate the transformation efficiency:
   Petri dish 1 efficiency = 430 colonies/0.0075 μg plasmid DNA ≈ 57,333 colonies/μg
   Petri dish 2 efficiency = 910 colonies/0.015 μg plasmid DNA ≈ 60,667 colonies/μg
   The average of the two values is about **59,000 colonies/μg**

# The Polymerase Chain Reaction

# 24



## 24.1 INTRODUCTION TO PCR

This chapter discusses some of the math calculations associated with running the polymerase chain reaction (PCR). This discussion is not intended to be a guide to performing PCR but rather explores the calculations you might encounter, particularly when optimizing a PCR reaction or setting up a PCR procedure. Chapter 25 continues our discussion by looking at the calculations associated with quantitative PCR.

PCR was first described by Kary Mullis in 1983 and since then has been adapted to become one of the most important techniques in the molecular biologist's toolkit. PCR allows analysts to select a specific, target sequence of DNA that is present in a sample in low amounts and then to make millions or even billions of copies of that particular sequence. Suppose, for example, that a scientist is studying the gene for a particular human trait and the gene is 1,000 base pairs (bp) long. The human genome contains about 3.2 billion bp, so if DNA is isolated from cells, the gene of interest will represent only about 0.00003% of the DNA isolated – not very much. PCR allows the scientist to make millions of copies of only the target gene. Or suppose forensic scientists are analyzing DNA from the saliva on a postage stamp. Only a miniscule amount of DNA is left on the stamp and so the DNA must be amplified millions of times to allow it to be analyzed. PCR is the tool for this task. Or suppose that clinicians need a diagnostic method to determine if a person is infected with a certain pathogen. One strategy is to look for DNA or RNA from that pathogen in a patient sample, such as blood or saliva. However, the pathogen's genetic information will only be a tiny, undetectable portion of any human sample. The vast majority of genetic material in the sample will be the patient's own DNA or RNA or will be genetic material from the varied microorganisms that normally coexist in human bodies. Therefore, diagnostic assays require significant amplification of the pathogen's DNA or RNA to detect it. PCR is again the tool for this task.

PCR is a laboratory method that mimics the cell's natural ability to replicate (reproduce) DNA using enzymes called DNA polymerases. Replication occurs naturally every time a cell

DOI: 10.1201/9780429282744-29

divides, for example, during wound healing and during growth. In PCR, the analyst simulates DNA replication by combining the required ingredients in a test tube and providing suitable conditions for a polymerase enzyme to synthesize new strands of the sample's DNA. The most common polymerase enzyme used in PCR is called *Taq* DNA polymerase. *The DNA from the sample is termed the* **template DNA**.

Although the PCR method simulates normal DNA replication, there are some differences between PCR and replication as it occurs naturally in a cell. One of these differences is that in PCR, only a short section of the DNA template is copied (typically up to around 10,000 base pairs). *The section of DNA that is replicated is the* **target sequence**, Figure 24.1.

How is it that in PCR the DNA polymerase enzyme only duplicates a target region rather than all of the DNA present? The answer lies in an important characteristic of DNA polymerases. These enzymes require a very short section of double-stranded DNA to initiate or *prime* synthesis. A **primer** *is a short piece of single-stranded DNA (or RNA) that is complementary to one end of a section of the DNA that is to be replicated.* Primers bind to single-stranded DNA creating a short double-stranded section. The DNA polymerase enzyme finds this double-stranded section and begins there to synthesize a new DNA strand. So, in PCR, there are primers that recognize and bracket the target region. The analyst controls the starting and ending points for DNA replication in PCR by the choice of specific primers. To design these primers, the analyst must know the DNA sequence of the target DNA or at least must know the DNA sequence of the ends of the target region.

The first step in PCR is to separate the two strands of original double-stranded DNA by subjecting the tube with the reaction ingredients, the reaction mixture, to a high temperature. Once the strands are separated, the primers can find their targets and bind, Figure 24.2. Observe in this figure that there is a short primer that is complementary to a sequence at the beginning of the target region on one strand of the DNA. There is a second short primer that is complementary to a sequence at the end of the target region on the opposite strand of DNA. Observe how the two primers thus recognize and bind to the ends of the target sequence so that they bracket the target portion of the DNA template that will be amplified. One of the primers is named the "forward" primer; the other is called the "reverse" primer.

A second important difference between PCR and natural DNA replication is that, in nature, replication occurs once when a cell divides. In the laboratory, during PCR, the target DNA is duplicated over and over again to generate millions of copies. This is accomplished by providing temperature conditions that promote repeated cycles of replication. After combining the components of the reaction mixture together in a tube, the analyst puts the tube in a device, called a **thermocycler**, *which subjects the mixture to a series of repeated temperature cycles.* As was shown in Figure 24.2, at the beginning of each cycle, step 1, the template DNA is separated into its two strands by subjecting the DNA to elevated temperatures. Next, step 2, the temperature is lowered enough to allow the primers to anneal (bind) to complementary regions of the target DNA (if the target is present). In the final step, step 3, the temperature is adjusted to allow the *Taq* DNA polymerase enzyme to work. The enzyme copies each strand starting from the primer on that strand. To do this, it pulls the needed nucleotide (an A, T, G, or C) from the reaction mixture and attaches it to the growing strand, Figure 24.3.

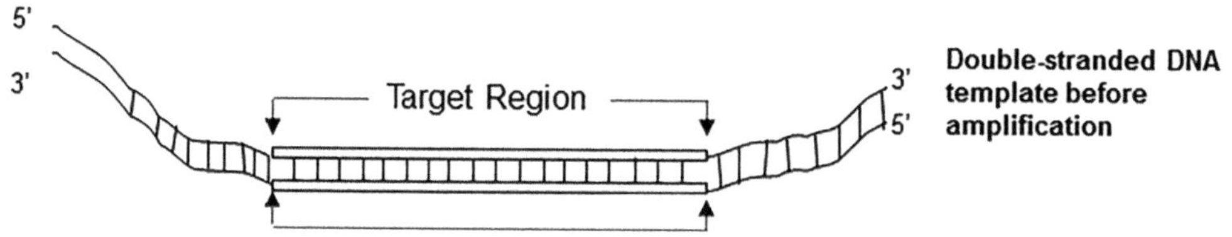


**FIGURE 24.1** A simplified sketch of double-stranded DNA before PCR amplification. The template DNA is isolated from the sample. This template DNA is actually much longer than is drawn here and extends out in both directions. In PCR, however, we are interested in only a short stretch of the template DNA, the target region. This target region might be, for example, a stretch of DNA that is characteristic of a pathogen or a stretch of DNA that is used to help distinguish one individual from another.

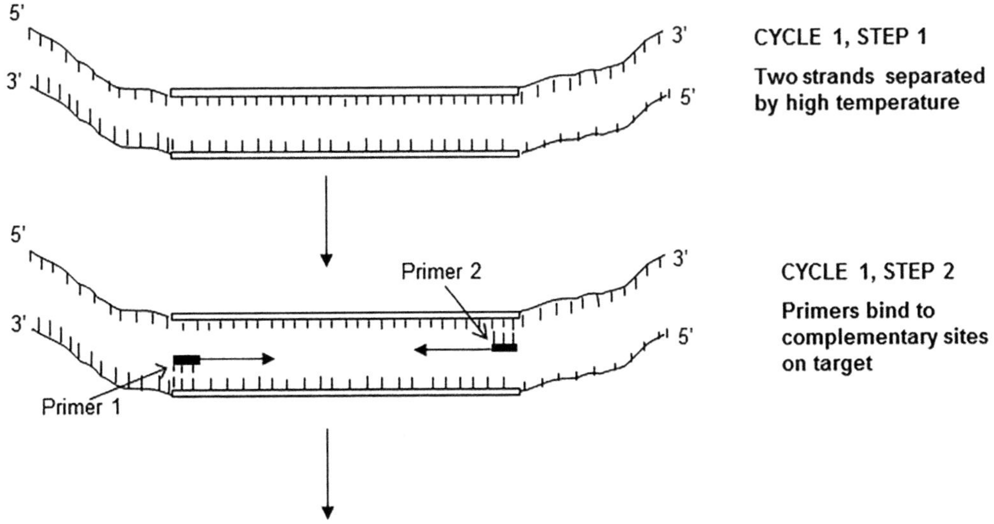


**FIGURE 24.2** The beginning of PCR. To begin a PCR reaction, the two strands of DNA are separated from one another using high temperature. Once they are separated, the two primers find their complementary (target) regions of DNA. One primer binds to one strand of DNA, the other primer to the other strand.

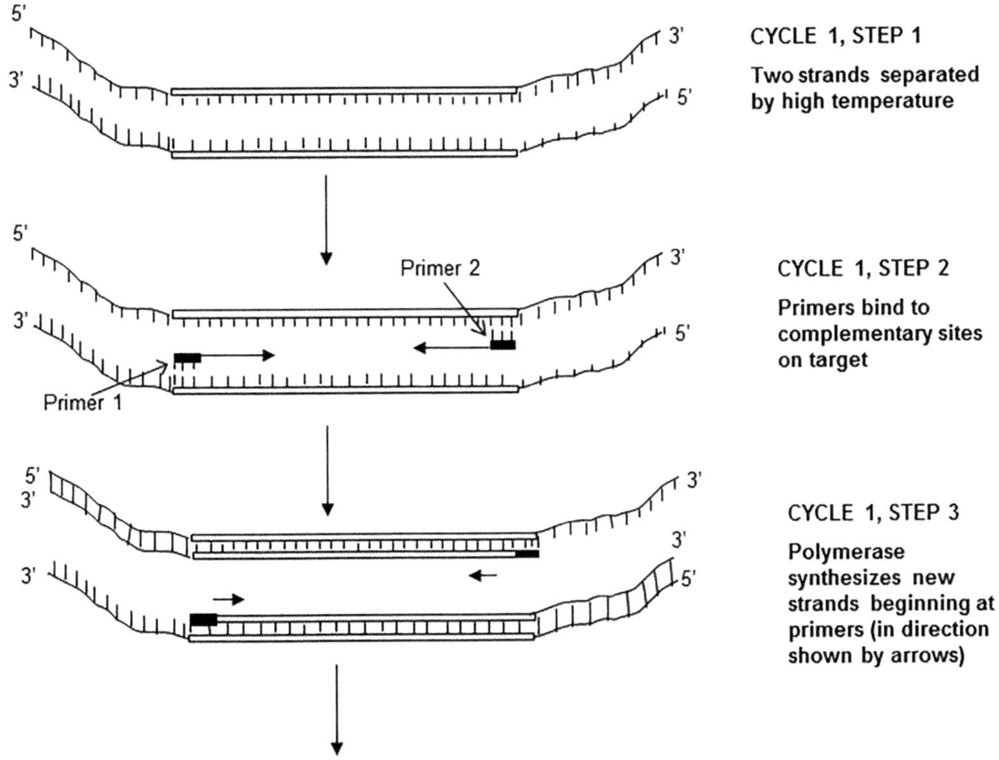


**FIGURE 24.3** One cycle of the polymerase chain reaction. In the first step of PCR, the two strands of the DNA template are separated by high temperature. Next, the temperature is lowered so that the primers complementary to the ends of the target sequence can bind to the template. In the final step of each cycle of PCR, the DNA polymerase enzyme builds new double-stranded DNA molecules by adding nucleotides complementary to the target sequence, beginning with each primer, and moving only in one direction, as shown by the arrows. This completes one cycle. This three-step process is repeated for 20–40 cycles; assuming 100% efficiency, the number of copies of the target sequence doubles after every cycle.

*The nucleotides are referred to as* **dNTPs** (deoxyribonucleotide triphosphates) to stand for any of the four types.

These three steps constitute one cycle of PCR at the end of which there are two double-stranded DNA molecules where originally there was only 1. Then, the process is repeated, resulting in four DNA molecules, and again to give eight, and so on. Usually the process is continued for 25–40 cycles until millions or even billions of copies of the target sequence have been created. Note that if the target sequence is not present in the DNA template, then the primers do not bind the template and no amplification occurs.

Note that PCR amplifies DNA – not RNA, *However, it is possible to convert RNA into DNA that has the same genetic information using an enzymatic reaction called* **reverse transcription,** sometimes abbreviated RT. *The DNA that is transcribed from RNA is called* **cDNA**. Thus, PCR is used to amplify DNA and also RNA that has been copied into DNA.

## 24.2 CONVENTIONAL, ENDPOINT PCR

In **endpoint PCR,** *the reaction is allowed to go through enough cycles to reach a plateau,* at which time the reactants are depleted and the maximum number of copies of target have been produced. This form of PCR provides a qualitative answer: is a particular target sequence present? In contrast, quantitative PCR (qPCR) provides information about the amount of target DNA initially present in the reaction mixture. qPCR will be introduced in Chapter 25.

In endpoint PCR, the tube containing the reaction mixture is removed from the thermocycler after all the desired cycles have been completed. If the amplification was successful, then there is a product, called the **amplicon,** consisting of millions of copies of the target sequence. The amplicon must then be detected. The conventional method of detection is to analyze a portion of the tube's contents using agarose gel electrophoresis followed by staining with the dye, ethidium bromide. (See Section 23.3 for information about electrophoresis.) Agarose gel electrophoresis separates DNA fragments based on differences in their sizes, with smaller fragments moving farther through the agarose gel than larger fragments. Ethidium bromide allows DNA to be visualized and photographed because it fluoresces when excited with UV light. PCR-amplified DNA is thus detectable as a band on the agarose gel, as in Figure 24.4.

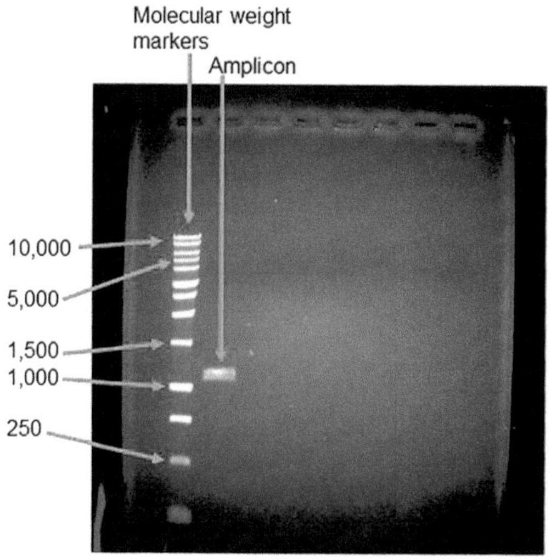


**FIGURE 24.4** Detecting a PCR product. The bright bands on the gel represent DNA fragments. Lane 1 (on the left) contains a MW marker consisting of a number of DNA fragments whose sizes are shown on the far left. The higher the band is on the gel, the larger the fragment. The band observable in lane 2 is a PCR product, the amplicon. In this experiment, the amplicon was expected to be 1,100 base pairs (bp) in size. The amplicon migrated a little less distance in the gel than the 1,000 bp fragment in the MW marker lane, which is consistent with the amplicon being 1,100 bp in size. This is therefore a positive result.

A molecular weight marker that contains DNA fragments of known sizes is run alongside the PCR samples during electrophoresis. The different fragments in the molecular weight marker move different distances through the gel. The size of the expected amplicon is known based on the length of the sequence bracketed by the primers, as was shown in Figure 24.2. If there is a band of DNA visible on the gel in the sample lane, then its mobility through the gel is compared to the mobility of the molecular weight markers. This allows the analyst to estimate the size of the amplicon in the sample. The sample must produce an amplicon of the expected size to be considered a positive result. If a band appears on a gel, but it is not the size expected for the amplicon, then the result is negative.

Endpoint PCR is qualitative. This type of PCR provides a yes or no answer; was the target DNA present in the sample? If the target was present, then a band is present on the gel. If the target was not present in the sample, then no band appears. Qualitative PCR is suitable to answer many important questions and is also a valuable method to produce ample quantities of target DNA to use for various purposes.

## 24.3 PCR IS AN ENZYMATIC REACTION

PCR is an enzymatic reaction and so a tube containing a reaction mixture is prepared for each sample. As with other reaction mixtures, the components of the reaction must each be present at the right concentrations. The primary constituents of the reaction mixture are: template DNA, enzyme, primers (both forward and reverse), and dNTPs, Table 24.1. There is also a buffer to keep the pH constant, and magnesium is a necessary cofactor for polymerase enzymes. The final reaction volume varies but is usually between 25 and 100 µL. Observe in Table 24.1 that there is variation in the exact concentrations of the various components of the mixture. This is because the optimal reaction concentrations depend on the samples to be amplified and the system being used. There are sometimes additional components, such as glycerol, that improve the results in a particular system.

**TABLE 24.1 The Main Components of a PCR Reaction**

| Component | Purpose | Final Amount or Concentration in Reaction Mixture |
|---|---|---|
| *PCR reaction buffer* | Controls the pH | 1X |
| *Magnesium, usually as $MgCl_2$* (may be combined in the reaction buffer) | A required cofactor for the polymerase enzyme | 1.5–2.0 mM |
| *DNA template* | The DNA containing the target that will be amplified | 0.001–1.0 µg (forensic analyses often use as little as 0.5–10 ng of DNA) |
| *Forward primer* | Oligonucleotide that recognizes the target sequence on one strand and initiates replication | 0.05–2 µM |
| *Reverse primer* | Oligonucleotide that recognizes the target sequence on the other strand and initiates replication | 0.05–2 µM |
| *Four dNTPs (dATP, dGTP, dCTP, dTTP)* | The subunits of DNA that are incorporated into the new DNA copies | 200 µM each is typical |
| *Thermostable DNA polymerase* | Enzyme that adds nucleotides to the new DNA strands | Between 0.01 units/µL and 0.05 units/µL (0.025 units/µL is common) |

## 24.4 SETTING UP A PCR AMPLIFICATION: OVERVIEW

Let us consider the simplest PCR situation. You have a PCR protocol that you are following, and you have stock solutions for all the components required by that protocol. Given that you have a protocol and stocks, this section shows a general procedure for preparing your reaction mixtures for your samples. Note that you will likely need to modify this procedure based on variations in the protocol used in your laboratory, but this section should still give you a sense of how PCR is performed. (The procedures in this chapter are based on those in: White, Bruce. *PCR Protocols: Current Methods and Applications (Methods in Molecular Biology).* Humana Press, 1993 and Burden, David, and Donald Whitney. *Biotechnology Proteins to PCR: A Course in Strategies and Lab Techniques*. Birkhäuser, 1995).

**Step 1. Determine Components of a Master Mix.**

Rather than adding each reaction component individually, one sample at a time, a "master mix" is usually prepared that pools the enzyme and other reaction components for all the samples. Once you decide what protocol to follow and how many samples you will be amplifying, you can make a table like Table 24.2a. This table shows each component of the PCR reaction mixture, the concentration of each stock solution, and the amount of each stock that will be added to each reaction mixture tube. The final column is blank and is filled in when you know how many samples you will be amplifying.

Suppose, for example, that you have nine samples (including controls) and so you plan to run nine reactions. This means you will have nine tubes, one for each sample, and each tube will contain all the necessary PCR components (template, dNTPs, etc.). It is good practice to make up some extra reaction mix to avoid being a little short at the end, so prepare enough reaction mixture for ten samples. Table 24.2b shows the last column of the table filled in for ten samples. For example, each tube requires 8 μL of dNTPs, you will be preparing enough mix for ten samples, so you need:

$$10 \text{ samples } (8\ \mu\text{L dNTPs/sample}) = \mathbf{80\ \mu L} \text{ of dNTPs}$$

Observe that the template DNA has been separated out in the table because it is added separately to each tube, one at a time. (Not every tube will have the same template DNA.)

**TABLE 24.2A Preparing Reaction Mixtures, PCR Protocol 1**

| Component | Stock Concentration | Amount to Remove for Each Reaction | Times the Number of Reaction Mixtures Required |
|---|---|---|---|
| *Reaction buffer with $MgCl_2$* | 10X | 10 μL | |
| *dNTPs* | Combined in one stock:<br>2.5 mM dATP<br>2.5 mM dTTP<br>2.5 mM dGTP<br>2.5 mM dCTP | 8 μL dNTP mix | |
| *Forward primer* | 50 pmol/μL | 1 μL | |
| *Reverse primer* | 50 pmol/μL | 1 μL | |
| *Taq DNA polymerase* | 5 units/μL | 0.5 μL | |
| *Water* | | Adjust so reaction volume is 100 μL in each tube (including template DNA) | |
| *Template DNA* | Between $10^5$ and $10^6$ copies in 10 μL buffer | 10 μL | |

**TABLE 24.2B Preparing Reaction Mixtures, PCR Protocol 1 With Amounts for Ten Samples**

| Component | Stock Concentration | Amount to Remove for Each Reaction | Assuming Ten Reaction Mixtures |
|---|---|---|---|
| *Reaction buffer with $MgCl_2$* | 10X | 10 µL | 100 µL |
| *dNTPs* | 2.5 mM each | 8 µL dNTP mixture | 80 µL of mixture |
| *Forward primer* | 50 pmol/µL | 1 µL | 10 µL |
| *Reverse primer* | 50 pmol/µL | 1 µL | 10 µL |
| *Taq DNA polymerase* | 5 units/µL | 0.5 µL | 5 µL |
| *Water* | | 69.5 µL | 695 µL |
| Template DNA | Between $10^5$ and $10^6$ copies in 10 µL buffer | 10 µL | 10 µL each tube |

**Step 2. Prepare the Master Mix**

Prepare a "master mix" that contains the ingredients in Table 24.2b, *except* the enzyme and the DNA template, that is, 100 µL of 10X reaction buffer, 80 µL of dNTP mixture, 10 µL of each primer, and 695 µL of water.

**Step 3. Dispense the Template DNA.**

Dispense 10 µL of template DNA (the samples) to each of 9 PCR tubes. The DNA template is added separately from the master mix to avoid having the reaction begin prematurely. Also, the DNA template will usually vary from tube to tube as different samples and controls are amplified.

**Step 4. Add the Enzyme to the Master Mix.**

Add the enzyme, in this case 5 µL, to the master mix, gently mix, and centrifuge to collect all the fluid.

**Step 5. Combine the Master Mix and the Template in Each Tube.**

Dispense 90 µL of the master mix to each of the nine PCR tubes, cap, mix gently, and spin briefly in a microcentrifuge. (Use a fresh tip to add master mix to each sample to avoid any possibility of contaminating one sample DNA with another.) All the components of the reaction are now together in each tube.

**Step 6. Place the Samples in the Thermocycler and Run the Amplification.**

The reaction mixtures are now amplified following the directions for your own thermocycler and using the times and temperature conditions given in your own protocol.

## 24.5 REACTION BUFFER

We have now looked at the overall procedure for PCR, assuming you have all the stock solutions you need for your protocol. In many cases you will have everything you need, and you will not have to perform many calculations to do PCR. Sometimes, however, you may need to prepare the stock solutions yourself and you may want to optimize the concentrations of various reaction components. If so, then you will need to understand the calculations that relate to each of the PCR reaction mixture components. The next sections of this chapter therefore discuss one by one the main components of the PCR reaction and the calculations associated with each.

PCR reaction buffer maintains the pH of the reaction mixture. It also often contains the magnesium that is required as a cofactor for the polymerase enzyme. (Magnesium is sometimes added separately from the reaction buffer.) The reaction buffer is usually made and stored as a 10X concentrated stock and then usually is diluted to 1X in the final reaction mixture. Typical components of the 10X and 1X buffer are:

| 10X Buffer | 1X Buffer |
|---|---|
| 100 mM Tris, pH 8.3 at 25°C | 10 mM Tris, pH 8.3 at 25°C |
| 500 mM KCl | 50 mM KCl |
| *15–20 mM $MgCl_2$ | *1.5–2.0 mM $MgCl_2$ |

* The ideal concentration of $MgCl_2$ varies depending on the system and is usually determined empirically (by trial and error). Too little $Mg^{2+}$ leads to low yields (or no yield) and too much $Mg^{2+}$ leads to nonspecific products (amplification of sequences that are not the target sequence). The $MgCl_2$ may be added separately from the buffer, particularly during experiments to optimize its concentration.

**Example Problem:**

You have prepared the following stock solutions (see Chapters 12 and 13 for more information about reagent preparation). How would you use these stock solutions to prepare 1,000 µL of 10X PCR reaction buffer?

| Stock Solutions | 10X PCR Buffer |
|---|---|
| 1 M Tris, pH 8.3 | 100 mM Tris, pH 8.3 |
| 1 M KCl | 500 mM KCl |
| 1 M $MgCl_2$ | 15 mM $MgCl_2$ |
| | Water to get 1,000 µL |

***Answer:***

This is a situation where you are going from a concentrated stock solution to a more dilute solution, and so the $C_1V_1 = C_2V_2$ equation applies. Use the equation three times, once for each component. (Note that 1 M = 1,000 mM.)

| | $C_1$ $V_1$ | | $C_2$ $V_2$ | |
|---|---|---|---|---|
| For Tris: | (1,000 mM) (?) | = | (100 mM) (1,000 µL) | ? = 100 µL |
| For KCl: | (1,000 mM) (?) | = | (500 mM) (1,000 µL) | ? = 500 µL |
| For $MgCl_2$: | (1,000 mM) (?) | = | (15 mM) (1,000 µL) | ? = 15 µL |

| | 10X PCR Buffer | |
|---|---|---|
| **Component** | **Volume** | **Concentration** |
| 1 M Tris, pH 8.3 | **100 µL** | 100 mM |
| 1 M KCl | **500 µL** | 500 mM |
| 1 M $MgCl_2$ | **15 µL** | 15 mM |
| Water | **385 µL** | |

The 10X buffer is a stock solution that is prepared and stored until needed. When it is time to run a reaction, the 10X stock is usually added to the reaction mixture in such a way that its final concentration is 1X.

**Example Problem:**

Suppose a final PCR reaction mixture volume will be 50 µL. How much 10X PCR reaction buffer should be added to the reaction mixture?

***Answer:***

This is a situation where you are going from a concentrated stock solution to a less concentrated solution, so the $C_1V_1 = C_2V_2$ equation applies.

$$C_1 \quad V_1 = C_2 \quad V_2$$

$$(10X)(?) = (1X)(50\ \mu L) \qquad ? = 5\ \mu L$$

So for a 50 µL reaction mixture, 5 µL of 10X buffer is used.

## 24.6 PRIMERS

Primers are single-stranded oligonucleotides, usually 15 to 28 bases (b) long (17 b is typical) whose sequences are complementary to the target DNA. Primers are required because the DNA polymerase enzymes synthesize new DNA strands beginning where primers are annealed to the template. The optimal concentration of primers varies; too much primer can result in amplification of sequences that are not the target, too little may result in an incomplete amplification. As shown in Table 24.1, the range of primer concentrations is generally from 0.05 to 2 µM.

Let us assume that you have primers that were synthesized by a commercial manufacturer. You will likely receive the primers lyophilized (freeze-dried) in a vial and you will receive a certificate with information about them. Dried primers must be reconstituted (dissolved) in water or buffer, aliquoted (put in individual tubes for storage), and stored in a freezer. How you reconstitute the primers depends on two things: the protocol you are following and the amount of primer you received in each vial.

As an example, assume you have purchased two primers whose certificate of analysis is shown in Figure 24.5. This certificate provides important information about the primers:

**CLEAN GENE PRIMER CERTIFICATE**

| Oligo Name | Oligo # | Length | MW | Tm | µg/OD | OD | µg | nmol | Sequence |
|---|---|---|---|---|---|---|---|---|---|
| forward | 23290 | 19 | 5716.7 | 61.2 | 31.8 | 12.9 | 410 | 72.0 | GCTCCTA CAAATGCC ATCA |
| reverse | 23291 | 20 | 6227.9 | 63.5 | 31.0 | 11.0 | 341 | 54.9 | GATAGTG GGATTGT GCGTCA |

**FIGURE 24.5** A certificate of analysis that accompanied two primers made by a commercial laboratory. The information in the certificate is described in the text.

- *The sequences of the primers are shown on the right.*
- *The molecular weight (MW) of each primer is shown.* This can also be calculated based on the sequence, as shown in Section 22.10.
- *The melting temperature of the primers, $T_m$, is shown.* Heat disrupts the hydrogen bonds holding together double-stranded nucleic acids. $T_m$ is the temperature at which half of the base pairs in a double-stranded nucleic acid have come apart to form single strands. In PCR, it is important to know the $T_m$ for the primers annealing to the template. If the temperature for the annealing step is too high, then the primers will not bind the template effectively. Conversely, if the temperature is too low, then the primers may bind non-selectively to DNA that is not their target.
- *Two columns relate to using spectrophotometry to quantify the amount of primer in each vial.* "µg/OD unit" is comparable to the estimates in Section 22.12. In that section, we said that an absorbance (absorbance is the same as OD) of 1 (at 260 nm) corresponds to 33 µg/mL of oligonucleotides. The value of 31.8 µg/OD is a comparable value but is more accurate because it is based on the actual sequence of the oligonucleotide. The µg/OD unit value is slightly different for the two primers because they have different sequences. The OD in the next column is the value that the manufacturer obtained when they tested a sample of the primer with a spectrophotometer. If you multiply the value in the column "µg/OD" times the OD reading, you get approximately the value in the next column, that is, the number of µg in your vial. The amount of primer DNA in the vial is important information.
- *The column labeled "nmol" lists how much of each primer you have in units of nmol.* You could calculate this value, based on the µg amount, and we will show this in a practice problem below. It is convenient that the manufacturer did this calculation for you.

To calculate how to prepare stock solutions of the primers, look at whatever protocol you will be following to do the PCR reaction. In PCR protocol 1, shown in Table 24.2, for example, the primers are each reconstituted to a stock concentration of 50 pmol/µL, and 1 µL of each primer stock is added to the reaction mixture when it is time to do a reaction. In PCR protocol 2, shown below in Table 24.3, the stock concentrations and the amounts of the primers are *not* specified. It is necessary for each user to decide how to make their own stock solutions and then to calculate how much of each primer stock should be added to get a final concentration between 0.1 and 1.0 µM. In the latter protocol, water is added as needed to bring the total volume to 50 µL; if more volume of primer is added, then less volume of water is needed and *vice versa*.

The two example problems below deal with primer calculations for the PCR protocols found in Tables 24.2 and 24.3.

**TABLE 24.3 PCR Protocol 2**

| Component | Amount to Add to Reaction Mixture | Final Concentration |
|---|---|---|
| *5X Reaction buffer with $MgCl_2$* | 10 µL | 1X |
| *dNTP Mix (10 mM each)* | 1 µL | 0.2 mM each dNTP |
| *Forward primer* | X µL | 0.1–1.0 µM |
| *Reverse primer* | Y µL | 0.1–1.0 µM |
| *Taq DNA polymerase (5 U/µL)* | 0.25 µL | 0.025 U/µL |
| *Template DNA* | Z µL | <0.5 µg/50 µL |
| *Water* | As needed to get 50 µL | |

**Example Problem:**

**This problem deals with calculating how to dissolve your primer when the stock concentration is to be 50 pmol/μL (as in PCR PROTOCOL 1, Table 24.2).**

Suppose that you have a vial from the manufacturer with 72 nmol of the first primer (as shown in the certificate of analysis in Figure 24.5). How could you prepare your lyophilized primer so as to have a concentration of 50 pmol primer/μL?

*Answer:*

You want to reconstitute the 72 nmol of primer in such a way that you have a stock solution with a concentration of 50 pmol primer/μL.

Begin by converting nmol to pmol:

$$72\text{ nmol} = 72{,}000\text{ pmol}$$

Next you can use a proportion: if you need a concentration of 50 pmol/1 μL, then how many μL are needed for your 72,000 pmol?

$$\frac{50\text{ pmol}}{1\,\mu\text{L}} = \frac{72{,}000\text{ pmol}}{?} \qquad \mathbf{? = 1{,}440\,\mu L}$$

So, you would reconstitute this primer in 1,440 μL of water or buffer. (The volume of the lyophilized primer is assumed to be insignificant.) When it is time to do a PCR reaction you would use 1 μL of this stock solution.

(There are 54.9 nmol of the second primer in this primer pair, Figure 24.5, so this vial of primer is dissolved in 1098 μL of buffer to get a stock concentration of 50 pmol/μL.)

**Example Problem:**

**This problem deals with calculating how to dissolve your primer when the final concentration is to be 0.1–1 μM (as in PCR PROTOCOL 2, Table 24.3).**

The PCR protocol in Table 24.3 does not specify the stock concentration for the two primers, so you must decide what concentration to make the stock solutions. It is convenient to express the stock concentrations in units of μM since the final concentration is specified to be between 0.1 and 1 μM. Suppose, for example, you choose 20 μM. (In some of their literature, Sigma Corporation recommends storing the primers they synthesize at a concentration of at least 20 μM because the primers are less stable when stored at lower concentrations.)

a. How would you dissolve 72 nmol of primer to get a 20 μM stock?
b. When it is time to do a PCR reaction, how much of each primer stock solution will you need for each reaction if you want a concentration of 1 μM?

*Answer:*

a. Begin by converting 72 nmol to μmol:

$$72\text{ nmol} = 0.072\,\mu\text{mol}$$

By definition, a 20 μM solution is 20 μmol in 1 L. (1 L = $10^6$ μL) Using proportions:

$$\frac{20\,\mu\text{mol}}{10^6\,\mu\text{L}} = \frac{0.072\,\mu\text{mol}}{?} \qquad \mathbf{? = 3{,}600\,\mu L}$$

So, if the dried primer is dissolved in 3,600 μL of water or buffer, you will have a 20 μM stock solution.

(There are 54.9 nmol of the second primer in this primer pair, Figure 24.5, so this vial of primer is dissolved in 2,745 μL of buffer to get a stock concentration of 20 μmol.)

b. When it is time to do a PCR reaction, how much of each primer stock solution will you need for each reaction if you want a concentration of 1 μM? (From Table 24.3, the final volume is 50 μL.) This again is a situation where you go from a concentrated to a dilute solution:

$$C_1 \quad V_1 = C_2 \quad V_2$$

$$(20\,\mu\text{M})\,(?) = (1\,\mu\text{M})\,(50\,\mu\text{L})$$

$$\mathbf{? = 2.5\,\mu L}$$

So you would add 2.5 μL of each primer to each reaction mixture.

## Practice Problems

1. ***For the first primer in Figure 24.5, show that 411.3 μg ≈ 72.0 nmol.***

2. ***For the second primer in Figure 24.5, show that 342.0 μg ≈ 54.9 nmol***

3. ***The primer stock concentrations in PCR protocol 1 are 50 pmol/μL. 1 μL of each primer stock is added in a 100 μL total reaction volume. What is the concentration of each primer in the reaction mixture in units of μM? Does this value fall in the range of primer concentrations in Table 24.1?***

## *Answers*

1. To convert a microgram amount to units of nmol, we need the MW of the primer. This is shown on the certificate in Figure 24.5; it is 5,716.7. It is also possible to calculate the MW based on the sequence of the primer, as was shown in Practice Problem 1, Section 22.10.

   A MW of 5716.7 means that 1 mole of this oligonucleotide weighs 5716.7 g
   1 nmol weighs $5716.7 \times 10^{-9}$ g = 5.7167 μg
   If 1 nmol is 5.7167 μg, then how many nmol is 411.3 μg?

$$\frac{1\,\text{nmol}}{5.7167\,\mu\text{g}} = \frac{?}{411.3\,\mu\text{g}} \qquad \mathbf{? \approx 72.0\ nmol}$$

   Alternatively, using the unit canceling strategy:

$$\left(\frac{411.3\,\cancel{\mu\text{g}}}{1}\right)\left(\frac{1\,\cancel{\text{mol}}}{5{,}716.7\,\cancel{\text{g}}}\right)\left(\frac{1\,\cancel{\text{g}}}{10^6\,\cancel{\mu\text{g}}}\right)\left(\frac{10^9\,\text{nmol}}{1\,\cancel{\text{mol}}}\right) \approx \mathbf{72.0\ nmol}$$

2. The MW of this primer is 6,227.9 as shown on the certificate in Figure 24.5. It is also possible to calculate the MW based on the sequence of the primer, as was shown in Practice Problem 2, Section 22.10.

A MW of 6,227.9 means that 1 mole of this oligonucleotide weighs 6227.9 g
1 nmol weighs $6227.9 \times 10^{-9}$ g = 6.2279 μg
If 1 nmol is 6.2279 μg, then how many nmol is 342.0 μg?

$$\frac{1\text{ nmol}}{6.2279\ \mu\text{g}} = \frac{?}{342.0\ \mu\text{g}} \qquad \mathbf{? \approx 54.9\ nmol}$$

3. By definition, 1 μM = 1 μmol/L
The concentration of each primer is 50 pmol/μL and 1 μL is added to the reaction mixture, so 50 pmol is added.
This 50 pmol is in 100 μL volume

$$\frac{50\text{ pmol}}{100\ \mu\text{L}} = \frac{50\times10^{-6}\ \mu\text{mol}}{100\ \mu\text{L}} = \frac{50\times10^{-6}\ \mu\text{mol}}{100\times10^{-6}\ \text{L}} = \frac{0.5\ \mu\text{mol}}{1\ \text{L}} = \mathbf{0.5\ \mu M}$$

This does fall in the range from Table 24.1.

## 24.7 NUCLEOTIDES

There are four dNTPs in each reaction mixture: dATP, dCTP, dGTP, and dTTP. The concentrations are always given for each dNTP. This means that a "2.5 mM dNTP mix" has 2.5 mM of each of the four nucleotides adding up to 10 mM total dNTPs. You can buy commercial preparations that combine all four dNTPs, or you can purchase them separately and make your own mixture.

Individual dNTPs are usually sold at a concentration of 100 mM. For PCR, they are usually combined into a stock solution so that the concentration of each is between 2.5 mM and 10 mM in the mixture. This combined stock solution is then aliquoted and stored until needed for a reaction. How is the combined solution prepared? Let us assume you want to make 20 μL of combined dNTPs, each at a concentration of 10 mM. Use the $C_1V_1 = C_2V_2$ equation:

$$\begin{array}{cccc} C_1 & V_1 = & C_2 & V_2 \\ (100\text{ mM}) & (?) = & (10\text{ mM}) & (20\ \mu\text{L}) \end{array} \qquad \mathbf{? = 2\ \mu L}$$

So, mix the following components:

| Purchased Component | Amount | Concentration in Stock |
|---|---|---|
| 100 mM dATP | 2 μL | 10 mM |
| 100 mM dGTP | 2 μL | 10 mM |
| 100 mM dCTP | 2 μL | 10 mM |
| 100 mM dTTP | 2 μL | 10 mM |
| Water | 12 μL | |
| | 20 μL | |

When it is time to run a PCR reaction, how much of the stored dNTP mixture will you need? Suppose your reaction volume will be 50 μL and you want the final concentration of each dNTP to be 200 μM. This is also a $C_1V_1 = C_2V_2$ problem. (Before plugging values into the equation, make sure the units of molarity match. 10 mM = 10,000 μM.)

$$C_1 \quad V_1 = C_2 \quad V_2$$

$$(10{,}000\,\mu M)(?) = (200\,\mu M)(50\,\mu L)$$

$$? = \mathbf{1\,\mu L}$$

## 24.8 ENZYME

*Taq* DNA polymerase is the polymerase enzyme most commonly associated with PCR, although there are other enzymes that are also used. Whatever polymerase enzyme is used, it must be stable at higher temperatures; otherwise, it would be destroyed every time the temperature was raised to separate the two DNA strands. If the enzyme were destroyed at every cycle it would need to be added over and over again, and the PCR method would not be nearly as valuable as it is.

Most often, *Taq* DNA polymerase is used at a concentration of 0.025 Units/μL. Too much enzyme can be detrimental to the reaction but if there is too little enzyme then less product may be made. Suppose your reaction volume is 50 μL and you have *Taq* DNA polymerase stock at a concentration of 5 U/μL. (Remember not to confuse the abbreviation for units, U, with the abbreviation for micro, μ.) You want 0.025 U/μL in your reaction mixture.

Use the $C_1V_1 = C_2V_2$ equation to calculate how much stock to add to a 50 μL reaction mixture:

$$C_1 \quad V_1 = C_2 \quad V_2$$

$$(5\,U/\mu L)(?) = (0.025\,U/\mu L)(50\,\mu L)$$

$$? = \mathbf{0.25\,\mu L}$$

It would be difficult to accurately add such a small volume, 0.25 μL, to each reaction tube. As you saw above, however, a "master mix" is usually prepared that pools the enzyme and other reaction components for all the samples. If a master mix is not prepared, then the enzyme stock will need to be diluted so that a volume greater than 0.25 μL is added to each reaction mixture.

**Practice Problem**

***What is the final concentration of the* Taq *DNA polymerase in PCR protocol 1, Table 24.2, and in PCR protocol 2, Table 24.3? Do they match each other, and do they match the final concentration in Table 24.1?***

***Answer***

Protocol 1: Add 0.5 μL of enzyme stock that is at a concentration of 5 U/μL. This gives 2.5 units in a reaction mixture that is 100 μL. So, there are 2.5 U/100 μL = **0.025 U/μL.**

Protocol 2: Add 0.25 μL of enzyme stock that is at a concentration of 5 U/μL. This gives 1.25 units in a 50 μL reaction mixture. So, there are 1.25 U/50 μL = **0.025 U/μL.**

Thus, the concentrations are the same in both protocols and they match the most common concentration as shown in Table 24.1.

## 24.9 TEMPLATE

The template for PCR can vary greatly. It might be DNA or RNA, plasmid, viral, or genomic DNA. It might be available in substantial quantities or it might be present in extremely low amounts, as in forensic samples and analyses of ancient samples. Depending on the situation, the target sequence might be a large proportion of the DNA added to the mixture or an extremely low proportion. For example, the template DNA might be a 4 Kb plasmid and the target site might be a sequence in that plasmid that is 1 Kb. In this situation, 25% of the input DNA is the target of interest. Conversely, a 1 Kb target sequence in the human genome ($3.2 \times 10^9$ bp) represents merely about 0.00003% of the DNA. About 800,000 times more human genomic DNA is needed to have the same amount of target DNA as in the plasmid example. It is thus easy to add too much DNA when working with plasmids and too little when working with genomic DNA. Reactions with too much DNA suffer from nonspecific amplification of nontarget regions while reactions with too little template may produce too little product.

Because the template for PCR can vary greatly, there is no standard concentration for the stock DNA template solution nor a specified amount of DNA that is usually added. Rather, there are guidelines that analysts usually follow:

- *The template volume should not be more than 1/10 the reaction volume (i.e., no more than 5 µL for a 50 µL reaction).*
- *Typically not more than 500 ng of human genomic DNA is added to a reaction.*
- *1–10 ng is usual for bacterial DNA.*
- *0.1–1 ng is typical for plasmid DNA.*
- *For forensic applications, as little as 0.5–10 ng of human DNA may be used. There are commercial kits and special protocols to optimize the amplification of these very low levels of human DNA.*

Observe in the guidelines above that the amount of template DNA is expressed in terms of nanograms. But the amount of DNA present in PCR is not always expressed in nanograms. It might be expressed in various other units, particularly "copies." For example, PCR protocol 1 (Table 24.2) specifies the number of copies of target to add: $10^5$–$10^6$ copies in 10 µL of buffer. It is therefore sometimes necessary to convert between copy number and a unit of weight. Chapter 22 introduced the ideas relating to this type of calculation; let us consider how they apply to PCR.

To figure out how many copies of a target gene sequence you have, you need to know how many molecules of template you have and also how many times a given target occurs in the template. Some human target sequences are only present once in the genome, Figure 24.6. Others are present more than once. For simplicity, in our calculations, we will assume that the target of interest is a single-copy gene.

Recall from Chapter 22 that it is possible to use conversion factors to convert between the length of DNA (in units of base pairs) and MW for DNA or RNA. A single nucleotide of DNA has a MW of, on average, 330 g/mole. Therefore, a single base pair (bp) has a MW of about 660 g/mole. (The conversion factor for a single nucleotide of RNA is slightly different and, on average, is about 339.5 g/mole.) With these conversion factors, it is possible to calculate the MW of the human genome, which is about $3 \times 10^9$ bp in length. The MW of the human genome is estimated to be:

$$\text{MW} = \frac{3 \times 10^9 \cancel{\text{bp}}}{1}\left(\frac{660\text{ g}}{1\text{ mol}\cancel{\text{ of bp}}}\right) = 1.98 \times 10^{12}\text{ g/mole}$$

Recall that 1 mole contains Avogadro's number of molecules. Avogadro's number is $6.0221 \times 10^{23}$. One mole of human DNA contains $6.0221 \times 10^{23}$ copies of the human genome, each one of which contains 1 copy of a single-copy gene of interest. We therefore determine the weight of DNA that contains one copy of our gene of interest by dividing the weight of 1 mol of the genome by Avogadro's number:

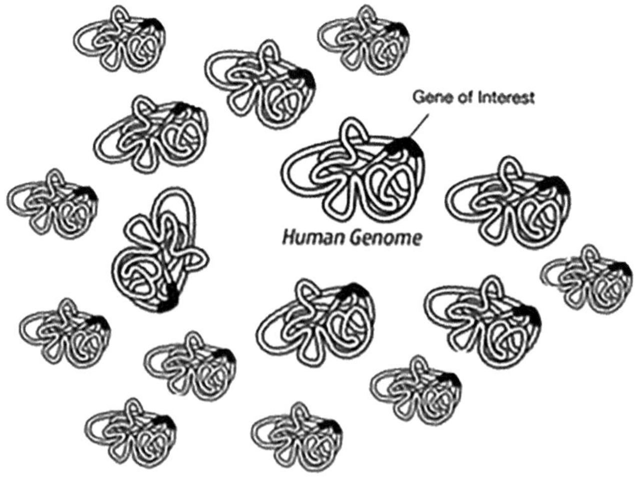


**FIGURE 24.6** A single-copy gene of interest is present one time in each copy of the human genome. Even though a picogram or nanogram is a very small weight, a picogram or nanogram of human DNA will contain many copies of the human genome, each of which will contain one copy of a single-copy gene of interest.

$$\left(\frac{1.98 \times 10^{12}\ \text{g}}{1\ \cancel{\text{mol}}}\right)\left(\frac{1\ \cancel{\text{mol}}}{6.0221 \times 10^{23}\ \text{molecules}}\right) \approx 3.3 \times 10^{-12}\ \text{g/molecule}$$

Thus the weight of DNA that contains one copy (molecule) of our gene of interest is about $3.3 \times 10^{-12}$ g or 0.0033 ng or 3.3 pg.

Suppose we have 100 ng of human DNA. How many copies of the gene of interest are contained in this amount of DNA? This can be solved by proportions:

$$\frac{1\ \text{copy}}{0.0033\ \text{ng}} = \frac{?}{100\ \text{ng}}$$

$$? \approx 3.03 \times 10^4\ \text{copies}$$

Here are some handy conversions you can use that are based on the logic we just demonstrated. These conversions assume that 1 molecule contains 1 copy of the target sequence of interest. (*From: Promega Protocols and Applications Guide.* Promega Corporation. Revision March 2011.)

- 1 µg of 1 Kb RNA $\approx 1.77 \times 10^{12}$ molecules
- 1 µg of 1 Kb dsDNA $\approx 9.12 \times 10^{11}$ molecules
- 1 µg of lambda DNA $\approx 1.9 \times 10^{10}$ molecules
- 1 µg of *E. coli* genomic DNA $\approx 2 \times 10^{8}$ molecules
- 1 µg of human genomic DNA $\approx 3.04 \times 10^{5}$ molecules

**Practice Problems**

1. ***RNase P is a gene found in all eukaryotic cells. This gene codes for a protein that cuts RNA as part of normal RNA processing in the cell. If human DNA is being tested, it is common for PCR kits to use RNase P as a positive control. When RNase P is used as a positive control, the reaction mixture includes primers that recognize this gene. Since human DNA always contains the gene***

***for RNase P, PCR should always provide an RNase P amplicon if everything works properly. If the RNase P control does not produce an amplicon, it might indicate that nucleic acids were not properly extracted from the samples or were degraded. It might also mean that the reaction was not set up properly. In any event, absence of an RNase P amplicon means the amplification did not work properly and any results are invalid.***

***Suppose that you want to prepare standards that contain specific numbers of copies of the RNase P gene. You purchase human DNA stock solution at a concentration of 100 ng/μL. How many microliters of this RNase P stock do you need to get 100,000 copies of the RNase P gene?***

2. ***Show that 1 μg of lambda DNA contains about $1.9 \times 10^{10}$ molecules. The length of a single lambda DNA molecule is 48,502 bp.***

3. ***Show that 1 μg of* E. coli *genomic DNA contains about $2 \times 10^{8}$ molecules. The genome of* E. coli *is about $4.6 \times 10^{6}$ bp.***

4. ***If you have 500 ng of template human genome DNA, how many copies of a target gene do you have, assuming it occurs once in the genome?***

5. a. ***The average MW of one RNA nucleotide is 339.5. The genome of the SARS-CoV-2 virus is 29,727 nucleotides in length (https://www.cdc.gov/sars/lab/sequence.html). This virus is the causative agent of the illness, COVID-19. What is the MW of this virus?***
   b. ***How much does one copy (molecule) of this virus weigh?***
   c. ***If you have 100 ng of this virus, how many copies do you have?***

## *Answers*

1. 1 μL of the purchased stock of human DNA contains 100 ng of DNA. 100 ng of human DNA was previously calculated to contain about 30,000 copies of each gene. Therefore, to get 100,000 copies requires:

$$\frac{1\ \mu\text{L}}{30{,}000\ \text{copies}} = \frac{?}{100{,}000\ \text{copies}}$$

$$\mathbf{? \approx 3.33\ \mu L}$$

2. Show that 1 μg of lambda DNA = $1.9 \times 10^{10}$ molecules.
   Recall from the practice problems in Section 22.11 that the MW of λ DNA is:

$$\left(\frac{660\ \text{D}}{1\ \cancel{\text{bp}}}\right)(48{,}502\ \cancel{\text{bp}}) \approx 3.201 \times 10^{7}\text{D}$$

   So, 1 mol ≈ $3.201 \times 10^{7}$ g. One mole contains $6.0221 \times 10^{23}$ molecules.
   How many moles are in 1 μg?

$$\frac{1\ \text{mol}}{3.201 \times 10^{7}\ \text{g}} = \frac{?}{1 \times 10^{-6}\ \text{g}} \qquad ? \approx 3.12 \times 10^{-14}\ \text{mol}$$

   If there are $3.12 \times 10^{-14}$ moles, how many molecules are present?

$$3.12 \times 10^{-14} \cancel{\text{mol}} \left( \frac{6.0221 \times 10^{23} \text{ molecules}}{\cancel{\text{mol}}} \right) \approx \mathbf{1.9 \times 10^{10} \text{ molecules}}$$

3. Show that 1 μg of *E. coli* genomic DNA contains about $2 \times 10^8$ molecules. The genome of *E. coli* is about $4.6 \times 10^6$ bp.

The MW of *E. coli* is:

$$\left( \frac{660 \text{ D}}{1 \cancel{\text{bp}}} \right) \left( 4.6 \times 10^6 \cancel{\text{bp}} \right) \approx 3.036 \times 10^9 \text{ D}$$

So one mole $\approx 3.036 \times 10^9$g and has $6.02214 \times 10^{23}$ molecules.
How many moles are in 1 μg?

$$\frac{1 \text{ mol}}{3.036 \times 10^9 \text{ g}} = \frac{?}{1 \times 10^{-6} \text{ g}} \quad ? \approx 3.294 \times 10^{-16} \text{ mol}$$

Then how many molecules are present in this many moles?

$$3.294 \times 10^{-16} \cancel{\text{mol}} \left( \frac{6.02214 \times 10^{23} \text{ molecules}}{\cancel{\text{mol}}} \right) \approx \mathbf{2 \times 10^8 \text{ molecules}}$$

4. If you have 500 ng of template human genome DNA, how many copies of a target do you have, assuming it occurs once in the genome?

Assuming 1 μg of human genomic DNA has about $3.04 \times 10^5$ molecules, how many molecules are in 500 ng?

$$500 \text{ ng} = 500 \times 10^{-3} \text{ μg} = 0.5 \text{ μg}$$

$$\frac{3.04 \times 10^5 \text{ molecules}}{1 \text{ μg}} = \frac{?}{0.5 \text{ μg}} \quad ? = 1.52 \times 10^5 \text{ molecules}$$

So there are **$1.52 \times 10^5$ copies of the target.**

5. a. MW of this virus is $29{,}727 \times 339.5$ g/mole $\approx$ **$1.01 \times 10^7$ g/mole**
   b. Divide $1.01 \times 10^7$ g/mole by Avogadro's number to determine weight in grams of one molecule (copy) of this virus:

$$\left( \frac{1.01 \times 10^7 \text{ g}}{1 \cancel{\text{mol}}} \right) \left( \frac{1 \cancel{\text{mol}}}{6.0221 \times 10^{23} \text{ molecules}} \right) \approx 1.68 \times 10^{-17} \text{ g/molecule}$$

   $1.68 \times 10^{-17}$ g/molecule = **$1.68 \times 10^{-8}$ ng/molecule**

   c. You can use proportions to calculate the number of copies present in 100 ng:

$$\frac{1 \text{ copy}}{1.6756 \times 10^{-8} \text{ ng}} = \frac{?}{100 \text{ ng}}$$

$$\mathbf{? \approx 6.0 \times 10^9 \text{ copies}}$$

# Quantitative PCR

# 25



## 25.1 WHAT DOES IT MEAN THAT PCR AMPLIFICATION IS EXPONENTIAL?

Chapter 24 introduced the basic principles of PCR and discussed calculations necessary when setting up a reaction mixture. This chapter will explore quantitation with PCR, which leads us into some of the math associated with exponential amplification, the hallmark of PCR.

In PCR, the number of copies of target DNA ideally doubles with each cycle. This means that the relationship between the cycle number and the number of copies of target DNA present is an exponential relationship, like the ones introduced in Chapter 17. In Chapter 17, we saw that the number of bacteria in a culture doubles at regular intervals; here, the number of DNA molecules doubles at each cycle. Assuming that a PCR reaction is perfectly efficient, Equation 25.1 is used to calculate how many copies of the target sequence will be present after a certain number of cycles:

$$N = 2^t (N_0) \qquad (25.1)$$

where:

$N$ is the number of copies of the target sequence after amplification
$t$ is the number of cycles
$N_0$ is the number of copies of the target sequence initially present in the reaction.

Observe that this equation is basically the same as the equation for bacterial growth shown in Chapter 17 because this is the same type of relationship. In Chapter 17, the equation for bacterial growth included a term, "t," for the number of generations that had elapsed. For PCR, the analogous term is still "t," but in PCR "t" is the number of cycles that have occurred.

DOI: 10.1201/9780429282744-30

For bacterial growth, there was a term "$N_0$," the number of bacteria present initially. For PCR, $N_0$ is the number of copies of the target sequence originally present in the sample. Thus, amplification in PCR and bacterial reproduction are mathematically analogous.

As is the case for bacterial growth, exponential DNA amplification cannot continue forever. There is eventually a plateau. The plateau is due to a number of factors influencing the reaction, most obviously the depletion of reactants. It is common for PCR reactions to begin to plateau after about 40 cycles.

Table 25.1 and Figure 25.1 illustrate the PCR relationship between copy number and cycles that have occurred when there are initially 100 copies of target present. Table 25.1 and Figure 25.1 show early cycles, before the reaction approaches the plateau.

**TABLE 25.1 The Relationship between Cycle Number and Copies of Target DNA Present ($N_0 = 100$)**

| Cycle Number | Copies of Target DNA Present |
|---|---|
| 0 | 100 |
| 1 | 200 |
| 2 | 400 |
| 3 | 800 |
| 4 | 1,600 |
| 5 | 3,200 |
| 6 | 6,400 |
| 7 | 12,800 |
| 8 | 25,600 |
| 9 | 51,200 |
| 10 | 102,400 |
| 11 | 204,800 |
| 12 | 409,600 |
| 13 | 819,200 |
| 14 | 1,638,400 |
| 15 | 3,276,800 |
| 16 | 6,553,600 |
| 17 | 13,107,200 |

**Example Problem:**

Twenty copies of a target sequence are present in a forensic sample. PCR is performed for 20 cycles. How many copies of the target sequence are theoretically expected at the end of PCR amplification?

***Answer:***

Apply Equation 25.1.

$$N = 2^t (N_o)$$

$$N = 2^{20}\,(20) \approx \mathbf{2.1 \times 10^7}$$

So, this PCR amplification theoretically results in millions of copies of DNA where originally there were only 20.

Observe in Table 25.1 that from cycle 0 to cycle 1, the number of copies of target DNA copies doubles. Equation 25.1 provides the same information.

$$N = 2^1\,(100) = 200$$

We can also say that the number of copies of target DNA increases "two-fold."

Between cycle 0 and cycle 2 the number of copies increases four-fold:

$$N = 2^2\ (100) = 400$$

Between cycles 0 and 3 the number of copies increases eight-fold:

$$N = 2^3\ (100) = 800$$

By cycle 4, the number of copies has increased 16-fold:

$$N = 2^4\ (100) = 1{,}600$$

Observe that this same pattern repeats over and over. For example, start at cycle 5. Between cycles 5 and 6, the number of copies increases two-fold. Between cycles 5 and 7, the number of copies increases four-fold. Between cycles 5 and 8, the number of copies increases eight-fold and between cycles 5 and 9 the number of copies increases 16-fold. You can start anywhere in Table 25.1 and find the same pattern.

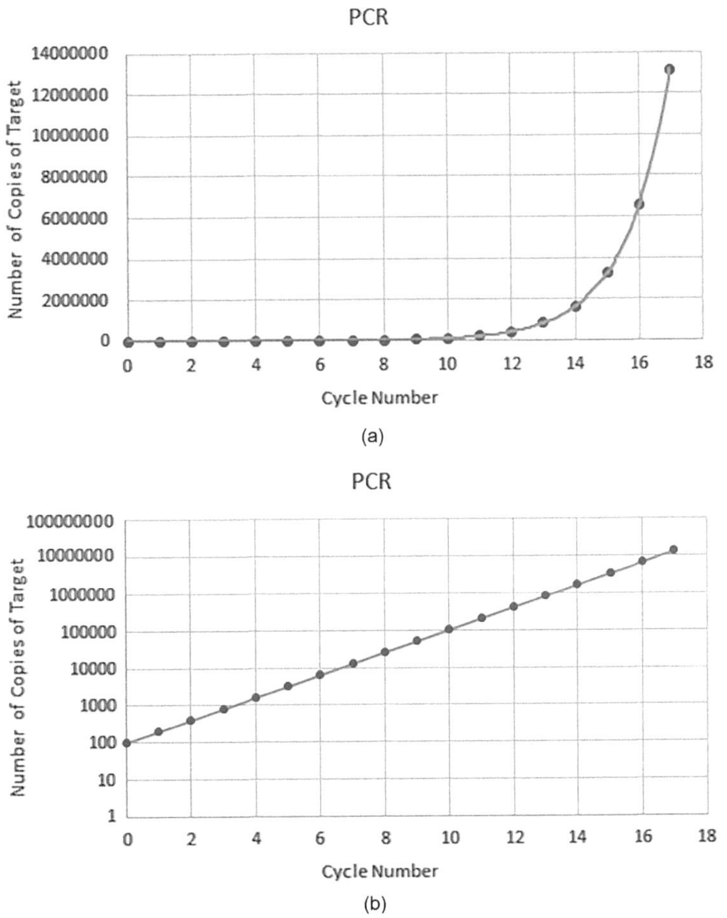


**FIGURE 25.1** The relationship between cycle number and DNA copies is exponential, although there is an eventual plateau. In this example, there were 100 copies of target initially, $N_0 = 100$. (a) The relationship between cycle number and number of copies of target DNA plotted on a linear scale. (b). The same relationship plotted on a semilogarithmic plot. Observe the similarity between these graphs and those of bacterial growth in Figures 17.3 and 17.4.

**Example Problem:**

1. How many fold does the copy number increase between cycles 10 and 11?
2. How many fold does the copy number increase between cycles 10 and 14?
3. How many fold does the copy number increase between cycles 20 and 21?
4. How many fold does the copy number increase between cycles 20 and 23?

***Answer:***

1. There is a two-fold increase between cycles 10 and 11.
2. When four cycles have elapsed, as is the case between cycles 10 and 14, the copy number increases 16-fold.
3. The copy number increases two-fold between cycles 20 and 21.
4. The copy number increases eight-fold between cycles 20 and 23.

How many cycles does it take for the copy number to increase ten-fold? This is not obvious. We know that the copy number takes three cycles to increase eight-fold and four cycles to increase 16-fold. We can reason that a ten-fold increase must require somewhere between three and four cycles. Tools from algebra allow us to calculate the actual number of cycles to obtain a ten-fold increase in copy number. The equation to calculate this is again Equation 25.1. Let us assume that $N_0 = 1$. Then:

$$\mathbf{10 = 2^x(1)}$$

We need to solve for the unknown, which is written here as x. You might recall from an algebra class that solving for an unknown when it is an exponent is performed by taking the log of both sides and rearranging the equation as follows:

$$\mathbf{\log 10 = \log 2^x}$$

$$\mathbf{\log 10 = x \log 2}$$

$$\mathbf{x = \frac{\log 10}{\log 2} \approx \frac{1}{0.30103} \approx 3.322}$$

Confirm on your calculator that 2 raised to the 3.322 power ≈ 10.

What is the significance of this? It takes about 3.322 cycles for the copy number to increase ten-fold in a PCR reaction *only if* the reaction is perfectly efficient. There is perfect efficiency *if* every template molecule replicates every cycle. In reality, PCR efficiency is often not perfect. Efficiency is therefore discussed in the next section.

## 25.2 PCR AND EFFICIENCY

The equation, $\mathbf{N = 2^t(N_0)}$, assumes that the PCR reaction is 100% efficient. But the PCR reaction is only 100% efficient if the reaction conditions are perfectly optimized with respect to the concentrations of reactants, the design of the primers, the absence of any inhibitory substances in the mixture, choice of temperatures, cycle times, and so on. Let us consider what occurs if the reaction is not 100% efficient. Suppose that we begin with 100 copies of the target sequence, $N_0 = 100$. If we plug 100 into Equation 25.1 and we have one cycle of replication, then:

$$N = 2^1(100) = 200$$

Thus, after one cycle, *if* the reaction is 100% efficient, the number of copies will double – 100 new copies will be made – and there will be 200 resulting copies of the target sequence in our test tube. But suppose that the reaction is only 50% efficient. This means that there will be half (50%) as many copies of the target sequence generated during a PCR cycle as we expect. We expect 100 new copies, but with 50% efficiency, only 50 new copies will be made. So, in this situation, after one cycle of replication, there will be 150 copies of the target sequence: the 100 copies with which we began plus 50 new copies.

Suppose that the efficiency is 80% (which is a more realistic figure for PCR efficiency than 50%). In this situation, there will be 80% of the expected copies generated by the reaction. We expect 100 copies to be produced, but with 80% efficiency, only 80 copies will be generated. Thus, after one cycle of replication at 80% efficiency, and with $N_0 = 100$, there will be 180 copies of target present. The Example Problem below further illustrates this concept.

**Example Problem:**

Twenty copies of a target sequence are present in a forensic sample. PCR is performed for 1 cycle.

a. How many copies of the target sequence are expected at the end of this cycle if the reaction is 100% efficient?
b. How many copies of the target sequence are expected at the end of this cycle if the reaction is 80% efficient?
c. How many copies of the target sequence are expected at the end of this cycle if the reaction is 90% efficient?

***Answer:***

a. $N = 2^1\,(20) = \mathbf{40}$
b. We expect 20 new copies to be made, but if the efficiency is 80%, then only $0.8 \times 20$ new copies will be made:

$$20 \times 0.80 = 16$$

So, we begin with 20 copies and get 16 new copies, for a total of **36** copies of target that will be present after one cycle of replication at 80% efficiency.

c. We expect 20 new copies to be made, but if the efficiency is 90%, then only $0.90 \times 20$ new copies will be made:

$$20 \times 0.90 = 18$$

So we begin with 20 copies and get 18 new copies, for a total of **38** copies of target that will be present after one cycle of replication at 90% efficiency.

The efficiency of PCR, abbreviated E, is typically expressed as a number between 0 and 1. If the reaction is perfect, with 100% efficiency, then $E = 1$. If the efficiency is 80%, then $E = 0.80$. Similarly, if $E = 0.90$, then the reaction is 90% efficient, and so on.

When the efficiency is not 100%, Equation 25.1 is no longer correct. Rather, the equation to determine the number of copies of target generated by PCR is Equation 25.2:

$$N = N_0(1+E)^t \qquad (25.2)$$

where:

N is the number of copies of the target sequence after amplification
t is the number of cycles
$N_0$ is the number of copies of the target sequence initially present in the reaction
E is the efficiency expressed as a number between 0 and 1.

To understand Equation 25.2, consider the situation where the efficiency is 100%. In that case, E = 1. The value within the parentheses then becomes 1+1, or 2. Thus, if the efficiency is perfect, then Equation 25.2 is the same as Equation 25.1. But if the efficiency is less than perfect, say, 80%, then E = 0.80 and the value in the parentheses is 1+0.80, or 1.80.

Suppose that we begin with 100 copies of target sequence, the efficiency is 80%, and we go through one cycle of PCR. Then, plugging into Equation 25.2:

$$N = 100\ (1+0.80)^1\ = 100\ (1.80) = 180$$

This is the same situation as described previously, but now we used an equation to find the answer. Consider what happens after ten cycles of PCR if $N_0$ is 100 and the efficiency is 80%:

$$N = 100(1+0.80)^{10} \approx 35{,}705$$

With 80% efficiency, if $N_0$ is 100, then ten cycles of PCR will produce about 35,705 copies of target. In contrast, if the efficiency is perfect, and if $N_0$ is 100, then after 10 cycles:

$$N = 100(2)^{10} = 102{,}400$$

Thus, with perfect efficiency, more than 100,000 copies of target will be produced, which is obviously preferable to the situation when the efficiency is only 80%. This tells us that optimizing the reaction conditions to improve efficiency is very important in PCR.

**Practice Problems**

1. a. ***If the efficiency of the PCR reaction is 87%, what is the value for E expressed as a number between 0 and 1?***
   b. ***If the efficiency of the PCR reaction is 75%, what is the value for E expressed as a number between 0 and 1?***
2. ***If the efficiency of a PCR reaction is 100% and you begin with 500 copies of target, how many copies will be present after three cycles? First, calculate the answer without applying Equation 25.1 or 25.2. Then use either equation to confirm your answer.***
3. ***If the efficiency of a PCR reaction is 100% and you begin with 250 copies of target, how many copies will be present after four cycles? First, calculate the answer without applying Equation 25.1 or 25.2. Then use either equation to confirm your answer.***
4. ***We can also express PCR results using DNA amounts or concentrations rather than copy numbers. If the efficiency of a PCR reaction is 100% and you begin with 1 ng of target, how much target will be present after three cycles? First, calculate the answer without applying Equation 25.1 or 25.2. Then use either equation to confirm your answer.***
5. ***If the efficiency of a PCR reaction is 100% and you begin with 50 pg of target, how much target will be present after three cycles? First, calculate the answer without applying Equation 25.1 or 25.2. Then use either equation to confirm your answer.***

6. ***Suppose that the efficiency of a PCR reaction is 100%, you begin with 5,000 copies of target, and the reaction goes through 22 cycles. How many copies of target do you expect to be produced?***
7. ***Suppose that the efficiency of a PCR reaction is 95%, you begin with 5,000 copies of target, and the reaction goes through 22 cycles. How many copies of target do you expect to be produced?***
8. ***Suppose that the efficiency of a PCR reaction is 80%, you begin with 5,000 copies of target, and the reaction goes through 22 cycles. How many copies of target do you expect to be produced?***

*Answers*

1. a. **0.87** b. **0.75**
2. After the first cycle, there will be 1,000 copies, after the second cycle 2,000 copies, and after the third cycle 4,000 copies.

$$N = 500 \text{ copies } (2)^3 = \mathbf{4{,}000 \text{ copies}}$$

3. After the first cycle, there will be 500 copies, after the second 1,000 copies, after the third 2,000 copies, and after the fourth 4,000 copies.

$$N = 250 \text{ copies } (2)^4 = \mathbf{4{,}000 \text{ copies}}$$

4. After the first cycle, there will be 2 ng, after the second 4 ng, after the third 8 ng.

$$N = 1 \text{ ng } (2)^3 = \mathbf{8 \text{ ng}}$$

5. After the first cycle, there will be 100 pg, after the second 200 pg, after the third 400 pg.

$$N = 50 \text{ pg } (2)^3 = \mathbf{400 \text{ pg}}$$

6. $N = 5{,}000\ (2)^{22} \approx \mathbf{2.1 \times 10^{10}\ copies}$
7. $N = 5{,}000\ (1+0.95)^{22} \approx \mathbf{1.2 \times 10^{10}\ copies}$
8. $N = 5{,}000\ (1+0.80)^{22} \approx \mathbf{2.1 \times 10^{9}\ copies}$

## 25.3 qPCR

In Section 24.2, we saw that in conventional or endpoint PCR, the reaction is allowed to go through enough cycles to reach the plateau region, at which time the reactants are depleted and the maximum number of copies of target have been produced. Electrophoresis and staining the gel are used to detect the resulting amplicon.

Endpoint PCR is qualitative. Qualitative PCR provides a yes or no answer; was the target DNA present in the sample? If the target was present, then a band is present on the gel. If the target was not present in the sample, then no band appears. Qualitative PCR is suitable to answer many important questions and is also a valuable method to produce ample quantities of target DNA to use for various purposes. However, there are times when a quantitative version of PCR is desirable.

**Quantitative PCR (qPCR)** *monitors DNA amplification as it occurs.* qPCR requires a method of making the amplified DNA visible as cycling proceeds. It would be impractical to run an electrophoresis gel after each cycle of PCR, so another means of detecting DNA is required. The solution is to use fluorescent dyes that label the DNA that is produced during the amplification and thereby make the DNA visible to a laboratory instrument. As PCR cycles, more DNA is produced, and more fluorescence is detected. Another name for qPCR is "real-time" PCR because the PCR amplification products are detected in "real time."

qPCR can provide quantitative information that can be important in many situations. For example, in food-related disease outbreaks, qPCR is often used to quickly determine how much (if any) of a specific pathogen is present in food samples suspected to be the cause of the outbreak, Figure 25.2. qPCR is used when scientists are researching the effects of different treatments on gene expression in cells. For example, scientists might be investigating the expression of a particular gene when cells are administered a drug at different doses. In this situation, qPCR can be used to look for the level (if any) of RNA that the cell produces when a particular gene is being expressed. (Recall that it is necessary to convert RNA into cDNA before running a PCR reaction.) Diagnostic PCR is another critically important application of this method. Millions of qPCR analyses have been performed (and thousands more tests are currently being performed daily) to test whether individuals are infected with the virus that causes COVID-19. It is essential to find infected people because they must be isolated from others and treated. Also, people who have been in contact with an infected individual must be quarantined to prevent further spread of the virus. For COVID-19 diagnosis, the value of qPCR is not usually its ability to provide quantitative information, but rather the fact that qPCR instrumentation is automated, the output is recorded directly by a computer, and many samples can be run simultaneously. qPCR is exquisitely sensitive and therefore low levels of viral genetic information can be detected in patient samples that primarily contain human (and bacterial) genetic information. When millions of samples are being analyzed, qualitative endpoint PCR, which is analyzed by running an electrophoresis gel, is impractical.

When PCR is used quantitatively, analysts want to detect how much of the target genetic information is in the samples at the *beginning* of the PCR reaction. In other words, analysts are either looking for the value of $N_0$ (in Equations 25.1 and 25.2) or they are comparing the values of $N_0$ among different samples. Observe that so far in this chapter, we have performed calculations in which we assumed that we knew the value for $N_0$. In reality, $N_0$ is unknown when we work with experimental samples.

Figure 25.3 shows the type of graph that is generated by a qPCR instrument. During qPCR, fluorescence is plotted on the Y-axis. In the early cycles of PCR, the amount of DNA present

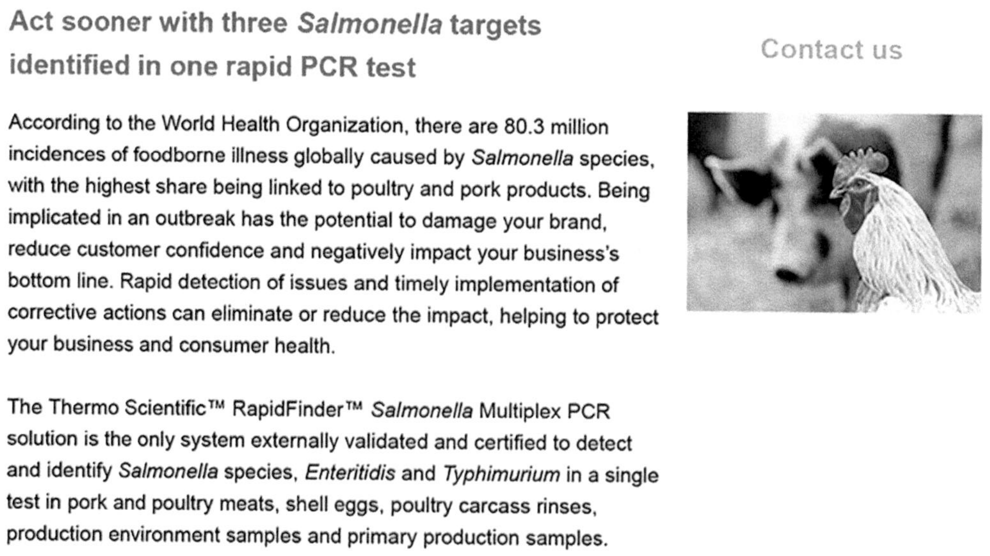


**FIGURE 25.2** Advertisement for a PCR test that rapidly detects the pathogen, ***Salmonella***, in food. There are a number of test kits, like this one, that use PCR to detect various pathogens in foods and also in clinical samples from patients. (Used by permission from Thermo Scientific.)

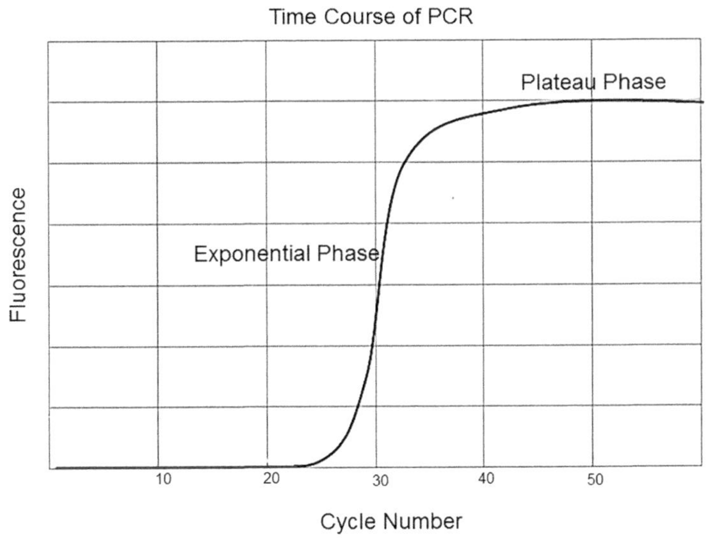


**FIGURE 25.3** The time course of PCR. Initially, the DNA present in the tube is not detectable. After a certain number of cycles enough DNA is present that it becomes visible and the exponential amplification of PCR is evident. Eventually, the reaction mixture is depleted and the system plateaus.

is doubling but its fluorescence is too low to be reliably detected. At a certain point, there is enough DNA present to be distinguished reliably from background fluorescence. After this point, the exponential increase in DNA is evident. However, after a certain number of cycles, all the primers and nucleotides in the reaction mixture are depleted, the DNA polymerase may lose some of its activity, and products may begin to break down. Eventually, there is no more increase in DNA product; this is the plateau region in the graph. When conventional (qualitative) PCR is used, what appears on an electrophoresis gel is the DNA present at the end of the process, in the plateau region. That is why conventional PCR, using gel electrophoresis for detection, is called "endpoint" PCR.

To understand how qPCR is used to obtain quantitative information, consider what happens when two samples are compared. One sample begins with a lot of target DNA ($N_0$ is higher), and the other sample has less. As you can see in Figure 25.4, the sample that begins with more DNA, shown in yellow, reaches a detectable level of fluorescence before the other sample, shown in black. The **threshold cycle ($C_t$)** *is the cycle where the fluorescence crosses a threshold and is bright enough to reliably detect.* The yellow sample has a $C_t$ value of about 19 and the black $C_t$ value is about 28. The more starting DNA that is present in a sample, the lower the $C_t$ value. Thus, ***$C_t$ values** provide a measure of the amount of target DNA initially present in a sample.* In this particular example, we do not know how much DNA was initially present in either tube; we only know that the sample shown in yellow began with more DNA than the sample shown in black. To determine the starting amount of target DNA in the samples in absolute terms, it is necessary to use standards with known amounts of target DNA. The $C_t$ values for the standards are then used to create a standard curve, as will be shown in Section 25.4.

Observe in Figure 25.4 that both the yellow and black samples reach the same endpoint (plateau) at the end of the run, even though the yellow sample began with more target DNA and reached the plateau sooner.

Let us further consider the meaning of the $C_t$ values. We know that if the efficiency is perfect, then the amount of DNA target doubles each cycle. Therefore, if the $C_t$ value goes down one unit, it means there was twice as much, two-fold, more DNA target originally present. For example, for a given plot, if the efficiency is perfect, a $C_t$ value of 19 represents twice as much starting material as a $C_t$ value of 20:

The fold difference in DNA present initially $= 2^{20-19} = 2^1 = 2$

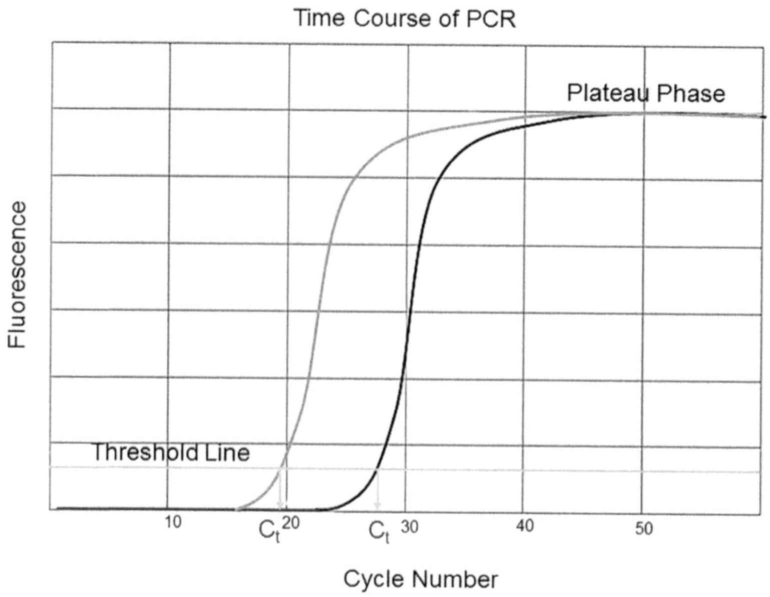


**FIGURE 25.4** qPCR run comparing two samples. Two samples both containing the target DNA of interest are shown. The sample drawn in yellow begins with a higher level of target DNA than the sample shown in black. Both attain the same number of DNA copies at the end of PCR, but the yellow sample does so more quickly. The $C_t$ value is the cycle number where the amount of DNA, and hence the fluorescence, crosses a threshold and can be reliably detected. The $C_t$ value for the yellow sample is lower than for the black sample. Thus, the $C_t$ value provides quantitative information about the amount of target DNA initially present in a sample.

A change of two $C_t$ units represents a four-fold difference in the amount of target DNA initially present:

The fold difference in DNA present initially $= 2^{20-18} = 2^2 = 4$

If the efficiency is perfect, a $C_t$ value of 19 represents eight times as much starting material as a $C_t$ value of 22:

The fold difference in DNA present initially $= 2^{22-19} = 2^3 = 8$

Thus:

A decrease in the $C_t$ value of 1 represents a $2^1$ (two-fold) higher $N_0$
A decrease in $C_t$ value of 2 represents a $2^2$ (four-fold) higher $N_0$
A change in $C_t$ values of 3 represents a $2^3$ (eight-fold) higher $N_0$
and so on.

Suppose the $C_t$ value does not so conveniently change by a whole number. For example, suppose that two samples are being compared, one with a $C_t$ value of 28.5 and the other with a $C_t$ value of 31.2. What does this difference mean in terms of the amount of DNA target that was present initially? To calculate this, we can use this logic:

The fold difference in DNA present initially $= 2^{31.2-28.5} = 2^{2.7} \approx 6.5$

## Practice Problems

1. ***Figure 25.5 shows the results of a qPCR run on a series of standards that began with known amounts of DNA. These samples contained the following concentrations of DNA (not listed in order of concentration):***

***5.0 ng/mL, 50 pg/mL, 50 ng/mL, 0.5 ng/mL, 5 pg/mL***

***Observe that each color is a different standard and there are 5 different $C_t$ values, $C_t1$, $C_t2$, $C_t3$, $C_t4$, and $C_t5$. Match the $C_t$ value with the standard:***
- ***5.0 ng/mL goes with which $C_t$ value?*** ________
- ***50 pg/mL goes with which $C_t$ value?*** ________
- ***50 ng/mL goes with which $C_t$ value?*** ________
- ***0.5 ng/mL goes with which $C_t$ value?*** ________
- ***5 pg/mL goes with which $C_t$ value?*** ________

2. ***qPCR assays for COVID-19 detect RNA from the virus that causes this disease, the SARS-CoV-2 virus. COVID-19 diagnostic assays generally do not report the $C_t$ values for individual patients. However, researchers are interested in determining whether $C_t$ values might provide useful information. Which of the following statements seems likely to be true?***
   a. ***A person with a low $C_t$ value on a COVID-19 test is more likely to be contagious than a person with a high $C_t$ value.***
   b. ***When a person is tested in the early stages of an infection, the $C_t$ value is likely to be low. Once the person is recovering, the $C_t$ value is likely to be high.***
   c. ***If many infected individuals in a community have COVID-19 tests with low $C_t$ values, it is likely that the disease is spreading in the community. Conversely, if many infected individuals have high $C_t$ values, it is likely the outbreak is waning.***
   d. ***Patients with low $C_t$ values are less likely to die of COVID-19 than those with high $C_t$ values.***

   ***(Information for this question was reported in:*** Service, Robert F. "A Call for Diagnostic Tests to Report Viral Load." *Science*, vol. 370, no. 6512, 2020, p. 22. doi:10.1126/science.370.6512.22.)

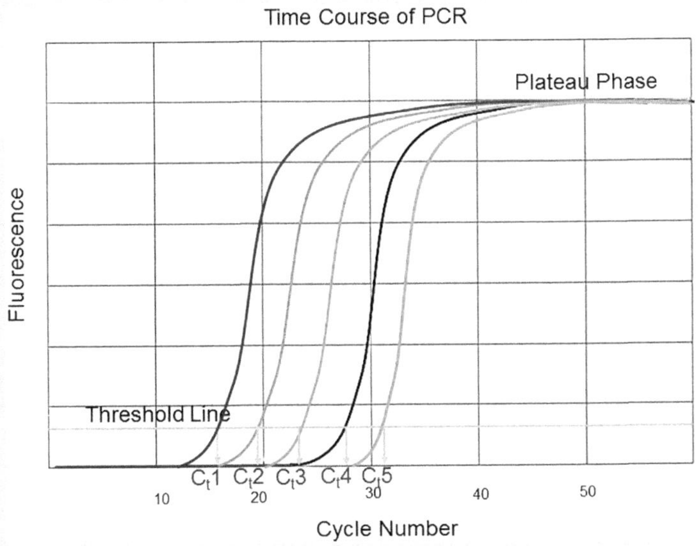


**FIGURE 25.5** qPCR run with five standards.

3. ***(This example is from Bio-Rad's Real-Time PCR Applications Guide, see reference at end of chapter.)***
   ***An experiment is being performed to compare the relative expression of a target gene, p53 in normal and cancerous ovarian cells. (When a gene is "expressed" it is turned on and the protein for which it codes is made. The gene, p53, codes for a protein that plays an important role in controlling cell division and cell death.) The researcher extracts total RNA from 1,000 normal and from 1,000 cancerous ovarian cells. The RNA from both samples is transcribed to cDNA and a qPCR assay for p53 is performed. The $C_t$ value for the normal cells is 15.0 and the $C_t$ value for the cancer cells is 12.0. What is the fold difference in expression between the two samples?***
4. ***The researchers repeat the experiment from problem 3, but this time they use cancer cells from a different patient source. They obtain a $C_t$ value of 15.4 for the normal cells and a $C_t$ value of 11.7 for the cancer cells. What is the fold difference in p53 expression in this experiment?***

*Answers*

1. Putting the standard values in order from lowest to highest:

   5 pg/mL, 50 pg/mL, 0.5 ng/mL, 5.0 ng/mL, 50 ng/mL

   The more original DNA present, the sooner the qPCR graph crosses the threshold and the lower the $C_t$ value. Thus, the standards that go with each $C_t$ value are as follows:

   **5 pg/mL <u>$C_t$ 5</u> 50 pg/mL <u>$C_t$ 4</u> 0.5 ng/mL <u>$C_t$ 3</u> 5.0 ng/mL <u>$C_t$ 2</u> 50 ng/mL <u>$C_t$ 1</u>**

2. a. Likely to be true, a low $C_t$ value indicates that more virus was present in the sample than if the Ct value is high. The more virus present in a person, the more contagious that person is likely to be.
   b. True. Once peoples' immune system mounts a vigorous response to the virus, the virus is eliminated, yielding a higher $C_t$ value.
   c. Likely to be true, if many infected individuals in a community have COVID-19 tests with low $C_t$ values, it is likely that the disease is spreading in the community. Conversely, if many infected individuals have high $C_t$ values, it is likely the outbreak is waning. Epidemiologists are investigating whether this can be useful in stemming outbreaks at the community level. If an outbreak seems to be on the rise, more aggressive contact tracing and quarantines may be helpful.
   d. False. Studies have shown that hospitalized patients with a low $C_t$ value are more likely to die than those with higher $C_t$ values.
3. Assuming that the efficiency was 100%, then the fold difference between the two samples is:

   $$2^{\text{Ct normal}-\text{Ct cancerous}} = 2^{15-12} = 2^3 = \mathbf{8}$$

   The expression of p53 is **eight-fold** higher in the cancer cells than the normal cells.
4. Assuming that the efficiency was 100%, then the fold difference between the two samples is:

   $$2^{\text{Ct normal}-\text{Ct cancerous}} = 2^{15.4-11.7} = 2^{3.7} \approx \mathbf{13.0}$$

   This time the fold difference is close to **13**.

## 25.4 PREPARING A STANDARD CURVE FOR PCR

In Chapter 16, we explored standard curves and how they are used in spectrophotometry. Standard curves are also used in many other types of quantitative analytical work, including qPCR. A standard curve for qPCR allows the analyst to determine how much target DNA was present originally in a sample. As discussed in Chapter 16, preparing a standard curve involves making a series of dilutions of a stock solution of the analyte of interest. In the case of qPCR, preparing the standard curve requires a stock of template DNA with a known concentration or amount of the gene of interest. This DNA stock is then serially diluted, for example, as shown in Figure 25.6. Typically, the standards are prepared in duplicate or triplicate and the results for each dilution are averaged.

The diluted standards are amplified by qPCR, and the results are graphed. The more DNA present in the standard, the sooner the fluorescence crosses the threshold where it can be detected and the lower the $C_t$ value. Thus, for the standards shown in Figure 25.6, the 100 ng/mL stock provides the lowest $C_t$ value, and the 0.01 ng/mL standard has the highest $C_t$ value. The $C_t$ value for each standard is recorded, Table 25.2, and these $C_t$ values are used to plot a standard curve, as shown in Figure 25.7. Observe that it is conventional to plot this standard curve with the *log* of the DNA concentration in the standards on the X-axis and the $C_t$ values on the Y-axis.

The standard curve can be used to estimate the concentration of DNA in unknown samples. qPCR of the unknown samples is performed along with the standards and their $C_t$ values are determined. For example, given the standard curve in Figure 25.7, suppose that the $C_t$ value for a sample is 29. Reading down to the X-axis, we see that this corresponds to a value of about –1.6. But recall that the scale on the X-axis is logarithmic. So, we need to know what concentration corresponds to a log value of –1.6. To calculate this, we need to take the antilog of –1.6; this will be the concentration of DNA in our original sample. The antilog of –1.6 is about 0.025, (e.g., $10^{-1.6} \approx 0.025$). This means that the $N_0$ for this sample is around 0.025 ng/mL of DNA. It is also possible to use the equation for the line shown on the standard

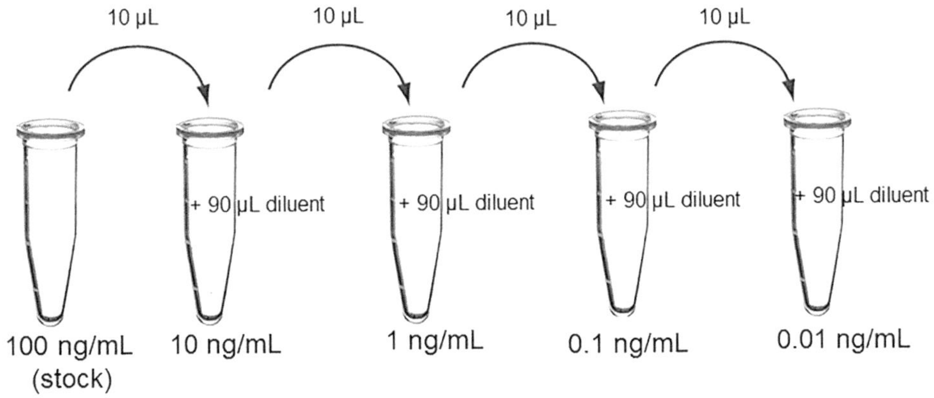


**FIGURE 25.6** A ten-fold dilution series for a quantitative PCR standard curve.

**TABLE 25.2 Example of DNA Standards Used to Prepare a Standard Curve**

| Concentration DNA in Standard (ng/mL) | Log Concentration DNA in Standard | $C_t$ |
|---|---|---|
| 0.01 | –2 | 30 |
| 0.1 | –1 | 27 |
| 1 | 0 | 24 |
| 10 | 1 | 20 |
| 100 | 2 | 17 |

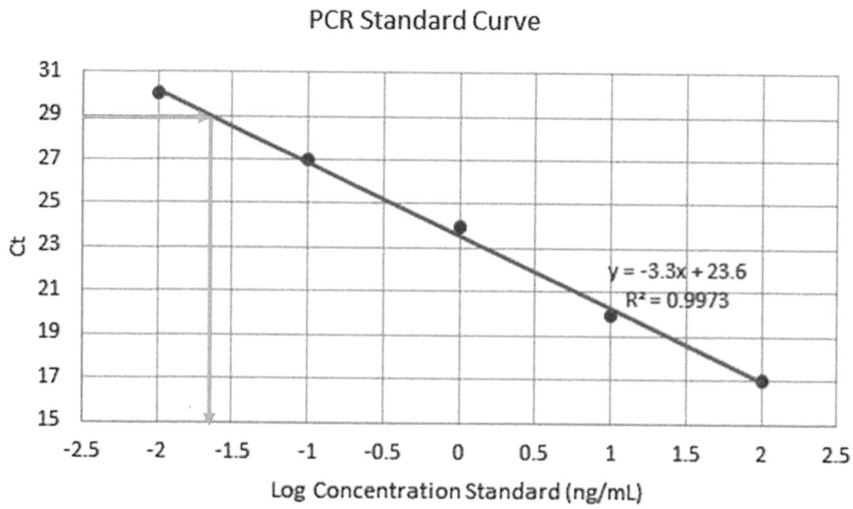


**FIGURE 25.7** A PCR standard curve. The logs of the DNA concentrations in the standards are graphed on the X-axis versus their $C_t$ values on the Y-axis. Using this standard curve, the concentration of DNA in a sample can be determined as described in the text. Observe that an R-squared ($R^2$) value is also shown on this graph. R-squared is a statistical measure of how closely the data fit the line that is shown. $R^2$ can vary between 0 and 1 or between 0% and 100%. The closer $R^2$ is to 1 (or 100%), the better. In our example, the change in $C_t$, that is, the Y-value, is almost entirely explained by changes in the standard concentration, the X-value. Hence, the data fit the line quite well and there is a high value for $R^2$, that is 0.9973. But $R^2$ is not exactly 1, so there is some variation in the Y-values that is explained by other factors. Perhaps there was a small amount of pipetting error or some fluctuation within the assay system.

curve graph to more accurately determine the concentration of DNA that corresponds to a $C_t$ value of 29:

$$29 = -3.3\ (x) + 23.6$$

$$5.4 = -3.3\ (x)$$

$$X \approx -1.636$$

$$\text{Antilog } -1.636 \approx \mathbf{0.023}$$

$$\text{or, } 10^{-1.636} \approx \mathbf{0.023}$$

This means the concentration of DNA in our original sample was about **0.023 ng/mL.**

Note that as is typical of all standard curves, there is only a certain range in which the standard curve is valid. It is not possible to accurately determine the amount of DNA originally in a sample if its $C_t$ value is outside the range of the $C_t$ values on the standard curve. In our example, the lowest $C_t$ value for any standard is 17 and the highest is 30. Therefore, if a sample has a $C_t$ value of 31 or 15, its value is outside the range of the standard curve and its DNA concentration should not be estimated using this standard curve.

## 25.5 USING THE STANDARD CURVE TO DETERMINE EFFICIENCY

A qPCR standard curve can be used to determine the efficiency of the amplification reaction, where efficiency is E, as discussed in Section 25.2 of this chapter. This is done based on the slope of the standard curve. If the slope of the line on the standard curve is about –3.322, the efficiency is 100%.

If you are curious as to why a slope of –3.322 represents perfect efficiency, recall from Section 25.2 that if the efficiency is perfect, it requires 3.322 cycles for the number of DNA copies to increase ten-fold. On a conventional qPCR standard curve graph, the X-axis is the log of the amount (or concentration) of amplified DNA. The X-axis is logarithmic, which means that moving from one major unit to the next on the graph represents a ten-fold increase in amplified DNA. Thus, with perfect efficiency, every 3.322 cycles there is a ten-fold change on the X-axis. The slope is a negative number (–3.322) because the slope goes down as we move from left to right, that is, the greater the amount or concentration of target DNA, the fewer cycles are required to reach detectable fluorescence.

Suppose that the slope of a qPCR standard curve is not –3.322. That means that the efficiency is not exactly 100%. What is the efficiency? To calculate this, we use Equation 25.3:

$$\mathbf{E = \left(10^{-1/slope} - 1\right)} \tag{25.3}$$

**or**

$$\mathbf{E = \left(10^{-1/slope} - 1\right)(100\%)}$$

where:

slope is the slope of a standard curve

E is the efficiency expressed as a number between 0 and 1, or as a percent.

To convince yourself that Equation 25.3 makes sense, try inserting the value –3.322 into it:

$$E = (10^{-1/-3.322} - 1) \approx \left(10^{0.3010} - 1\right) \approx 2 - 1 = 1$$

As expected, if the slope is –3.322, this equation gives an efficiency of 1 or 100%.

For the example in Figure 25.7, Equation 25.3 yields:

$$E = \left(10^{-1/-3.3} - 1\right)(100\%) = \left(10^{0.30303} - 1\right)(100\%) \approx 101\%$$

For qPCR, the efficiency should be close to 100%, generally between 90% and 105%. Low efficiencies may be due to poor primer design or reaction conditions that have not been optimized. An efficiency above 100% may indicate pipetting errors or the presence of nonspecific amplification products. An efficiency of 101% is probably close enough to 100% to assume that the efficiency of the PCR reaction is perfect. Each laboratory's quality control procedures must specify how close the efficiency must be to 100% to be acceptable.

**Practice Problems**

1. ***If the slope of a qPCR standard curve is –3.436, what is the efficiency?***
2. ***If the slope of a qPCR standard curve is –3.361, what is the efficiency?***
3. ***A standard curve is to be prepared. In this example, the number of copies of the target gene of interest in the standards is used. Plot the standard curve with the log of DNA copy number on the X-axis and $C_t$ value on the Y-axis and determine the efficiency of the system.***

| DNA Copy Number | Log DNA Copy Number | $C_t$ |
|---|---|---|
| 10 | | 36 |
| 100 | | 32.1 |
| 1,000 | | 28.9 |
| 10,000 | | 25.2 |
| 100,000 | | 21.8 |
| 1,000,000 | | 18.3 |

***Answers***

1. $E=\left(10^{-1/-3.436}-1\right)(100\%)\approx(1.9545-1)(100\%)\approx\mathbf{95.45\%}$
2. $E=\left(10^{-1/-3.361}-1\right)(100\%)\approx(1.9839-1)(100\%)\approx\mathbf{98.39\%}$
3. Figure 25.8 shows the standard curve.

$$\text{Efficiency} = E=(10^{-1/-3.5171}-1)\approx\left(10^{0.2843}-1\right)\approx 1.9245-1=\mathbf{0.9245\ or\ 92.45\%}$$

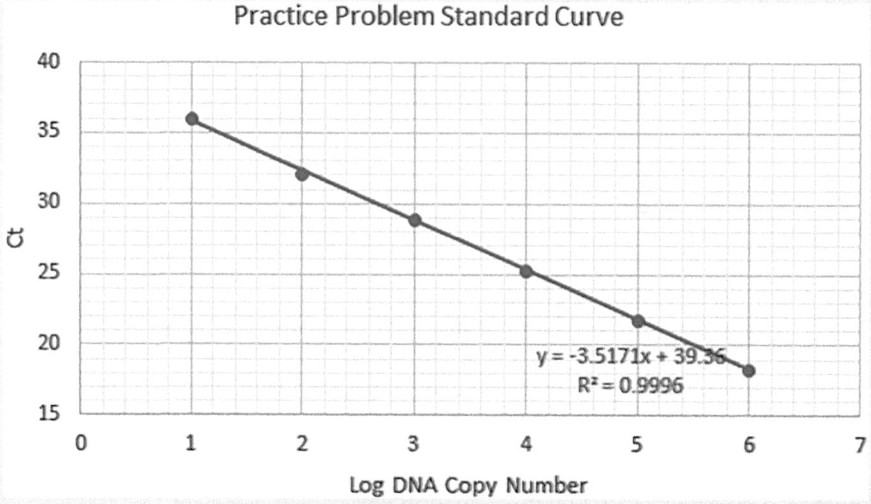


**FIGURE 25.8** Standard curve for Practice Problem.

## 25.6 FINDING THE MATH: CASE STUDY, GNOMEGEN COVID-19 qPCR DETECTION KIT

### 25.6.1 BACKGROUND

There are a number of commercially produced test kits that use qPCR to look for SARS-CoV-2 RNA. If the SARS-CoV-2 viral RNA is present in a patient sample, it indicates that the person is infected and has COVID-19 (although the disease may be present with few, if any symptoms). In this case study, we use data for a qPCR COVID-19 test kit that is sold by the company Gnomegen. Similar data are available from other companies and could be used to further explore qPCR calculations. While we will use these data to explore some quantitative calculations, note that the Gnomegen COVID-19 RT-qPCR Detection Kit is intended for the *qualitative* detection of RNA.[1]

The Gnomegen qPCR test kit contains primers that recognize two regions of the gene that codes for the virus's nucleocapsid (N) protein. The nucleocapsid protein plays an important role in allowing the virus to invade human cells. The two regions are called "N1" and "N2." The test kit also contains primers that recognize the human RNase P gene. These primers are included as a positive control (as was explained in Practice Problem 1 in Section 24.9.)

Note that since the SARS-CoV-2 virus has an RNA genome, RNA extracted from patient samples is transcribed into cDNA before the qPCR cycles begin.

[1] The information in this case study is derived from the "Gnomegen COVID-19 RT-qPCR Detection Kit Instructions for Use." The FDA required this information before approving the Gnomegen qPCR test kit for emergency use during the COVID-19 pandemic. The full document is available at https://www.fda.gov/media/137895/download.

## 25.6.2 LIMIT OF DETECTION AND GNOMEGEN DATA

When a company requests permission from the FDA to market a COVID-19 test kit, they must provide data that describe the performance characteristics of their assay. One of these performance characteristics is the **limit of detection (LoD)**, *the lowest amount or concentration of target DNA that can be reliably detected.* The FDA defines LoD as the lowest concentration at which approximately 95% of all true positive samples test positive. Gnomegen describes their procedure for determining the LoD as follows: "To determine the LoD, 5 upper respiratory samples ... from healthy donors were pooled and individually spiked with serially diluted quantified whole viral genomic RNA extracted from cells infected with SARS-CoV-2 obtained from a COVID-19 positive specimen ... to prepare a simulated, contrived clinical matrix. Contrived clinical matrix with viral spike-ins were individually purified and tested. Samples were extracted [to obtain RNA] ... Purified RNA was tested using the Gnomegen COVID-19 RT-qPCR Detection Kit ... [which includes transcribing RNA into cDNA.]. The approximate LoD was identified by testing 10, 5 and 2-fold serial dilutions of the characterized stock of purified whole viral RNA. For each dilution, a total of 3 replicates were tested."

By "contrived clinical matrix," Gnomegen means that known amounts of viral RNA were spiked (added) into human tissue of the type that would be present if a swab were taken from the respiratory tract of a patient being tested for COVID-19.

A portion of the Gnomegen results is shown in Table 25.3.

### Questions

1. RNase P is a positive control. Suppose the RNase P samples did not have fluorescence above background. What would this mean?
2. Based on the data in Table 25.3, what is the LoD of the Gnomegen assay for N1 and N2?
3. Suggest a serial dilution strategy to obtain the dilutions shown in Table 25.3. Assume that you have a stock solution with $4\times10^4$ copies of the viral genome/μL, which is the concentration Gnomegen scientists used. Note that when the qPCR assay is run, 5 μL of each standard or sample is added to the reaction mixture. For example, as shown in Table 25.3, the first standard has 2,000 copies of the viral genome. (2,000

**TABLE 25.3 Data from Gnomegen Assay**

| Number Copies Viral RNA in Reaction | N1 $C_t$ | N2 $C_t$ | RNase P $C_t$ | # of Positive N1 Target Samples | # of Positive N2 Samples |
|---|---|---|---|---|---|
| 2,000 | 26.62 | 27.67 | 32.61 | 3/3 Samples | 3/3 Samples |
| 2,000 | 26.90 | 28.03 | 33.15 | | |
| 2,000 | 26.90 | 28.02 | 32.63 | | |
| 200 | 29.87 | 30.87 | 33.24 | 3/3 Samples | 3/3 Samples |
| 200 | 29.91 | 31.24 | 33.02 | | |
| 200 | 30.23 | 31.39 | 33.29 | | |
| 20 | 33.36 | 32.66 | 30.73 | 3/3 Samples | 3/3 Samples |
| 20 | 33.97 | 34.86 | 32.18 | | |
| 20 | 33.34 | 33.61 | 30.93 | | |
| 10 | 33.46 | 34.96 | 32.20 | 3/3 Samples | 3/3 Samples |
| 10 | 35.40 | 36.00 | 30.68 | | |
| 10 | 33.61 | 36.33 | 32.30 | | |
| 2 | Undetermined | Undetermined | 30.39 | 1/3 Samples | 1/3 Samples |
| 2 | Undetermined | Undetermined | 31.18 | | |
| 2 | 34.91 | 38.93 | 42.28 | | |
| 1 | Undetermined | Undetermined | 31.15 | 2/3 Samples | 0/3 Samples |
| 1 | 35.54 | Undetermined | 32.54 | | |
| 1 | 35.57 | Undetermined | 32.40 | | |

copies is an *amount*.) These 2,000 copies must have been contained in a volume of 5 µL. Therefore, the *concentration* of RNA in the dilution tube must have been $4 \times 10^2$ copies/1 µL. The next dilution tube must have had a *concentration* of $4 \times 10^1$ copies/1 µL to provide 200 copies in 5 µL and so on.

4. Use the data for N1 in Table 25.3 to graph a standard curve. Note that only the standards with 2,000, 200, 20, and 10 copies can be used for this purpose. (Why?) Note also that three replicates of each dilution were tested. Take the average of the three replicates to make your graph.
5. Based on the standard curve, what is the efficiency of the reaction?
6. If a patient sample has a $C_t$ value of 28, what is $N_0$ for that sample?

## Answers

1. If the RNase P positive control does not have detectable fluorescence, it means something went wrong and the assay is invalid. A lack of detectable fluorescence in the positive control can indicate that RNA was not successfully extracted from the samples or the transcription of RNA into cDNA did not work. Whatever the cause, trouble shooting is required.
2. Based on the data in Table 25.3, the LoD for this assay is ten copies/reaction for both N1 and N2. If there are fewer than ten copies, the assay did not provide a positive result ≥ 95% of the time.
3. There is more than one strategy that will work to prepare these dilutions with the constraints specified. Figure 25.9 provides one strategy
4.

| Number Copies Viral RNA in Reaction | Log Number Copies Viral RNA in Reaction | Average N1 $C_t$ |
|---|---|---|
| 2,000 | 3.3 | 26.81 |
| 200 | 2.3 | 30.00 |
| 20 | 1.3 | 33.56 |
| 10 | 1 | 34.16 |

Figure 25.10 shows the standard curve for these data.

5. Based on the standard curve, the efficiency is:

$$E = \left(10^{-1/-3.2703} - 1\right) \times 100\% = \left(10^{0.30578} - 1\right) \times 100\% \approx \mathbf{102\%}$$

6. If a patient sample has a $C_t$ value of 28, what is $N_0$ for that sample?

$$28 = -3.2703\ X + 37.591$$

$$X \approx 2.93$$

Taking the antilog of this X-value gives ≈ **857 copies** of viral genome were in the patient sample.

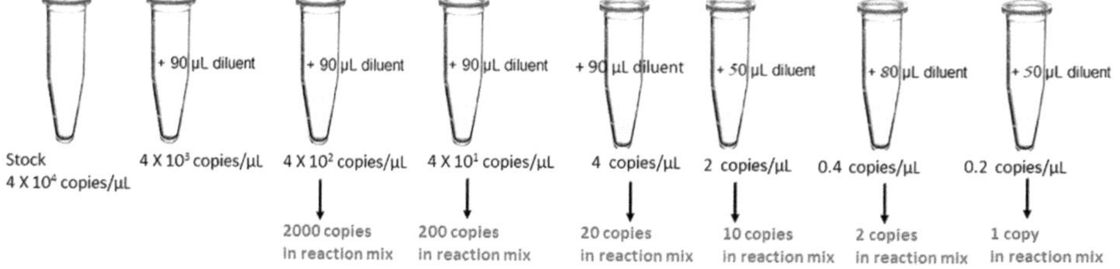


**FIGURE 25.9** A strategy for serial dilutions to make the required dilutions of viral RNA.

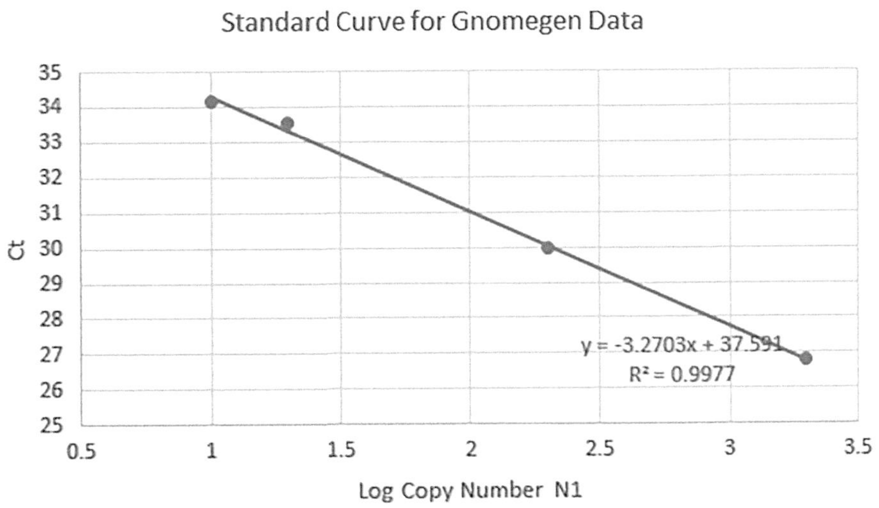


**FIGURE 25.10** Gnomegen data standard curve.

## ADDITIONAL REFERENCES

If you wish to probe more deeply into the math of qPCR, this article is helpful:

Rutledge, R. G. "Mathematics of Quantitative Kinetic PCR and the Application of Standard Curves." *Nucleic Acids Research*, vol. 31, no. 16, 2003, pp. 93e–93. doi:10.1093/nar/gng093.

Bio-Rad, a manufacturer of supplies for PCR, has a useful "Applications Guide to Real-Time PCR, Bulletin 5279." It is currently downloadable at www.bio-rad.com/webroot/web/pdf/lsr/literature/Bulletin_5279.pdf.

Here are two calculators for converting between nanograms or bp length and copy number:

"DNA Copy Number Calculator, Thermo Fisher Scientific – NL." www.thermofisher.com/nl/en/home/brands/thermo-scientific/molecular-biology/molecular-biology-learning-center/molecular-biology-resource-library/thermo-scientific-web-tools/dna-copy-number-calculator.html. Accessed 18 April 2021.

"Copy Number Calculator for Realtime PCR, Science Primer." www.scienceprimer.com/copy-number-calculator-for-realtime-pcr. Accessed 18 April 2021.

# Calculations Relating to Protein Purification and Analysis

26



## 26.1 INTRODUCTION

Proteins are biological molecules that perform a wide array of tasks in cells. For example, **antibodies** *are proteins that protect cells from foreign invaders.* **Transcription factors** *are proteins that turn genes on and off at the proper times.* **Enzymes** *are proteins that catalyze the thousands of chemical reactions that occur in cells.* Recall from Chapters 22 to 25 that enzymes also are used as essential tools that allow biotechnologists to manipulate nucleic acids. Proteins are important in the research laboratory and in biotechnology companies where they are produced in large quantities for medical and industrial applications.

The functional diversity of proteins is possible because they are structurally diverse. As with the English language, where an immense number of words with varied meaning are formed using only 26 letters, diverse proteins are formed using primarily 20 different amino acid subunits. A protein consists of amino acid subunits that are linked together into a chain, which then folds into various structures. Every protein has a different sequence of amino acid that determines its final structure and function.

Proteins are relatively large molecules. For comparison, recall that the molecular weight of NaCl is 58.44. The molecular weight of hemoglobin, a protein that carries oxygen in our cells, is about 64,000. β-galactosidase, an enzyme that is important in molecular biology applications, has a molecular weight of about 465,400.

Like other molecules discussed previously in this text, the concentration of proteins in a solution can be expressed in various ways. Concentration can be expressed in terms of molarity. Researchers often express protein concentration in units of mg/mL. In biotechnology production environments, where large amounts of proteins are produced as drugs or for other purposes, protein concentration might be expressed in terms of grams of

DOI: 10.1201/9780429282744-31

protein produced per liter of suspended cells. The calculations associated with these various expressions will be familiar to you because we have encountered them in various places throughout this text.

**Example Problem**

It is relatively simple to convert between concentration expressed in terms of molarity and concentration expressed in terms of mg/mL. Let us see why this is so. As an example, consider NaCl with a MW of 58.44.

$$\text{For NaCl, by definition}: 1\,\text{M} = \frac{58.44\,\text{g}}{1{,}000\,\text{mL}}$$

Divide the numerator and denominator by 1,000:

$$1\,\text{M} = \left(\frac{0.05844\,\text{g}}{1\,\text{mL}}\right) = \left(\frac{58.44\,\text{mg}}{1\,\text{mL}}\right)$$

This means that, for any compound:

$$\textbf{Concentration in mg / mL} = (\textbf{molarity})(\textbf{MW})$$

This leads to Equation 26.1.

**EQUATION 26.1: Conversion between Concentration in Molarity and mg/mL**

$$\textbf{Concentration in mg / mL} = (\textbf{molarity})(\textbf{MW})$$

**Example Problem**

Suppose you have a 0.75 M solution of NaCl. Express this concentration in terms of mg/mL.

***Answer:***

Using Equation 26.1:

$$\text{Concentration in mg/mL} = (\text{Molarity})(\text{MW})$$

$$\text{Concentration in mg/mL} = (0.75\,\text{M})(58.44)$$

$$= \textbf{43.83 mg/mL}$$

**Example Problem**

Suppose you have a 0.1 mM solution of β-galactosidase (FW = 465,400). Express this in terms of mg/mL.

***Answer:***

First, 0.1 mM = 0.0001 MUsing Equation 26.1:

$$\text{Concentration in mg/mL} = (0.0001\ \text{M})(465{,}400) = \mathbf{46.54\ mg/mL}$$

**Practice Problems**

1. ***A protein with a MW of 65,000 is present in a solution at a concentration of 1 × $10^{-3}$ M. Convert this to units of mg/mL.***
2. ***The MW of bovine serum albumin (BSA) is 66,463 D. A solution of BSA is present at a concentration of 100 μg/mL. Convert this to:***
   a. ***Units of mg/mL***
   b. ***Units of %***
   c. ***Units of M***
   d. ***Units of mM***

***Answers***

1. Using Equation 26.1:

$$\text{Concentration in mg/mL} = (\text{molarity})(\text{MW}) = (0.001\ \text{M})(65{,}000) = \mathbf{65\ mg/mL}$$

   We can also solve this as follows:
   For this protein, a 1 M solution has a concentration of 65,000 g/1000 mL.
   A 0.001 M solution has a concentration of 65 g/1000 mL.
   Divide the numerator and denominator by 1,000 to obtain **65 mg/1 mL.**
2. The MW of BSA is 66,463. A solution of BSA is present at a concentration of 100 μg/mL. Convert this to:
   a. 100 μg/mL = **0.1 mg/mL**
   b. 100 μg/mL = 0.0001 g/mL = 0.01 g/100 mL = **0.01%**
   c. Using Equation 26.1:

$$\text{Concentration in mg/mL} = (\text{Molarity})(\text{MW})$$
$$0.1\ \text{mg/mL} = (?)(66{,}463)$$
$$? \approx \mathbf{1.50 \times 10^{-6}\ M}$$

   d. 1.50 × $10^{-6}$ M = **1.50 × $10^{-3}$ mM**

## 26.2 DETERMINING PROTEIN CONCENTRATION BY UV SPECTROPHOTOMETRY

When working with proteins, it is necessary to have assays to:

- detect the proteins
- quantify the amount and concentration of protein in a preparation
- determine the activity (function) of the protein
- determine the degree of purity of a specific protein.

There are a number of methods that are used to assay proteins. For example, in Chapter 23 we introduced electrophoresis, a method commonly used in protein analysis. In Section 16.7, we introduced ELISAs, another common method of analyzing proteins. Spectrophotometric methods, as introduced in Chapter 16, are also important when working with proteins. Spectrophotometric assays are relatively fast, simple, and inexpensive and thus are common in all types of biotechnology settings. Spectrophotometric assays are therefore the major emphasis of this chapter.

The simplest method to estimate the concentration of protein in a sample is to measure its absorbance in a spectrophotometer at a wavelength of 280 nm. (This requires a spectrophotometer that can measure absorbance of light in the ultraviolet (UV) range.) This method works because certain amino acids absorb light at 280 nm. Therefore, as the concentration of a protein increases, its absorbance of light at this wavelength also increases. This spectrophotometric method is analogous to the estimation of nucleic acid concentration that was discussed in Section 22.12. However, proteins are much more diverse in structure than nucleic acids. Therefore, there is considerable variability in the degree to which each protein absorbs UV light. Sometimes the very general approximation is used: that protein at a concentration of 1 mg/mL will have an absorbance of 1 at 280 nm under standard conditions. However, given the variability from protein to protein, this is not a particularly accurate method of assaying protein concentrations.

A more accurate way to use absorbance at 280 nm to estimate protein concentration is to use the absorptivity constant for that specific protein. Recall from Section 16.4 that an absorptivity constant is a measure of a compound's inherent tendency to absorb light of a particular wavelength. (Absorptivity constants are introduced in Section 16.4, and it might be helpful to review that section now.) In many cases, it is possible to find the absorptivity constant for a specific protein using a web browser or reference book (for example, Lundblad, Roger, and Fiona Macdonald. *Handbook of Biochemistry and Molecular Biology*. 5th ed., CRC Press, 2018.) Once an absorptivity constant has been determined for a particular protein with its distinct amino acid composition, the protein's concentration in a solution can be estimated based on its absorbance. For example, for the protein BSA, the absorptivity constant is such that a 0.1% solution at a wavelength of 280 nm has an absorbance of 0.66. (This value assumes a standard, 1 cm cuvette, that is, sample holder.) This absorptivity value for BSA would likely be expressed in the literature as "$A^{0.1\%}{}_{280} = 0.66$."

Suppose a BSA solution has an absorbance at 280 nm of 1.346 (with a standard cuvette). What is its concentration? This can be readily calculated using a proportion equation:

$$\frac{0.1\%\ \text{BSA}}{0.66} = \frac{?}{1.346}$$

$$? \approx 0.20\%$$

$$0.20\% = 0.20\ \text{g}/100\ \text{mL} = 0.002\ \text{g/mL} = \mathbf{2\ mg/mL}$$

As was noted in Section 16.4, absorptivity constants have units. For proteins, it is common for analysts to report the constants for a 1% solution, a 0.1% solution, or to use molar absorptivity constants. Therefore, pay attention to the units when using absorptivity constant values reported in the literature.

Using a published absorptivity constant at 280 nm to calculate the concentration of a protein in a solution provides only an approximate answer. This is because the degree to which a protein absorbs light depends on the pH and ionic concentration of the solution, what impurities (if any) are present, and the calibration of the spectrophotometer. Still, it is more accurate to estimate protein concentration using an absorptivity constant for that particular protein than it is to use the broad generalization that 1 mg/mL of protein has an absorbance of 1.

### Practice Problems

***For all these problems, assume that conditions are standard and a 1 cm cuvette is used.***

1. ***The $A^{0.1\%}{}_{280}$ value for BSA is 0.66. This means that a 0.1% solution of pure BSA under standard conditions is expected to have an absorbance of 0.66 at 280 nm. If the absorbance of a pure BSA solution under these standard conditions is 1.00, what is its approximate concentration in units of mg/mL?***
2. ***The $A^{0.1\%}{}_{280}$ for IgG (a protein that composes antibodies) is 1.38. If an IgG solution has an absorbance at 280 nm of 1.00, what is its approximate concentration in units of µg/mL?***
3. ***The $A^{1\%}{}_{280}$ value for β-galactosidase is 19.1. This means that a 1% solution of pure β-galactosidase solution under standard conditions is expected to have an absorbance of 19.1 at 280 nm. (This is a theoretical value. No spectrophotometer can read such a high absorbance value.) If a β-galactosidase solution has an absorbance of 0.500 at 280 nm, what is its approximate concentration in units of mg/mL?***
4. ***The molar absorptivity constant of a protein is 6.0 × 10⁴/M-cm. The protein has a molecular weight of 75,000. What absorbance at 280 nm is predicted for a solution of this protein with a concentration of 0.1 mg/mL?***
5. ***The molar absorptivity constant for BSA at 280 nm is reported to be 43,824/M-cm. Show that this is equivalent to an $A^{0.1\%}{}_{280}$ value of 0.66. Recall that the FW of BSA is 66,463.***

### *Answers*

1. The $A^{0.1\%}{}_{280}$ value for BSA is 0.66. If the absorbance of a pure BSA solution under these standard conditions is 1.00, then:

$$\frac{0.1\%\ \text{BSA}}{0.66} = \frac{?}{1.00}$$

$$? \approx 0.1515\% = 0.1515\ \text{g} / 100\ \text{mL} = \mathbf{1.515\ mg / mL}$$

2. The $A^{0.1\%}{}_{280}$ for IgG is 1.38. If an IgG solution has an absorbance at 280 nm of 1, then:

$$\frac{0.1\%\ \text{IgG}}{1.38} = \frac{?}{1.00}$$

$$? \approx 0.07246\% = 0.07246\ \text{g} / 100\ \text{mL} = \mathbf{724.6\ \mu g / mL}$$

3. The $A^{1\%}{}_{280}$ value for β-galactosidase is 19.1. If a β-galactosidase solution has an absorbance of 0.500 at 280 nm, then:

$$\frac{1\%\ \beta\text{gal}}{19.1} = \frac{?}{0.500}$$

$$? \approx 0.0262\% = 0.0262\ \text{g} / 100\ \text{mL} = \mathbf{0.262\ mg / mL}$$

4. The molar absorptivity constant of a protein at 280 nm is $6.0 \times 10^4$/M-cm. The protein has a molecular weight of 75,000. What absorbance at 280 nm is predicted for a solution of this protein with a concentration of 0.1 mg/mL? One way to think about this is as follows:

   Step 1. Convert 0.1 mg/mL to molarity. Using Equation 26.1:

$$\text{Concentration in mg/mL} = (\text{Molarity})(\text{MW})$$

$$0.1\ \text{mg/mL} = (?)(75{,}000)$$

$$? \approx \mathbf{1.333 \times 10^{-6}\ M}$$

   Step 2. Plug values into Beer's equation:

$$\text{Absorbance} = (\text{Absorptivity constant})(\text{path length in cm})(\text{concentration})$$

$$? = \left(6.0 \times 10^4 / \cancel{\text{M-cm}}\right)\left(1\ \cancel{\text{cm}}\right)\left(1.333 \times 10^{-6}\ \cancel{\text{M}}\right)$$

$$? \approx \mathbf{0.080}$$

   So, this solution is expected to have an absorbance of about 0.080.

5. The molar absorptivity constant for BSA at 280 nm is reported to be 43,824/M-cm. Show that this is equivalent to an $A^{0.1\%}{}_{280}$ value of 0.66. The FW of BSA is 66,463.
   One way to think about this is as follows:
   Step 1. Convert 0.1% to molarity.
   0.1% = 0.1 g/100 mL = 1 g/1,000 mL
   Using proportions:

$$\frac{\dfrac{1\ \text{M}}{66{,}463\ \text{g}}}{1{,}000\ \text{mL}} = \frac{\dfrac{?}{1\ \text{g}}}{1{,}000\ \text{mL}}$$

$$? \approx 1.505 \times 10^{-5}\ \text{M}$$

   So, for BSA:

$$0.1\% \approx 1.505 \times 10^{-5}\ \text{M}$$

   Plug these values into Beer's equation and see if the answer is 0.66.
   Beer's law:

$$\text{Absorbance} = (\text{Absorptivity constant})(\text{path length in cm})(\text{concentration})$$

$$\text{Absorbance} = \left(\frac{43{,}824}{\cancel{\text{M-cm}}}\right)\left(1\ \cancel{\text{cm}}\right)\left(1.505 \times 10^{-5}\ \cancel{\text{M}}\right) \approx \mathbf{0.66}$$

## 26.3 SPECTROPHOTOMETRIC COLORIMETRIC ASSAYS OF TOTAL PROTEIN

The method of using absorbance at 280 nm to measure protein concentration is quick, easy, and is commonly applied. However, this method provides only an estimation of protein concentration, and it requires a spectrophotometer with the capability of working in the UV range. There are other spectrophotometric protein assay methods that are sensitive to nearly all proteins that can be used with a (less expensive) spectrophotometer that works only in the visible light range and that provide more accurate concentration results. One of these assay methods, the Bradford assay, will be discussed as an example. (Bradford, Marion M. "A Rapid and Sensitive Method for the Quantitation of Microgram Quantities of Protein Utilizing the Principle of Protein-Dye Binding." *Analytical Biochemistry*, vol. 72, no. 1–2, 1976, pp. 248–54. doi:10.1016/0003-2697(76)90527-3.)

The basis of the Bradford assay is the observation that certain amino acids found in most proteins selectively bind a dye, Coomassie Brilliant Blue G-250, also called Bradford reagent. When the dye binds amino acids under the proper conditions of temperature and pH, it changes color from reddish-brown to blue. The more protein present, and therefore the more of these amino acids there are to bind the dye, the more blue color appears in the solution. This color change can be quantified using a spectrophotometer at 595 nm. *This type of assay that involves a colored product is called a* **colorimetric assay.** The Bradford assay can be used for samples whose protein concentration is between about 1 and 1,500 µg/mL.

**Protein without color + Bradford Reagent** ⟶ **Blue Product**

To perform a Bradford assay, one first prepares standards that consist of a protein solution that is diluted to known concentrations. The standards and the samples are reacted with the Bradford dye reagent and their absorbances are measured. The standards are used to construct a standard curve with protein concentration on the X-axis and absorbance on the Y-axis, as we saw in Chapter 16. Based on the standard curve, the concentration of protein in the samples is determined.

Ideally, when a protein assay is performed, the standards should be prepared using the protein of interest. For example, if you are a researcher studying protein CD30, then protein CD30 is the protein of interest and you should make a standard curve using it. (CD30 is a marker for certain blood cancers.) However, this requires that you have a stock solution of the protein of interest (CD30 in this example) with a concentration of protein that is known based on another (non-spectrophotometric) assay. Such a standard is often not available or is too expensive to use routinely. For example, it costs hundreds of dollars to get 100 µg of purified CD30. For some proteins of interest, it is difficult or impossible to obtain a pure preparation with a known concentration. Therefore, it is common practice to use a protein other than the protein of interest as the standard. BSA is commonly used as standard in protein assays because it is readily available with high purity at a moderate cost.

The use of BSA as a standard when performing protein assays has an issue of which you should be aware. Different proteins often have different reactivities with the dye reagents used in protein assays. Thus, at a given concentration, BSA might develop more or less color than your protein of interest when each is reacted with Bradford reagent. For this reason, when using BSA as a standard, the results provided by a protein assay are *relative*, not *absolute*. What do we mean by relative and absolute in this context? Suppose you are using the Bradford assay to compare the amount of protein between various experimental groups. In each experiment, you use BSA as the standard. Suppose that based on a protein assay, experimental sample 1 has 10 mg/mL protein and experimental sample 2 has 20 mg/mL protein. You can reasonably conclude that experimental sample 2 has twice as high a concentration of protein as experimental sample 1. You are making a **relative** comparison between the two groups. But you cannot be sure that experimental group 1 has an actual – **absolute** – concentration of 10 mg/mL protein or that experimental group 2 has an absolute concentration of 20 mg/mL. This is because your protein of interest may react with the Bradford reagent more or less strongly than does BSA. Thus, you cannot make an **absolute** determination of the protein of interest concentration in your experiments when using BSA as the standard. In practice, relative comparisons are often perfectly acceptable. Later in this chapter, we will consider the purification of a protein using a series of steps that sequentially remove more and more contaminants from the protein of interest. In a protein purification procedure, the protein concentration at each step is compared with the concentration at the previous step. In this situation, relative (not absolute) results are required.

Box 26.1 provides an overview of the Bradford assay procedure, which is then discussed in Example Problems below.

**BOX 26.1: The Bradford Protein Assay**

Step 1. Prepare at least 5 standards with known concentrations of the protein of interest. Alternatively, if the quantity of protein of interest is limited, use bovine serum albumin. Standard concentrations should span the range of concentrations expected in samples.

Step 2. Prepare the samples. The samples must have concentrations in the range of the standards. It is therefore advisable to prepare several dilutions of each sample. Prepare the blank, a preparation that does not contain the analyte.

Step 3. Add Braford Reagent to standards, samples, and blank.

Step 4. Measure absorbances of standards and samples. Prepare a standard curve.

Step 5. Use the standard curve to determine the concentration of protein in each sample.

**Example Problem:**

**Step 1: Prepare the Standards.**

The first step is to prepare protein standards by diluting a stock protein solution to known concentrations.

You begin with a protein (BSA) stock solution at a concentration of 1.0 mg/mL and you want to make a series of five dilutions in buffer with final concentrations ranging from 1 to 25 µg/mL. Each dilution should have a volume of 2.0 mL. The table below is designed to help you with your dilutions. Fill in the blanks in the table.

| Tube Number | Final BSA Concentration (µg/mL) | Volume of Stock Solution | Volume of Buffer |
|---|---|---|---|
| 1 | 1.0 | 2 µL | 1.998 mL |
| 2 | 5.0 | ____ | ____ |
| 3 | 10.0 | ____ | ____ |
| 4 | 20.0 | ____ | ____ |
| 5 | 25.0 | ____ | ____ |
| Blank | 0.00 | 0 | 2.000 mL |

*Answer:*

This is yet another situation where you have a concentrated stock solution that needs to be diluted to particular concentrations. To determine the amount of stock you will need to make the desired final protein concentrations, use the $C_1V_1 = C_2V_2$ equation, where $C_1$ and $C_2$ are the concentrations of the stock and the diluted sample respectively and $V_1$ and $V_2$ are the volumes of the stock and the diluted sample.

For example, for the first standard:

$$C_1V_1 = C_2V_2$$

$$(1{,}000\ \mu g/mL)(?) = (1\ \mu g/mL)(2\ mL)$$

$$? = 0.002\ mL = 2\ \mu L$$

Add buffer to make 2 mL total volume.

| Tube Number | Final BSA Concentration (µg/mL) | Volume of Stock Solution (µL) | Volume of Buffer (mL) |
|---|---|---|---|
| 1 | 1.0 | 2 | 1.998 |
| 2 | 5.0 | 10 | 1.990 |
| 3 | 10.0 | 20 | 1.980 |
| 4 | 20.0 | 40 | 1.960 |
| 5 | 25.0 | 50 | 1.950 |

**Example Problem:**

**Step 2: Prepare the Samples.**

Prepare the samples whose protein concentration is to be determined. In order for the assay to be valid, the samples need to have concentrations in the same general range as the standards (in this example, 0–25 µg/mL). Since you do not know the concentration of protein in the samples, it is advisable to prepare several dilutions of each sample with the idea that the protein concentration in one or more of the dilutions will lie in the same concentration range as the standards. A blank is also prepared with 2 mL of buffer.

How would you prepare 2 mL of a 1/5 and a 1/10 dilution of a sample? (If necessary, refer to Chapter 14 for a discussion of dilutions.)

*Answer:*

Proportions can be used to solve this problem. For the 1/5 dilution:

$$\frac{1}{5} = \frac{?}{2\ mL} \qquad ? = \mathbf{0.4\ mL}$$

So, take 0.4 mL of the sample protein solution and add 1.6 mL of buffer.

For the 1/10 dilution:

$$\frac{1}{10} = \frac{?}{2\ mL} \qquad ? = \mathbf{0.2\ mL}$$

So, take 0.2 mL of the sample protein solution and add 1.8 mL of buffer.

**Step 3: Add the Bradford Reagent.**

At this point you should have five standards and several dilutions of each sample. Remove the same volume of each standard, sample, and the blank, for example, 0.8 mL, and place them in separate test tubes. Add the Bradford reagent to each tube, in this example, use 0.2 mL. Mix the tubes thoroughly and wait a set amount of time. The samples with protein should change to a blue color; the more protein present, the more intensely blue they should be.

**Step 4: Prepare a Standard Curve Based on the Absorbances of the Standards.**

"Blank" the spectrophotometer and read the absorbance of each of the standards using a spectrophotometer at 595 nm. Prepare a standard curve based on the absorbances of the standards. Plot the concentration of protein on the X-axis, absorbance on the Y-axis.

**Step 5: Determine the Concentration of Protein in Each Sample.**

Read the absorbance of each sample with all its dilutions. Use the standard curve to determine the concentration in each sample. Those samples that are too concentrated or too dilute to fall on the standard curve should not be used. To determine the concentration in the diluted samples, it is necessary to multiply by the reciprocal of the dilution.

**Example Problem:**

Determine the concentration of protein in the samples prepared in step 2 above, based on the standards prepared in step 1 above.

The absorbances of the standards, step 1, and the samples, step 2, are:

| Standard or Sample | Protein Concentration (µg/mL) | Absorbance |
|---|---|---|
| Standard 1 | 1.0 | 0.076 |
| Standard 2 | 5.0 | 0.378 |
| Standard 3 | 10.0 | 0.810 |
| Standard 4 | 20.0 | 1.610 |
| Standard 5 | 25.0 | 1.920 |
| Sample, undiluted | ? | 3.600 |
| Sample, 1/5 dilution | ? | 1.600 |
| Sample, 1/10 dilution | ? | 0.750 |

The standard curve, based on the values for the standards above, is:

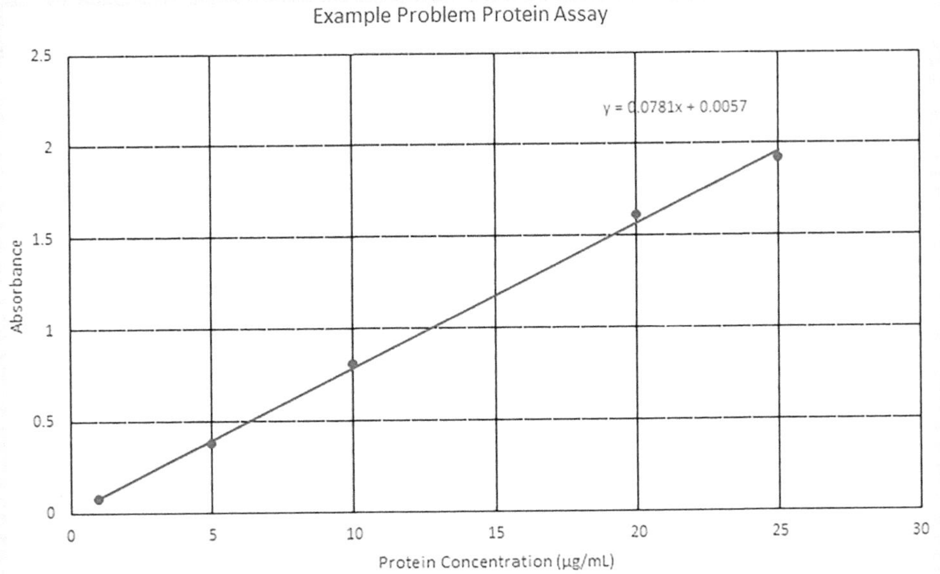


**FIGURE 26.1** Example problem protein assay.

***Answer:***

Reading off the graph, Figure 26.1, or using the equation for the standard curve line, the concentrations are:

| Sample | Absorbance | Concentration |
|---|---|---|
| Undiluted sample | Too high to be meaningful | — |
| Sample, 1/5 dilution | 1.600 | ≈ 20.4 μg/mL |
| Sample, 1/10 dilution | 0.750 | ≈ 9.53 μg/mL |

The value from the 1/5 dilution must be multiplied by 5 (because of the dilution):

$$20.4\ \mu g/mL \times 5 \approx 102.0\ \mu g/mL$$

The value from the 1/10 dilution must be multiplied by 10:

$$9.53\ \mu g/mL \times 10 = 95.3\ \mu g/mL$$

An average of the two values gives **98.7 μg/mL** as the value for the concentration of protein in the sample.

## Practice Problems

1. ***Fill in the following table for preparing standards. Assume that you have a stock solution of protein at a concentration of 0.500 mg/mL and you want 2 mL final volume for each standard.***

| Tube Number | Final BSA Concentration (µg/mL) | Volume of Stock Solution | Volume of Buffer |
|---|---|---|---|
| 1 | 1.0 | ___ | ___ |
| 2 | 3.0 | ___ | ___ |
| 3 | 7.0 | ___ | ___ |
| 4 | 15.0 | ___ | ___ |
| 5 | 20.0 | ___ | ___ |
| Blank | 0.00 | 0 | 2.000 mL |

2. ***Show how would you prepare 2.0 mL of a sample with the following dilutions:***
   a. ½
   b. ¼
   c. *1/8*
   d. *1/10*
3. ***The following values are obtained for the standards. Prepare a standard curve based on these values.***

| Tube Number | Final BSA Concentration (µg/mL) | Absorbance |
|---|---|---|
| 1 | 1.0 | 0.07 |
| 2 | 3.0 | 0.22 |
| 3 | 7.0 | 0.51 |
| 4 | 15.0 | 1.06 |
| 5 | 20.0 | 1.42 |

4. ***Suppose that you obtained the absorbances below for the diluted samples. What is the concentration of protein in the samples based on the standard curve from problem 3?***

   ***Sample, dilution 1/2*** ***Too high to read***
   ***Sample, dilution 1/4*** ***Above the values for the standards***
   ***Sample, dilution 1/8*** ***0.88***
   ***Sample, dilution 1/10*** ***0.69***
5. ***Suppose you are performing an assay for the concentration of your protein of interest using the Bradford method. You are using BSA to create your standard curve. In this scenario, suppose that BSA reacts more strongly with the Bradford reagent than does your protein of interest. The standard curve for BSA is shown below. On the same graph, indicate what it might look like if you had a stock solution of known concentration of your protein of interest and used it to create the standard curve.***

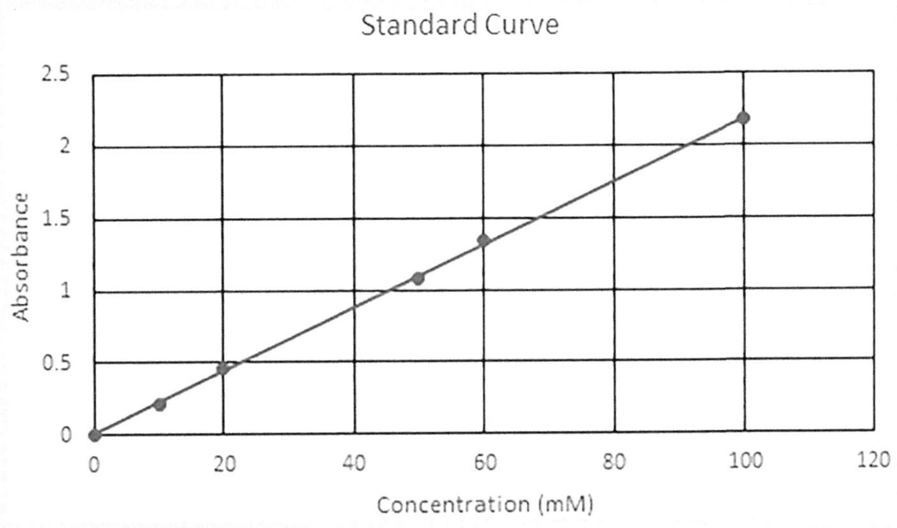


*Answers*

1.

| Tube Number | Final BSA Concentration (μg/mL) | Volume of Stock Solution (μL) | Volume of Buffer |
|---|---|---|---|
| 1 | 1.0 | **4.0** | **1996.0 μL** |
| 2 | 3.0 | **12.0** | **1988.0 μL** |
| 3 | 7.0 | **28.0** | **1972.0 μL** |
| 4 | 15.0 | **60.0** | **1940.0 μL** |
| 5 | 20.0 | **80.0** | **1920.0 μL** |
| Blank | 0.00 | **0** | **2.000 mL** |

2. a. To prepare 2.0 mL of a 1/2 dilution:

$$\frac{1}{2} = \frac{?}{2.0\ \text{mL}} \quad \mathbf{? = 1.0\ mL}$$ **So, use 1 mL of sample and add 1 mL of buffer**

b. To prepare 2.0 mL of a 1/4 dilution:

$$\frac{1}{4} = \frac{?}{2.0\ \text{mL}} \quad \mathbf{? = 0.5\ mL = 500\ \mu L}$$

**So, use 500 μL of sample and add 1,500 μL of buffer**

c. To prepare 2.0 mL of a 1/8 dilution:

$$\frac{1}{8} = \frac{?}{2.0\ \text{mL}} \quad \mathbf{? = 0.25\ mL = 250\ \mu L}$$

**So, use 250 μL of sample and add 1,750 μL of buffer**

d. To prepare 2.0 mL of a 1/10 dilution:

$$\frac{1}{10} = \frac{?}{2.0\ \text{mL}} \quad \mathbf{? = 0.2\ mL = 200\ \mu L}$$

**So, use 200 μL of sample and add 1800 μL of buffer**

3.

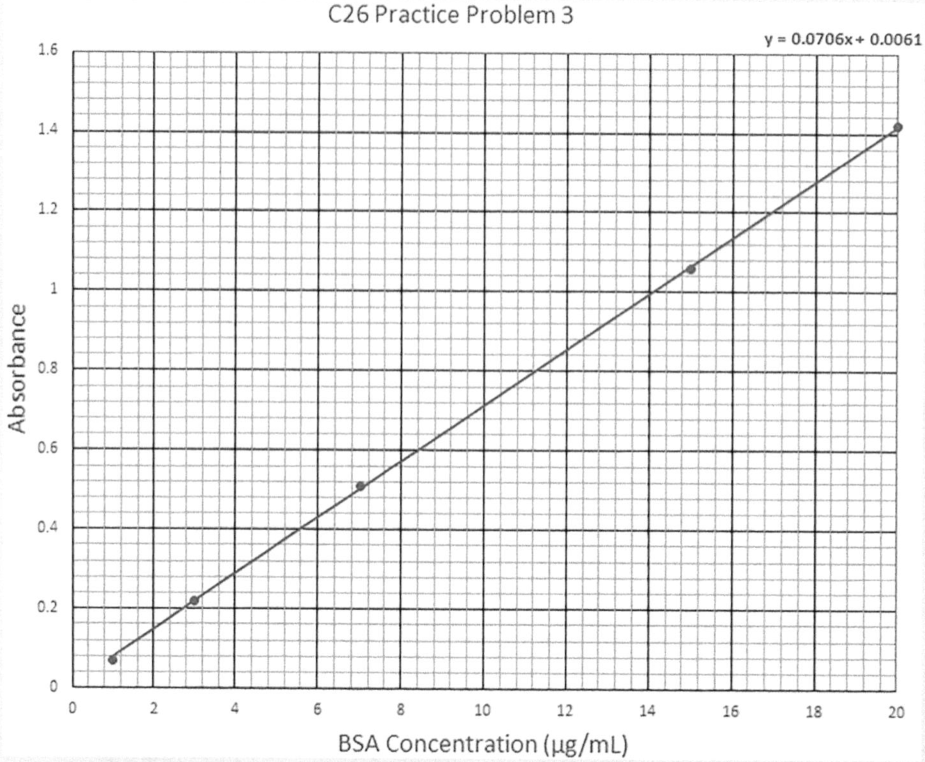


4. Sample, dilution 1/8

0.88 absorbance corresponds to concentration of about 12.37 µg/mL. This must be multiplied by reciprocal of dilution, so the concentration of protein in the sample was about **99.0 µg/mL.**

Sample, dilution 1/10

0.69 absorbance corresponds to concentration of about 9.69 µg/mL. This must be multiplied by the reciprocal of the dilution, so the concentration of protein in the sample was about **96.9 µg/mL.**

Average ≈ **97.9 µg/mL**

5.

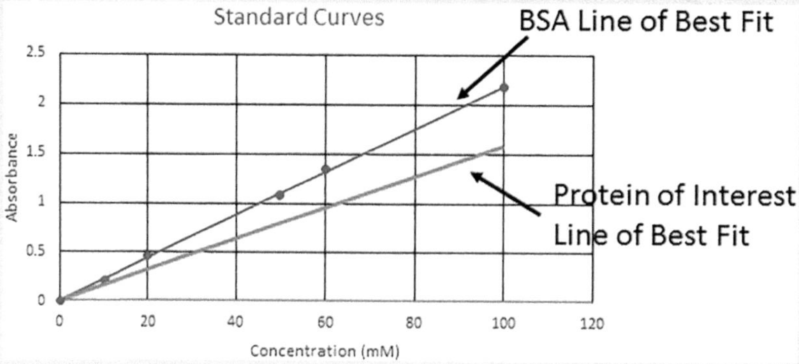


The protein of interest has a less steep slope than BSA because it reacts less intensely with the dye than does BSA.

## 26.4 ASSAYS FOR SPECIFIC PROTEINS

The Bradford assay and other total protein assays like it do not distinguish one protein from another because they are sensitive to almost all proteins. Most of the time, we are interested in a particular protein that does a particular job, and so we need additional assays that are sensitive to only the protein of interest. The most obvious way to look for a particular protein is to test for its activity. Thus, antibodies, which attack their foreign targets by binding to them, are assayed by looking for that binding. ELISA assays, introduced in Chapter 16, are commonly used to test for specific antibodies and for other proteins as well. Enzymes, which catalyze chemical reactions, are assayed by looking at the chemical reaction they catalyze. Let us consider enzyme assays in more detail.

Enzymes catalyze reactions. This means that they help convert starting compounds, called substrates, into ending compounds, called products:

$$\text{Substrate(s)} \xrightarrow{\text{Enzyme}} \text{Product(s)}$$

To assay an enzyme, one usually measures its activity by looking either for the disappearance of substrate or the appearance of product.

Enzyme activity is expressed as "units." There are various definitions of the term "unit." The **International Unit (IU) of enzyme activity** *is a commonly used definition and is the amount of enzyme required to catalyze transformation of 1.0 µmole of substrate to product per minute under optimal conditions* (such as a particular temperature and pH). The **SI unit of enzyme activity** *is another common definition and is the amount of enzyme necessary to transform 1.0 mole of substrate to product per second under optimal conditions.* Manufacturers often define the activity of their enzyme products using their own definition of a unit that is conveniently measured in the laboratory.

**Example Problem:**

An assay for enzyme Q measures the disappearance of substrate. In 15 minutes, 12 mmoles of substrate are converted to product. What is the activity of the enzyme preparation in International Units?

***Answer:***

$$12\ \text{mmoles} = 12{,}000\ \mu\text{moles}$$

The rate of conversion of substrate to product is 12,000 µmoles in 15 minutes = 800 µmoles/minute, so the preparation contains **800 IU** of enzyme.

**Example Problem:**

The enzyme DNA Polymerase I is used to catalyze the synthesis of DNA from nucleotide subunits. A manufacturer of this enzyme defines a unit as "the amount of enzyme that incorporates 10 nmol of deoxyribonucleotides into...[a nucleic acid] in 30 minutes...". Suppose that you want to incorporate 1 µmol of deoxyribonucleotides into a strand of DNA in a 30 minute reaction. The enzyme comes from the manufacturer at a concentration of 7 U/µL. How many µL of the enzyme will you need?

*Answer:*

1 µmol = 1,000 nmol. If 1 unit incorporates 10 nmol of dNTPs in 30 minutes, then how many units are needed to incorporate 1,000 nmol of dNTPs in 30 minutes?

$$\frac{1\text{ unit}}{10\text{ nmol}} = \frac{?}{1{,}000\text{ nmol}} \quad ? = 100\text{ units}$$

100 units are required and the concentration of the enzyme is 7 U/µL. So, how many µL are required to get 100 units?

$$\frac{7\text{ U}}{1\,\mu\text{L}} = \frac{100\text{ U}}{?} \qquad ? \approx \mathbf{14.3\ \mu L} \quad \text{Rounded up, this is } \mathbf{15\ \mu L} \text{ of enzyme.}$$

**Practice Problems**

1. ***An assay for the imaginary enzyme biotechase measures the disappearance of substrate. In 10 minutes, 15 mmoles of substrate is converted to product. What is the activity of the enzyme preparation in International Units?***
2. ***An assay for enzyme Y measures the disappearance of substrate. In 30 minutes, 21 mmoles of substrate is converted to product. What is the activity of the enzyme preparation in International Units?***
3. ***You have received a vial of enzyme that is labeled as containing four SI units of enzyme. How many IU of enzyme are in the vial?***
4. ***The enzyme called "RQ1 RNase-Free DNase" is used to destroy DNA when one is working with RNA and DNA is an unwanted contaminant. The manufacturer defines a unit as "the amount of enzyme required to completely degrade 1 µg of DNA in 10 minutes at 37°C, and in 50 µL of a buffer containing.... [specific components]". The enzyme is supplied at a concentration of 1 U/µL. If you think you have about 500 ng of DNA contaminating your RNA preparation, what would be the minimum number of µL of the RQ1 RNase-Free DNase that you would use? Assume you plan a 10 minute incubation.***

*Answers*

1. The rate of conversion of substrate to product is 15,000 µmoles in 10 minutes = 1,500 µmoles/minute, so the preparation contains **1,500 IU of enzyme**.
2. 21 mmoles = 21,000 µmoles. The rate of conversion of substrate to product is 21,000 µmoles in 30 minutes = 700 µmoles/minute, so the preparation contains **700 IU of enzyme**.
3. Four SI units convert 4 moles of substrate to product in a second. This is the same as $4 \times 10^6$ µmol per second and $240 \times 10^6$ µmol/minute = $\mathbf{2.4 \times 10^8}$ **IU**.

   Alternatively, using a unit canceling strategy:

$$\left(\frac{4\ \cancel{\text{mol}}}{1\ \cancel{\text{second}}}\right)\left(\frac{60\ \cancel{\text{second}}}{1\text{ minute}}\right)\left(\frac{10^6\ \mu\text{mol}}{1\ \cancel{\text{mol}}}\right) = \frac{2.4\times10^8\ \mu\text{mol}}{1\text{ minute}} = \mathbf{2.4\times10^8\ IU}$$

4. 500 ng = 0.5 µg. If 1 unit degrades 1 µg of DNA in 10 minutes, then how many units are needed to degrade 0.5 µg? Let us use the unit canceling strategy:

$$0.5\ \cancel{\mu g}\left(\frac{1\ \text{unit}}{1\ \cancel{\mu g}}\right) = \mathbf{0.5\ unit}$$

0.5 U requires 0.5 µL. It is unlikely that you would try to pipette out only 0.5 µL. More likely you would add 1 µL of the enzyme, containing 1 unit, and you would have a surplus of the enzyme.

## 26.5 AN EXAMPLE OF A SPECIFIC ENZYME ASSAY: THE β-GALACTOSIDASE ASSAY

Recall from Chapters 22 to 25 that enzymes are used to manipulate nucleic acids. In the problems in those chapters, and in some of the problems in this chapter, the activity of the enzymes is provided by the manufacturer, usually expressed as U/µL. How do the manufacturers of enzyme products know how many units they are providing in each microliter? The answer is that they test each enzyme preparation with an assay specific for the enzyme of interest. Here, we will demonstrate such an assay using the enzyme β-galactosidase as an example.

β-Galactosidase is an enzyme with many applications in the molecular biology laboratory. Scientists created an assay specifically for β-galactosidase by taking advantage of its biological activity. In nature, β-galactosidase cleaves the bonds between the two sugars found in a family of disaccharides (carbohydrates composed of two sugar subunits) known as β-galactosides. The bacterium, *E. coli*, makes the enzyme β-galactosidase and is therefore able to utilize lactose, a disaccharide found in milk, as an energy source. In *E. coli*, the reaction catalyzed by β-galactosidase looks like this:

$$\text{Lactose} \xrightarrow{\beta\text{-galactosidase}} \text{Glucose + Galactose}$$

After this cleavage occurs, the bacterium uses the resulting individual sugars as energy sources.

The substrate in the naturally occurring reaction catalyzed by β-galactosidase is lactose, and the products are glucose and galactose. Both the substrate and products of this natural reaction are colorless. But, in a test tube, β-galactosidase will also cleave a synthetic sugar, called o-nitrophenyl-β-galactoside or ONPG. The product of this cleavage is o-nitrophenol, abbreviated ONP, and galactose:

$$\textbf{ONPG} \xrightarrow{\beta\text{-galactosidase}} \text{ONP + Galactose}$$

ONPG is colorless, but ONP is yellow; therefore this test tube reaction can be followed by looking for the appearance of yellow color. If ONPG is added to a tube with a sample and if β-galactosidase is present in the sample, then the ONPG will be converted to ONP and a yellow color will appear in the tube. The more β-galactosidase in the sample, the more yellow color will appear. The amount of yellow color present can be quantified with a spectrophotometer. Thus, ONPG provides a means to specifically assay a sample for the presence of β-galactosidase. One unit of β-galactosidase is defined as the amount of enzyme that will convert 1 µmole of ONPG to ONP in 1 minute at 37°C.

This β-galactosidase assay can be performed by preparing a standard curve with ONP. However, in practice most analysts use a shortcut and do not prepare a standard curve each time the assay is performed. Instead, analysts take advantage of a published molar absorptivity constant for ONP. (See Section 16.4 for an explanation of absorptivity constants.

See also the note at the end of this chapter, Section 26.9, that explains the derivation of the equation below.) While this shortcut is not as accurate as preparing a standard curve each time the reaction is run, it does allow an analyst to compare one sample preparation to another, and most of the time, such comparisons are all that is required.

Based on the absorptivity constant, the units of β-galactosidase are calculated using Equation 26.2:

**EQUATION 26.2 β-Galactosidase Activity**

$$\text{Units of } \beta\text{-galactosidase} = \frac{(A_{420})(0.38)}{\text{Minutes at } 37°\text{C}}$$

**where $A_{420}$ is the absorbance of the solution at a wavelength of 420 nm**

Box 26.2 provides an overview of the β-galactosidase assay, which is subsequently described in more detail.

**BOX 26.2: The β-Galactosidase Assay**

Step 1. Dilute samples.

Step 2. Add small volume of diluted sample to assay buffer.

Step 3. Equilibrate to 37 °C.

Step 4. Add substrate, ONPG, to samples and blank.

Step 5. Incubate at 37 °C to allow reaction to occur.

Step 6. Stop the reaction.

Step 7. Read sample absorbances.

Step 8. Calculate the units of enzyme activity using Equation 26.2.

**Step 1: Dilute the Samples with Buffer.**

This assay is very sensitive to low concentrations of enzyme. Therefore, the first step is usually to dilute a small amount of the preparations to be assayed. For example, one might make a 1/100 dilution by removing 1 µL of a sample preparation and adding 99 µL of buffer.

**Step 2: Remove a Small Volume of Diluted Sample and Add to 1 mL of Assay Buffer.**

A small volume of each diluted sample, for example, 10 µL, is removed and is added to 1 mL of assay buffer. A blank is prepared at the same time that contains 10 µL of buffer instead of sample.

**Step 3: Equilibrate to 37°C.**

The β-galactosidase assay is done at 37°C because this is the temperature at which the enzyme works in nature. The sample and the substrate are therefore brought to 37°C.

**Step 4: Add the Substrate.**

0.2 mL of the substrate, ONPG, is added to the sample(s) and blank.

**Step 5: Allow the Reaction to Occur.**

The sample(s) and blank are incubated at 37°C to allow the reaction to occur. During the incubation the enzyme, β-galactosidase cleaves the ONPG, yielding galactose and ONP. As ONP is produced, a yellow color appears.

**Step 6: Stop the Reaction.**

The reaction will keep going until all the substrate is converted to product. However, we want the reaction to continue only long enough to get enough color to easily read in a spectrophotometer. Therefore, the reaction is stopped by adding stop solution when enough color has developed. The time when the reaction is stopped is recorded. In this method, 0.5 mL of stop solution is added.

**Step 7: Read the Absorbance(s).**

The sample(s) absorbance(s) is read in a spectrophotometer at a wavelength of 420 nm.

**Step 8: Calculate the Units of Enzyme Activity.**

The units of enzyme activity are calculated using Equation 26.2.

**Example Problem:**

β-Galactosidase is being purified for use in the laboratory and you want to determine the enzyme activity in a preparation. You do the following:

1. Dilute the preparation by removing 1 µL and adding it to 99 µL of buffer.
2. Remove 10 µL of the diluted preparation and add it to 1 mL of reaction buffer.
3. Equilibrate the sample and substrate to 37°C.
4. Add 0.2 mL of ONPG to the mixture and incubate at 37°C until ample yellow color appears.
5. Stop the reaction at the end of 11 minutes by adding 0.5 mL of stop solution.
6. Read the absorbance of the sample at a wavelength of 420 nm. The absorbance is 0.412.
   a. What is the enzyme activity in the diluted sample preparation?
   b. What is the enzyme activity in the original preparation expressed as U/mL?

***Answer:***

a. The $A_{420}$ in this example is 0.412 and the time is 11 minutes. Plugging into the Equation 26.2:

$$\text{Units of } \beta\text{-galactosidase} = \frac{(0.412)(0.38)}{11\text{ minutes}} \approx 0.0142\text{ units}$$

These 0.0142 units were in 10 µL of sample. We can use proportions to determine how many units would be in 1 mL:

$$\frac{0.0142\text{ units}}{10\ \mu\text{L}} = \frac{?}{1{,}000\ \mu\text{L}} \qquad ? \approx \mathbf{1.42\ units}$$

So, the enzyme activity is **1.42 units/mL.**

b. Now we need to remember that the sample was diluted 1/100 in Step 1. Therefore, multiply (1.42 units/mL) (100) = 142 U/mL. So, the β-galactosidase activity in the undiluted preparation is **142 U/mL.**

**Practice Problems**

1. ***β-galactosidase is being purified for use in the laboratory and you want to determine the enzyme activity in a preparation. You perform the following steps:***
   - ***Dilute the sample 1/50.***
   - ***Remove 10 μL of the diluted preparation and add it to 1 mL of reaction buffer.***
   - ***Equilibrate to the proper temperature for the reaction.***
   - ***Add 0.2 mL of ONPG to the mixture and incubate for 13 minutes at 37°C.***
   - ***Stop the reaction with 0.5 mL of stop solution.***
   - ***Read the absorbance at 420 nm.***
   - ***The absorbance is 0.982.***

   ***What is the concentration of enzyme in the original preparation expressed as units/mL?***
2. ***β-galactosidase is being purified for use in the laboratory and you want to determine the enzyme activity in a preparation. You perform the following steps:***
   - ***Dilute the sample 1/200.***
   - ***Remove 20 μL of the diluted preparation and add it to 1 mL of reaction buffer.***
   - ***Equilibrate to the proper temperature for the reaction.***
   - ***Add 0.2 mL of ONPG to the mixture and incubate for 19 minutes at 37°C.***
   - ***Stop the reaction with 0.5 mL of stop solution.***
   - ***Read the absorbance at 420 nm.***
   - ***The absorbance is 1.482.***

   ***What is the concentration of enzyme in the original preparation expressed as units/mL?***
3. ***β-galactosidase is being purified for use in the laboratory and you want to determine the enzyme activity in a preparation. You perform the following steps:***
   - ***Dilute the sample by removing 5 μL of sample and adding it to 145 μL of buffer.***
   - ***Remove 15 μL of the diluted preparation and add it to 1 mL of reaction buffer.***
   - ***Equilibrate to the proper temperature for the reaction.***
   - ***Add 0.2 mL of ONPG to the mixture and incubate for 21 minutes at 37°C.***
   - ***Stop the reaction with 0.5 mL of stop solution.***
   - ***Read the absorbance at 420 nm.***
   - ***The absorbance is 0.562.***

   ***What is the concentration of enzyme in the original preparation expressed as units/mL?***
4. ***β-galactosidase is being purified for use in the laboratory and you want to determine the enzyme activity in a preparation. You perform the following steps:***
   - ***Dilute the sample by removing 5 μL of sample and adding it to 200 μL of buffer.***
   - ***Remove 20 μL of the diluted preparation and add it to 1 mL of reaction buffer.***
   - ***Equilibrate to the proper temperature for the reaction.***
   - ***Add 0.2 mL of ONPG to the mixture and incubate for 13 minutes at 37°C.***
   - ***Stop the reaction with 0.5 mL of stop solution.***
   - ***Read the absorbance at 420 nm.***
   - ***The absorbance is 0.876.***

   ***What is the concentration of enzyme in the original preparation expressed as units/mL?***

5. ***β-galactosidase is being purified. You have 200 mL of a crude preparation of the enzyme. You perform the following steps:***
   - ***Dilute the sample by removing 1 μL of sample and adding it to 999 μL of buffer.***
   - ***Remove 20 μL of the diluted preparation and add it to 1 mL of reaction buffer.***
   - ***Equilibrate to the proper temperature for the reaction.***
   - ***Add 0.2 mL of ONPG to the mixture and incubate for 16 minutes at 37°C.***
   - ***Stop the reaction with 0.5 mL of stop solution.***
   - ***Read the absorbance at 420 nm.***
   - ***The absorbance is 0.786.***
     a. ***What is the concentration of β-galactosidase in the diluted sample expressed as units/mL?***
     b. ***What is the concentration of β-galactosidase in the undiluted sample expressed as units/mL?***
     c. ***How much activity is there in the entire 200 mL of the crude preparation expressed as units?***

*Answers*

1. The $A_{420}$ in this example is 0.982 and the time is 13 minutes. Plugging into Equation 26.2:

$$\text{Units of } \beta\text{-galactosidase} = \frac{(0.982)(0.38)}{13 \text{ minutes}} \approx 0.0287 \text{ units}$$

These 0.0287 units were in 10 μL of sample. We can use proportions to determine how many units would be in 1 mL:

$$\frac{0.0287 \text{ units}}{10\ \mu\text{L}} = \frac{?}{1{,}000\ \mu\text{L}} \qquad ? \approx 2.87 \text{ units}$$

So, the enzyme activity is 2.87 units/mL.

The sample was diluted 1/50 so multiply 2.87 units/mL times the reciprocal of the dilution.

(50) (2.87 units/mL) ≈ **144 U/mL**. This is the β-galactosidase activity in the undiluted preparation.

2. The $A_{420}$ in this example is 1.482 and the time is 19 minutes. Plugging into Equation 26.2:

$$\text{Units of } \beta\text{-galactosidase} = \frac{(1.482)(0.38)}{19 \text{ minutes}} = 0.02964 \text{ units}$$

These 0.02964 units were in 20 μL of sample. We can use proportions to determine how many units would be in 1 mL:

$$\frac{0.02964 \text{ units}}{20\ \mu\text{L}} = \frac{?}{1{,}000\ \mu\text{L}} \qquad ? = 1.482 \text{ units}$$

So, the concentration is 1.482 units/mL.

The sample was diluted 1/200. Therefore, multiply 1.482 units/mL by the reciprocal of the dilution, which = **296.4 U/mL**. Therefore, the β-galactosidase activity in the undiluted preparation is about 296.4 U/mL.

3. The $A_{420}$ in this example is 0.562 and the time is 21 minutes. Plugging into Equation 26.2:

$$\text{Units of } \beta\text{-galactosidase} = \frac{(0.562)(0.38)}{21 \text{ minutes}} = 0.010169524 \text{ units}$$

These 0.010169524 units were in 15 µL of sample. We can use proportions to determine how many units would be in 1 mL:

$$\frac{0.010169524 \text{ units}}{15\,\mu\text{L}} = \frac{?}{1{,}000\,\mu\text{L}} \qquad ? = 0.677968254 \text{ units}$$

So there are 0.677968254 U/mL

The sample was diluted 5/150 = 1/30. Therefore, after multiplying by the reciprocal of the dilution, 30, we see that the β-galactosidase activity in the undiluted preparation is about **20.3 U/mL.**

4. Plugging into Equation 26.2:

$$\text{Units of } \beta\text{-galactosidase} = \frac{(0.876)(0.38)}{13 \text{ minutes}} = 0.025606 \text{ units}$$

$$\frac{0.025606 \text{ units}}{20\,\mu\text{L}} = \frac{?}{1{,}000\,\mu\text{L}} \qquad ? \approx 1.280 \text{ units} \quad \text{So there are } 1.280 \text{ U/mL}$$

The sample was diluted 5/205 = 1/41. Therefore, the β-galactosidase activity in the undiluted preparation is about **52.5 U/mL.**

5. a. Plugging into Equation 26.2:

$$\text{Units of } \beta\text{-galactosidase} = \frac{(0.786)(0.38)}{16 \text{ minutes}} = 0.0186675 \text{ units}$$

$$\frac{0.0186675 \text{ units}}{20\,\mu\text{L}} = \frac{?}{1{,}000\,\mu\text{L}} \qquad ? = 0.933375 \text{ units}$$

So there are **0.933375 U/mL** in the diluted sample.

b. The sample was diluted 1/1,000. Therefore, the β-galactosidase activity in the undiluted preparation was **933.375 U/mL.**

c. This can be solved by proportions. We know there are 933.375 units in 1 mL, so how many are in the entire 200 mL of the crude preparation?

$$\frac{933.375 \text{ units}}{1 \text{ mL}} = \frac{?}{200 \text{ mL}} \qquad ? = \mathbf{186{,}675 \text{ unit}}$$

## 26.6 SPECIFIC ACTIVITY

**Specific activity** is a convenient way of expressing the purity of a particular protein. *It is calculated as the amount (or units) of the protein of interest divided by the total amount of all proteins in a sample.* When a protein preparation is very pure, all the protein in the preparation is the protein of interest and the specific activity is high. When the protein of interest is contaminated by other proteins, the specific activity is lower. The more the contaminants, the lower the specific activity.

Calculating specific activity requires performing two assays: a total protein assay (like the Bradford assay) and an assay specific only for the protein of interest. Based on these two measurements, it is possible to calculate the specific activity of a protein using Equation 26.3:

**EQUATION 26.3 Specific Activity**

$$\textbf{Specific activity} = \frac{\textbf{Activity of the protein of interest in units / mL}}{\textbf{mg of total protein / mL}}$$

**or**

$$\textbf{Specific activity} = \frac{\textbf{Activity of the protein of interest in units}}{\textbf{mg of total protein}}$$

Observe that these two forms of the equation are basically the same, except that the first is expressed in terms of *concentrations* and the second in terms of *amounts*.

**Example Problem:**

You have a preparation of an enzyme. You test its activity using an enzyme assay specific for that protein and get a value of 142 units/mL. You also do a protein assay and find you have 0.6 mg/mL of total protein. What is the specific activity for this preparation?

***Answer:***

$$\textbf{Specific activity} = \frac{\textbf{Activity of the protein of interest in units / mL}}{\textbf{mg of total protein / mL}}$$

$$= \frac{142 \text{ units/mL}}{0.6 \text{ mg/mL}} \approx \textbf{237 units / mg}$$

**Practice Problems**

1. ***You have a preparation that you test for enzyme activity and for total protein. The activity assay gives you 250 units/mL, and the total protein assay yields 15 mg protein/mL. What is the specific activity of this preparation?***
2. ***β-Galactosidase is being purified for use in the laboratory and you want to know the specific activity of a preparation. You run a Bradford assay first. You make a 1/10 dilution of this preparation and a 1/20 dilution. Based on your standard curve, the Bradford assay results are:***
   ***In a sample diluted 1/10, there are 50 µg/mL of protein.***
   ***In a sample diluted 1/20, there are 23 µg/mL of protein.***
   - ***You also run a β-galactosidase enzyme assay as follows:***
   - ***You dilute the sample by removing 5 µL of sample and adding it to 195 µL of buffer.***
   - ***You remove 20 µL of the diluted preparation and add it to 1 mL of reaction buffer.***

- ***You equilibrate to the proper temperature for the reaction.***
- ***You add 0.2 mL of ONPG to the mixture and incubate for 14 minutes at 37°C.***
- ***You stop the reaction with 0.5 mL of stop solution.***
- ***You read the absorbance at 420 nm.***
- ***The absorbance is 0.389.***

***What is the specific activity of this preparation?***

3. ***You need to purchase enough enzyme Z to perform 100 reactions. You determine that this will require ~8,000 units of enzyme. The catalog from your favorite supplier offers the following choices:***

***1 unit of enzyme activity catalyzes the conversion of 1 µmole of A to B in 1 minutes at 25°C at pH 7.5.***

| | | | |
|---|---|---|---|
| *Grade 1* | *From aardvark liver* | *100 mg* | *$50* |
| | *activity 10,000 Units/g* | *500 mg* | *$200* |
| | | *1 g* | *$350* |
| *Grade 2* | *From aardvark liver* | *100 mg* | *$200* |
| | *activity 50,000 Units/g* | *500 mg* | *$700* |
| | | *1 g* | *$1,500* |
| *Grade 3* | *From aardvark liver* | *1 g* | *$30* |
| | *activity 2,000 Units/g* | *5 g* | *$110* |
| | | *10 g* | *$250* |

a. ***What enzyme grade would be your best choice if your main priority is to find the least expensive option?***

b. ***Which of these products has the highest specific activity?***

4. ***You are working with stem cells and require a reagent called "stem cell detachment reagent" in order to perform the procedure. A portion of the protocol you are following is shown below. Figure 26.2 shows a label from the vial of lyophilized (freeze dried) stem cell detachment reagent that you purchased from a manufacturer. How would you prepare this reagent?***

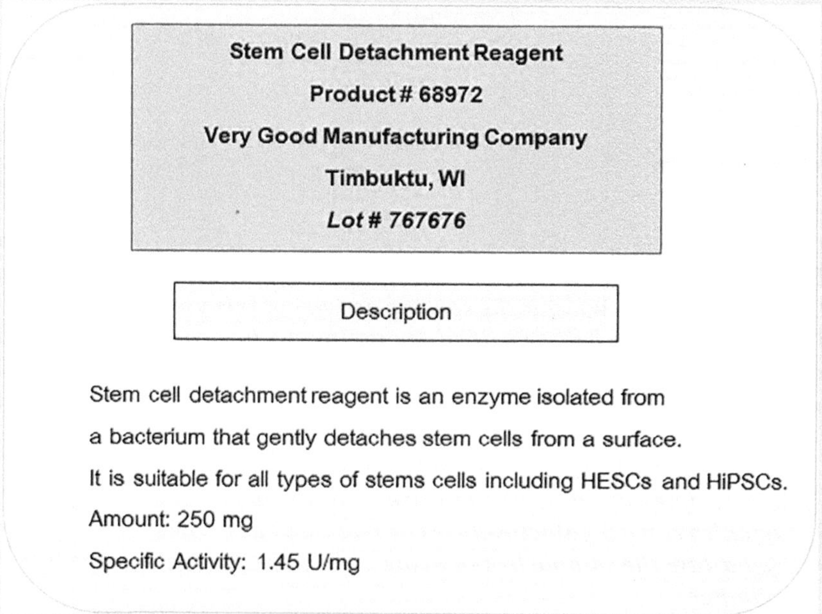
Stem Cell Detachment Reagent
Product # 68972
Very Good Manufacturing Company
Timbuktu, WI
Lot # 767676
Description
Stem cell detachment reagent is an enzyme isolated from
a bacterium that gently detaches stem cells from a surface.
It is suitable for all types of stems cells including HESCs and HiPSCs.
Amount: 250 mg
Specific Activity: 1.45 U/mg

**FIGURE 26.2** Label from stem cell detachment reagent.

**2. Prepare Stem Cell Detachment Reagent.**

**2.1. Prepare 40 mL of 0.5 U/mL working solution.**

**2.1.1. Lyophilized proteins tend to be hygroscopic. Once opened, the vial should be stored desiccated.**

**2.1.2. Bring the vial to room temperature before opening. The vial should not be cool to the touch.**

**2.1.3. Weigh out and dissolve the appropriate amount of stem cell detachment reagent in cell culture medium to obtain 40 mL of a 0.5 U/mL solution.**

**2.1.4. Filter sterilize through a 0.22 μm filter.**

**2.1.5. Aliquot and store at −20°C for up to 3 months.**

**2.1.6. Avoid repeated freezing and thawing.**

**2.1.6.1. Thawed aliquots can be stored between −2 and −4°C for up to 2 weeks.**

## *Answers*

1. $$\text{Specific activity} = \frac{\text{Activity of the protein of interest in units/mL}}{\text{mg of total protein/mL}}$$

$$= \frac{250\ \text{U}/\text{mL}}{15\ \text{mg}/\text{mL}} \approx \mathbf{16.7\ U/mg}$$

2. From the Bradford assay for total protein:

$$(10)(50\ \mu\text{g/mL}) = 500\ \mu\text{g/mL}$$

$$(20)(23\ \mu\text{g/mL}) = 460\ \mu\text{g/mL}$$

$$\text{The average} = 480\ \mu\text{g/mL of total protein} = 0.480\ \text{mg/mL}$$

From the β-galactosidase enzyme assay:

Plugging into Equation 26.2:

$$= \frac{(0.389)(0.38)}{14\ \text{minutes}} \approx 0.010558571\ \text{units}$$

$$\frac{0.010558571\ \text{units}}{20\ \mu\text{L}} = \frac{?}{1{,}000\ \mu\text{L}} \qquad ? \approx 0.5279\ \text{units so, there are } 0.5279\ \text{U/mL}.$$

The sample was diluted 5/200 = 1/40. Therefore, the β-galactosidase activity in the undiluted preparation is about 21.1 U/mL.

$$\text{Specific activity} = \frac{\text{Activity of the protein of interest in units/mL}}{\text{mg of total protein/mL}}$$

$$= \frac{21.1\ \text{U}/\text{mL}}{0.480\ \text{mg}/\text{mL}} \approx \mathbf{44\ U/mg}$$

3. First, you want to consider the specific activities of each enzyme grade and determine what quantity you need to purchase:

Grade 1: At a specific activity of 10,000 units/g, you will need 0.8 g to provide the 8,000 activity units needed. This will require eight 100 mg vials for a total of $400 or 1 g for $350.

Grade 2: At 50,000 units/g, you will need 160 mg or 2 × 100 mg for $400.

Grade 3: At 2,000 units/g, you will need 4g of protein at 4 × 1g for $120 or 5g at $110.

a. **The most cost effective option is grade 3, which is the least pure.**
b. **The highest specific activity and therefore the most concentrated activity is found in grade 2.**

4. You will need to thaw the vial and weigh out a portion of the lyophilized material. To calculate how much to weigh out, you want 40 mL at a concentration of 0.5 U/mL. So you need:

$$(40\,\text{mL})(0.5\,\text{U/mL}) = 20\ \text{units.}$$

From Figure 26.2, the specific activity of the reagent is 1.45 U/mg. Using a proportion expression:

$$\frac{1.45\,\text{U}}{1\,\text{mg}} = \frac{20\,\text{U}}{?}$$

$$? \approx 13.79\,\text{mg} = \mathbf{0.01379\,g}$$

Carefully weigh out this amount of the powder.

Measure out **40 mL** of cell culture medium and dissolve the powder in the medium. (This type of solution is probably not brought to volume because the amount of powder is so small as to have little effect on the volume.)

Filter sterilize.

Aliquot (divide into small volumes for storage in freezer).

Store remaining lyophilized powder in a desiccator.

## 26.7 CALCULATIONS OF PURIFICATION FACTOR AND YIELD

Imagine that a particular protein is being isolated from a natural source, such as bacterial cells, plant cells, or animal cells. This protein of interest is only one of a great many proteins found in that cellular source. The protein of interest must be separated from all the other proteins present. Typically, the protein of interest will be isolated in a series of steps. If all goes well, after each step the amount of contaminating proteins should decrease. At the same time, the percentage of the protein in the preparation that is the protein of interest should increase, because the protein of interest is becoming more and more pure. Thus, the specific activity should increase in a multistep purification process. Unfortunately, there is inevitably some loss of the protein of interest in almost any purification process. So, while the protein of interest becomes increasingly pure, there tends to be less of it.

We will discuss three calculations that relate specifically to a protein purification procedure: purification factor, yield, and percent yield. The **purification factor** *is a comparison of the specific activity at some point in a purification procedure to the specific activity at the beginning of the purification process.* The purification factor is calculated as Equation 26.4:

**EQUATION 26.4: Purification Factor**

$$\textbf{Purification factor} = \frac{\textbf{Specific activity at a particular step}}{\textbf{Specific activity at the beginning of the purification process}}$$

Since the specific activity should increase with each separation step, the purification factor should be >1. The purification factor has no units, because the units cancel.

**Example Problem:**

The protein concentration from the Bradford assay at the beginning of a purification process is 1,000 mg/mL, and the enzyme activity is 30,000 units/mL. After the first purification step, the protein concentration from the Bradford assay is 100 mg/mL and the enzyme activity is 25,000 units/mL. What is the purification factor?

***Answer:***

The specific activity at the beginning of the purification process is:

$$\frac{30{,}000\ \text{U/mL}}{1{,}000\ \text{mg/mL}} = 30\ \text{U/mg}$$

The specific activity after the first purification step is:

$$\frac{25{,}000\ \text{U/mL}}{100\ \text{mg/mL}} = 250\ \text{U/mg}$$

The purification factor is:

$$\frac{250\ \text{U/mg}}{30\ \text{U/mg}} \approx \mathbf{8.33}$$

So, the purity has improved by a factor of 8.33. Or, to say it a different way, the protein is 8.33 times purer after the first purification step than it was to begin with.

Yield is the total amount of a protein of interest at a particular step. For enzymes, yield is best expressed as the total number of units of enzyme activity. Yield will decrease in a multistep purification process because some loss of the protein of interest occurs with each step, Figure 26.3. Yield is not expressed as a concentration because this does not tell you how much protein you have altogether. For example, if you are a strawberry farmer and you have 18 bushels of strawberries per row, what is your yield if you have 50 rows? The answer is 900 bushels. If you report that you have 18 bushels per row, no one will know the yield since they do not know how many rows you have. Similarly, yield is reported as the total number of activity units, not as a concentration. Enzyme yield is calculated using Equation 26.5:

**EQUATION 26.5: Yield**

$$\textbf{Yield of enzyme in activity units} = (\textbf{Total number of mL})\left(\frac{\textbf{Units}}{\textbf{mL}}\right)$$

**Example Problem:**

Your enzyme activity in a particular preparation is 142 U/mL and you have 100 mL of preparation. What is the yield?

***Answer:***

$$(100\text{ mL})(142\text{ U/mL}) = \mathbf{14,200\ units}$$

Percent yield compares the total amount of the protein of interest present at a particular step in a purification process to the total amount of that protein that was present at the very beginning. We know that this number should go down because of the inevitable loss of protein that occurs during purification. To calculate the percent yield, use Equation 26.6:

**EQUATION 26.6: Percent Yield**

$$\textbf{Percent yield} = \frac{\textbf{Total amount of the protein of interest at a particular step}}{\textbf{Total amount of the protein of interest initially}} \times \mathbf{100\%}$$

**Example Problem:**

At the very beginning of a purification process you have 125,000 units of an enzyme of interest. You go through three purification steps at the end of which there are a total of 52,000 units of this enzyme remaining. What is the percent yield?

***Answer:***

$$\frac{52,000\text{ units}}{125,000\text{ units}} \times 100\% = \mathbf{41.6\%}$$

**Practice Problems**

1. ***Based on the data in Figure 26.3, what is the ultimate % yield for this protein of interest (that is, percent of the protein of interest that was originally present that remains after step 4)?***
2. a. ***If there were initially 250,000 U of target protein present, about how many units were present at the end of step 2?***
   b. ***If there were initially 250,000 U of target protein present, about how many units were present at the end of step 4?***
3. ***Which step removed the most impurities?***
4. ***Which step reduced the yield of the target protein the most?***

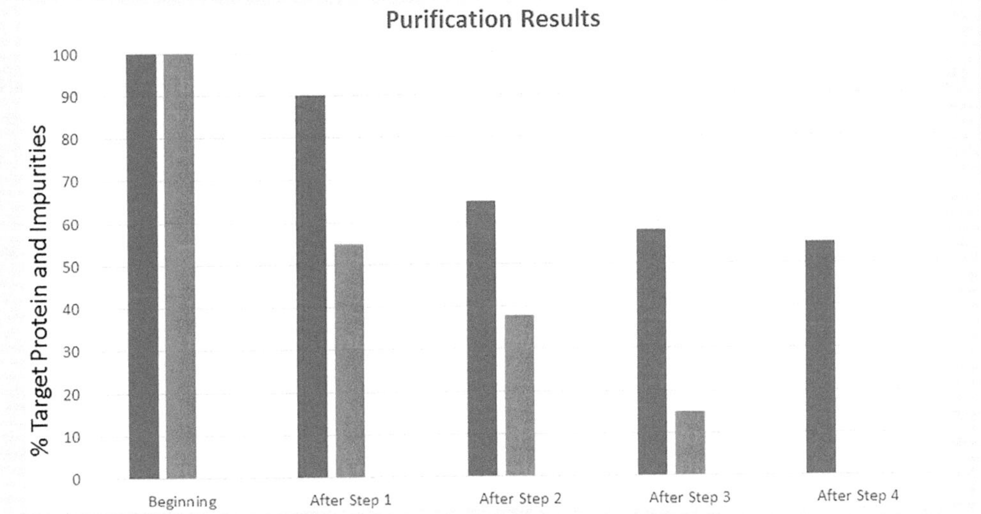


**FIGURE 26.3** As purification proceeds, yield decreases but purity increases. This graph illustrates a protein purification strategy with four steps, labeled on the X-axis. The blue-colored bars represent the amount of target protein present, expressed as a percent, and the orange bars are the impurities present, also expressed as a percent. Initially 100% of the target protein and its impurities are present. After the first purification step, some of the target protein is lost. The blue bar is lower indicating that about 90% of the original amount of target protein is present. After each step, the yield of the protein of interest decreases, but its purity, and therefore specific activity, increases.

***Answers***

1. Based on the data in Figure 26.3, the ultimate yield was about 55%.
2. a. At the end of step 2 about 65% of the target protein remained. So the number of units remaining was about:

$$(0.65)(250{,}000\text{ U}) = \mathbf{162{,}500\ U}$$

   b. At the end of step 4, about 55% of the target protein remained. So the number of units remaining was about:

$$(0.55)(250{,}000\text{ U}) = \mathbf{137{,}500\ U}$$

3. Step 1 removed about 45% of the impurities. Other steps removed fewer impurities.
4. Step 2 removed about 25% of the target protein and so reduced the yield of target protein more than any other step.

## 26.8 SUMMARIZING THE RESULTS OF A PURIFICATION PROCEDURE

In a multistep purification procedure, a protein is isolated from a source and is then purified in a series of steps. As shown in Figure 26.3, at each step we expect the following:

1. There should be less and less contaminating protein as the purification proceeds. Therefore, the specific activity should increase.

2. Some of the protein of interest will be lost along with the contaminating proteins. Therefore, the yield will decrease at each step.

The following example shows a scheme in which a protein is purified in a step-by-step process. After each step, the specific activity of the protein is measured, and the yield is calculated.

**Example Problem:**

The enzyme, β-galactosidase was purified from a culture of bacteria in a series of steps as follows:

1. 10 L of cells were grown in nutrient broth.
2. The 10 L were centrifuged to separate the cells from the broth. The result was a pellet containing the bacterial cells.
3. The cell pellet was resuspended in buffer and the cells' walls were broken apart to release the cellular contents. The resulting suspension was centrifuged again resulting in a pellet at the bottom of the tube and a supernatant (liquid above the pellet). *The pellet and the supernatant were assayed for β-galactosidase activity.* Enzyme activity was detected only in the supernatant, so the pellet was set aside to be discarded. The supernatant is called the "crude extract".
4. The crude extract was treated with salt to precipitate the β-galactosidase. The precipitated enzyme was collected by centrifugation and was resuspended in buffer. *The resulting β-galactosidase preparation was assayed for enzymatic activity and for total protein.*
5. Salt was removed from the β-galactosidase solution using a method called dialysis. The resulting β-galactosidase preparation was assayed for β-galactosidase activity and for total protein.
6. The β-galactosidase preparation was next passed through a chromatography column, another purification step that separated the β-galactosidase from a number of impurities. *The resulting enzyme preparation was assayed for β-galactosidase activity and for total protein.*

   The results of the protein and enzyme assays are shown in the table below.

   a. Fill in the blanks in the table.
   b. What happened to the specific activity as the purification proceeded?
   c. What happened to the percent yield as the purification proceeded?

**Purification of β-Galactosidase from Bacteria**

| Purification Activity Step | Total Protein (mg) | Total Activity (units) | Specific Activity (units/mg) | Yield (%) |
|---|---|---|---|---|
| Crude Ex. | 2,140 | 1,360 | 0.64 | 100 |
| After salt precipitation | 760 | 1,350 | ____ | 99 |
| After dialysis | 740 | ____ | 1.80 | ____ |
| After chromatography | 390 | 1,240 | ____ | ____ |

### *Answer:*

a. Specific activity equals the amount of activity of the protein of interest divided by the total amount of protein present. Percent yield is the percent of the amount of starting activity that is still present after each purification step. In this example, 1,360 units represent 100% yield.

| Purification Step | Total Protein (mg) | Total Activity (units) | Specific Activity (units/mg) | Yield (%) |
|---|---|---|---|---|
| Crude Ex. | 2,140 | 1,360 | 0.64 | 100 |
| After salt precipitation | 760 | 1,350 | **1.78** | 99 |
| After dialysis | 740 | **1,332** | 1.80 | **98** |
| After chromatography | 390 | 1,240 | **3.18** | **91** |

b. As the purification proceeded, the β-galactosidase became purer; therefore, the specific activity increased.
c. As we would predict, some of the β-galactosidase was lost at each step and the percent of total activity remaining (yield) decreased as the purification proceeded.

### Practice Problems

1. ***You are presented with the following data from a series of purification steps for the enzyme "comatase". Fill in the blanks in the table.***

| Purification Step | Total Protein (mg) | Total Activity (units) | Specific Activity (units/mg) | Yield (%) |
|---|---|---|---|---|
| Crude Ex. | 12,350 | 9,000 | ____ | 100 |
| Extraction | 10,233 | 8,289 | 0.81 | 92.1 |
| Salt precipitation | 3,860 | ____ | 1.65 | ____ |
| Dialysis | 1,140 | 5,625 | ____ | 62.5 |
| Chromatography | 386 | 4,688 | 12.15 | ____ |

2. ***You are interested in an enzyme produced by a particular bacterium.***
   - ***You grow 10 L of the microorganism.***
   - ***You centrifuge the 10 L to obtain a pellet of cells.***
   - ***You resuspend the cell pellet in 20 mL of buffer, break open the cells, and remove the cellular debris by centrifugation. The enzyme of interest is in the supernatant. (Assume there are 20 mL of supernatant.) The supernatant is the crude extract.***
   - ***You remove 0.5 mL of the crude extract and perform an enzyme assay. You find there are 645 units of enzyme activity in the 0.5 mL sample of crude extract.***
   - ***You take another 0.5 mL sample of crude extract and perform a protein assay. You find there are 34 mg of protein present in the 0.5 mL of crude extract.***

   a. ***Draw a flow chart of this procedure.***
   b. ***What is the specific activity of enzyme in the crude extract?***
   c. ***How many units of enzyme activity were in the original 10 L (assuming no loss of activity occurred)?***

3. Fill in the table below:

**Practice Problem, Purification Procedure: Summary**

| Purification Step | Enzyme (units/mL) | Total Protein (mg/mL) | Volume (mL) | Units in Total Volume | Yield (%) | Specific Activity (units/mg) | Purification Factor |
|---|---|---|---|---|---|---|---|
| Crude | 500 | 10.0 | 40 | | 100 | | 1 |
| After salt precipitation | 2,000 | 20.0 | 5 | | | | |
| After dialysis | 800 | 4.0 | 10 | | | | |
| After chromatography | 500 | 0.5 | 6 | | | | |

## *Answers*

1.

| Purification Step | Total Protein (mg) | Total Activity (units) | Specific Activity (units/mg) | Yield (%) |
|---|---|---|---|---|
| Crude Ex. | 12,350 | 9,000 | 0.729 | 100 |
| Extraction | 10,233 | 8,289 | 0.810 | 92.1 |
| Salt precipitation | 3,860 | 6,369 | 1.65 | 70.8 |
| Dialysis | 1,140 | 5,625 | 4.93 | 62.5 |
| Chromatography | 386 | 4,688 | 12.15 | 52.1 |

2a.

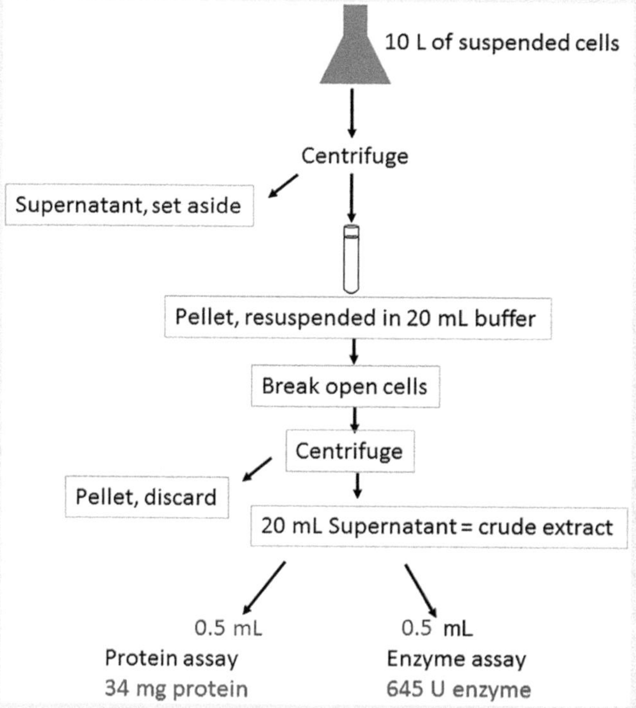


b. The specific activity in the crude extract was 645 U/34 mg ≈ **18.97 units/mg** protein
c. If there were 645 units/0.5 mL of supernatant, then there were **25,800 units** in the entire 20 mL, which is the amount in the original 10 L (assuming no loss of activity during the various steps up to this point).

3.

**Practice Problem, Purification Procedure: Summary**

| Purification Step | Enzyme (units/mL) | Total Protein (mg/mL) | Volume (mL) | Units in Total Volume | Yield (%) | Specific Activity (units/mg) | Purification Factor |
|---|---|---|---|---|---|---|---|
| Crude | 500 | 10.0 | 40 | 20,000 | 100 | 50 | 1 |
| After salt precipitation | 2,000 | 20.0 | 5 | 10,000 | 50 | 100 | 2 |
| After dialysis | 800 | 4.0 | 10 | 8,000 | 40 | 200 | 4 |
| After chromatography | 500 | 0.5 | 6 | 3,000 | 15 | 1,000 | 20 |

## 26.9 FOOTNOTE: THE β-GALACTOSIDASE EQUATION

This note shows the derivation of Equation 26.2:

$$\textbf{Units of } \beta\textbf{-galactosidase} = \frac{(\mathbf{A_{420}})(\mathbf{0.38})}{\textbf{minutes at 37°C}}$$

By definition:

1 unit of activity = amount of enzyme that will convert 1 μmol of substrate to product in 1 minute.

Therefore, we need to know how many μmol of product (ONP) appeared in the test tube in the time the reaction took place. This derivation begins with Beer's law.

**1.** $\mathbf{A_{420} = \alpha\, b[ONP]}$ Beer's law

where:

$A_{420}$ is the absorbance at a wavelength of 420 nm

the brackets [ ] mean "concentration"

α is the absorptivity constant (in this case use molar extinction coefficient)

b is the path length (assume 1 cm)

**2.** Molar extinction coefficient for ONP is: $\dfrac{4{,}500\ \text{L}}{\text{mol}\cdot\text{cm}}$

*This is known from previous studies. See Section 16.4 for an explanation of absorptivity constants.*

**3.** $A_{420} = \left(\dfrac{4{,}500\ \text{L}}{\text{mol}\cdot\cancel{\text{cm}}}\right)(1\ \cancel{\text{cm}})[\text{ONP}]$

*Substituting the molar extinction coefficient into Beer's equation and assuming 1 cm pathlength. The cm cancel.*

**4.** $\dfrac{(A_{420})(\text{mol})}{4{,}500\ \text{L}} = [\text{ONP}]$

*Dividing both sides by 4,500 L/mol*

**5.** $\left(\dfrac{(A_{420})(\text{mol})}{1\ \text{L}}\right)\left(\dfrac{1}{4{,}500}\right) = [\text{ONP}]$

*Rearranging the equation*

**6.** $\left(\dfrac{(A_{420})(10^6\ \mu\text{mol})}{1{,}000\ \text{mL}}\right)\left(\dfrac{1}{4{,}500}\right) = [\text{ONP}]$

*Substituting 1 mol = $10^6$ μmol and 1 L = 1000 mL*

7. $\left(\frac{(A_{420})(1\,\mu\text{mol})}{10^{-3}\text{ mL}}\right)\left(\frac{1}{4{,}500}\right)=[\text{ONP}]$

*Dividing numerator and denominator by $10^6$*

8. $\left(\frac{(A_{420})(1\,\mu\text{mol})}{1\text{ mL}}\right)\left(\frac{1000}{4500}\right)=[\text{ONP}]$

*Multiply numerator and denominator by 1,000 to get answer to be per 1 mL*

9. $\frac{(A_{420})(\mu\text{mol})}{1\text{ mL}}(0.222222)(1.7\text{ mL})=\text{Amount of ONP in }\mu\text{mol}$

*The equation in step 8 will give the concentration of ONP in the test tube in units of μmol/mL, but we want to know the amount (in units of μmol) of product. The volume in the tube is 1.7 mL. So, we multiply the concentration, which is in units of μmol/mL × 1.7 mL. (volume = 1 mL reaction buffer + 0.2 mL ONPG + 0.5 mL stop solution)*

10. $(A_{420})(0.3777\,\mu\text{mol})=\text{Amount of ONP}$

11. $(A_{420})(0.38\,\mu\text{mol})=\text{Amount of ONP}$

*0.3777 is rounded to 0.38*

12. $\frac{(A_{420})(0.38\,\mu\text{mol})}{\text{minute}}=\frac{\mu\text{mol of ONP formed}}{\text{minute}}=\text{Units of }\beta\text{-galactosidase}$

*Need to divide by number of minutes the reaction proceeded to get the answer on a per minute basis.*

# Index

Note: **Bold** page numbers refer to tables and *italic* page numbers refer to figures.

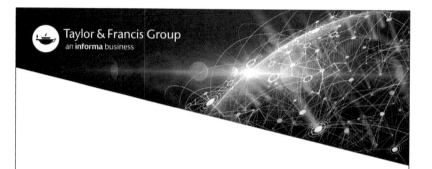

9780367244804